Nursing

Administration

A Micro/Macro Approach for Effective Nurse Executives

Phillip J. Decker, PhD
Associate Professor of Management
Barney School of Business and
Public Administration
University of Hartford
West Hartford, Connecticut

Eleanor J. Sullivan, RN, PhD, FAAN
Dean and Professor
School of Nursing
University of Kansas
Kansas City, Kansas

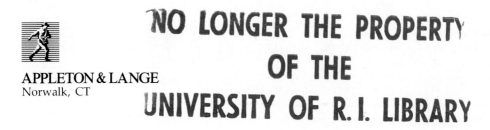

APPLETON & LANGE
Norwalk, CT

Copyright © 1992 by Appleton & Lange
A Publishing Division of Prentice Hall

92 93 94 95 96 / 10 9 8 7 6 5 4 3 2 1

Prentice Hall International (UK) Limited, *London*
Prentice Hall of Australia Pty. Limited, *Sydney*
Prentice Hall Canada, Inc., *Toronto*
Prentice Hall Hispanoamericana, S.A., *Mexico*
Prentice Hall of India Private Limited, *New Delhi*
Prentice Hall of Japan, Inc., *Tokyo*
Simon & Schuster Asia Pte. Ltd., *Singapore*
Editora Prentice Hall do Brasil Ltda., *Rio de Janeiro*
Prentice Hall, *Englewood Cliffs, New Jersey*

Library of Congress Cataloging-in-Publication Data

Nursing administration : a micro/macro approach for effective nurse
    executives / [edited by] Phillip J. Decker, Eleanor J. Sullivan.
        p.   cm.
    Includes index.
    ISBN 0–8385–7073–9
    1. Nursing services—Administration.   I. Decker, Phillip J.
    II. Sullivan, Eleanor J.
    [DNLM: 1. Nurse Administrators.   2. Nursing Services—organization
    & administration.   WY 105 N97315]
    RT89.N7639 1992
    362.1'73'068—dc20
    DNLM/DLC
    for Library of Congress   91–33327

Acquisitions Editor: William Brottmiller
Production Editor: Elizabeth Ryan
Designer: Janice Barsevich
Production: Tage Publishing Service

ISBN 0-8385-7073-9

9 780838 570739
90000

CONTENTS

CONTRIBUTORS

General Clara L. Adams-Ender
Commanding General
Ft. Belvoir, Virginia

JoAnn S. Alexander, BSN, MSN
Associate Professor, School of Nursing
University of Evansville
Evansville, Indiana

Captain Margaret Armstrong
Deputy Director, Navy Nurse Corps,
   Reserve Affairs
Bureau of Medicine and Surgery
   (OONCR)
Washington, DC

Lieutenant Colonel Claudia Bartz
Chief, Department of Nursing
196th Station Hospital
SHAPE, Belgium

Marjorie V. Batey, RN, PhD
Professor, Community Health Care
   Systems
School of Nursing
University of Washington
Seattle, Washington

H. John Bernardin, PhD
University Research Professor
College of Business and Public
   Administration
Florida Atlantic University
Boca Raton, Florida

Lieutenant Colonel Joanne M. Black
Clinical Nursing Research Consultant
Office of the Surgeon General
Bolling Air Force Base, DC

Diane K. Boyle, RN, PhD
Assistant Professor
School of Nursing and Department of
   Nursing Administration
The Medical College of Georgia
Augusta, Georgia

Jim Breaugh, PhD
Professor, Management
School of Business Administration
University of Missouri
St. Louis, Missouri

Rita Clifford, RN, PhD
Assistant Dean for Student Affairs
School of Nursing
University of Kansas
Kansas City, Kansas

Helen Connors, RN, PhD
Associate Professor
School of Nursing
University of Kansas
Kansas City, Kansas

James P. Cooney, PhD
Dean, College of Health Sciences
Georgia State University
Atlanta, Georgia

Donna M. Costello-Nickitas, RN, PhD
Graduate Program Coordinator,
    Nursing Administration
Hunter College-Bellevue School of
    Nursing
New York, New York

Susan Crissman, RN, MNEd
Senior Vice President
Memorial Hospital
South Bend, Indiana

Phillip J. Decker, PhD
Associate Professor of Management
Barney School of Business and Public
    Administration
University of Hartford
West Hartford, Connecticut

Dennis Dossett, PhD
Associate Professor, Management
School of Business
University of Missouri
St. Louis, Missouri

Pam Duchene, RN, DNSc
Executive Vice President of Clinical
    Services
Mississippi Methodist Hospital and
    Rehabilitation Center
Jackson, Mississippi

Sandra R. Edwardson, RN, PhD
Associate Professor, School of Nursing
University of Minnesota
Minneapolis, Minnesota

J. Kevin Ford, PhD
Associate Professor
Department of Psychology
Michigan State University
East Lansing, Michigan

Linda Fournier, RN, MS, ND
Assistant to the Director
Nursing Services Research and
    Support
Rush Presbyterian-St. Luke's Medical
    Center
Chicago, Illinois

Mary Ann F. Fralic, RN, DrPH, FAAN
Senior Vice President, Nursing
Robert Wood Johnson University
    Hospital
and Clinical Associate Dean
Rutgers University College of Nursing
New Brunswick, New Jersey

Germaine Freese, RN, MS
Assistant Head Nurse
North Memorial Medical Center
Robbinsdale, Minnesota

Douglas Fugate, PhD
Professor, Marketing
College of Business Administration
Western Kentucky University
Bowling Green, Kentucky

Brigadier General Barbara Goodwin
Chief, Air Force Nurse Corps
HQ/USAF
Bolling Air Force Base, DC

David P. Gustafson, PhD
Associate Professor, Management and
  Organizational Behavior
School of Business Administration
University of Missouri
St. Louis, Missouri

Jim Guthrie, PhD
Professor, Human Resource
  Management
School of Business
University of Kansas
Lawrence, Kansas

Rear Admiral Mary F. Hall
Director, Navy Nurse Corps
Bureau of Medicine and Surgery
Washington, DC

Sandra M. Handley, RN, PhD
Research Fellow, School of Nursing
University of Kansas
Kansas City, Kansas

Sue T. Hegyvary, PhD, FAAN
Dean, School of Nursing
University of Washington
Seattle, Washington

**Mary Kay Hermann, RN, MA, MSN,
  EdD**
Professor, School of Nursing
University of Evansville
Evansville, Indiana

Colonel John M. Hudock
Retired, US Army
Falls Church, Virginia

Tonda Hughes, RN, PhD
Research Associate, Department of
  Psychiatric Nursing
College of Nursing
University of Illinois at Chicago
Chicago, Illinois

Judith Jezek, RN, EdD
Associate Professor, College of
  Nursing
Rush University
Chicago, Illinois

Liz Johnson, RN, PhD
President
Link Inc.
Irving, Texas

Charles L. Joiner, PhD
Professor and Senior Associate Dean
School of Health Related Professions
The University of Alabama at
  Birmingham
Birmingham, Alabama

Jeffrey S. Kane, PhD
Professor, Department of Management
  and Marketing
University of North Carolina at
  Greensboro
Greensboro, North Carolina

Kimberly F. Kane, PhD
Associate Professor
Babcock Graduate School of
  Management
Wake Forest University
Winston-Salem, North Carolina

Thomas B. Keal, BS
Principal, Gemini Management
  Associates
Scottsdale, Arizona

Joan T. Kiely, BSN, MSN
Associate Professor
School of Nursing
University of Evansville
Evansville, Indiana

Roger O. Lambson, PhD
Vice Chancellor of Administration
University of Kansas Medical Center
Kansas City, Kansas

Captain Sandra S. Lindelof
Assistant for Policy to Director, Navy
  Nurse Corps
Bureau of Medicine and Surgery
Washington, DC

Diana J. Mason, RN, PhD, FAAN
Associate Director of Nursing for
  Education and Research
Beth Israel Medical Center
New York, New York

Ann Minnick, RN, PhD
Director, Nursing Services and
  Support
Rush Presbyterian-St. Luke's Medical
  Center
Chicago, Illinois

Glenda S. McGaha, RN, PhD
Associate Professor, School of Nursing
University of Alabama at Birmingham
Birmingham, Alabama

Raymond A. Noe, PhD
Associate Professor, Industrial
  Relations
Industrial Relations Center
University of Minnesota
Minneapolis, Minnesota

Steven D. Norton, PhD
Associate Professor, Management
School of Business and Economics
Indiana University at South Bend
South Bend, Indiana

Mary K. Pabst, RN, MS
Assistant to the Director, Nursing
  Services Research and Support
Rush Presbyterian-St. Luke's Medical
  Center
Chicago, Illinois

Sharon L. Pontious, RN, PhD
Information Systems and Clinical
  Research Scientist
Division of Nursing Services
St. Louis Children's Hospital
St. Louis, Missouri

Colonel Patricia Porter
Chief Professional Nursing Programs
Office of the Surgeon General
HQ/USAF
Bolling Air Force Base, DC

**Tim Porter-O'Grady, RN, EdD, CS,
  CNAA, FAAN**
Senior Partner
Affiliated Dynamics, Inc.
Atlanta, Georgia

Scott D. Ramsey, MUP
Assistant Director of
  Telecommunication
Dept. of Information Technology
University of Kansas Medical Center
Kansas City, Kansas

Sandra Robertson, RN, MS
Associate Director, Nursing Services
Research and Support
Rush Presbyterian-St. Luke's Medical
  Center
Chicago, Illinois

Phyllis Schultz, RN, PhD
Associate Professor, Community
  Health Care Systems
School of Nursing
University of Washington
Seattle, Washington

Karen Kelly Schutzenhofer, RN, EdD
Director, Center of Nursing Excellence
St. Louis Children's Hospital
St. Louis, Missouri

Sandra R. Shelley, DNSc
Senior Manager
Ernst & Young
Chicago, Illinois

John J. Short, MM
Assistant Vice President,
  Administrative Support Services
Rush Presbyterian-St. Luke's Medical
  Center
Chicago, Illinois

Carolyn H. Smeltzer, RN, EdD, FAAN
Vice President, Nursing
University of Chicago Hospitals
and Clinical Professor
Marcella Niehoff School of Nursing
Loyola University of Chicago
Chicago, Illinois

Marlene K. Strader, RN, PhD
Associate Professor, Nursing
University of Missouri
St. Louis, Missouri

Eleanor J. Sullivan, RN, PhD, FAAN
Dean and Professor
School of Nursing
University of Kansas
Kansas City, Kansas

Roma Lee Taunton, RN, PhD
Associate Professor, School of Nursing
University of Kansas
Kansas City, Kansas

FOREWORD

Change, change, change . . . reading about it, seeing it and feeling it ignites sparks of excitement of entering a new era. Nursing administration is entering a new era and this book captures the excitement and possibilities of this chapter in our history.

The nursing administration of the past is not the nursing administration of the future. Like other parts of organizational development and management, nursing administration in the past has centered heavily on top-down mechanistic views of organizations. The challenge to bridge operational and clinical components of health care organizations too often was not built on a sound foundation of theory and research.

Also, like many other types of organizations, health care organizations are learning the necessity of integrating the macro and micro levels of organization. In nursing administration, this change means setting and managing the environment for caring. Strategic planning reflects not only the overall organizational goals, but those goals as translated in day-to-day care of patients and clients. Quality control is not just an issue of structure, but one of theory-based practice, reflecting complex interrelationships among all levels of the organization.

Health care often has been behind other parts of society in organization design and development. Health care organizations have tended to cling devotedly to bureaucratic models of organization even after many other human service organizations were changing to more open system models. Gareth Morgan in his book, *Images of Organization* (Sage Publications, 1986) describes the bureaucratic model as predicated on the view of organizations as machines. While that view seems contradictory to the goals of health care, in fact the structure and function of hospitals and other health care facilities still tend to reflect this mechanistic perspective.

Nursing administration is in a critical position to change that perspective and the functioning of health care organizations. It stands at the interface of operations and clinical practice. It addresses macro level issues of the organization with full knowledge of issues and problems at micro level, that is, practitioner, patient, and family. Issues of cost, control, and competition in the market place are blended with those of caring for individuals and families. The use of authority, rules, and procedures in decision making are blended with the necessity for clinical judgment and the worth and satisfaction of employees.

Nursing administration is a tall order. This book portrays the excitement as well as the challenge and importance of being on the threshold of a new era.

Sue T. Hegyvary, PhD, FAAN

Nurse executives in health care settings have a responsibility to ensure that patients receive the health care that they need to lead active, productive lives. To offer quality nursing services it is essential to provide nursing leadership and effective administration. This book focuses on the skills of the nurse executive, and the theory and knowledge needed by nursing executives to function in today's health care institutions. This book presents the competitive nature of the health care industry, the economics of nursing service in institutions, the problems associated with and the shortage of professional health care personnel, and the emphasis on quality outcomes and consumerism in health care today.

The health care environment is constantly changing and will continue to do so at a very rapid pace in the future. This change will be demanded not only by government entities but by the consumers who use health care. Consumers include both patients, family physicians and third party payers. Businesses will have more impact on health care in the future than they have had in the past. We may also see increasing interest in nationalized insurance of health care. Consequently, the economic pressures on health care institutions is intense. Because nursing constitutes the largest group of employees and the largest labor cost in most health care institutions, the demand on nursing executives for quality, efficiency, and effectiveness will increase. The aim of this book is to analyze the theory, systems, and processes that will ensure nursing executive efficiency, and ultimately the effectiveness of nursing service within health care institutions.

This book is designed to help all nursing executives, nursing managers, and nurses aspiring to those positions. It is also designed for masters level courses in nursing administration taught in a nursing service setting. Staff nurses who wish to understand more fully the institutions in which they work may also find this text a useful resource about nursing service and health care institutions.

To learn about health care organizations, their administration, and the administration of nursing services, it is essential that students and executives have a firm grasp of the conceptual models and theories that explain how these organizations work. Action based on this understanding is also required. The philosophy of this book, then, is to present both the theory and the practical application of that theory. Although most texts are concerned primarily with the micro (individual behavior) view, it is our intent to describe both the macro (organizational) and the micro aspects of administration. It is our aim to present practical theories that work and translate them into action. We believe that the interconnection between both the theoretical and the practical is needed in nursing administration. Not only will the reader understand the theory behind organizations and organizational behavior in organizations, but we expect the reader to also learn what practicing administrators do to influence organizational dynamics to facilitate organizational effectiveness. From the very first chapter, positive, organizational outcomes and organizational effectiveness are stressed. This philosophy is expanded in the introduction where we describe the organizing model for the book. This organizing model has organizational effectiveness as its primary dependent variable.

Most nursing care today exists in institutions. If nursing care is to be successful, the institution must be successful. On the other hand, if the institution is to be successful, nursing must be efficient and successful. Thus, we see the two as inexorably linked. The complexity of nursing, the complexity of health care, and the complexity of organizations and their environments makes it unlikely that any one theory or process will provide a definitive answer to all of the questions about how nurses and health care organizations behave or should behave. We focus on diverse theories and facets of behavior, but ultimately, we focus on the effectiveness of nursing service because we think that the effectiveness of nursing service is the key element to health care in the future of America.

The text is divided into eight sections for ease of use. Section I introduces nursing administration, nursing organizational theory, and the power and politics of nursing and health care. The second section discusses strategic planning, culture, and the basic elements of effectiveness in setting the direction of nursing service within the organizational context. The third section deals with organizing the organization and discusses organizational structure, environment, change, and communication systems. This section also includes a chapter about military executive nursing systems because many graduate nurses pursue military careers. Organizing human resource management systems are discussed in the fourth section, and the fifth section deals with the issues of organizing people, including training, group theory, managing problem employees, and collective bargaining. The sixth section is not typically found in nursing administration books; it deals with the technology, physical facilities, and other issues that surround the production of nursing service. Organizing the Work, the seventh section, deals with staffing, scheduling, control systems, conflict management and project management. The last section, Optimizing the Organization, deals with optimizing nursing service. The chapters of this section include marketing, institutional research, and innovation.

The contributors to this text represent a wide perspective of nursing service in health care organizations. The contributors come from nursing administration, schools of nursing, schools of business, industrial psychology, and health care administration. They also include military nurses and hospital executives. In short, we have gathered a mix of authors that is unique in a nursing administration book. Most of the chapters have been written by teams of individuals who represent differing viewpoints about nursing service. This book is further strengthened in that many of the authors come from schools of business, health care administration, and from administration of hospitals. The contributions of these management and administration experts are not often readily available to nursing managers and administrators. The combination of theoretical knowledge and practical experience with the diverse authorship of this text provides a rich blend of content, integrating administration skills and concepts appropriate for the effective nursing executive in daily practice. Furthermore, each contribution has been carefully edited by the authors to conform to the basic goals of the book, which is to provide a complete micro/macro view of nursing service effectiveness for both the nursing executive and the prospective masters student pursuing a nursing administration career.

The authors wish to acknowledge the contributors to this book. We also wish to thank the Appleton & Lange editors involved in this project, including William Brottmiller, Marion Welch, Eileen Burns, Tony Caruso, and Elizabeth Ryan. We owe a special debt of gratitude to the many reviewers who made comments and suggestions at various stages of the process of producing this book. Their experience and insight have been essential to enhancing the quality and usefulness of this text. We would also like to thank our various secretaries who have participated in this book, particularly Michelle Wethington, Kathleen Sloan, Marcia Pressly, and Patricia Walters. We would like to thank Sandra Handley for her help in editing and fine-tuning this text. Thanks also go to the students in graduate nursing administration courses taught at the School of Nursing at the University of Kansas for their helpful comments and review. Finally, this book could not have been completed without the wonderful support and understanding of our families. Book writing can be hard on families and our families responded with grace and generosity.

We owe a debt of gratitude to Shirley Martin, Dean, School of Nursing, University of Missouri, St. Louis, who brought us together and who can take pride that this book and others are now reality.

Phillip J. Decker   Eleanor J. Sullivan

INTRODUCTION

Both effectiveness and efficiency are important to administrative and managerial performance. Effectiveness is goal attainment. An effective administrator selects appropriate goals and strategies and accomplishes them or, alternatively, accomplishes institutional goals assigned. Efficiency, on the other hand, is a technical concept that indicates the ratio of output to input. The goal is to obtain the greatest output from the least amount of input. For example, several engines might be evaluated by the ratio of their power output to their fuel input. The one that both outputs the most power *and* uses the least fuel is the most efficient. The efficiency of a human service operation may be established in similar fashion. An efficient administrator maximizes the level of goal achievement with a minimum of inputs (human, physical, and financial).

Although efficiency and effectiveness are both important, Peter F. Drucker[1] argues that effectiveness is the critical criterion for organizational success. He states that the pertinent question is not how to do things right, but how to do the right things. It is senseless to accomplish inappropriate ends efficiently. For example, the advent of the automobile made the carriage obsolete. It then made no sense for a firm to continue manufacturing carriages, no matter how efficiently the company could do it. It also is possible to be effective without being efficient. John F. Kennedy, in 1960, set a goal to put a person on the moon before the end of the decade. The goal was accomplished but because of many safety redundancies and cost overruns, NASA was inefficient in doing it.

Although the need for efficiency must never be overlooked by an administrator, effectiveness is the pre-eminent criterion for us in promoting nurse executive development in this book. We define effectiveness as goal attainment. We view the process of establishing organizational goals and objectives and of strategic planning as the means to define the mission and objectives of the organization. Accomplishing these goals and objectives, therefore, becomes the definition of effectiveness. To accomplish goals efficiently is to conserve resources that then become available to be used for other goal attainment.

---

[1]Peter F. Drucker. *Managing for Results.* New York: Harper & Row. 1964, p. 5.

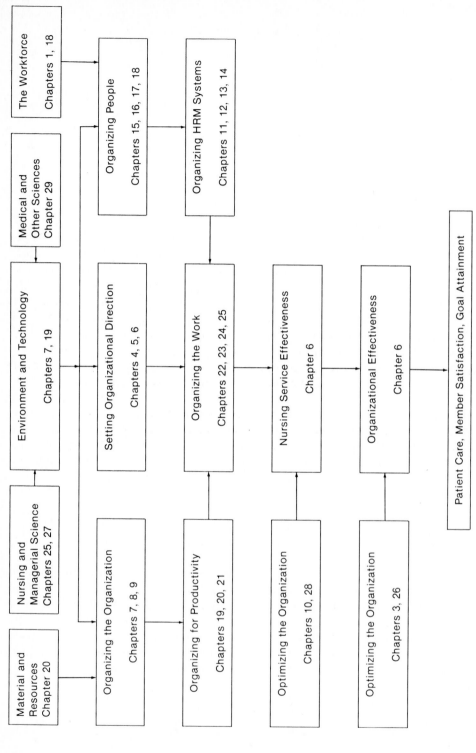

Figure 1. Integrating Model

The term *organizational effectiveness* is used in a variety of ways. Some have equated it with profit or productivity, others view it as member job satisfaction, still others see it as providing for societal good. Each of these is valued, but it is important to see that effectiveness is best assessed by those whose goals are congruent and tied to the mission of the organization. Various groups have a stake in any organization's success; consequently, it is necessary to take a multiple constituency approach in planning for success. While our focus is on the nursing constituency and on nursing service effectiveness, we recognize that nursing service exists in a larger institution and a larger environment.

The overall focus of this book, therefore, becomes the influences on nursing service effectiveness. Organizational effectiveness is influenced by four major categories of variables: environmental characteristics, organizational characteristics such as structure and technology, employee characteristics, and managerial policies and practices including nursing, science, and practice (see Fig. 1).

All health care institutions have a number of important constituencies, which include physicians, nurses, other health care providers, technical services, and the managerial and administrative components of that institution. Health care institutions are unique because of this unusual configuration of constituencies. Most organizations have a chain of command from the top executive to the lowest employee. Health care institutions often have different chains of command across administration, nursing, and medicine. In addition, medicine has a power base in institutions because physicians, by virtue of their referral of patients, are often the customers rather than employees of the institution.

It is apparent that health care institutions are very complex, and there are many variables across the different power bases that affect nursing service effectiveness. Figure 1 illustrates how the sciences of management, nursing, and organizations lead to practices that affect nursing service effectiveness. Each is discussed in greater detail in the pages that follow, but let this model guide the overall conceptual framework of this text, which uses science as the primary independent variable and nursing service and institutional effectiveness as the dependent variables.

An Introduction to Nursing Administration

CHAPTER 1

Nursing Administration: The Next Decade

Mary Ann F. Fralic

Key Concept List

The health care revolution
Nursing executive responsibilities
Contemporary health care payment systems
Nursing administration functions
Multidimensional organizations
Nursing's entrepreneurial component
Research and theory development in nursing
Effectiveness: The goal of the administrator

The nurse administrator is responsible for the acquisition and deployment of resources to support patient care. Just as the success of an organization is dependent on the competence of its managers, the nursing division is dependent on the competence and skill of the nurse administrator. Increasingly complex health care organizations require a continually enhanced level of sophistication in nursing administration. The purpose of this chapter is to provide a conceptual framework for viewing the entire panorama of the chief nurse executive's work and the context in which that work is accomplished. The terms, chief nurse executive, chief nursing officer, nurse executive, vice president of nursing and nursing administrator will be used interchangeably throughout the text.

Complicating the nurse administrator's work is the fundamental change in the nature of the health care industry that is occurring and the rapid change that will continue (Vaill, 1989). Thus a highly destabilized context surrounds nurse executive practice. Our work world is undergoing continuous reshaping, and each of us faces relentless and almost simultaneous changes. Vaill uses the analogy that the periods of calm still water are now few and far between in nursing. In fact, it is suggested that we live in a world of "permanent white water" (Vaill, p 2). The metaphor conveys a sense of constant energy, rapid movement, and uncertainty. Intelligence, experience, and skill are essential within this continuously changing context.

THE HEALTH CARE REVOLUTION: NURSING IN THE MAELSTROM

Today's nurse executive evolved from white uniform to business suit in the 1960s and 1970s, and moved from director to vice-president and senior vice-president during the 1980s. "The status, autonomy, and authority of hospitals' chief nursing officers is greater now than in the past" (*Modern Healthcare*, 1988, p 15). The 1990s should be even more promising. Perry (1989) notes that "nurse executives are increasingly managing a wider range of hospital services, attending high level meetings, and are better educated and better paid" than their predecessors (p 92). There is increased importance accorded to the role of the nurse executive as a member of the senior management team in health care organizations. Salary, title, and perquisites reflect that importance. All of this brings with it the requirement for transition from circumscribed responsibility to full accountability, as well as all the expected threats and opportunities. Nurse executives have to account for and be responsible for the performance of others. *Hospitals* magazine (October 5, 1989, p 5) describes the job of today's vice-president of nursing as one of the most difficult jobs in the hospital—and therein lies the challenge and excitement. Those who are successful in these positions will have unprecedented influence on the design, effectiveness, and quality of nursing practice systems. Additionally, they will have a tangible and increasingly significant impact on the total organization.

Nurse executives practice across all health care settings and across all specialties. There are models for single hospitals, multihospital corporations, consortia, vertically and horizontally integrated organizations, and highly centralized or fully decentralized organizations with matrix design. The organizational structure in each of these environments may differ. However, despite some functional variations, certain basic tenets apply. In some settings the nurse executive may be asked to assume corporate responsibilities, for example, as an officer of a subsidiary corporation. This function would be assumed in addition to the essential institutional responsibilities as a senior officer of the primary organization. Additionally, and most central to the nurse executive's position, is full responsibility for the performance of the nursing division.

In each of these areas, the nurse executive will have responsibilities that are (1) strategic, (2) fiduciary, and (3) operational. There are also professional and developmental (research and development) responsibilities that are inherent in the leadership of the nursing division. Thus, even though practice settings differ for nurse administrators, there are basic areas of commonality in management practice and responsibility. Additionally, there is the key interface in all instances with the chief executive officer of the organization, chief medical officer, often a chief operating officer, and possibly a chief academic officer in a university health center. These officers, along with the other senior level colleagues of the nurse executive, constitute the institution's leadership team. The chief nursing officer must perform as an integral, effective, and maximally functioning member of that team.

THE NEW HEALTH CARE SCENARIO

The evolutionary environment in which health care occurs is a highly dynamic practice market dominated by a prospective payment system, active competition for consumers, and the significant influence of technology. There is a growing need for specialized personnel, and a major impact from diminished nurse supply and increasingly expensive professional nurses. Nurse administrators must have expert skills to function effectively in this complex practice market (Hechenberger, 1988). Fundamental and often traumatic change must be managed, and this will be one of the key determinants of success for nurse administrators.

Prospective payment methodologies have become the norm and continuing pressure mounts to reduce the escalating cost of health care. Reimbursement mechanisms frequently direct and shape health care. Managed care systems (HMOs, PPOs, IPAs, etc) were organized with health care cost reduction as a major objective. Alternative practice models and care delivery methods have evolved as attempts to respond to the contemporary health care environment. These models take various forms, and case management, differentiated practice, and restructured work environments are examples (Tonges, 1989). They are designed to be responsive to the environmental realities of diminishing resources, while attempting to maximize quality (Brett & Tonges, 1990; Bair et al, 1989). Nursing has taken leadership in many of these areas and developed highly viable systems (Gamble, 1989).

Results of Contemporary Payment Systems

A key concept is that health care exists within a market-driven economy and has itself become market-driven. Competition among health care providers and health care institutions has been stimulated by market forces. Productivity enhancement is focused on offering better quality at lower prices (Katz, 1988). To do this, we must move beyond process and also measure results—what happens to patients, good or bad, based on nursing intervention. We must design quantitative systems to precisely track nursing intervention costs and patient outcomes that are attributable to nursing action. To be effective in any market-driven environment, one must know the customer (the patient) and one must know the product (nursing care). Successful future nursing systems will focus on those areas.

Complicating the harsh realities of contemporary and projected future health care reimbursement systems is the steadily shifting change in case mix and acuity that is reflected, for example, by a higher intensification of nursing care needs by patients in hospitals and other settings. Increasing demand for services compounds this problem. The combination of higher volume and intensity and diminished financial resources creates serious personnel issues. Health care institutions utilize professional, technical, and support personnel who must have appropriate credentials, training, and experience. Shortages may exist at any time in any or all of these categories, and may range from mild to acute. The nurse executive must see that all levels of qualified personnel are available, since they are essential to the support of quality nursing practice, and to the success of the overall institution.

Nursing Education Trends

The majority of registered nurses continue to be prepared in associate degree programs, with fewer prepared in baccalaureate programs, and very few in diploma schools (Rosenfeld, 1990). There has been a dramatic increase, however, in the number of associate degree or diploma RNs who return to school to earn the baccalaureate degree (American Association of Colleges of Nursing (AACN) Survey, 1988). There is also a substantial increase in the number of nurses enrolled in master's level (10 percent increase in the past 4 years) and doctoral programs (62 percent increase) (AACN, 1988). These figures depict an increasingly better educated professional work force.

This work force demands specific employment conditions. Graduating baccalaureate nurses rank-ordered items of importance to them in selecting their first place of employment in a survey by Orr (1989). Factors identified as most important included quality of patient care, professional recognition, adequate staffing, an environment of open communication, and sensitivity to individual needs and values. This supports the belief that nurses remain committed to the quality aspects of patient care and professionalism. These factors are encouraging in that one can expect and look forward to an increasingly better prepared professional work force that maintains the values of excellence in patient care. Expert nursing management systems will be required to develop and maintain the organizational and clinical environments to support these nurses in quality practice.

HOW TODAY'S NURSE ADMINISTRATOR FUNCTIONS

First and foremost, nursing organizations are being designed and structured for competence. Hall's concept of competence (1988) is that people are driven by a need to do things well, combined with the basic human desire to accomplish what needs to be done. This drive for excellence is the basis for the competence process. In Hall's view, we must "appreciate competence as a generalized human trait, as a widespread capacity to do what needs to be done. Convention would often have us equate competence with the possession of some special expertise, but such a posture promotes a narrow view of the human potential available in our organizations" (Hall, p 31). Personal competence is continually enhanced by learning how to deal with and solve any number of problems, how to innovate, how to continue to learn, and how to profit from our experiences (Hall, 1988).

Competence is essential for nurse administrators if they are to achieve true executive stature within a corporate environment. Executive level business skills are required. To think conceptually, to view their area of responsibility as part of the larger whole, is crucial. Nursing is viewed contextually and realistically as part of the health care organization and the greater health care system. A clear understanding of the realities external to the organization is required. Every organization is dependent on certain types of resource exchanges (eg, information, dollars, people, equipment) for its operation. All organizations are vulnerable to extraorganizational influence (Pfeffer & Salancik, 1978)—that is, influencing factors that derive from the external environment. Awareness of business, societal, financial, and professional trends and issues is mandatory.

Successful nurse executives are well credentialled, experienced, and they have built a solid "track record." They can work behind the scenes to get goals met, and they can manage many relationships simultaneously. Balancing the intricate needs of the nursing staff, the administration, and the medical staff with the needs of the patient is a constant challenge. Yet, successfully balancing these multiple and often competing and conflicting relationships is paramount for success in nurse executive practice.

Effective nurse leaders build high performance teams, and they are decisive. It has been estimated that 80 percent of the business decisions that one is faced with should be made on the spot, 15 percent need to mature, and 5 percent need not be made at all (Calano & Salzman, 1988). The power of decisiveness becomes an art to be mastered.

Because of environmental realities, nurse administrators function effectively in highly competitive situations. They know the system and know how to operate within it. They are able to confront in a nonconfrontational mode. They can translate goals into action. They are acutely aware of the fact that there are few things that managers can accomplish alone, and they rely on the support, cooperation, or approval of a large number of people (Uyterhoeven, 1989). Successful nurse executives know that credibility and trust are the foundation of managerial effectiveness, since our actions are always scrutinized. Personal credibility permits executives to be effective as well as to fail on occasion. Trust, integrity, and credibility are indispensable and intertwined in management, and must never be underestimated. Boardroom behavior, sound governing board relations, and "bottom-line skills" are also essential attributes. The professional executive image is projected. Simply stated, one must look and act the part consistently.

Those who would be successful in nursing administration welcome and thrive in changing, uncertain, pressure-filled environments. Key indicators of success include management prowess, competence, consistency, integrity, as well as equanimity and imperturbability. Another indispensable attribute is a sense of humor and the ability to not take oneself quite so seriously, despite very serious responsibilities. "Some women who interview for key management roles exhibit an exhausting intensity. Lighten up . . . keep your life in balance by combining hard work and play in every week. Boards are not seeking grim workaholics for senior management roles" (Vergara, 1989, p 27). Understanding and practicing concepts of self-care, one brings the highest level of physical and mental resources, balance, and enthusiasm to one's professional activity.

To summarize how today's nurse administrators function, first remember that management is decision making. Next, all of one's personal and professional resources and experiences are utilized to effectively make those decisions. Then, the quality of those decisions will be the final delineator of effectiveness. To quote Uyterhoeven, "a managerial record . . . is established through the cumulative impact of a series of decisions. . . . If these decisions can be related not only to the demands of each separate issue, but also to an overall philosophy and master plan, their internal consistency and cumulative impact will establish a strong and cohesive organizational fabric. This is the landmark of an effective and successful manager" (p 145).

OPERATING WITHIN COMPLEX MULTIDIMENSIONAL ORGANIZATIONS

The nurse administrator operates as executive, consultant, peer, subordinate, role model, coach, adjudicator, and more. Thus, there are complex roles within equally complex organizations. All of these dimensions of the nurse executive role are put into play to address the paramount economic issues. Managing the serious financial issues is key to balancing quality patient care with often stark and ominous budget realities. Savvy managers do not dissipate energy by wishing for resources that simply will not and cannot be provided. Rather, they ask the question "How can I make the best use of the resources that I now have?" Additionally, the ethical dimensions of patient care demand keen attention by the nurse executive in resource-constrained, technology-driven systems.

Business Skills

Since the work of the nurse executive is the acquisition and deployment of resources for patient care, the requisite skills are essential. Solid contemporary business approaches are required for the design and presentation of any new service or concept. The nurse executive knows how to write successful business plans. Vestal's definition (1988) of a business plan is that it is ". . . a written document that spells out in detail the proposed business venture and the expectations of that business over a specified number of future years. The plan serves as a guide for efficient project operation and management; an information source; and a document that will facilitate decision making, motivation, and the measurement of performance" (p 121). Any commonly used format for a professionally developed business plan is acceptable, provided it follows established business protocols. All programs, whether they be clinical or nonclinical, need and deserve careful planning and proposal development if the idea is to be supported. All projects require the support of the organization, planned resources, funding, and evaluation to ensure both the clinical and the economic success of the proposed activity (Johnson, et al, 1988). A businesslike format for all programs, ideas, and concepts should become the requirement for all nurse administrators so that the organization views the overall management of the nursing division as highly professional from both clinical and business perspectives. This credibility is essential in gaining support and resources for patient care.

Cost accounting is another integral managerial technology to be learned. The cost of nursing services and the cost per unit of service is determined in a precise and clear manner that is readily understandable to the finance division of the organization. Various approaches can be used to determine the cost of nursing care, and these include the per diem method, diagnosis based methods (the DRG approach), cost per unit of intensity, or cost per nursing unit based on patient classification systems (Huckabay, 1988). Appropriate methods are selected for each unique institutional environment, and appropriate to the financial methods used in the organization. Being the largest single cost center has both privileges and responsibilities. Thus, nursing data track expenditure of the significant resources and measure the appropriate and effective utilization of those resources.

Regulation and Documentation

Regulatory requirements also command a significant segment of the nurse administrator's time and attention. Nursing divisions operate with the approval and accreditation of various and multiple licensing bodies, such as state health departments, boards of nursing, and the Joint Commission for Accreditation of Healthcare Organizations (JCAHO). Additional evaluations and surveys may be required, depending on the nature and type of the health care organization. The underlying principle of all evaluation procedures is the assessment and analysis of adherence to quality standards. This focus has become sharpened in recent years. For example, JCAHO's nursing standards for the 1990s have been developed to measure the outcomes of nursing practice, rather than to focus on the process of care. This trend also is reflected in the clinical indicator approach to judging the overall effectiveness of patient care. Nursing systems are being developed to capture the outcome of nursing activity and measure its effectiveness. For example, the rigorous, detailed and prescriptive nature of nursing care plans is being replaced by documentation systems designed to reflect the planning process for patient care. Monitoring systems of the future will be targeted toward maximizing information in concise formats while, at the same time conserving the professional's time.

Documentation systems also are responsive to the reality of today's patient populations—high acuity and shorter lengths of stay in hospitals. In this situation, one cannot require rigid copious documentation systems. Nurse administrators will see that systems are in place that are responsive to all regulatory requirements and professional resources and realities, and compliant with professional standards.

The Corporate Culture

Effective managers are always cognizant of the culture and politics in today's complex organizations. O'Donnell notes that "anyone who has worked for more than one employer knows that there truly is such a thing as a corporate culture, or personality, that permeates it. This culture is revealed by an attitude of the employees and how they deal with customers as well as with each other" (O'Donnell, 1989, p 44). The attitude or culture of an organization originates with the chief executive officer, and, in the nursing division, it originates with the chief nursing officer. The corporate culture is a composite of the attitudes, the beliefs, and the philosophy of the institution, and a composite of the type of people that are hired and retained, and who share the values that fit the culture. Organizations with strong, positive corporate personalities have an easier time attracting and retaining very high quality people, despite shifts in market supply and demand. Well-thought-out strategies and long-range plans are continuously kept in the forefront of consciousness, and all decisions are made based on the mission of the organization, its culture, and its goals and policies (Kerfoot, 1988).

Managing Your Boss

Effective managers know that the key relationship that they have in an organization is with their boss in that the boss enables one to be successful in an organization. Managing your boss is a term that Gabarro and Kotter (1980) use to describe the process of consciously working with your superior in a way that will yield the best possible results for the organization, for your boss, and for you. The term does not refer to political maneuvering or so-called apple polishing. ''Good managers recognize that a relationship with a boss involves mutual dependence and that, if it is not managed well, they cannot be effective in their jobs. Effective managers see managing a relationship with a boss as part of their job. As a result, they take time and energy to develop a relationship that is consonant with both persons' styles and assets and that meets the most critical needs of each'' (p 92). Drucker (1977) clarifies that one does not really manage a boss; rather, you work with the human being, and you learn how to do this based on the unique nature of each boss-subordinate relationship. He cautions that you have a responsibility to make certain that the boss understands what it is that you are trying to do. You also have a serious requirement to manage the time that the boss allots to you, and to ensure that it is productive time. Think through the best way to use the boss's time. The simple approach is to recognize that bosses represent a critical resource, and they each have their own objectives about what they hope to achieve. Successful subordinates know what these objectives are and do everything possible to help the boss to achieve them. After all, this is what we all expect from our own subordinates.

THE ENTREPRENEURIAL COMPONENT

Today's nurse administrator must possess entrepreneurial qualities; that is, the ability to design a new and different tomorrow. That may sound ambitious, but it is exactly what must be done. Rather than become intimidated by the enormity of the task of designing new patient care systems and approaches, let us first take a backward look to our rich professional heritage and Florence Nightingale. She is the paramount model for each of us in that, with virtually no resource except herself, she literally designed a plan and future for professional nursing. An old History of Nursing text (Griffin & Griffin, 1965) describes Miss Nightingale's singular contribution in the following way: ''. . . with her powerful personality, her vision, and her practical organizing ability, she took the lead [in the movement to train professional nurses], placed it on a high powerful foundation of organization, sound educational principles, and high ethics, and inspired it with an enthusiasm that gave it an impetus under which it is still progressing. A few years before Miss Nightingale's time there was no such thing as professional nursing. At the time of her death nursing was a profession, administered by women and offering them nursing and educational opportunities, formerly unthinkable'' (p 135). Each of us is asked not to perform on a level of magnitude such as this, but our task is nonetheless substantial. It is time to again redesign the work of patient care and to restructure the environments in which patient care is provided. There must be a fundamental rethinking of nursing work. Hospitals that focus primarily on issues of compensation, without making serious efforts to optimize the potential of existing nursing resources, will not maintain the competitive edge that will be needed for success in future environments. And high quality nursing definitely provides a competitive edge for organizations.

Tomorrow's Nurse Manager

One cannot discuss restructuring the work environment without considering the essential concept of developing nurse managers to direct tomorrow's work force. Much of the current literature describes efforts to enhance the staff nurse role with little discussion of the inevitable changes in the middle manager's role as a result of this shifting of power from the nurse manager to the staff nurse. The staff nurse of the future will have greater autonomy, more active decision making and self-direction which will result in managers doing less decision making, supervising, and directing. New approaches to nursing management are inevitable with new nursing practice system designs. For example, new categories and types of workers, matrix reporting relationships between departments, redesigned jobs, restructured work environments, and new and expanded performance expectations all require different managerial skills. Managers for the future will need to learn techniques for instilling collaboration, cooperation, self-direction and commitment. As tomorrow's restructured environments are adapted to accommodate new categories and types of workers, coordination, communication and team building will be essential managerial skills (Kanter, 1990; O'Boyle, 1990).

Drucker (1980) states that managers are paid to enable people to be fully productive and that the job of the boss is to be a resource, to support employees in meaningful work, and to provide exposure to continuous learning. He identifies these characteristics as necessary elements in the management of knowledge workers and integral to the productivity of the human resource. Contemporary nurse administrators are well versed in these areas and will master the new fundamentals in the management of people.

The entrepreneurial nurse administrator will see that nursing work is carefully analyzed and evaluated. All elements of that work will be identified and considered, with attention focused on all things that are done, asking if in fact they should be done, and, if so, who is presently doing them, and then who should be doing them. Such analysis will reveal, in most settings, extraordinarily disproportionate time involved in indirect nonnursing activity by nurses, as compared to direct patient care activity. This is a clear example of the benefit of work analysis and the need to redirect the time of scarce, finite, and increasingly expensive nurse professionals. Such activity leads to creative designs for patient care, with new clinical and nonclinical support systems provided for the professional nurse. Thoughtful nursing work redesign will be the responsibility of tomorrow's nurse manager and will facilitate the utilization of every resource in a manner that maximizes and preserves the quality of the patient care system.

Information System Design

Another key entrepreneurial trait is the ability to design and utilize automated information systems. The term "nursing informatics" has entered our lexicon which is defined as the use of computers to store, analyze and transmit data and communication. Holzemer (1988) refers to the "triangulation of informatics, nursing, and patient care" (p 469). The appropriate use of informatics will enable us to reshape administrative, clinical, education, and research systems. Computer technology that is properly designed can yield impressive results in understanding the cost and quality of patient care, in managing the delivery of patient care services, and in recruiting and retaining staff. Also, computer technology can be a significant labor-saving device for those who provide patient care. Automated charting and documentation systems and rapid accessibility to clinical data are exceptionally useful to the practicing nurse. Point of care capability such as bedside computers promise to greatly enhance nursing productivity.

Information systems that support nursing administrative practice and provide essential decision support also are being developed and utilized. Staffing and scheduling systems, quality monitoring results, precise cost information, and utilization reports are examples of data and systems that support administrative decision making. A strategic plan, developed and adopted within each organization, enables the organization to adequately plan for the incorporation of appropriate information systems and technologies. This process, which requires adequate time and attention, is well worth the investment. Comprehensive information systems can provide a distinct competitive advantage in enhancing managerial and clinical performance.

RESEARCH AND THEORY DEVELOPMENT

There is no dispute that clinical research is critical to validating practice and developing theory. Nurse administrators are acknowledging their roles as contributors to research and theory development by asking cause-and-effect questions about the situations that they encounter in practice (Anderson, 1989) and by supporting clinical nursing research in their setting. As research is designed that shows clinical nursing activity directly improves patient outcomes and thus reduces the cost and length of stay, the cost-benefit of clinical nursing research will be evident. Approaches such as this will yield tangible results and enthusiastic support for funding research activity within the nursing division.

In addition, nursing administration research is urgently needed as we are continuously and scientifically examining relationships that exist between certain actions and certain predictable outcomes. Today's challenge is to continuously improve patient outcomes in compressed periods of time, at lower cost, and with no compromise in quality. Nursing administration research must be aimed at developing systems to isolate, highlight, and manage cost while measuring quality in defensible and readily understood terms. Administrative research also will be important for system design and validation. For example, data about the parameters associated with a change in care delivery models (cost, patient and staff satisfaction, length of stay, quality measures) are necessary in order to analyze critically the results of the change. Nurse executives are continuously asked to make decisions that have long-range implications and significance. Decision support systems are needed for nurse administrators so that actions are built on a solid, tested information base. Decisions are better, they are more solidly based, and they are supported more readily when they are quantitatively focused. Today's issues are too complex, the stakes are too high, and the demands are far too pressing not to have a continually developed base of information upon which to evaluate actions and proposals (Fralic, 1989).

NEW DIRECTIONS

Tomorrow's nurse administrator must deal smoothly and effectively with all categories of colleagues. The institution's medical leadership is one crucial area that requires successful relationships and interaction. Other division or department heads also are key colleagues requiring effective interactions. In addition, the nurse administrator must be able to work effectively with unionized work groups if that is part of the work environment. Unions may represent professional, technical, or support level workers. Appropriate participation and demeanor during the negotiating process, reasoned decisions, and subsequent contract administration also are essential skills that must be cultivated.

Today's work force, as described by Drucker (1980), is two-pronged. One segment is composed of "knowledge workers" with fairly advanced education who perform highly specialized tasks and enjoy almost unlimited mobility. The other segment consists of "service workers," many with limited schooling and skills. Even though there are many commonalities, each group requires different management approaches, policies, and practices. Each group responds to a different organization of work and expectations and needs for recognition and reward differ. Values between the two groups also may differ greatly. The effective nurse administrator is sensitive to these distinctions and is appropriately responsive.

Managing the new-breed professional brings with it the requirement for new competencies. There has been and will continue to be a required major revamping in the way organizations attract employees and design benefits. Demands of the new breed professional include flexible scheduling, self-governance and participative management systems, career ladders, job sharing, selection among multiple benefit choices, child care, elder care, among others. The *Wall Street Journal* (January 9, 1990, p B1) reported that American employers are entering a new era of employer-employee relations. Companies are responding with benefits that cater to employees' "life stages," providing different benefit choices for each phase of a worker's life. The objective is to increase job satisfaction and retain valued employees. Contemporary nurse administrators will see nurses as highly valuable resources and will be comfortable with a professional staff that requires a highly challenging work environment, different compensation structures, consideration for their family responsibilities and personal lives, and also for their need to share in the decision-making process relative to patient care.

Assessment and Incorporation of Technology

The rapid advancement of technology in health care has raised serious issues of ethics and cost. New medical technology has extended life and often dramatically increased expenditures, thus stirring vigorous debate in health care circles about the proper application of technology and equitable access. Technological developments will undoubtedly impact and shape future clinical practice. For example, newly developed technical machines will require new skills and often new categories of workers to operate and maintain them; future implantable medication delivery methods will require different nursing systems; newer and more portable dialysis equipment will dramatically alter care regimens for renal patients; the development of new immuno-suppressant drugs is stimulating rapid advancement in the scope of organ transplantation; genome research and other biotechnological advances will reshape disease processes as we know them today. Nurse administrators must be prepared to analyze all emerging technology for the impact on practice, cost, and the ethical dimension surrounding the application of such technology.

New equipment developments can often be considered labor-saving devices. For example, devices that provide automated blood pressure and blood gas readings directly conserve nursing time. The ability of cardiac monitoring equipment to automatically download data to bedside computer systems eliminate data entry or documentation by nurses. Managing technology—that is, the right choice of technological tools and the knowledge of how to use them—will distinguish the nurse administrator of the 1990s.

Other Trends

Over the next decade, nurse administrators will face many demands, including a renewed focus on strategic planning and the ability to incorporate substantive high-level planning into relatively compressed time frames of intense activity. This concept is called Compression Planning (Nettles, 1989). "Compression planning requires a team of key people determined to resolve their issue—within hours or days, not weeks or months. . . . Today's fast-paced competition makes it difficult to tolerate talk-it-to-death intellectualizers who drain energy from organizations. High speed, collaborative, and decisive action is demanded in order to succeed" (p 34).

Marketing the nursing product is another skill that is commanding increased importance. The quality and caliber of the nursing product is a distinct marketing edge to an institution and the savvy nurse executive knows how to showcase that strength. All the while, in each of these areas, the nurse executive is managing fast-paced and inexorable change. Competencies such as these will be the hallmarks of success.

MANAGEMENT LEVELS AND NECESSARY SKILL AREAS

Simon's (1976) extensive work in decision making serves as the basis for the thesis that management is decision making. Charns and Schaefer's premise (1983) is that decision making in the interest of improved organizational performance is the work of nurse managers at all levels of management. The next step is to identify the requisite skill areas and competencies that nurse managers must possess.

Katz (1974) classified observable skills of managers and identified three basic skill areas: conceptual, human, and technical. He states that all successful managers must possess these skills in varying degrees, according to the levels of management position that they hold.

Conceptual skill enables one to think of "relative emphasis and priorities among conflicting objectives and criteria; relative tendencies and probabilities (rather than certainties); rough correlations and patterns among elements (rather than clear-cut, cause-and-effect relationships)" (Katz, p 101). Katz observes that the ability to conceptualize may best be viewed as an innate ability. This is perhaps true, since one can look at a group of staff nurses in action, and a certain few will demonstrate the ability to see beyond their own patient assignment, and to view the entire work unit, and then to see that work unit as part of the larger whole of the nursing division. These nurses are the innate conceptualizers.

The concept of human skill is divided into leadership ability within the manager's own unit and skill in intergroup relationships. Katz notes that "internal intragroup skills are essential in lower and middle management roles and that intergroup skills become increasingly important in successively higher levels of management" (p 101).

Technical skill implies "an understanding of, and proficiency in, a specific kind of activity, particularly one involving methods, processes, procedures, or techniques" (Katz, p 91). The technical category can be modified by dividing technical skill into nursing management technology and nursing practice technology. Most managers are more comfortable with practice technology since it is more concrete and familiar. But management technology also consists of skills that can be applied in specific situations, such as, coaching, disciplining or appraising employees. The amount and type of technical skill required varies according to the size and scope of the management position held.

The mix or blend of conceptual, human, and technical skill requirement is variable and this provides a useful conceptual base for viewing nursing management work. For example, head nurses require the highest level of nursing practice technology since they supervise the direct work of patient care. Conversely, the role of chief nursing officer requires the least level of nursing practice technology and the highest level of conceptual skill, since that person is farthest removed from direct work, but is responsible for linking all subunits of the nursing division and then linking the division to the total organization. Assessing the level of conceptual, human, and technical skill is valuable in evaluating nurse managers or prospective nurse managers.

How Nursing Services are Organized

There is much variation in how nursing divisions are organized. However, certain titles and basic levels occur in most organizations; some may have only one or two of these levels, and others may have all of them. However, the top nursing position in health care organizations is the chief nurse executive (can be known as senior vice-president, vice-president, or other titles consistent with other senior level positions in the organization). That person has overall responsibility for the quality of the nursing service and the cost and productivity of the resources utilized in providing that service. Next is the associate/assistant administrator level, also known by a wide variety of titles. This position may or may not be present in smaller organizations. The next level frequently found is the clinical directors of nursing, commonly designated to certain clinical services (eg, director of critical care nursing, medical or surgical nursing). This person often manages multiple units within a nursing division. A supervisor may or may not be present, or may only be present on the evening and night shifts. The head nurse manages a specific unit and reports directly to a respective clinical director of nursing.

This description depicts typical nursing service hierarchies although infinite variety occurs across organizations. Flatter organizational designs appear to be most responsive to current environments. The mission of the organization, philosophy of its leadership and of the nursing division, and the complexity of its patient care systems will determine the type and nature of the management hierarchy and structure. Very new and different management structures surely will develop over the next decade, driven by evolving institutional models, matrix and service line structures, the nature and scope of nursing work, span of control, and evolving characteristics of the work force. The continuing challenge for the nurse executive will be to consistently evaluate all elements within the nursing division to determine the type, nature, and structure of management and supervision that will be appropriate and effective for each institution.

EFFECTIVENESS: THE GOAL OF THE NURSE ADMINISTRATOR

One can be considered to be effective when stipulated goals and objectives are met. The success of the nurse executive is the sum total of personal, group, and organizational performance. Wise managers know that they cannot be successful unless their subordinates succeed. The collective strength and performance of individual work units creates the successful manager.

How does one maintain the essential skills needed to be effective and to operate within dynamic managerial environments? One answer is that the nurse administrator must have a systematic plan and program for continuous self-development. Comprehensive reading is essential. In addition to the clinical nursing and nursing administration literature, an effective administrator also reads the business and health care and hospital literature.

The sheer volume of required professional reading can be overwhelming and requires a manageable approach. The Current Journal Index can help manage this task. A librarian compiles all of the table of content pages for a particular set of journals each month. The administrator, along with senior staff, selects key journals from any literature source (nursing, business, health care) to review on a monthly basis. The librarian puts the table of content pages into a packet and circulates them. Administrators scan the topics in all of the key publications each month obtaining copies of articles of particular interest to read. This technique far surpasses the traditional method of creating stacks of journals that continue to grow, outdate, and seldom get read. By using a Current Journal Index, administrators can keep abreast of all of the key publications in nursing and related fields by being able to scan everything from, for example, the *Harvard Business Review,* to *Medical Economics,* to *Modern Healthcare,* to the *Journal of Nursing Administration,* to the *American Journal of Nursing.* The administrator can keep current on issues and topics and has access to the latest information.

Additional Administrative Functions/Skills

Successful administration obviously requires the ability to manage large budgets by utilizing expert financial skills. Planning capability (long-term, short-term, and operational planning) is a literal cornerstone of managerial competence. The ability to measure the cost and quality of the nursing product cannot be overemphasized. Every facet of the new environment will require that the highest quality product be delivered at reasonable and competitive cost.

A new focus on the customer and orientation to the market also is required. As Hymowitz suggests (*Wall Street Journal,* March 20, 1989) "managers will be intimately hooked to suppliers and customers and well versed in competitors' strategies. Swift product design and marketing decisions will be essential. Instant performance will be the norm and incompetence will be difficult to hide" (Hymowitz, 1989, p B1). The nurse administrator must be able to translate these ideas from the corporate world to the world of patient care.

Other skills and abilities that the nurse administrator must possess include analyzing the ethical and legal dimensions of nursing practice, structuring the organization for productivity and quality, and planning for innovation (the research and development function). Then the nursing division can be poised to move forward in new, demanding, and ever-changing environments.

Another necessary skill is facilities planning. Nurse administrators bring operational realities to physical plant projects, contributing a needed dimension to the design of environments in which patient care will occur. Chapter 19 describes and explains effective planning of physical facilities.

The ability to function in an intra- and inter-professional manner is another element needed for success in nurse administration. Constant and productive interaction with other professions is necessary. One also feels the responsibility to contribute actively to the profession of nursing, adding to its prominence and visibility, since nurse executives represent literally hundreds of nurses within their organizations.

How does one find time to fill all of these myriad roles and to acquire all of these skills and attributes? Oncken and Wass (1974) provide wonderful insight as to how managers create available time, in their classic article entitled "Management Time: Who's Got the Monkey?" They analyze boss-imposed time, system-imposed time, and self-imposed time, and observe that the management of time necessitates that managers get control over the timing and content of what they do. Their "monkey-on-the-back" analogy focuses on the category of subordinate-imposed time and gives clear direction to managers on how to reconceptualize and reallocate the hours available to them. It is instructive and humorous reading, and recommended for all serious managers.

CONCEPTUALIZING NURSING ADMINISTRATION

Now, having visualized the entire panorama of the present and future field of nursing administration, it is useful to conceptualize the management work to be done, particularly in fast moving and often tumultuous environments. Contingency models are particularly well suited for these environments, since they are not prescriptive, but rather are contingent on situational factors and are wholly responsive to the environment. Charns and Schaefer (1983) present a useful example of a theory-based contingency model predicated on the premise that management is decision making. They identify three critical areas in which all managers make decisions:

- The interface of the organization with the environment
- Organizational design
- Managerial strategies

Management decisions that concern the organization's interface with the environment pertain to the external environment and the organization's mission, purpose, and goals. Decisions that involve the design of the organization relate to (1) the work, (2) the people, (3) the structure, and (4) coordination. Managerial strategies are viewed as either formal managerial technologies (eg, budget systems, position descriptions) or informal management processes (eg, power and influence, leadership). The effective administrator is required to make decisions in each of these areas and the quality of the decision will be largely determined by the nature, scope, and caliber of the information on which the decision is based.

The Charns and Schaefer model (1983) enables one to view the entire spectrum of management work. One can conceptualize every arena in which managers must act. A nursing administrator can utilize this model daily as a vehicle for the consideration, analysis, and synthesis of data, and subsequently as the basis for decision making. Conceptualizing management enables one to visualize and then properly compartmentalize the many elements of the work to be done and decisions to be made. Critical decision areas that all nurse administrators must consider are depicted in Figure 1–1 which is based on the Charns and Schaefer framework.

THE FUTURE

The nurse executive in the future will be more accountable, more influential, more corporate in mindset, and more competitive in acquiring resources for patient care. This nurse executive will function in a variety of single and multi-institutional models and structures, and will be able to effectively manage a diverse and multicultural work force. This person will be responsive to the increasing demand for higher qual-

I. Environmental Interface
  A. External Environment
    1. The Organization
      a) the overall organization
      b) intra-division
        (1) manpower supply (professional/nonprofessional)
        (2) the contemporary worker
        (3) technology
        (4) institutional history
      c) inter-department
        (1) the contemporary worker
        (2) technology
        (3) institutional history
      d) medical staff
        (1) the contemporary physician
        (2) patient care
        (3) research
        (4) technology
        (5) institutional history
    2. The Government
      a) accrediting, regulatory, and legal bodies
      b) political relations
      c) economic forces
    3. The Profession
      a) professional nursing practice issues
      b) nursing education systems
      c) student relationships (formal/informal)
    4. The Society
      a) health care trends and issues
        (1) general population demographics
        (2) societal and economic forces
        (3) emerging technologies (medical/non-medical)
      b) public relations
        (1) community relations
        (2) societal and economic forces
  B. Mission, Purpose, and Goals
    1. Organizational
    2. Divisional
    3. Unit Level
      a) philosophy
      b) objectives
II. Organizational Design
  A. Work
    1. Analysis
      a) patient care
      b) research support
  B. People
    1. Type
      a) preparation
      b) knowledge
      c) capability
      d) tenure
    2. Numbers
    3. Mix
  C. Structure
    1. Division of Work
    2. Allocation of Decision Making
    3. Design of Variable Approaches for Varying Degrees of Uncertainty
      a) imitative
      b) innovative
  D. Coordination
    1. What requires coordination
    2. How is it best coordinated
    3. Inter-System Dependencies
      a) inter-unit
      b) non-nursing support systems
      c) medical care systems
      d) research systems
III. Managerial Strategies
  A. Formal Managerial Technologies
    1. standards of care
    2. quality of care indexes
    3. audits
    4. position descriptions
    5. performance appraisal
    6. reward system
    7. educational system
    8. scheduling/assignments
    9. procedures
    10. planning technologies
    11. research
    12. committees
    13. policies
    14. work rules
    15. budgetary processes
    16. information systems
  B. Informal Managerial Processes
    1. Power
    2. Status
    3. Influence
    4. Leadership
    5. Committees
    6. Allocation of Informal Rewards
    7. Relationships
      a) unit level RN/MD
      b) staff
      c) peer collaboration

Figure 1-1. Critical Decision Areas for Nurse Managers *(Source: Reprinted by permission of the JB Lippincott Company. An exhibit from Fralic MF, O'Connor A, A Management Progression System for Nurse Administrators, Part 1,* Journal of Nursing Administration. *April 1983, 9–13.)*

ity, lower cost, and precise resource tracking systems, recognizing that these are nursing's strong suits. These strengths will be developed, showcased, and interpreted in systematic quantitative ways.

The nurse executive will be actively involved in preparing the next generation of nurse administrators and in influencing their curriculum and educational experiences. Practicing nurse executives will collaborate closely with faculty to assure that there is an appropriate blend and integration of academia and the practice world, and that a rigorous curriculum and pace is established to reflect the realities of the work place.

The nurse executive of today and tomorrow will work assiduously to accomplish two things. First, to acquire and sharpen every skill that will be needed to perform competently in the 1990s and second, to assure that those who follow will be ready, enthusiastic, and well prepared to face every challenge that the future will surely present. Nurse executives of the next decade will treat these responsibilities seriously, will be challenged and stimulated by them, and will know with certainty that the quality and integrity of patient care systems will be their contribution to the future.

REFERENCES

American Association of Colleges of Nursing. Special Report: RN Baccalaureate Nursing Education (1986–1988). Washington, DC, American Association of Colleges of Nursing. (ERIC Document Reproduction Service No. ED-299-866) 1988

Anderson R. A theory development rose for nurse administrators. *Journal of Nursing Administration.* 19:5, 23 May 1989

Bair NL, Griswold JT, Head JL. Clinical RN involvement in bedside-centered case management. *Nursing Economics.* 7:3, 150, May–June 1989

Brett JL, Tonges MC. Restructured patient care delivery: Evaluation of the ProACT model, *Nursing Economics.* 8:1, 36, January/February 1990

Calano J, Salzman J. The power of decisiveness. *USAir.* 58, June 1988

Charns MP, Schaefer MJ. *Health Care Organizations—A Model for Management.* Englewood Cliffs, NJ, Prentice-Hall, 1983

Drucker PF. *Managing in Turbulent Times,* New York, Harper & Row, 1980

Drucker PF. How to manage your boss. *Management Review,* 9, May 1977

Fralic MF. Decision support systems: Essential for quality administrative decisions. *Nursing Administration Quarterly.* 14:1, 1989

Gabarro JJ, Kotter JP. Managing your boss. *Harvard Business Review* 92, January–February 1980

Gamble SW. Changing roles in the '90s: Will RNs manage MDs? *Hospitals.* 42, November 20, 1989

Griffin GJ, Griffin HJ. *Jensen's History and Trends of Professional Nursing,* 5th ed. St. Louis, MO, C V Mosby Co, 1965

Hall J. *The Competence Connection—A Blueprint for Excellence.* The Woodlands, TX: Woodstead Press, 1988

Hechenberger NB. The future of nursing administration education. *Journal of Professional Nursing.* 4:4, 279, 1988

Holzemer WL. Nursing informatics: Remembering our future. *Nursing & Health Care.* 469, November/December 1988

Huckabay L. Allocation of resources and identification of issues in determining the cost of nursing services. *Nursing Administration Quarterly.* 72, 1988

Hymowitz C. Day in the life of tomorrow's manager. *Wall Street Journal.* March 20, 1989

Johnson JE, Sparks DG, Humphreys C. Writing a winning business plan. *Journal of Nursing Administration.* 18:10, 15, October 1988

Kanter RM. When giants learn to dance. New York, Simon and Shuster, 1990

Katz DR. Coming home. *Business Month.* 57, October 1988

Katz RL. Skills for an effective administrator. *Harvard Business Review.* 90, September/October 1974

Kerfoot KM. Thinking administratively: A must for the effective nurse manager. *Nursing Economics.* 6:3, 139, May-June 1988

Nettles J. Compression planning. *USAir.* 34, February 1989

O'Boyle TF. From pyramid to pancake. *Wall Street Journal.* R-37, June 4, 1990

O'Donnell KP. Shared values, corporate culture foster good hiring, *Modern Healthcare.* 19(44), November 3, 1989

Oncken W Jr, Wass DL. Management time: Who's got the monkey? *Harvard Business Review.* 52:6, 75, November/December 1974

Orr P. Factors important to BSN graduating seniors and employment decisions. *Nursing Management.* 20:6, 68, 1989

Perry L. Nurse executives managing more executive services, solidifying their roles—survey. *Modern Healthcare.* 92, March 10, 1989

Pfeffer J, Salancik GR. *The External Control of Organizations.* New York, Harper & Row, 1978

Rosenfeld P. *Nursing Student Census, 1989.* New York, NLN, 1, 1990

Simon HA. *Administrative Behavior: A Study of Decision Making Processes in Administrative Organization.* 3rd ed. New York, Free Press, 1976

Tonges MC. Redesigning hospital nursing practice: The professionally advanced care team (ProACT) Model, Part 1. *Journal of Nursing Administration.* 19:7, 31, July/August, 1989

Uyterhoeven H. General managers in the middle. *Harvard Business Review.* 136, September/October 1989

Vaill PB. *Managing as a Performing Art.* San Francisco, CA, Jossey-Bass, 1989

Vergara GH. Playing the cover game by the rules. *Health Care Executive.* 27, Vol. 4:6, November/December 1989

Vestal KW. Writing a business plan. *Nursing Economics.* Vol. 6:3, 121, May–June 1988

CHAPTER 2

Synthesis of Nursing and Organizational Theories

Phyllis Schultz

> ## Key Concept List
>
> Definition of an organization
> Types of organizations providing health care
> Nursing theories
> Administration theories
>   the mechanistic perspective
>   the organismic perspective
>   the potentiating perspective
> Organization design

From birth to death, it is commonly acknowledged that human experience is lived mostly through organizations. From 35 to 60 percent of adults' waking hours are spent in some type of organization—most of it in employment. Although some types of paid work involves working out of one's home, more than 90 percent of society's needs for goods and services are met through simple or complex organizations (Hall, 1986). *Organizations are systems of coordinated actions done by groups of people toward common goals under some form of leadership or coordination.*

The nature of work and employment are changing substantially as the nation's economy is based more on information and services than on the production of materials and goods. These are revolutionary changes Drucker describes as the "post-business knowledge society" and Kanter calls the "post-entrepreneurial society"

(Drucker, 1989, p 173; Kanter, 1989, p 9). Organizations are changing to adjust to these societal trends and the manner in which they are managed is changing as well.

With few exceptions, most nursing care is provided through some type of organization. Even in home care settings, families and friends rely on assistants and professionals to whom they gain access primarily through nursing and health care organizations of some type.

A principal reason for the pervasiveness of organizations is that greater achievements and efficiencies can be gained by pooling the talents, knowledge and skills of many persons. In addition, people enjoy interacting with others and finding ways to realize their individual goals through collective efforts. To accomplish the benefits of coordinated effort, organizations must be coordinated. This is the responsibility of administrators and managers. Yet, for all their beneficial qualities, organizations often leave persons feeling dehumanized, frustrated, angry, and demoralized. Blocked communications, dictatorial decisions, arbitrary application of rules, and punitive actions undermine peoples' sense of accomplishment, threaten productivity and thwart creativity.

Administrators of organizations are held responsible for how people experience organizations, both by those who work in them and those who come in contact with them. As a result, all administrators, including nurse administrators, must understand how organizations are formed, how decisions are made, how tasks and skills are organized, and how organizations grow, change, decline, and, sometimes, die.

FOUNDATIONS OF ADMINISTRATIVE PRACTICE

The practice of administration is the actions administrators take, based on their own knowledge and other information, to create and sustain organizations for achieving shared goals. The foundation for this practice is knowledge of organizations as uniquely human phenomena. Both descriptive (empirical) and prescriptive (normative) knowledge are required. The foundation for administration is experience *and* knowledge gleaned from nursing, and behavioral, social, organizational sciences (Blair, 1989).

Nursing science—theories and research on which to base practice—has been developing for more than a century. Nursing theories, with the exception of Nightingale's writings, appeared in the literature as early as 1952. They originated primarily from nurses' reflections on their clinical care of individuals, families and groups. While Nightingale advised that the management of nurses in hospitals was to be by a "trained nurse" who understood how to organize care (Nightingale, 1858), development of nursing science for administrative practice has lagged behind clinical.

Organizations became the focus of systematic study in the twentieth century. Scott identified the late 1940s as the time when the study of organizations appeared as a "specialized field of inquiry within the discipline of sociology" (Scott, 1987, p 7–8). Consequently, there is available a large body of literature in many disciplines for understanding the formation, maintenance, growth, change, and death of nursing organizations. The aim here is to integrate that of nursing and business.

DEFINITIONS OF ORGANIZATION

Systematic study of organizations led to definitions of the concept. Definitions helped to distinguish formally structured and legally recognized organizations from various other collectivities such as gatherings of individuals for social events, transient group-ings for political demonstrations, or rescue efforts following a disaster. Scott (1987) suggested that many available definitions of the concept of organization reflect a theo-retical perspective. Organizations defined as goal-directed, for example, hierarchi-cally structured enterprises are used which emphasize a rational, efficiency-driven perspective. Other definitions reflect a view of organizations as natural, organic sys-tems focused on survival. Still others consider the influence of internal and external environments with organizations defined as coalitions of political interest groups with conflicting and differing types and degrees of power. Morgan (1986) summa-rized a wide range of literature to define organizations in metaphorical images: ma-chines, organisms, brains, cultures, political systems, psychic prisons, beings in flux and transformation, and instruments of domination. These metaphors draw attention to the many facets of experience in organizations. They bring to awareness supportive or troublesome aspects that tend to be taken for granted. Organizations are dynamic collectivities of human social interaction continually recreated and sustained through dynamic processes of coordination and conflict enacted by members who share a common mission and who pool their talents and energies toward individual and or-ganizational achievement.

CURRENT TYPES OF ORGANIZATIONS
FOR PROVIDING HEALTH CARE

The changing economic base of society and the range and complexity of health ser-vices have given rise to many types of organizations. One way to categorize the health care organizations is across the lifespan on a continuum from primary care to long-term care (see Fig. 2–1).

At one end of the continuum are organizations through which primary or first access care is provided. At the other end are organizations through which long-term care in homes is provided. Organizations between the two ends of the continuum include alternatives to hospitals, hospital care, and posthospital centers (eg, highly specialized diagnostic, surgical and rehabilitation centers). Hospital care includes small community hospitals, regional hospitals, and large community and teaching hospitals. Posthospital care is provided through highly specialized home visits, reha-bilitation hospitals, and long-term care facilities that may include several levels of care. With the exception of the highly specialized centers and the highly technological

Primary care	Alternatives to hospitals	Hospital care	Posthospital care	Long-term care

Clinics
  private
  public health
  HMO'S
  PPO'S
	Diagnostic
	  centers
		Small community
		  hospitals
		
		Regional hospitals
			High tech/
			  acute
			  home care
				Home care

	Surgical
	  centers
		Large community
		  hospitals
				Long-term
				  facilities

Occupational health		Teaching hospitals		

School clinics	Rehabilitation
	  centers
		Specialty
		  hospitals
			Rehabilitation
			  hospitals	

Prison clinics				
[- - - - - - outpatient - - - - - -]			[- - - - - outpatient - - - - - -]	
[© © © © © © © © © inpatient © © © © © © © © ©]				

Figure 2-1. Continuum of Health Care: Types of Health Care Organizations[a]

[a]Health care organizations vary by type of ownership, managerial control, payment sources, type of environment, and market control.

home care, inpatient care is characteristic of the organizations listed in the midsection of the continuum.

TYPES OF ORGANIZING STRUCTURES

In addition to the complexity of types of care represented on the continuum, health care organizations vary according to several dimensions (eg, ownership, size, managerial control, environments, and market). For example, primary care organizations may be privately owned medical or public health clinics, outpatient offices of health maintenance organizations (HMOs), or consortia of private medical corporations. They may vary in size and administrative structure from small groups of specialty physicians or nurses in public health clinics with one administrative level, to multidepartment outpatient clinics in teaching hospitals.

The types of ownership and managerial control of health care organizations also varies considerably. They may be owned by a single individual or a partnership with little formal structural differentiation or coordination between those who provide the care and those who manage. Another type is the large national or multinational investor-owned corporations with divisional structures in which management is part of the corporation. These health care organizations are characteristic of the ''managerial model'' commonly observed in corporations in other sectors of society (Scott, 1982). Still others include locally owned corporations, often with traditional ties to church groups or community-based philanthropic organizations. The structures may be divisional, matrix or some combination. The management of these organizations may be part of the corporation or may be under contract with another organization specializing in health care management (Shortell & Kaluzny, 1988). A "heteronomous model" of management may evolve in these organizations to give a competitive edge through a partnership of professionals and managers (Scott, 1982). Health care corporations may be owned by a cooperative and have a multidivisional structure to provide care across the entire continuum from primary care through tertiary hospital to long term facility and home care (Conrad, Mick, Madden, & Hoare, 1988). These vertically integrated systems control many aspects of the health care market, reducing the uncertainty and turbulence of their environments.

In addition to variations in intra-organizational patterns of ownership and structure, administrators of health care organizations may join with other organizations in various types of interorganizational arrangements to coordinate efforts and provide a broad spectrum of services (Rogers & Whetten, 1982; Conrad, Mick, Madden & Hoare, 1988). The systematic study of organizations has revealed a continuum of interorganizational relationships (IOR) ranging from little or no relationship to varying types and complexities of control and consolidation: They include organizational agreements, contracts, unification to consolidation into multicorporate holding companies. The types of goals, numbers of persons served, the number and type of resources used, complexity of care, formalization of rules, the nature of the power distribution, and degree of control over decision-making influence the type of IOR (Rogers & Whetten, 1982).

Exchange of information to facilitate care is all that is required in referral relationships (Morrissey, Hall, & Lindsey, 1982). If, however, personnel or other resources are to be exchanged, formal agreements may need to be drawn up. If one organization provides an entire service—high risk maternity and/or neonatal care, for example—a contract that specifies policies as well as exchange agreements is needed. These types of agreements may result in a "set of organizations" with one focal organization involved in dyadic agreements with other organizations, or a "network" of organizations designed to attain self-interest goals or provide services to a specific population (Morrissey, Hall, & Lindsey, 1982). A more middle-range type of IOR is some form of overarching governing agreement within which the previously independent organizations or units carry out their interdependent activities. Finally, the most inclusive and controlling form of IOR is the purchase of one organization by another. When this type of agreement is transacted, the IOR reverts to an intra-organizational structure. Starkweather referred to the variations in IOR arrangements as "affiliation," "management contract," "umbrella corporation," or "merger consolidation" in his study of hospital mergers (Starkweather, 1981).

Recent rapid changes in organizational structure in health care have been stimulated by economic factors in the environment—(eg, market competition, government regulation, rising costs) (Conrad, Mick, Madden, & Hoare, 1988). Fixed forms of intra-organizational vertical and horizontal integration (Scott, 1987) such as divisions and matrices have given way to combinations of structures that mix intra-organizational and interorganizational forms within a single organization (Thompson, 1967). Control of operations is increasingly decentralized to units where critical operations occur even as initiatives for strategic innovation are centralized. The purpose of these emerging forms is to improve a health care organization's ability to respond to fluctuations in the environment by controlling more components of the continuum of care without increasing the transaction costs (Conrad, Mick, Madden & Hoare, 1988).

NURSING CARE

Nursing is part of the services provided in all health care organizations represented on the continuum of care (Fig. 2–1). The extent to which nursing is the principle service varies as does the type and complexity of nursing care. Concurrently, the educational and skill level of nursing personnel also vary. These variances require the ability to deal with a wide range of organizational complexity. Nurse administrators manage organizations that range from small to very large size, from one or two dimensions of formal structure to several levels of hierarchy and multiple divisions, from the supervision of one or two office staff to the direction of multiple types of professional and support personnel with varying degrees of educational preparation and skills, from a few hundred clients per year to hundreds of thousands, from budgets of a few thousand to millions of dollars.

Given the variations and complexities of health care organizations, administrators face situations of uncertainty, change, and conflicts that demand performance that is more than a set of technical skills. They must hold the mission of the organization in their consciousness even as they oversee the technical performance of the smallest units. They must inspire creativity and innovation in people even as they insist on high productivity (Kanter, 1989). To confront these challenges, administrators need to possess a guide to action that is based on more than the expediencies of the moment (Schon, 1987). Such a guide is theory.

USE OF THEORY IN PRACTICE

Stevens notes that nurse administrators theorize, whether they realize it or not "by virtue of the structures they employ to place patients and staff, to distribute the work to be done, and to tell how it is to be accomplished" (1984, p 125).

Argyris and Schon (1974) call such theories "theories-in-use," which are to be distinguished from espoused theories. Espoused theories are what someone says they would do in a particular set of circumstances. An individual's espoused theories may or may not be compatible with their theories-in-use. To put it plainly, actions speak louder than words!

Why Theories for Practice?

"A practice is a sequence of actions undertaken by a person to serve others who are considered clients" (Argyris & Schon, 1974, p 6). It is more than skills and completion of tasks. A practice is a mosaic of beliefs, values, knowledge and intentions that result in an excellence of performance of intrinsic worth that extends beyond tangible outcomes (MacIntyre, 1985). Job design is a skill; managing an organization is a practice. Conflict management is a skill; inspiring people to work together for a common good is a practice.

Just as many nursing theories evolved from clinical practice, theories of nursing administration can be generated from practice. Reflective scholarship and research by practicing nurse administrators and nurse researchers also can generate nursing administration theories. They are needed to ground the specialty practice of nursing administration squarely in the nursing discipline even as it incorporates knowledge from the organization sciences (Henry, 1989; Orem, 1989).

Theories stimulate practitioners to consider the assumptions and values they hold about their clients and to become more intentional in the actions they take (Argyris & Schon, 1974). A clear understanding of the client is essential for identifying theories to guide administrative actions.

The Client in Nursing Administration

Traditionally, in nursing, the client has been identified as a person, family, or group with whom individual nurses interact to restore, promote, or maintain health. Systematic concept analysis of the term client in nursing revealed that nurse administrators focus on several clients at once. Furthermore, the nature of their client is threefold: (1) persons who receive nursing care regardless of setting; (2) persons who deliver nursing care; and (3) nursing care organizations as social interactional units (Schultz, 1987). Some examples of group (1) are those who receive care—inpatients, outpatients, families, or community groups. Examples of group (2) are those who provide care, support staff who support the direct care providers, and administrative staff who direct, facilitate and coordinate delivery of care. Some components of the social interactional whole of the nursing organization (3) include resources, costs of providing care, quality of care, subunit interaction, and the social and technical work environment (Schultz & Miller, 1990).

This extended definition of client requires that other central concepts of nursing, (eg, environment, health, and nursing processes) be specified and congruent with it. The nursing process enacted by nurse administrators may include organizational assessment, corporate policy analysis and development, delivery system design, and program development and evaluation as well as individual-level nursing assessment. Theories of nursing administration explicate the unique relationships among nursing's central concepts when the client is both client, provider, and the organization.

How Theories Help

Paradoxes, rapid change, and conflicting demands are the trademarks of organizations today (Kanter, 1989). Theories help practitioners of all types deal with the ''unique, uncertain, conflicted situations of practice'' (Schon, 1987, p 22). Furthermore, repeated actions based on theory give rise to what Schon has called ''professional artistry'' or that excellence of performance which has an aesthetic and moral quality to it that is more than the specific tasks involved. Particular procedures can be combined with skills to accomplish tasks, but theory combined with experience gives rise to the exemplary competence of the "expert practitioner" (Benner, 1984). The goal of expert practitioners is that their espoused theories and their theories-in-use are compatible and consistent. One way for nurse administrators to achieve this goal is to examine the theoretical foundations of their actions by becoming familiar with and integrating theories from nursing and organization science into their practice.

INTEGRATED THEORIES FOR NURSING ADMINISTRATIVE PRACTICE

Inspired by Morgan's use of metaphors to "read organizations" (1986, p 11) and by Henry's categorization of nursing theories according to Morgan's metaphors (Henry, 1989), key concepts from organization science and nursing are brought together to form beginning guides to practice. The formulations are intended to illustrate a synthesis of the nursing and organization sciences.

Classification of Theories

Three major perspectives—the mechanistic, the organismic, and the potentiating are presented in the following sections. Key concepts germane to each perspective are listed in Table 2–1 along with the organization and nursing theorists with which they are associated.

The Mechanistic Perspective—The Classics

Development of the theories that contribute to the mechanistic perspective paralleled the transformation of America from an agrarian to an industrial society. Organiza-

TABLE 2-1. SYNTHESIS OF ORGANIZATION AND NURSING THEORIES FOR NURSING ADMINISTRATIVE PRACTICE

	Key Concepts	Organization Theories	Nursing Theories
Mechanistic	Structure Function Resources Efficiency	Weber Fayol Taylor/Gilbreth Drucker	King Johnson
Organismic	Needs Adaptation Environment Boundary spanning Differentiation Integration Contingency Effectiveness	Maslow/McGregor Herzberg Katz and Kahn Kast and Rosenzweig Lawrence and Lorsch Trist Thompson	Erickson, Tomlin and Swain Roy/Levine Nightingale Orem
Potentiating	Holism Open inquiry Learning to learn Self-organizing Contradictions Mutual causality	Morgan and Ramirez Simon/Cyert and March Argyris and Schon Herbst/Susman Benson/Weick Maruyama	Neuman Rogers Newman Parse

tions are viewed as closely articulated, tightly functioning, efficient enterprises involving clearly stated goals, instrumental rationality (fixed design for decision making), hierarchy, strict lines of communication, clear lines of authority and control, routine, efficiency, and productivity (Morgan, 1986). The organization is considered closed to the outside world and environment and a fixed structure for differentiating tasks and coordinating the work between units is used to achieve organizational goals. Four concepts are especially characteristic: hierarchy (structure), routine (function), efficiency (use of resources), and productivity (goals). A statement of the relationships among these concepts (called a proposition) illustrates the essence of this perspective. It is: *Organizational productivity is a product of hierarchy, routine and efficiency.* The principal proponents of this perspective in organization science are Weber (1947), Fayol (1949), Taylor (1911), Gilbreth (1911), and Drucker (1954).

Although this theoretical perspective tends to view people as instruments rather than as thinking, feeling, creative beings, the key concepts of several nursing theories are mechanistic. For example, King included several mechanistic concepts as the basis of her theory: goal attainment, communication, authority, control, structure, resources, and function (King, 1989). Four of these parallel those from the early classics in organization science: structure (hierarchy), function (routine), resources (efficiency) and goals (productivity). Using King's concepts, a guiding proposition for nursing administrative practice can be formulated: *Goal attainment for the nursing organization is achieved through structure, function and resources.*

The goal for nursing organizations from this perspective is efficient use of people and materials to maintain a high degree of productivity through a fixed structural design for rational decision making (Johnson, 1980). Time-and-motion studies of nursing tasks to improve efficiency, clear lines of command and authority, and control through centralized monitoring of nursing activities contribute to the realization of individual and organizational goals.

Nurse administrators using this perspective will be especially attuned to patient problems and may systematically use patient classifications to describe case mix and costs of care. With an orientation toward efficient use of resources, patients who demand a heavy outlay of nursing resources may be judged to be more than the organization can afford (eg, patients with care requirements more costly than those reimbursed under DRG guidelines). If structural differentiation and coordination in nursing units do not result in improved productivity, strategic planning will direct the nurse administrator to restrict admission of these types of patients and market the organization's services to populations with problems that can be dealt with more efficiently, thereby increasing earnings.

The Organismic Perspective—Open Systems

By midcentury, students of complex organizations and managers had become increasingly aware of two features of organizations ignored by the classical theorists: the importance of meeting the needs of workers for rewards and affiliation (Maslow, 1968; McGregor, 1960) and the influence of forces from the environment impinging on the organization (Katz & Kahn, 1978). It became clear that organizations were not closed but open systems and that organizational survival in an environment was a major force to study. To assure survival of the organization, administrators pay attention to changing factors in the external environment and design the organization so that its subsystems can adapt to environmental demands. Effectiveness is of equal, if not greater, importance than efficiency and is defined as the adaptation of the organization to internal and external environments through contingent rationality (Morgan, 1986). The contingent rationality of the organismic perspective is contrasted with the instrumental rationality of the mechanistic. Contingent rationality means making decisions about organizational design in response to shifting environmental factors rather than in accordance with a predetermined design of people and tasks (Thompson, 1967). More than one design may be required among the subunits of the organization.

Key concepts of the organismic perspective are needs, adaptation, environment, boundary spanning, differentiation, integration, contingency and effectiveness (see Table 2–1) and Chapter 7. Characteristic of this perspective is the concept: *Organizational survival is determined by adaptation to the environment through boundary spanning, structural variation (contingency) and role differentiation.* Lateral communication between units facilitates integration thereby enhancing effectiveness. Integrated exchanges between strategic, technological, human–cultural and structural subsystems and the environmental suprasystem satisfy needs for survival and bring about adaptation (Morgan, 1986, p 49).

Fluctuations in the task environment, which includes sources of system inputs, markets for outputs, competitors and regulators, give rise to uncertainty and dependency. Dimensions of uncertainty include complexity, diversity, variability, threat, isolation, and coordination of these components. Scarcity and dispersion are the dimensions of organizational dependence on resources in the environment. Scanning the task environment is an essential managerial skill within this perspective. The patterns give rise to many middle range propositions which can guide further study and as clues to interventions for organizational survival.

Several nursing theorists incorporate the concepts of need (Erickson, Tomlin, & Swain, 1983), adaptation (Roy, 1984; Levine, 1973), environment (Nightingale, 1858), and boundaries (Orem, 1989) in their theories. Recently, Roy and Anway (1989) have explicated the Roy Adaptation Model for use in nursing administrative practice. It is the most thorough attempt to date to develop a theory essentially organismic and focused on individuals that can describe and explain organizational phenomena. The Roy Adaptation Model for Administration (RAMA), articulates the focus of nursing, whether the client is an individual person or an organization, as comprised of five elements: the person(s), goals, health, environment, and nursing activities. Each element is analogous with an organizational component. These elements are outlined in Fig. 2–2.

According to Roy, the goal of nursing is the adaptation of persons to their environments. The analogous goal for organizations as clients is adaptation to their environments and resources. The concept, environment, is defined as the world in and around the person or as the conditions internal and external to the organization. Health is being and becoming an integrated, whole person or being and becoming an integrated organizational system continuously adapting to environmental demands. Nursing activities include two complementary processes: the nursing process for individual persons as clients and the managerial process for organizations.

CLIENT AS PERSON	CLIENT AS ORGANIZATION
Social interactional being	Social interactional collective
GOAL (OF THE THEORY)	GOAL (OF THE THEORY)
adaptation of persons to their environments	Adaptation of organizations to their environment and resources
ENVIRONMENT	ENVIRONMENT
The world in and around the person	Conditions internal and external to the organization
HEALTH	HEALTH
Being and becoming an integrated, whole person	Being and becoming an integrated system continuously adapting to environmental demands
NURSING ACTIVITIES	NURSING ACTIVITIES
Nursing process	Managerial process
assessing	planning
diagnosing	organizing
implementing	leading
evaluating	controlling
ADAPTIVE SUBSYSTEMS	ADAPTIVE SUBSYSTEMS
Physiologic mode	Physical components
basic life needs	basic resources:
bio-physiological systems	personnel, physical plant, security and fiscal systems
Self-concept	Image and culture
beliefs and feelings about one's self in part from response from others	how organization members perceive themselves from environmental feedback
Role	Role
individual's behavior in society	functions to accomplish the work of the organization
Interdependence	Interdependence
satisfying relationships with others	intra- and interorganizational relationships

Figure 2–2. Using Roy's Client-Centered Theory for Organizations *(Adapted from: Roy C, Anway R. Roy's adaptation model: Theories for nursing administration. In: Henry B, Arndt C, DiVincenti M, Marriner-Tomey A. Dimensions of Nursing Administration: Theory, Research, Education, Practice. Cambridge, MA, Blackwell Scientific Publications, 1989, 75–88)*

The adaptive subsystems of persons have their counterpart for organizations. For example, the adaptive physiologic mode for the person includes the biophysiological systems through which basic life needs are met. Similarly the physical components of an organization are the physical plant, the personnel, security and fiscal systems that are basic to its survival. The image and culture of an organization is analogous to the self-concept of the person. The role subsystem has to do with an individual's behavior in society. The role subsystem of an organization differentiates the work to accomplish tasks. Finally, the interdependence subsystem of the person is the satisfying relationships individuals have with other persons. For an organization, intra-organizational relationships are the strategies for achieving integration and lead to effectiveness. Relationships between organizations bring about integration of the organization with sectors of the environment (eg, hospitals with their suppliers of materials, their managed care contractors, their arrangements with physician-owned professional corporations).

An example of a proposition for guiding action using Roy's model is: *The health of a nursing organization, as a social interactive collective of persons, is determined by effective integration of adaptive subsystems through the application of nursing administration activities to achieve the goal of adaptation to its environment and resources.* The proposition can apply to a nursing unit, to a division in a multidivisional health care corporation, or to a free-standing home health care agency with few members. Definitions of the concepts and the proposition direct the administrator to evaluate the functioning of various organizational subsystems in relation to fluctuations in the environment. For example, the increasing number of elderly, chronically ill members of an HMO could represent a change in the external environment of a home care agency and stimulate negotiation of a new service contract between the agency and the HMO. The contract brings about an alteration in the basic resources (physical subsystem) of the home care agency. To accommodate to the change in the physical subsystem, the role subsystem may have to include more boundary spanners. Information processing procedures may be streamlined, a change in the interdependence subsystem. The image and culture of the home care agency may change from one in which agency members perceive themselves as a relatively small, independent organization to the image of an important actor in an interorganizational network.

The Potentiating Perspective—An Emerging View

The third major theoretical perspective on organizations is an emerging view of organizations as information processing entities in continuous change and metamorphosis (Cyert & March, 1963; Simon, 1947). From this perspective, organizations are viewed holistically as more than the sum of their machinelike parts and more than the whole of their interactive adaptive subsystems (Morgan & Ramirez, 1984). Members of organizations are more than passive responders to environmental opportunities and constraints; they are active players in a dynamic energy field, generating and shaping resources, vigorously pursuing interests, and creating new possibilities. There is no fixed, predetermined structure. Boundaries between units and departments and between the organization and its environment are fluid. They are created and recreated by the people who carry out the essential activities of the organization and their supporting colleagues. From the potentiating perspective, structure evolves from the engagement of members in the internal dynamics of the organization and with its environment as they interact with it directly. It might be characterized as mature and professional.

The potentiating perspective features two themes. The first is from decision-theory suggesting that organizations are uniquely human enterprises with capabilities for handling vast amounts and types of information and for dealing with complexity, uncertainty and ambiguity in much the same way individual humans do. The second theme is that the design of organizations must facilitate these information processing capabilities (Morgan & Ramirez, 1984).

The potentiating perspective also suggests that organizations are in a continuous process of flux and transformation which are not only self-organizing but are self-producing through circular patterns of interaction with various sectors of their environments. Transformation occurs as a dialectical process between opposing and conflicting demands. It involves a mutual causality which must be understood and its dynamic quality in some sense managed. Conflicting demands in health care, such as taking time to treat the whole person, contradict the demand for increased efficiency and high productivity. Coming to terms with these conflicts requires organizational transformation—new approaches to organizing care and a potentiating perspective.

One proposition that exemplifies the potentiating perspective is: *Open inquiry is essential to members' ability to learn and grow which results in self-organizing for dealing with contradictory, multiple, and mutual causal forces internal and external to the organization.*

Current changes in nursing reflect the dynamics of this perspective. For example, members of nursing units design information systems more responsive to the care needs of patients, change unit operating norms, and design their division of labor so that each nurse can practice nursing as an aesthetic and moral whole rather than a set of tasks. The nursing division epitomizes the holistic practice of nursing even as each nurse reflects that practice. In response to changes in nursing, other components of the organization are energized to examine their own assumptions (learn to learn); the resulting dynamism is what Kanter has called ''churn—the continuous regrouping of people and functions and products to produce unexpected, creative new combinations'' (1989, p 354).

Decision making is more responsive to the needs of people and the configuration of circumstances of the moment. This is markedly different from the fixed rules of decision making of the mechanistic perspective (instrumental rationality) or decisions contingent on environmental factors characteristic of the organismic perspective (contingent rationality).

Nursing theories that encompass the potentiating perspective are of recent origin and tend to be quite controversial. Newman's theory of health as expanding consciousness (1986) and Parse's theory of ''unfolding possibilities'' (1981) are congruent with the potentiating view of organizations. Newman defined health as a process of ''increasing complexity, growth, transformation, and evolution of consciousness'' (1986, p 19). Within each person is the potential for growth and evolving consciousness.

By analogy, many people associated with an organization have the potential for growth through self-organizing forms that facilitate creativity. There is positive energy exchange between individuals, between the components of the organization, between the parts and the whole, and between the organization and the environment.

According to Newman, the nursing process focuses on pattern recognition as the basis for a plan of care. The nurse helps clients bring their underlying patterns to consciousness in relation to their goals (1986). Health is expanding consciousness, that is, a gathering in of information as the stimulus for evolving new patterns. Consciousness is the interaction of time, movement and space.

By extrapolation, nurse administrators who use this perspective to guide their practice will ''read the organization'' to discover the patterns of contradiction and mutual causality in relation to time, movement and space (Morgan, 1986). Administrative initiatives and policies are designed to facilitate self-organization. A characteristic proposition of a Newman perspective in nursing administration may be: *Self-organization will result in increased consciousness of organizational members, release of creativity, and transformation of the entire organization.*

In Parse's theory (1981), three major ideas are emphasized which provide a depth of understanding of the processes of self-organizing, self-producing transformation of organizations. First, persons structure "personal meaning from experiences at various levels of the universe simultaneously (multidimensionally)" (Parse, 1989, p 70). They do this through communicating (languaging), the sense they make of everyday experiences (imaging), and confirming their beliefs about the choices that are made (valuing). Second, persons "cocreate rhythmical patterns that are paradoxical in nature" (p 70): revealing-concealing, enabling-limiting, and connecting-separating. These are the contradictions embedded in the experiences of persons relating to one another. Third, persons "move beyond the 'now' with envisioned dreams and hopes of what is not yet" (p 70).

Persons in organizations enact the processes Parse described and through them, the organization is created and recreated—transformed as a uniquely human enterprise. Persons make sense of their experiences in an organization, coming to terms with organizational contradictions through similarly paradoxical patterns of relating to each other. These patterns of relating enable persons to transcend the current reality of the organization—the now—and envision the organization as they would like it to be. This envisioning empowers persons to originate change which, in turn, transforms the organization.

Nurse administrators who understand organizations from this perspective recognize the patterns of persons relating to one another as the dynamics of any human enterprise. The dynamics cannot be controlled, manipulated or constrained without risk of undermining the very creativity and potentiality that makes the organization responsive to its environment and positioned for success. Nurse administrators who hold the potentiating perspective participate in the processes of organizational transformation (Rogers, 1980). They facilitate envisioning and help to smooth the inevitable conflicts that arise from differing visions across various interrelating groups.

Taking a Different View Altogether

The three theoretical formulations presented above represent only a few of several perspectives on organizations. Other views may appeal to nurse administrators better articulating their experiences in organizations. Henry (1989) has categorized several nursing theories according to these images: organizations as cultures, organizations as political systems, organizations as psychic prisons, and organizations as instruments of domination.

Organizations as Cultures

Viewing organizations as cultures introduces the idea that organizations reflect the values and meanings of the members. Through the socialization of the members to shared norms and values, organizations are socially constructed realities. Setting the values and establishing the norms is understood to be the special prerogative of the chief executive, although others may be invited to participate. Whether planned or serendipitous, the organization takes on a unique character that sets it apart. This perspective is rapidly taking its place among the prevailing theories of organization and is covered in Chapter 5.

Organizations as Political Systems

The tendency on the part of members of organizations to form groups and coalitions on the basis of their interests has led to the view of organizations as political systems. Through this perspective, health care organizations are seen as competing blocks of physicians, administrators, investors and insurers who jockey for control of technology, resources, dividends, or market share. Nurses may be passive bystanders to the power struggles or unwitting collaborators for the goals of one or more other groups. Increasingly, however, nurses identify their own interests in the organization. They are beginning to find ways to insert their interests into the political arena, to identify their sources of power, and to engage in resolving conflicts in positive ways for realizing patients' and therefore nursing's goals. For example, collective bargaining units strive to improve nurses' salaries and working conditions while shared governance increases nurses' input into decision making.

Organizations as Psychic Prisons

There is an emerging view of organizations as places where people act out latent emotional drives and unconscious strands of their personalities. Morgan (1986) termed organizations that result from these behavioral patterns as psychic prisons. From this perspective, behavior of members of organizations are a continuance of roles learned in the family (eg, parent and child interactions, dependence and codependence). These roles perpetuate the feelings of powerlessness and dependence on the authority of childhood. The analogy in health care organizations is the playing out of the physician as father, the nurse as mother, and the patient as child (Melosh, 1982; Reverby, 1987).

Organizations as Instruments of Domination

The last alternative theory is a view of organizations as instruments of domination. Proponents of this theory of organizations suggest that conflicting interests be arranged into rigid social structures devised by classes: owners, managers, and workers. With this perspective, hospitals are viewed as the laboratories of physicians exclusively under physician control with other members, especially nurses, as subservient. More recently, however, economic pressures and the increasing influence of administrators have weakened this hegemony and opened health care organizations to the influences of multiple interests which carry the seeds of change. Insofar as organizational structures perpetuate power imbalances rather than empower all persons in the organization to realize their potential, they contribute to domination rather than to shared aims and goal achievement.

These alternative views of organizations have their counterparts in nursing theories, according to Henry (1989). Readers may find them useful for developing their own unique synthesis as reflective of their practice and as self-conscious guides to future actions.

USING THEORY FOR ORGANIZATIONAL DESIGN

Organizational design is the way by which authority, responsibility, work flow, and information are arranged for a particular organization (see Chapter 7). Efforts to change an organization's design can be focused at several levels. The smallest level is for individual positions such as support staff or clinicians. Other levels include design for work groups, clusters of work groups, an entire organization, a network of organizations, or entire systems of organizations within a societal sector such as human services. For nurse administrators, design at all levels will be required in their practice.

Nurse Administrator as Active Design Maker

Nurse administrators as organizational designers originate from nursing's values and mission in society tempered by economic and productivity challenges. Their designs are influenced further by their synthesis of nursing and organization science which is the unique perspective they bring to the design enterprise. As strategic plans are formulated, nurse administrators can influence the mission and shape of the entire health care organization based on the nursing and organization science perspectives they hold.

View of Persons

Nurse administrators' views of persons vary according to their theoretical perspectives. From the mechanistic perspective, for example, persons are likely to be viewed as finely tuned instruments to be coordinated to achieve fixed goals. Each staff member and group plays a specific part which, when each part works well, results in high productivity and standardized quality.

Organismically, persons are understood to be subsystems of organizational systems which are in constant interaction with their environments. Personal goals and survival are interdependent with the survival and success of the entire organization. Similarly, the nursing division is interdependent with the larger health care organization.

Administrators' View of Organizations

The nursing organization as a social interactional unit will be viewed differently by nurse administrators based on their theoretical perspective. Nurse administrators who hold a mechanistic perspective will implement a fixed design within which persons are valued for their ability to fit in and perform tasks with precision for high efficiency and high productivity. This approach would be especially appropriate for alternative surgical centers where the technology is more certain and the tasks more routine than home care, for example. In this system, organizational success results from the tight fit of design and skill for precision and efficiency.

By contrast, the organismic perspective guides nurse administrators to design various components of the organization contingent on environmental demands. It might be appropriate to decentralize some operations to small, autonomous units so decisions are timely, functions modified, and tasks specified to meet changes in the case mix of patients. Shortages of professional and support personnel coupled with fluctuations in census have necessitated designs that locate staffing decisions at the patient care unit level, abbreviate communications, and establish reward structures to meet staff needs without sacrificing organizational goals. Here organizational success is the flexible use of resources to adapt to environmental change and fluctuations.

The potentiating perspective extends the organismic contingency design to maximize the talents and skills of every member as a reflection of the organization as a whole. Organizational health is enhancing the self-organizing, self-producing and envisioning tendencies of persons in the organization through the processes of learning to learn and toward an ever expanding consciousness of what the organization can become through growth and change in individuals and groups.

MANAGING ORGANIZATIONS FOR NURSING CARE

Nurses, who administer organizations are challenged to provide leadership, to recruit and retain nursing personnel, to enhance staff and manager potential, to manage conflict between individuals and interest groups, and to encourage growth and creativity of all members of the organization. These administrative problems require different skills based on various theoretical perspectives and on characteristics of the staff being managed. For example, some health care personnel are confident of their skills, have specific jobs, and meet their needs for growth and change outside the work place. They require a stable and efficient leader who adheres to policies, is fair, and is able to be a buffer between themselves and environmental demands. Administrators who can employ the mechanistic approach with these staff face little conflict and will be able to recruit and retain staff where these staff are assigned. High quality care will be sustained by these personnel. Their effectiveness will be based on a high degree of coordination among members, efficient use of time and resources, and high performance of skills.

The organismic perspective alerts nurse administrators to the different stages of maturity and accountability of their personnel and to changes in situational opportunities and constraints. Particular work groups within the organization may vary in their ability to coordinate efforts within their own groups and to integrate their work with other units. These developmental and situational differences will give rise to conflicts which, if not managed, can affect the quality of care, impede continuing positive growth, and can lead to high turnover. Administrative actions can be directed toward giving increasing responsibility and self-direction to individuals and groups as they gain experience, and toward delegating to individuals specific projects that challenge them to expand their skills and experience.

Conflict, recruitment and retention, quality of care, and entrepreneurship assume different qualities from the potentiating perspective. The turmoil of change is recognized as the outward manifestations of an underlying pattern of creativity in need of expression. Leadership, then, is the ability to recognize these patterns and help the members of the organization to understand and use such energy to encourage positive growth. The emergence of entrepreneurial initiatives by individuals and groups can affect the entire organization making it more unique and competitive.

NEW ORGANIZATIONS FOR NURSING CARE

As knowledge for nursing practice of all levels and roles continues to develop, nurses are becoming clearer about how to organize nursing services to realize the mission of their profession in society. Historically the Frontier Nursing Service exemplified an effort to create and maintain an organization explicitly to provide nursing care. A more recent example of organizing to provide nursing care is the Loeb Center where rehabilitation of patients was designed with professional nursing as the major therapy based on Hall's theory of nursing. Hall saw nursing as "promoting healing through a holistic combination of clinical, technical, psychosocial and teaching skills" (Alfano, 1988, p 34). Some departments of nursing have adopted a particular nursing theory to serve as the organizing framework for the department and for planning care, nursing interventions, and patient care documentation.

Community Nursing Centers
For more than a decade, nursing centers have originated in a variety of settings and under a variety of auspices. Designed to offer nursing services directly to the public without medical or other corporate jurisdiction, these centers feature nurse management and control to provide home care, education and health promotion to particular groups at risk such as the elderly or low income groups, to provide outreach services to underserved groups, and to provide opportunities for faculty to model exemplary nursing practice (Nursing Centers, 1990). These centers will become increasingly important as society comes to terms with current issues of access to care.

Nursing Corporations
Nursing organizations owned and incorporated by nurses for the purpose of providing nursing care in homes, clinics or hospitals, or as a basis for consulting or psychotherapy have been formed in recent years. Through these organizations, nurses (individually or collectively) offer their services directly to the public, and control their practice within the boundaries of state nurse practice acts and reimbursement regulations.

Holistic Healing Centers
Similar to nurse-owned corporations, nurses are increasingly initiators of centers for health care based on nontraditional theories and methods of restoring, maintaining

and promoting health. Based on a rejection of the separation of mind, body, and spirit inherited from seventeenth century scientific thought and modern allopathic medical treatment, these centers provide nurses and others with opportunities to organize care and do research according to more holistically oriented nursing and other human science theories (Quinn, 1988).

How Synthesis of Theories Suggests New Forms

As nurse administrators examine their "espoused theories," their "theories-in-use," and the perspectives of traditional and emerging theories, inadequacies of current organizational forms for providing nursing care becomes clearer. Designing organizations so nurses can realize their full potential can lead to nurses working with individuals and groups to realize their full potential. A culture of creativity and innovation can be created. Initiative from nursing can enhance entire health care organizations. Through such transformation, health care organizations can realize their missions of improving the health of society.

SUMMARY

Given the ubiquity of organizations in modern life and the dependence of nurses on organizations as the means through which nursing care is provided, knowledge of organizations as well as nursing is essential to the practice of nursing administration. The size and complexity of organizations with which nurses are associated ranges from the small and simple to the large and complex. The client in nursing administration practice is definable as both the persons associated with organizations and organizations themselves as social interactional units. Consequently, the most important knowledge nurse administrators bring to their practice is their view of the fundamental nature of persons and organizations. Theoretical perspectives of nurse administrators can be discerned by their actions, whether their views result from lived experiences and values or are consciously espoused frameworks which they can articulate, evaluate and re-examine. Several views are summarized which synthesize nursing and organization science. Two currently prevailing views and one emerging perspective are outlined with implications for the design of nursing organizations and administrative processes: the mechanistic, the organismic and the potentiating. Of these three, the mechanistic and organismic perspectives are useful for designing nursing organizations to meet specific types of nursing needs. The potentiating perspective is the most congruent with nursing's espoused assumptions, values, and intentions as reflected in the nursing literature but is the most difficult to actualize in current health care organizations.

REFERENCES

Alfano, GJ. A different kind of nursing. *Nursing Outlook.* 36:1, 34, 1988
Argyris C, Schon DA. *Theory in Practice: Increasing Professional Effectiveness.* San Francisco, CA, Jossey-Bass Publishers, 1974

Argyris C, Schon DA. *Organizational Learning: A Theory of Action Perspective.* Reading, MA, Addison-Wesley,1978

Benner P. (1984). *From Novice to Expert: Excellence and Power in Clinical Nursing Practice.* Menlo Park, CA, Addison-Wesley, 1984

Blair EM. Nursing and administration: A synthesis model. *Nursing Administration Quarterly.* 13:2, 1–11, 1989

Conrad DA, Mick SS, Madden CW, Hoare G. Vertical structures and control in health care markets: A conceptual framework and empirical review. *Medical Care Review,* 45:1, 49, 1988

Cyert RM, March JG. *A Behavioral Theory of the Firm.* Englewood Cliffs, NJ, Prentice-Hall, 1963

Drucker PF. *The Practice of Management.* New York: Harper and Row, 1954

Drucker PF. *The New Realities: In Government and Politics/in Economics and Business/in Society and World Views.* New York, Harper and Row, 1989

Erickson HC, Tomlin EM, Swain MA. *Modeling and Role-modeling: A Theory and Paradigm for Nursing.* Englewood Cliffs, NJ, Prentice-Hall, 1983

Fayol H. *General and Industrial Management.* London, Pitman, 1949

Gilbreth FB. *Motion Study.* New York: Van Nostrand, 1911

Hall RH. *Dimensions of Work.* Beverly Hills, CA, Sage Publications, 1986

Henry B. Epistemological approaches to interdisciplinary inquiry for nursing administration. In: Henry B, Arndt C, Di Vincenti M, Marriner-Tomey A. *Dimensions of Nursing Administration: Theory, Research, Education, Practice.* Cambridge, MA, Blackwell Scientific Publications, 1989, 235–246

Johnson DE. The behavioral system model for nursing. In: Riehl JP, Roy C, Eds. *Conceptual Models for Nursing Practice,* 2nd ed. New York, Appleton-Century-Crofts, 1980

Kanter RM. *When Giants Learn to Dance.* New York, Simon and Schuster, 1989

Katz D, Kahn RL. *The Social Psychology of Organizations.* New York, John Wiley, 1978

King IM. King's systems framework for nursing administration. In: Henry B, Arndt C, Di Vincenti M, Marriner-Tomey A. *Dimensions of Nursing Administration: Theory, Research, Education, Practice.* Cambridge, MA, Blackwell Scientific Publications, 1989, 35–46

Levine ME. *Introduction to Clinical Nursing,* 2nd ed. Philadelphia, PA, FA Davis, 1973

MacIntyre A. *After Virtue: A Study in Moral Theory.* Notre Dame, IN, University of Notre Dame Press, 1984

Maslow AY. *Toward a Psychology of Being.* New York, Van Nostrand, 1968

McGregor D. *The Human Side of Enterprise.* New York, McGraw-Hill, 1960

Melosh B. *"The Physicians's Hand": Work, Culture, and Conflict in American Nursing.* Philadelphia, PA, Temple University Press, 1982

Morgan G. *Images of Organization.* Beverly Hills, CA, Sage Publications, 1986

Morgan G, Ramirez R. Action learning: A holographic metaphor for guiding social change. *Human Relations.* 37, 1, 1984

Morrissey JP, Hall RH, Lindsey ML. *Interorganizational Relations: A Sourcebook of Measures for Mental Health Programs.* Rockville, MD, US Department of Health and Human Services (ADM)82–1187, 1982

Newman M. *Health as Expanding Consciousness.* St. Louis, CV Mosby, 1986

Nightingale F. (1858). Subsidiary notes as to the introduction of female nursing into military hospitals. In: Seymer LR, *Selected Writings of Florence Nightingale.* New York: Macmillan, 1954

Nursing Centers: Meeting the Demand for Quality Health Care. New York, National League for Nursing Publication 21:2311, 1987

Orem D. Nursing administration, A theoretical approach. In: Henry B, Arndt C, Di Vincenti M,

Marriner-Tomey A. *Dimensions of Nursing Administration: Theory, Research, Education, Practice.* Cambridge, MA, Blackwell Scientific Publications, 1989, 55–62

Parse RR. *Man-Living-Health: A Theory of Nursing.* New York, John Wiley & Sons, 1981

Parse RR. (1989). Parse's man-living-health model and administration of nursing service. In: Henry B, Arndt C, Di Vincenti M, Marriner-Tomey A. *Dimensions of Nursing Administration: Theory, Research, Education, Practice.* Cambridge, MA, Blackwell Scientific Publications, 1989, 69–74.

Quinn JF. Building a body of knowledge: Research on therapeutic touch, 1974–1986 (review). *Journal of Holistic Nursing.* 6:1, 37, 1988

Reverby SM. *Ordered to Care: The Dilemma of American Nursing, 1850–1945.* Cambridge, Cambridge University Press, 1987

Rogers DL, Whetten DA. (1982). *Interorganizational Coordination: Theory, Research and Implementation.* Ames, IA, Iowa State University Press, 1982

Rogers ME. A science of unitary man. In: Riehl JP, Roy C, eds. *Conceptual Models for Nursing Practice,* 2nd ed. New York, Appleton-Century-Crofts, 1980

Roy C. *Introduction to Nursing: An Adaptation Model,* 2nd ed. Englewood Cliffs, NJ, Prentice-Hall, 1984

Roy C, Anway R. (1989). Roy's adaptation model: Theories for nursing administration. In: Henry B, Arndt C, Di Vincenti M, Marriner-Tomey A. *Dimensions of Nursing Administration: Theory, Research, Education, Practice.* Cambridge, MA, Blackwell Scientific Publications, 1989, 75–88

Schon DA. *Educating the Reflective Practitioner: Toward a New Design for Teaching and Learning in the Professions.* San Francisco, Jossey-Bass, 1987

Schultz PR. When client means more than one: Extending the foundational concept of person. *Advances in Nursing Science.* 10:1, 71, 1987

Schultz PR, Miller KL. Nursing administration research, Part one: Pluralities of persons. *Annual Review of Nursing Research,* 8: (in press).

Schultz PR. Milestones in the success of nursing as an emerging discipline. Paper presented at the annual meeting of the American Association of Colleges of Pharmacy, Salt Lake City, July 10, 1990

Scott WR. (1987). *Organizations: Rational, natural and open.* Englewood Cliffs, NJ: Prentice-Hall, Inc.

Shortell SM, Kaluzny AR. and Associates. *Health Care Management: A Text in Organization Theory and Behavior.* New York: John Wiley & Sons, 1988

Simon HA. *Administrative Behavior.* New York, Macmillan, 1947

Scott WR. Managing professional work: Three models of control for health organizations. *Health Services Research,* 17:213, 1982

Starkweather DB. *Hospital Mergers in the Making.* Ann Arbor, MI, Health Administration Press, 1981

Stevens BJ. *Nursing Theory: Analysis, Application, Evaluation.* Boston, MA, Little, Brown & Co, 1984

Taylor FW. *Principles of Scientific Management:* New York: Harper and Row, 1911

Thompson JD. *Organizations in Action.* St. Louis, MO, McGraw-Hill, 1967

Weber M. *The Theory of Social and Economic Organization.* London: Oxford University Press, 1947

CHAPTER 3

Power and Politics in Health Care Organizations

Donna M. Costello-Nickitas
Diana J. Mason

Key Concept List

Power
Politics
Coalition building
Networking
Support base

Whether leading a unit, a department, or an institution, nurse administrators must be effective at influencing decision making in the workplace. As leaders within the nursing profession and the health care system, nurse administrators also must be able to influence decision making regarding professional, health, and social policies. Wielding influence in any of these arenas requires power and political savvy. The nurse administrator who effectively uses influence and persuasion to establish new policies or practices, manages both personnel and conflict, and portrays an image of savvy and success will quickly be recognized as a powerful person—one to whom others will come for support and leadership.

This chapter discusses the relevance of power and politics for the nurse administrator, explains the various dimensions of power and politics, and discusses how the nurse manager can develop power and astutely influence the decisions and events in health care organizations.

POWER AND POLITICS IN HEALTH CARE ORGANIZATIONS: TRANSFORMING VISIONS INTO REALITIES

In a study of how nurse managers in a southwestern city viewed power, Heineken (1985) reported that nurse executives were more likely than first level nurse managers (head/charge nurses) to believe that one needs to ''be political'' to get and keep power. She noted that if this discrepancy in values between the two groups of nurse managers exists, it may interfere with nurses' ability to plan strategies for change:

> Nurse executives will be striving to cultivate and maintain political alliances. Head nurses and charge nurses will not . . . If head nurses place less value on the need to ''be political,'' they may miss unique opportunities to gain broad-based support for their ideas, proposals, and programs . . . If head nurses are not using their own political influence within the health-care setting, staff have little opportunity to learn these behaviors from their role models (p 38).

One would expect to find some differences between nurse executives and head nurses in terms of their views of politics, given the differences in their roles, authority and span of control. Of importance here is the extent to which political thinking and behavior is valued, supported and fostered within the nursing department. The importance of politics for the nurse manager may be obvious to some; however, discussions of power and politics are difficult for many nurses. Predominantly women, nurses are not necessarily socialized or educated to openly attest to wanting power or to learn how to use it. Additionally, politics tends to be viewed as a tainted, almost unethical, endeavor, particularly as scandals in government continue to make headline news. It thus becomes imperative for nurse administrators to recognize that power and politics are predominantly means to an end (Stevens, 1980). What one does with the power and politics is as important as the means one uses to achieve the end.

While both nurse executives and staff nurses share a vision for quality patient care, how that quality is defined and provided may differ. For example, the nurse executive must define quality within a context that includes considerations of cost and the health of the institution. It is particularly critical for leaders in nursing and health care to examine their ends or visions. Certainly the crisis in the health care system in the United States and the nursing shortage demand that nurses be clear and articulate. The times also demand that nurses develop a vision that is macroscopic, ie, one that reflects an understanding of the broader systems and issues in health care and society. Daily work reinforces a vision that tends to be microscopic, that focuses only one one's immediate area of responsibility. The successful nurse administrator can effectively manage that immediate area within the context of the larger system and be able to influence both.

When the Vision Isn't Enough

While many nurses have a vision of nursing and health care that is humanistic and altruistic, influencing others toward a shared vision is often thwarted by misunderstanding change. One often thinks that others should be persuaded purely by the facts that support one's vision. Failure to distinguish between the facts and the politics of the matter can doom an important change to failure.

In nursing and health care, there is abundant evidence that facts alone do not always produce needed change. For example, the American Academy of Nursing (1983) conducted a study of the factors that promote recruitment and retention of nurses. The Magnet Hospital Study documented factors such as decentralization of nursing departments to enhance the authority of staff nurses to match their responsibility, elimination of non-nursing tasks, and participation in policy-making committees within the institution. In spite of this documentation, such changes were not adopted on a widespread basis in hospitals throughout the country. Prior to this study, the Joint Commission on Collaborative Practice demonstrated that practice models that support nurse-physician collaborative practice increases the professional satisfaction and shared decision making of both providers. Again, such practice models were not widely adopted. Thus, in 1988, when the acute shortage of nurses lead to a national study of its causes, the Secretary's Commission on Nursing reported that factors contributing to the shortage included outdated practice models, lack of control over daily practice affairs, and failure of institutions to include nurses in institutional policy-making. Having the facts had not changed the willingness of health care institutions to do what was necessary to promote nurses' job satisfaction, improve patient care, and increase retention.

UNDERSTANDING POLITICS AND POWER

Politics can be defined as influencing; specifically, it is influencing the allocation of scarce resources and the decisions of others (Mason & Talbott, 1985; Stevens, 1980). Politics is inherent in any system where resources are absolutely or relatively scarce and where there are competing interests for those resources (Zaleznik, 1979). Politics is largely an interpersonal endeavor that requires coalition building and astute analytic and communication skills.

While politics is usually associated with the world of government, it is a part of every sphere of a nurse's world. Mason and Talbott (1985) defined four spheres for nurses' political action: the workplace, government, organizations, and communities. The bulk of this chapter discusses politics of the workplace; however, it is important for nurse administrators to understand the relevance of the other three spheres to their effectiveness in the workplace.

Most nurse administrators have firsthand experience with the effect of government on nursing and health care. The financing of health care is increasingly being driven by federal policies and regulations. Governments set standards for inspecting and licensing health care facilities and home health agencies, define the legal scope of nursing practice, and establish and monitor public health policy. The government also is a major employer of nurses, as in state mental health facilities, veterans hospitals, and public health departments (Mason & Talbott, 1985).

In spite of these and many other ways in which the sphere of government directly or indirectly influences the workplace, Archer and Goehner (1981) reported that 94 percent of a national sample of the top nurse administrators from a variety of health care institutions and agencies believed nurses are not as politically active [as they could be]. The primary reasons they gave for this lack of participation were lack of preparation, apathy, and failure to realize the importance of political participation. However, Klein (1984) and others (MacKinnon, 1982; Ridd & Calloway, 1987) noted that women's involvement in politics often arises from their personal needs and experiences. Increasing nurses' involvement in the politics of government may be dependent upon the nursing community's ability to articulate and make visible the connections between what government does and what nurses do in their everyday practice, as well as what supports nurses need in their personal lives.

Professional organizations provide a mechanism for nurses' voices to collectively be heard. National, state, and district, and other nursing organizations monitor governmental regulations and lobby public officials on a regular basis. They also work together to influence how the public views nursing, set standards for nursing practice, and participate in interdisciplinary efforts to shape public policy. These organizations can often publicize issues and call for strategies that the nurse administrator cannot publicly address.

As any member of a dynamic nursing organization can attest, politics also is an inherent part of the organization's operations. Nurses are a diverse group. Selecting and electing representatives for organizations, setting organizational policies, and developing a professional agenda and priorities all require skill to enable many voices to be head as one. The community is a sphere of politics that encompasses all of the other spheres. Community leaders sit on hospital boards of trustees, exert pressure to influence public policy, and define priorities for their communities. The nurse who is visible and influential in the community can often enhance power in the workplace and has the potential to mobilize community support for an issue or concern in the workplace.

Public and Workplace Policy

Nurse administrators often help and implement workplace policies on a daily basis, and can be active players in the development of public policy. Unfortunately, studies of the nursing shortage have repeatedly documented that nurses have not been as visible in the policy-making processes of government and the workplace as they could be (Secretary's Commission on Nursing, 1988). This requires an understanding of what policy is and how it is developed.

The dictionary defines policy as "a principle, plan, or course of action, set by governments, organizations, and institutions." Diers (1985) defines policy as dealing with the "shoulds and oughts," distinguishing it from politics, which she sees as conditioning or influencing policy development. However, defining the "shoulds and oughts" is a value-laden process, around which agreement can be difficult. Indeed, MacPherson (1987) argues that nursing's voice represents values of caring that conflict with those of the dominant voice in American society, including competition, efficiency, and individualism. Nursing has the opportunity to help society see caring as a social responsibility and to recognize the cost-effectiveness of such an ethic. An enhanced nursing voice in the development of public and workplace policies can significantly alter which policies are developed and what they will espouse.

Policy is developed in both the public and private sectors. The Robert Wood Johnson and Pew Trust Foundations are examples of private philanthropic corporations that have influenced health policy through their funding of demonstration projects that address major problems in health care delivery, including the organization of hospital nursing services.

The policy process begins with identifying the problem and "getting on the agenda" (Diers, 1985). Whether nursing's issues are on the agenda depends on whether nurses help set the agenda, whether the climate is right for the issue to be of interest to policy makers, and whether nursing has the resources and skills to make the issue a chief priority. For example, it has been known that hospital practice arrangements were inadequate for promoting job satisfaction among nurses and interdisciplinary decision making. It was not until the nursing shortage became so severe that it was crippling the safe delivery of patient care that the public and private entities began to discuss providing support to explore alternative practice models. The crisis has made the climate right for rewriting hospital policies related to practice arrangements. Additionally, the nursing community was united and positioned to call for the federal government to study the shortage and issue recommendations to address this long-standing problem. The nursing community had developed the power and influence within the federal government to move the issue onto the agenda. Now is the time all nurses to seize the opportunity that the shortage presents for getting on the agenda.

Once on the agenda, one must find an audience and develop strategies needed for moving the issue (Center for Women in Government, 1984). The audience should include those people and groups whom the problem affects (nurses, physicians, hospital administrators, third party payors, patients and their families), as well as potential allies and adversaries (health advocacy groups, the media, senior citizen's groups, organized medicine, health-related foundations and organizations).

Developing appropriate policy for an issue or problem requires thoughtful analysis based on data and an exploration of alternative responses to the problem. Today computerized nursing information systems improve the availability and usability of data to support development of nursing and health related policies. The costs, benefits, effects, and feasibility of alternative responses to care needs must be analyzed.

Part of developing policy is determining who will implement and evaluate it. Issues related to responsibility, authority, and accountability arise here. While developing policy appears to be straightforward and logical, in actuality it is usually a complex and circular process that involves politics from beginning to end.

The regulatory and legislative processes of government demonstrate the interaction between policy and politics. Hundreds or thousands of bills may be drafted during the legislative session of a state government. Few of these bills become law. Many do not get beyond the purview of a committee because the "audience" they address is too narrow. Often a committee chair will schedule hearings on a piece of legislation or the issue it addresses. The hearings may be a legitimate attempt to stimulate input and recommend developing policy for the issue; however, they also can be orchestrated affairs to create the appearance of a supportive audience for the legislator's agenda. In addition, the final piece of legislation may reflect extensive compromises to account for the values and concerns of diverse audiences.

Once legislation becomes law, regulations must be developed to implement the policy. Nurses often ignore this important policy arena. Regulations may be issued on a nursing or health related policy that have had little or no input from the nursing community, although most state nurses associations work diligently to monitor this process. When "regs" are written, they must be made public and an opportunity provided for public comment. Again, hearings may be held that may or may not be legitimate attempts to address the public's concerns.

Because of policy makers' leadership positions and firsthand experience with many issues and problems, it is imperative that nurse administrators become actively involved in the process of making health policy. The first step is to learn the legislative and regulatory structure and processes in the federal, state, and local governments and identify other public and private entities that develop nursing and health related policy. The League of Women Voters and local or state governments often publish documents on the structure and process of government. However, attending a public hearing, lobbying legislators, or observing a legislative session can provide the firsthand experience that allows one to truly begin to "know" how policy is formally made.

The second step is to know policy makers. In government, this means legislators, their staff, and both elected and appointed members of the executive branch of government. Not only visit these government officials and personnel but also attend the elected officials' fundraisers to make stronger connections to some policy makers (Mason & Talbott, 1985). Certainly nurses know the importance and how-to's of establishing relationships with patients. These are the same skills that one uses to establish relationships with policy makers.

To position oneself to be a policy maker or have significant influence with those who make policy is the third step. This step requires that one excel at step two and become recognized by the policy maker as an expert on health. Sending the policy maker relevant literature on a current policy issue, sharing one's expertise during a visit and through letters, offering to develop a candidate's position on health care issues while organizing nurses to participate in the campaign, are all techniques that can be used.

These same steps apply to moving into positions of influence in the policy-making process of the workplace. To maximize one's power in the workplace, the nurse administrator must develop connections and influence within the other spheres of government, organizations, and communities. This requires a long-term plan for developing power.

PERSPECTIVES ON POWER AND POLITICS

Before examining how to acquire and use power and political skills, a discussion of the context in which these skills have been developed and embraced is needed. As a predominantly female profession, it is incumbent on nurses to understand how gender has influenced what society believes and how it behaves. This is particularly so in discussing the public sphere of a nurse's life. Although such an understanding can enlighten how one perceives one's private life, the public world is the one in which the nursing community has been struggling for recognition and legitimacy.

Gilligan (1982) and others (Chodorow, 1978; Donovan, 1985) suggest there are different sets of values and perspectives about the world than the dominant ones by which society operates. Gilligan noted that while the highest forms of moral reasoning had been held to be based on an ethic of justice in which rights and autonomy are valued (Kohlberg, 1981), research supporting this theory had been done largely by men studying men. When women were studied using Kohlberg's theoretical framework, they were found to be unable to move beyond the third stage of a six-stage process of moral development and were held to be morally immature. Gilligan, using a qualitative approach to uncovering the processes women used to make ethical decisions, discovered a different process of moral reasoning that is based on an ethic of caring and responsibility that arises out of the experience of connection and attachment. Under Gilligan's framework, the context of the moral dilemma is of prime consideration in the process of moral reasoning.

Gilligan points out that the ethic of caring is not gender-specific; however, her framework was consistent with the experience and work of other feminist theorists and researchers who view women as having different values, perspectives, and experiences that are often negated by a male-dominated world. Some women espouse values of the dominant system, and some men hold values that reflect an ethic of caring. What is important is that there are many voices in society. Rather than having one voice dominate society's policies and practices, these multiple voices should be encouraged and integrated into public debates and policy making.

Gilligan's perspective has been embraced by a growing number of nurses who have written about nursing's voice of caring being diminished in the work world, in science, and in society where the dominant voices have been those that do not value women's perspectives. Nursing is based on an ethic of caring that is not usually consistent with the ethic of institutional politics and decision making. Thus, the nurse administrator often is caught between two worlds, trying to increase nursing influence in the male-dominated administrative world, while attempting to maintain a connection to and loyalty from the antithetical and largely female world of nursing. Thus, one hears staff nurses complain about the nurse administrator who has "forgotten nursing," who appears to have been co-opted into adopting the values and beliefs of the dominant system that is seen as valuing efficiency and product, rather than caring and process.

Certainly, the public world of power and politics has long been dominated and defined by values not often based on a caring ethic. The prime example of this is the literary classic *The Prince*, by Machiavelli, where eliminating one's potential enemies was a primary rule for political success. Many rules of power and politics reflect this Machiavellian passport for acquiring and using power. It may be another reason why many nurses are averse to embracing the role of politics in their everyday work.

As Gilligan is quick to point out, the aim of hearing and understanding these "different voices" is not to discredit traditional voices but rather to put them in their proper perspective. Thus, it becomes important for nurse administrators to first value their own voices, to critically examine traditional voices, and identify ways to blend the best of each. For some, the fit between the nurse and the organization is too disparate to be blended.

Most nurse administrators are in health care organizations that are run by or modeled after traditional models of hierarchical power. To move into a position of power in these institutions requires knowing the rules of the game as set by the game makers, developing the skills necessary to play the game, and using the skills wisely. Nursing needs leaders who can play the game with skill and savvy. However, nursing also needs for the nurse winners in the game to respect the ethic of caring on which nursing is based, and to integrate it into one's methods of operating whenever possible. Few would disagree with the notion that health care and the systems and society in which it is provided need to reflect an ethic of caring to a greater extent than is currently evident.

Most of the political skills described have been developed within traditional male-dominated systems. Some reflect an ethic of caring and connection to a greater extent than others. Each nurse administrator must evaluate these and other techniques for developing power and political action, to determine which are appropriate for use, and begin to develop alternative ways of influencing decision making in the public sphere more consistent with an ethic of caring.

It becomes important that nurse administrators, many of whom are women, realize both the importance and the difficulty of pursuing power and political action while committing to an ethic of caring.

Empowerment and Nurse Administrators

"Empowerment" has become an over-used word in recent years. It has been used in social work, nursing, community, and even business literatures (Kanter, 1983; Block, 1987; Conger & Kanungo, 1988) with increasing frequency. However, the concept of empowerment as "power-sharing" arises from the feminist literature.

Miller (1976) suggests that women indeed have demonstrated the capacity to share power, and may be more comfortable with this model. This is why the term empowerment has been used as a more appropriate approach to power than the traditional model of power-grabbing—ie, seizing power at any cost and holding it close to oneself. Miller further suggests that women bring a unique perspective to understanding and using power, and therefore can easily support the empowerment of others.

In keeping with the commitment to an ethic of caring that embodies nursing, nurse administrators need to examine the current models of power. Most health care organizations operate from traditional hierarchical models that will be discussed later. It is proposed here that nurse administrators explore and develop a model of empowerment or power sharing. The overall theme for empowerment for nurse administrators lies in taking action on behalf of oneself, one's colleagues, one's staff and one's patients.

EMPOWERMENT

Empowerment is "... a process aimed at ... changing the nature and distribution of power in a particular cultural context" (Bookman & Morgen, 1988). It requires an attentive listening to our own senses as well as listening to others, consciously taking in and forming strength (Wheeler & Chinn, 1989). Empowerment involves enabling others to recognize their talents and contributions to the organization as well as experiencing a sense of one's own personal power. Fostering the development of others is power sharing.

For nurse administrators to experience empowerment, Stuart (1986) suggests that they increase connections with other subunits within the workplace, create conditions that make them irreplaceable, and participate in high-level decision making. In this case, one's actions to empower oneself are based on the understanding of the existence of traditional power-grabbing models that predominate in health care organizations. One must first get the power to be able to share it with others. Therefore, the nurse administrator needs to know both traditional power grabbing techniques, as well as begin to develop the nontraditional techniques for power sharing.

Beck (1983) identified three dimensions of empowerment as:

1. Developing a positive and potent self esteem
2. Developing self-efficacy with skills needed to attain personal and collective goals
3. Consciousness raising regarding the web of political and social realities that provide a context for one's life circumstances

The dimensions of empowerment are not mutually exclusive but rather overlap each other. They also are not linear, but rather interactive. Development of one dimension is contingent upon developing the other two dimensions. Empowerment involves commitment to develop self as well as others. Improving one's self-esteem occurs when one uses power strategies to act on one's behalf, or when one recognizes that holding an oppressed position, either by the nature of one's gender or role in society, is not one's own fault. By understanding the socio-political context of one's position in society, the constraining forces of oppressive conditions can be counteracted and rejected. As nurse administrators acknowledge and appreciate their own abilities and strengths and share these with others, a commitment toward empowerment is made. Empowerment mobilizes one's resources and enables change in constructive and creative ways. To be empowered is to experience a sense of hope, excitement, and energy.

A prerequisite to empowerment is a plan to unify and commit oneself, as well as those who follow, to develop politically astute skills for change. This sense of commitment and teamwork toward producing change goes far beyond the nurse administrator and followers. It includes peers, superiors, other health providers, patients—all those who must support the vision. Kanter (1983) suggests that the effect of enabling others to act is to make them feel strong, capable, and committed. Empowerment develops a feeling of ownership and is more likely to increase one's energies to produce extraordinary results.

Exemplary nurse administrators will encourage collaboration, build teams, and empower others. As a skillful politician, the nurse administrator must acknowledge the structure and function of the system in which he or she seeks to empower. By using a political approach that concentrates on both vertical and horizontal power as well as the relationship between groups or subgroups within the system, the nurse administrator will have the ability to operate within a power grabbing system when it cannot be changed, and use power sharing approaches, or empowerment, whenever possible. It is the ability to build teams and empower others that will enable nurses to fully develop their strengths, abilities and personal power.

Power

The intense, competitive environments of today's health care organizations present difficult challenges for the nurse administrator. The scarcity of human and fiscal resources forces the nurse administrator to continually justify nursing costs relative to patient acuity and diagnostic related group, to make budget-driven decisions that compete with professional values, and to answer tough questions about nurse productivity versus cost.

Using power to acquire the needed resources and to influence others in the health care organization is an essential function of the nurse administrator. Power is a critical component of organizational life. The forces of power are inevitable and emerge in organizations because administrators depend on others to perform effectively. Being dependent means being needful of others for resources, assistance, information, approval, time, and money (Kotler, 1984). Increasingly, the nurse administrator uses power and political clout to provide the best care allowed by the limited resources available. The ability to effectively use power can make the difference in an administrator's success or failure. Therefore, the effective nurse administrator is knowledgeable and skillful at acquiring and using power.

Power has been defined as an individual's ability to influence others or the behavior of others. For the nurse administrator, defining power must include the potential to achieve goals and the ability to get things done through others in effective and competent ways. This definition of power connects the concept of influence with the achievement of organizational goals. By the nature of their positions, nurse administrators can manage by using a wide variety of influencing skills. The real skill to influence others, however, is the ability of the nurse administrator to produce a desired effect without directly using one's authority and making a command. The ethical and skillful use of power is important. Here the nurse administrator's influencing skills involve the use of formal authority, relationships, and access to information to attain organizational goals but not for self-serving means.

Creating the Power Image

The acquisition and use of power must be enhanced by an image that portrays organizational status and success. A nurse administrator will be perceived and acknowledged as powerful by others when displaying political savvy and by accumulating multiple power bases and organizational networks. A successful nurse administrator goes beyond positional power to influence others or to go along with one's "vision."

Creating a power image includes increasing one's visibility, forming coalitions and learning to bargain effectively.

Increasing one's visibility is key to having control of valued resources. Being at the right place at the right time with the right people will lead to access and influence of actual or potential resources. Gaining control over scarce resources, controlling information and gaining access to top policy makers in the organization can all be established through alliances with friends and foes, superiors and subordinates. All are needed to support and win over to favorable or not so favorable decisions.

When attempts to influence or convince others are blocked or when faced with a conflict of interest, the nurse administrator must either move to form a coalition or bargain. In forming a coalition one temporarily joins with others with a similar position to succeed in obtaining a desired end. If on the other hand, a tradeoff can be made where something of equal value can be exchanged, then bargaining is the route of choice. In either case the nurse administrator seeks to create a powerful personal image and not solely use positional power of authority.

Personal power can be enhanced by good interpersonal relations. An effective administrator creates an air of cooperation and positivity, as well as a sense of obligation towards the organization, while avoiding obtrusive and defensive behavior toward the competition. Courteous relations can serve to develop a support base that can be mobilized at a later time. Courtesy is a powerful strategy that makes others feel good and leads them to believe that you are fair and just. However, do not be blinded or too near-sighted to think that the competition will not strike back. Always be prepared and make the first move. Do not be surprised and, when necessary, be first to make the peace offering be it network, coalition, bargaining, or tradeoff.

Additional Sources of Power

The ability to influence and exercise power over others is accessible through the formal organizational structure, making it legitimate for nurse administrators to use their official authority. According to French and Raven (1960) power holders are accorded power because of the number of power bases they establish. The six bases of power identified by French and Raven are: reward, expert, informational, positional or legitimate, coercive, and connection. By building multiple power bases, the nurse administrator develops an effective power image within the organization. The ability to develop multiple power bases rests on the administrator's acquisition of power and political savvy.

Having the resources and abilities to bestow rewards and acknowledge excellence increases power. It is a positive means that can serve to empower one's staff. While one tends to think of rewards in terms of money and status, rewards also can include publicizing the achievements of staff, thanking staff and other personnel for a job well done, accommodating staff requests for time off and other perquisites. The more creative the administrator, the greater can be the repertoire of rewards.

Nurse administrators can capitalize on their influence of positional power to meet their goals. Through developing a deeper understanding of the dynamics of power and using the skills of communication, persuasion, negotiation, leadership, and networking, nurse administrators can develop new strategies to meet the current trends.

A nurse administrator who is able to put available information to work becomes more powerful in forecasting nursing services vis-à-vis hospital census as well as in calculating how best to reduce capital and personnel costs.

The power of professional expertise offers the surest way of establishing and sustaining nursing's power base in health care (Fagin, 1982). By using expert power, the nurse administrator can be a policy maker and organizational influencer who sets the rules rather than abides by them. The degree to which the nurse administrator is perceived by others as having special knowledge or skill is an important factor in influencing others.

Control of information is another effective power strategy. A nurse administrator is able to influence others because of access to accurate information and the ability to communicate effectively with others. An important component of resource allocation is accurate information. By sharing accurate information, the nurse administrator can lead discussions and effect decisions that demonstrate nursing's cost effectiveness. For example, an astute nurse administrator sees the trends in health care finance or diminished resources as opportunities to transfer power of decision making into the hands of staff nurses who commit to excellence in caring.

By cultivating multiple sources of power, nurse administrators can develop effective methods of collective action, mutual support, and interdependence. By acknowledging their own professional expertise and that of their staff, nurse administrators increase the power of all nurses. Thus, in fostering an ethic of care governed by a philosophy of power sharing and expertise, the nurse administrator as well as staff are empowered by encouraging cooperation and by sharing information, expertise, and collaboration. Only through the use of varied power bases can the nurse administrator generate an image and status of importance, authority and prestige. Status and material success of the nurse administrator often includes such basics as salary, an office next to the hospital administrator's office, secretary, furnishings, parking space, and budgetary control of departmental resources.

Positional power in and of itself does not promise power over others. To be perceived as powerful and have an image of success the nurse administrator must assume the traits or behaviors that others in the organization interpret as powerful. Chief among these traits or behaviors is the ability to create a positive "can do" attitude which communicates a message that anything is possible and every problem has a solution. The message is clear—powerful people get things done. Being visible and available, dressing accordingly, and communicating effectively sends a powerful signal.

Using Power

Power is only the means by which a nurse administrator gets things done; it is not the ends. When power is used wisely, it can promote the achievement of goals and objectives. Therefore, power must be accepted, understood and used (del Bueno & Freund,1986). To control and decrease abuse of power, the nurse administrator must acknowledge that power is a part of organizational life and seek to understand its nature and use. To survive the power plays and politics of the organization, it pays to know the rules. Is power grabbed or shared within the organization? Del Bueno and Freund (1986) implied that women frequently make the mistake of withdrawing from power plays and politics and uncover too late that they have been left out of important decisions. To prevent being left out in the cold, the nurse administrator must determine whether the waters are shark-infested (del Bueno & Freund, 1986) or calm. Swimming with sharks refers to cut-throat politics by which one eliminates the opposition and cultivates support through fear. If this is how power is played, then it is best if the nurse administrator recognizes this as power grabbing. Understanding the fundamental principles of this play will prepare the nurse administrator for the attack.

In a power grabbing atmosphere the nurse administrator can assume that strangers are the enemy or competitors until proven to the contrary. Move to counter any aggression promptly with overt retaliation. Do not seek to appease or be conciliatory. Be sure to anticipate aggression and make the first move. Try at all costs to take your competitor by surprise. Plan an organized attack by starting internal dissension. Deflect personal attacks by introducing an issue or gossip that sets your competitors fighting among themselves. And finally, do not show your loss in public. On the other hand, when the organization promotes an atmosphere of power sharing and fosters an image of power as positive and productive, the nurse administrator must advocate ways that enhance power as a means to cultivate and maintain organizational alliances. Sharing of information and expertise helps to build a power base which contributes to the whole of the organization, not just one part. Acting as role model and demonstrating power as a source of influence, the administrator attempts to show how power can be seen as helpful in persuading other members of the health care team, patients, and families. By using power connections to influence decisions and actions, nurse administrators gain broad-based support for ideas, proposals, and plans. Understanding the importance of power as well as the acceptable and unacceptable uses of power, the nurse administrator is in a position to establish unity, strength and cohesiveness in the health care organization. Power sharing supports an ethic of care which promotes concern for the self as well as others but not at the expense of devaluing or deceiving another.

Successful nurse administrators manage problems and the competition by using foresight—power that comes from strategic planning. Planning allows for the opportunity to gather power and resources to solve problems. Strategic planning provides for smoother operations. However, sometimes the best of plans must be ignored and crisis intervention put in motion. This may mean personally dealing with the situation (Costello-Nickitas, 1985) which allows for an assessment of details and an avenue for ideas and opinions to be discussed openly.

Despite the belief that power has the potential to create cooperation, collaboration, and change, those who feel uncomfortable with the notion of having and using power remain (Heineken, 1985). The negative image of power causes some to shy away from acknowledging the benefits of using personal and professional power. Power is neither good nor bad; it is a neutral force. When individuals use power to manipulate or coerce others to accomplish some personal gain, then power is abused. When used appropriately in meeting goals of the organization, coercion is usually used only with those who only respond to force or punishment.

It is easy to induce fear and punishment in others who fail to conform to desired change, assignments or rules. By using the authority obtained through one's positional power to gain compliance, the nurse administrator risks losing respect and trust. It is far better to establish credibility through knowledge, skill, and expertise than coercion.

Given the complexities of health care organizations and the uncertainty of where the needed resources are to be obtained, the nurse administrator must use power as a means of controlling information and gaining access to key policy makers. Having formulated channels through which information can be shared, data accessed, and decisions made, the nurse administrator can then calculate the risks in using power strategies to increase one's power base.

APPLICATION OF POWER AND POLITICS FOR THE NURSE ADMINISTRATOR

Knowing the System

The way to uncover the values, norms, languages, priorities or even hidden agendas of the organization is to observe its members in action. Observing others allows for determining what are acceptable versus unacceptable behaviors. It is important to quickly learn the limits of each of these behaviors so as not to fall prey to someone else's objective. By knowing the values and beliefs of the organization, the nurse administrator can pursue behaviors or strategies that comply and not violate the established rules. Each organization has its own norms, values, and sacred cows which the culture or social reality of life within the organizational community. By being able to identify and understand this social reality, the nurse administrator develops sensitivity toward individual needs, vested interests, and hidden agendas. Knowing the system can ensure compliance and avoid conflict with the norms and values of the organizational culture.

Assessing Formal and Informal Structures and Process

Knowing how to use the formal and informal organizational structures can expand and enhance the nurse administrator's power and influence. An examination of what the organization looks like on paper and how it behaves in reality can reveal a great deal about its values and commitments. For example, by reading the written documents that govern the organization's mission, philosophy, goals, and objectives, the nurse administrator easily can determine what are the priorities—eg, patient care, research or medical education. By examining the organizational chart, the nurse administrator can quickly identify one's location in the pecking order and chain of command.

A thorough look at the policies and procedures that govern human resources informs the nurse administrator how the organization values and cares for its members. If these policies and procedures reflect current trends in health care, then the organization is progressive in supporting its personnel. Looking into the financial status of the organization and determining its financial health can be informative and educational. Knowing if you are on a sinking ship by reading the organizational's annual report will prove insightful if you desire to initiate a special project. Tracking how the organization spends and allocates monies will help direct your efforts when attempting to influence others to support your ideas and visions.

Once a thorough assessment has been made of the organization's formal structures, the nurse administrator is ready to identify informal structures and processes. The informal structure of the organization is not always easy to uncover. A prerequisite is being an insider and knowing the informal networks of the key members who influence decisions in the organization. To gain access to this informal system, the nurse manager must expand interactions with both superiors and subordinates for information and communication. This means taking time away from desk work and walking around the organization to meet and greet personnel. By reaching out to others in an informal manner, the nurse administrator sends a message that one is approachable and ready to listen.

Learning the advantages of developing informal communication can benefit the nurse administrator inside and outside the organization. Using social situations to meet and speak with potential power brokers can provide an opportunity to share knowledge and expertise. Attending office promotion parties, holiday celebrations, or farewell affairs provides informal ways to conduct sound business and establish professional networks and coalitions.

Knowing the Power Brokers

To be perceived as powerful and successful at accomplishing organizational goals, the nurse administrator must be able to accurately assess who has power and who gets what, as well as when and how it is gotten. Connection power is valuable when the nurse administrator seeks to use this influence of knowing people in high places to receive support or resources on proposed projects. Therefore, it is essential that the nurse administrator be able to identify and associate with the power brokers of the organization. By understanding where the power lies, attempts can be made to consolidate efforts toward the right people at the right time. Power brokers have access to such varied resources as money, personal and positional connections, and property. To gain access to these resources the nurse administrator must network with powerbrokers. To establish effective networking relationships, the nurse administrator must take the time and effort needed to recognize and cultivate both the formal and informal power brokers in the organization.

Power brokers are easy to recognize. They are usually assertive and have a positive self-image. The personal attributes of power brokers are amplified by their confident gait, good eye contact, and high visibility, all of which help create the image of power. Powerful people possess not only the knowledge and expertise to accomplish goals but have control over their physical body by looking healthy and physically fit. Being in control of mind and body promotes self-confidence and a determination to succeed. Success is powerful and influential and is what creates a true power broker.

Knowing the Suprasystem

Once the organization has been fully assessed and understood, nurse administrators can expand their horizons by focusing on people and events outside the organization to the larger community. This community might include local, state, or federal influences and even the local community where the organization is geographically located. Knowing the issues or concerns of the greater community can only serve to protect and enhance the interests of the nurse administrator. Without knowledge of the bigger picture, the nurse administrator misses opportunities to promote professional issues as well as learn about the trends and concerns of others who might appreciate support. The nurse administrator is encouraged to engage in community affairs to promote a positive image of the organization and to allow opportunities to be sensitive to the needs of the suprasystem.

Developing a Support Base

Even if one operates solely on the basis of positional power and authority, a support base is necessary to ensure that one's decisions or stances are enabled and given the fullest chance of being operationalized. A support base consists of all possible avenues of support. Too often, it is assumed that cultivating one's boss is the primary means for obtaining support for one's positions. Recognizing and cultivating the connections that flow among all elements in a system also provide support for one's positions. Such a perspective embraces developing connections among diverse constituencies that vary from the people cleaning the hospital floors to the media brokers in the community.

Additionally, how one develops this support base may differ according to one's perspectives and ethics. Traditional models of developing support bases rely on doing favors and expecting paybacks, retribution for nonsupport, and "swimming with the sharks." On the other hand, women have generally relied on other skills that emphasize developing connections among people in ways that are mutually supportive and that rely on active listening, demonstration of concern for the person, kindness, and lack of confrontation. This latter method becomes ineffective if used repeatedly by the nurse executive. When used with deliberation, however, it can be effective. A blending of the methods of the dominant model of power and politics with some of the traditional ways to cultivate interpersonal relationships may provide the nurse executive with the most visionary and effective means for developing a support base.

A primary technique for developing these connections is networking (Puetz, 1985). Networking requires that one identify constituencies to be developed and put oneself in the position of meeting and connecting to them. For example, networking with the people who clean the floors may include simply introducing oneself to housekeeping personnel on an individual basis while making rounds, acknowledging the person at subsequent meetings, and showing an interest in that individual as a fellow worker and contributor to the institution's goals. Networking with other administrators may include attending social functions that enable people to develop a more personal connection than occurs when one connects across a meeting table. Networking with media may require attending a meeting of a business organization that features a panel of media specialists. Of course, simply attending this meeting is not sufficient. Introducing oneself, exchanging business cards, and suggesting a follow-up lunch with key contacts to discuss an issue of mutual concern will enable the connection to develop.

Clearly, networking is time-consuming. A deliberative and prioritized plan for networking and integrating networking into one's daily life is necessary. Assessing what connections one ought to have or does not need to have, what connections one actually has, and ways to develop connections constitute the basis for a long term plan for networking. Integrating networking into one's professional life requires an understanding of a basic premise of networking: by knowing each other, we can help each other. This requires that one look for ways to help others, respond to requests for help when possible, and know when and how to ask for help from others.

Networking can be seen as the foundation for coalition building. A coalition is a formal or informal group representing diverse constituencies for the purpose of moving toward a goal of interest to all parties in the coalition. Physicians and nurses may disagree about many issues, but there are many others with which they can and should unite, including issues that address patient care. Similarly, other administrators, social workers, psychologists, housekeeping staff, and community health advocacy groups can align with nursing around particular issues of common concern. Building and working with coalitions requires that one agree to disagree on other issues.

Informal coalitions can be formed prior to meetings for the purpose of moving an item on the agenda in a particular direction. They also can be formed around issues on which the nurse administrator needs broad-based support. Whether formal or informal, coalition building requires the ability to identify and capitalize on others' interests on an issue. As with networking, this is not a one-sided affair. One must be prepared to support others' interests on this and other issues. This stance is consistent with feminist perspectives that value cooperation and sharing over competition. Since feminist perspectives and values do not predominate in health care institutions, however, one must be careful that one's presence and position within a coalition of interests is not misrepresented or abused.

Developing a support base requires that one nurture and develop one's connections both within and outside of nursing. Again, this approach must become a part of one's daily professional work style. While it is possible to develop a support base in a crisis situation, it is best to have support available and nurtured prior to its use. Operating from a framework of empowerment suggests that one is continually involved in engaging others to participate in decision making which in itself can foster supportive relationships.

One must know which constituency to call in for support and when to call it, depending on the issue and its political context. One also must know that one's support base will provide the support that is advantageous and consistent. For example, if a director of nursing is fired by the CEO and wants her position restored, she must be assured that if she mobilizes the nursing staff in her defense, they will act in ways she believes will be appropriate for the situation. An unsigned petition to the mayor of the city to restore the director to her post in a private institution is cause for embarrassment and may jeopardize the director's effort at reinstatement. This means that one must truly "know" one's constituencies, have access to them directly or indirectly, and be able to mobilize them when needed.

A support base also provides one with a constituency for collective action. Change is rarely easy. When change is planned as a shared or collective effort, it can be creative, enduring, and energizing. As empowerment demonstrates, the process for change can be as important to nursing as the change itself.

Choosing the Issue

While one should be continually developing and nurturing a support base, choosing the issue to influence requires equal attention. There are many issues that one can take on during the course of one's professional day. Taking on all problems is neither wise nor expedient. Deciding which to influence can be difficult and involve deciding how important the problem is and its political context, including one's own political standing.

Analyzing the importance of the problem requires that one evaluate values and perspectives from which "importance" is determined. Importance can be determined from bottomline economic survival or from concern about quality of patient care. These two perspectives can and often do collide. One also can consider the short and long-term consequences of the problem, its resolution or its persistence. A clear analysis of whether the climate is conducive for the problem to be resolved, whether it can be resolved at the present time, and what resources it will take to manage the problem versus its resolution must all be considered. Chief among these resources are one's own time and energies required.

The political context of the problem must be analyzed. What factors impinge on the issue, within the institution and in the community and society? Today, if an issue is concerned with cost containment, the political climate is ripe for support from certain segments of society, including the government and business community. Who has a vested interest in the problem that may conflict with yours? What will involvement in the issue do to your own political standing? Will you be put at odds with another power broker in the institution? Will you be viewed as defending important principles or causes? What will losing the issue do to your image and effectiveness within the institution? How will you be affected if you are unable to win on the issue? Will involvement in this issue, whether winning or losing, provide you with a stronger support base (eg, will it unite and mobilize an otherwise apathetic nursing staff)? Is your involvement in the issue more for the sake of the issue or is it for increasing your power base. Sometimes what appear to be crucial issues are really struggles for power, particularly when two power brokers are intently in direct conflict with each other on an issue with neither side willing to negotiate a compromised solution.

Oftentimes, the importance of the issue conflicts with political considerations of choosing to be involved in the issue. One may decide to take on a seemingly unimportant issue because it is important to the nursing staff and the staff's perception of themselves as able to make change. Sometimes, one takes a chance on getting involved in an issue. Once involved, retreat may or may not be possible. Thus is it helpful to separate the issue from its political context. It is also important to count mistakes as learning experiences and recognize that politics is rarely clear-cut and absolute. A sense of humor helps put any situation in perspective.

Developing the Issue

Analyzing the issue or problem requires that one first clearly define the problem and, its causes and contributing factors. If the data are not available to support logical deductions about the extent of the problem and its causes or contributing factors, one must weigh the costs to acquire it versus not having the information. Specific data also are needed when analyzing alternative solutions to the issue or problem. What are the costs and benefits of alternatives?

Additionally, one needs to analyze the values and beliefs of various constituencies affected by the issue. How can the issue or problem be "sold" to these constituencies? For example, the nurse administrator who has an innovative model that promotes greater job satisfaction and quality care for nursing practice will need to address the potential cost effectiveness of the model to sell the idea to the boss. One also may need to find the bottom line that makes the issue of concern to physicians or social workers in order to mobilize their support for the plan. This "hook" may not be the primary reason for instituting the model, but will be the words that will arouse the attention and interest of those whose support is wanted.

Selling one's position or plan requires an awareness and anticipation of opposing arguments and preparation to argue away the opposition. A good position paper is one that includes opposing arguments and discusses why these arguments are unimportant, false, or insufficient.

Developing an issue also entails analyzing how the issue should be promoted. Is it an issue that should be managed behind the scenes on an informal basis? Is a formal position paper needed? Do groups and/or individuals need to be sensitized to the issue through articles in an in-house publication that can then put the issue "on the agenda" or through a leak to a contact in the media who can raise the problem as a public issue? What method of presentation of an issue or plan will be most successful with each constituency? Standard marketing techniques should be brought into play on major issues or problems. Once the issue is developed, one must continually evaluate how to move the issue or how to address any problems.

Moving the Issue

Timing. Regardless of the issue, the nurse administrator must be sensitive to timing as a significant factor in moving an issue or planned change. The best presentation can fail to gain full recognition if timing is too early or late. Knowing when to act or withhold the issue can influence success toward problem resolution. The key in moving an issue is careful timing and planning with clear vision and scope of the issue as well as choosing the right place to introduce the issue.

Using Outside Experts. When looking for key figures to lend support, it is sometimes best to go outside the organization. By using outside experts with no vested interest, the soundness and fit of the issue is more credible. Outside experts tend to be less threatening and often provide professional pressure to persuade the nonbelievers. An effective authority on the issue is critical to successful presentation of your case. By maintaining contact with outside experts, the nurse administrator gains a personal support system to pursue the issue as well as special assistance when needed.

Selectively Communicating Information. Once a time has been chosen to present the issue, the nurse administrator must determine who in the organization might lend support to the projected plan. Potential supporters should be listed and plans made to create a coalition. This selective art of communication allows the nurse administrator to rally a preselected base of support persons who have been briefed about the risks and liabilities of the projected plan. By selectively seeking support and actively communicating, the nurse administrator has preassessed the marketing plan and is ready to proceed.

Marketing the Issue

To market one's projected plan is to identify needs and wants of others through creating and exchanging values and products. Kotler (1984) suggests that marketing is a social process whereby individuals or groups obtain what they want through an exchange process. Knowing the needs and wants of your market presupposes that the nurse administrator has identified individuals or groups where there exists a potential exchange relationship. These relationships might include physicians, patients, peers, and other personnel within the organization. If the projected plan includes a market outside the organization, the nurse administrator must seek to establish community-based relationships with individuals or groups, such as legislators, regulators, volunteers or potential consumers of the organization.

When seeking to influence a potential marketing group, the nurse administrator's approach must include a thorough understanding of market's values, needs, and wants. For the appeal to be successful, the nurse administrator's strategy should be based on a well-developed plan with identified goals and objectives. If necessary, a survey or other research plans might be required to assess the market.

Working the Committee. As the opportunity draws closer for the issue to be presented, the nurse administrator must promote the issue by attending to the needs and wants of committee members. Plans should be made to brief each member on the issue to ensure that each member knows the specific issue and supports the organizational goals. Addressing their key concerns about the issue reduces potential opposition from growing and gives the nurse administrator time to consider the comments and make adjustments if needed. In addition, the nurse administrator must be ready to ask key members to speak in support of the issue when discussion begins. Gaining support by identifying members as advocates or neutrals can help the nurse administrator plan accordingly. When advocates stand together there is a cumulative strength that can potentially be used against adversaries. The nurse administrator also must know the strength of adversaries and their arguments as well as be prepared to diffuse the opposition. All attempts should be made to use whatever resources are available to move the issue in one's favor. Using your support base can enhance the perceived importance of the issue as well as result in a win-win outcome for all.

Negotiation and Compromise. In reality not all projected plans are perfect on the first introduction. What then are the possible alternatives to moving the issue? Can the nurse administrator find acceptable compromises? If so, to what ends can an acceptable solution be negotiated and with whom? Learning the art of negotiation and compromise is critical if the nurse administrator is to be a team player. Knowing the long- and short-term objectives of what you want will allow for temporary sacrifices needed occasionally. Sometimes half a loaf is better than none at all.

If you must compromise on an issue be sure the stakes are not too high. The concession should be of equal or less value. Remember to keep a scorecard on the number of compromises or concessions made during the negotiation process. The purpose behind this is that you can explain to the opposition just how much you have surrendered to move toward resolution. However, try not to make the first concession but use a tradeoff, such as "If I do that for you, what will you do for me?" After all, the art of negotiation is being able to fulfill both parties needs so that the solution is win-win.

SUMMARY

Nurse administrators will be exposed to politics in every aspect of their organization life. It is crucial to acquire highly developed, politically astute skills to influence and obtain available resources. A successful nurse administrator is a good politician and a team player. To "wheel and deal" with others to gain access to limited resources does not imply that nurse administrators adopt behaviors or the traditional model of power grabbing. They bring unique skills from the caring ethic that can be used to add power-sharing strategies to traditional power grabbing techniques. With a focus on power sharing, nurse administrators can bring to light this ethic of care in health care organizations. As leaders in health care organizations, nurse administrators can effectively garner support of their followers and colleagues while modeling empowerment to all.

Using political savvy and effective power strategies, the nurse administrator can help other nurses appreciate the importance of political action for developing the health care organization, health policies and to the profession. By applying political knowledge and skill to bring about change in the health care organization, the nurse administrator empowers the system to respect its members and work together on its differences. Empowerment allows nurse administrators to recognize that by caring for one's self or one's interests the whole organization benefits.

Lobbying for the needs of patients, staff, and health policies brings attention to needed changes in health care delivery. By developing a personal plan to enhance one's political skills and power, a commitment is made to transform the workplace where power is valued and the art of influence is just as important as communication, cooperation and collaboration. The ultimate goal of power and politics in the health care organization is to improve its quality of care and environment.

REFERENCES

American Academy of Nursing. *Magnet Hospitals: Attraction and Retention of Professional Nurses.* Kansas City, MO, American Nurses Association, 1983

Archer SE, Goehner PA. Acquiring political clout: Guidelines for nurse administrators. *Journal of Nursing Administration.* 11:49, 1981

Beck B. *Empowerment: A Future Goal for Social Work. Working Papers in Social Policy.* New York, Community Service Society, 1983

Block P. *The Empowered Manager.* San Francisco, Jossey-Bass, 1987

Bookman A, Morgan S. *Women and the Politics of Empowerment.* Philadelphia: Temple University Press, 1988

Center for Women in Government. *Women and Public Policy.* Albany, NY: The Center, 1984

Chodorow N. *The Reproduction of Mothering.* Berkeley, University of California Press, 1978

Conger JA, Kanungo RN. The empowerment process: Integrating theory and practice, *Academy of Management Review.* 31, 1988

Costello-Nickitas D. One manager's strategies for creating a supportive work environment. In: Mason DJ, Talbott SW, eds. *Political Action Handbook for Nurses: Changing the Workplace, Government, Organization and Community.* Menlo Park, CA, Addison Wesley, 1985, 261–263

del Bueno DJ, Freund CM. *Power and Politics in Nursing Administration: A Casebook.* Owings Mills, MD, National Health Publishing, 1986

Diers D. Policy and politics. In: Mason DJ, Talbott SW, eds. *Political Action Handbook for Nurses: Changing the Workplace, Government, Organizations and Community.* Menlo Park, CA, Addison Wesley, 1985, 53–60.

Donovan J. *Feminist Theory: The Intellectual Traditions of American Feminism.* New York: Ungar, 1985

Fagin C. Nursing's pivotal role in American health care. In: Aiken L, Gortner S, eds. *Nursing in the 1980's: Crisis, Opportunities, Challenges.* Philadelphia: Lippincott, 1982

French J, Raven B. The bases of social power. In: Cartwright D, ed. *Studies in Social Power.* Ann Arbor: University of Michigan Press, 1960

Gilligan C. *In A Different Voice.* Cambridge, MA, Harvard University Press, 1982

Heineken J. Power: Conflicting views. *Journal of Nursing Administration.* 15:11, 36, 1985

Kanter RB. *The Change Masters.* New York: Simon & Schuster, 1983

Klein E. *Gender Politics.* Cambridge, MA, Harvard University Press, 1984

Kohlberg L. *The Philosophy of Moral Development.* San Francisco: Harper and Row, 1981

Kotler P. *Marketing Management: Analysis, Planning and Control,* 5th ed. Englewood Cliffs, NJ, Prentice-Hall, 1984

MacKinnon C. Feminism, marxism, method and the state: An agenda for theory. *Signs.* 7:515, 1982

MacPherson K. Health care policy, values and nursing. *Advances in Nursing Science.* 9:1, 1987

Mason DJ, Talbott SW, eds. *Political Action Handbook for Nurses: Changing the Workplace, Government, Organizations, and Community.* Menlo Park, CA, Addison-Wesley, 1985

Miller JB. *Towards a New Psychology for Women.* Boston: Beacon, 1976

Puetz B. Networks. In: Mason DJ, Talbott SW, eds. *Political Action Handbook for Nurses: Changing the Workplace, Government, Organizations, and Community.* Menlo Park, CA, Addison-Wesley, 1985, 190–194

Ridd R, Calloway H. *Women and Political Conflict: Portraits of Struggle in Times of Conflict.* New York: New York University Press, 1987

Secretary's Commission on Nursing. Final report. Washington, DC, Department of Health and Human Services, 1988

Stevens B. Power and politics for the nurse executive. *Nursing and Health Care.* 1:4, 208, 1980

Stuart GW. An organizational strategy for empowering nursing. *Nursing Economics.* 4:2, 69, 1986

Wheeler CE, Chinn PL. *Peace and Power: A Handbook of Feminist Process,* 2nd ed. New York: National League for Nursing, 1989

Zaleznik A. Power and politics in organizational life. *Nursing Dimensions.* 7:2, 64, 1979

SECTION II

Setting Organizational Direction

CHAPTER 4

Strategic Management in Nursing Administration

Liz Johnson

> ## Key Concept List
>
> Strategic management
> Planning
> Mission, objectives, and goals
> Information analysis

Over the decades of the 1970s and 1980s, the concept of corporate strategy became an "idea in good currency" in America's private industry. Both in the business literature and in practice, one can find evidence of capital budgeting, long-range planning, strategic planning, and, more recently, strategic management. Movement in this direction evolved from concern about diminished profitability of American businesses. There is now recognition that sound corporate strategy is a prerequisite for long term success. And yet, corporate strategy has created only limited success for American businesses. The primary reason is that more emphasis has been placed on strategy *formulation* than on strategy *implementation*. A second reason is that most organizations are still operating on a short-term focus. Corporate strategy has had less than widespread use in the American health care industry and almost none in nursing. This chapter presents a methodology for formulating and implementing strategy for nursing.

The reader will find answers to the what as well as the how-to of strategic management. Specifically, what is pursued is:

1. An in-depth explanation of the nature of strategic management—its scope, its meaning, its components, and concepts peculiar to it.
2. A methodology for strategy formulation and strategy implementation.

WHY STRATEGIC MANAGEMENT IS IMPORTANT

Strategic management is important because it can give nursing the tools for strengthening both its desire and ability to design its own future through the formulation and implementation of sound strategy. Strategic management also is important because it is one of the key areas of responsibility for all executives. Executives, including nurse executives, have three major spheres of administrative responsibility: day-to-day operations, management of the culture of their organization, and management of strategy. No one area can be sacrificed for the other. Rather, all three must coexist and synergize each other. When managed, the outcome of their interplay will be greater than the sum of their individual contributions. It is too often the case that nurse executives spend most of their time on operational issues of the present moment. Little time remains for managing the culture within nursing (see Chapter 5) and even less time is spent planning future strategy. Thus, strategy is often excluded from mainstream activity. And yet, growing challenges signal the need for nursing to have a well-articulated strategy for the future. There is the challenge of the critical shortage of resources—personnel, money, support services, and time. There is the phenomenal growth in technology capable of enhancing both the quality of patient care and productivity of staff but often unattainable for a variety of reasons. There is the expectation that nurse leaders apply sophisticated business knowledge to maintain high productivity and low costs. There are increasing accountability challenges. There are changes in the culture of professional nursing. There is the need to manage, not simply monitor, the quality of services delivered. All of this means that nursing and all other professions are today required to operate by new rules.

Operating by new rules requires maintaining a balance among daily operations, the culture, and planning for the future. It is no longer acceptable to do one to the exclusion of the others. They all must be done simultaneously. If the nurse executive places too much emphasis on operational issues of today, the emphasis on the future required by the new rules is overlooked. If the nurse executive maintains the cultural norm of status quo, opportunities to maximize the use of information, new insights, and creativity may be overlooked. If the nurse executive fully embraces the future with little regard for the present and past realities, important continuities can be compromised. The tools of strategic management encourage a proper combination of all three executive responsibilities.

WHAT IS STRATEGIC MANAGEMENT?

Strategic management in nursing is actualizing a plan to bring about future goals. This plan is based on the best information about:

1. Nursing's consumers
2. Forces in nursing's environment
3. Nursing's unique competencies that give it a competitive advantage

This strategic plan is designed to help nursing (and its containing organization) achieve pre-eminence in the marketplace. Additionally, such a strategic plan minimizes the possibility that nursing will be faced by abrupt surprises. Finally, the strategic plan can produce innovations in service delivery, improvements in quality of care, enhancements in the quality of work life, and enhancement of reputation, among other advantages.

STRATEGIC MANAGEMENT

Definitions of strategic management typically have at least five common features. They are:

1. Administrative in nature
2. Systematic
3. Environment related
4. Future oriented
5. Sensitive to the correct positioning of an organization (or a department within) in its environment

Administratively, strategic management involves a great deal of planning, organizing, and coordinating activities to assure achievement of positive outcomes. When executed appropriately, these activities, coupled with appropriate execution, can create a dynamic supporting framework for turning future plans into reality. It is important to administer the strategic management process so that the goals of the nursing department and the institution are compatible. In organizing and directing the strategic management process, it is important to incorporate principles of the change process. In controlling, outcome targets must be developed early in the process and effective supervisory techniques used to assure achievement of the targets. This is discussed in more depth later.

The systematic nature of strategic management is reflected in the orderliness and thoroughness with which it should take place. Preparing a nursing department to use its best capabilities and to have the best reputation is not accidental; it is systematically orchestrated. The best interests of the nursing department and its members are not served when issues relating to its future are mentioned only casually in a periodic meeting, after an unfavorable finance report is distributed, or when the annual planning retreat is being organized. Planning for nursing's future requires continuous refinement of the best thinking of those who have a vested interest in nursing's future. Those who participate in the decision making about nursing's future can do their best thinking and planning only if an organized process of strategic planning is instituted. This process should extend to all levels of the nursing organization. The environmental emphasis of strategic management recognizes that nursing is an open system, embedded in and in continuous interaction with its environment. The environment can be conceptualized as having several layers as one moves beyond nursing, to its containing organization, to the environment beyond the organization. The environment also can be conceptualized as having several dimensions which must be considered as nursing plans for its future. Examples of these dimensions are patient volume/acuity/demand, physician preferences, and regulatory/legal requirements (see Fig 4–1). The undeniable presence of these forces in nursing's environment means that a nursing department cannot operate as though it is a closed system. It must acknowledge these forces and utilize them in planning strategically for its de-

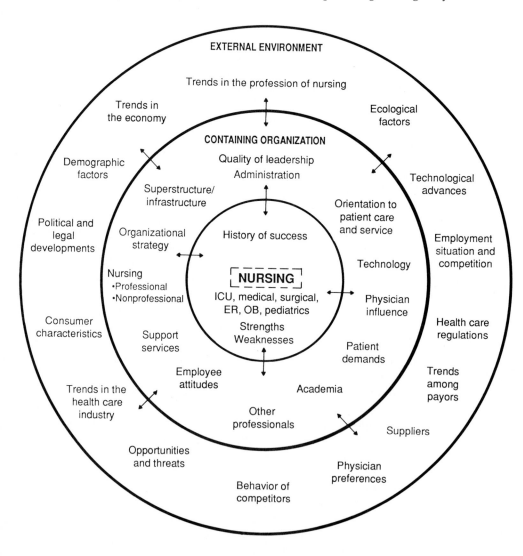

Figure 4–1. Nursing in its Environments

sired future. *One of the most common deficiencies seen in strategic management is that the strategic plan does not demonstrate an appreciation of environmental forces.*

Strategic management's emphasis on the future requires that the nursing department make the best decisions today in order to achieve desired objectives in the future. In the words of Peter Drucker, "Strategic management deals not with future decisions but with the futurity of present decisions." (Drucker, 1974) The essence of this thought is put into action when a nursing department creates and maintains a continuous process for deciding how nursing would function if the members could have it the way they desire it in the future. The fundamental notion undergirding such a process is the collective belief that the nursing department can create an image of a desired future and design ways to bring it about. Strategic management's emphasis on correct positioning within the environment reflects the need to identify areas of excellence that will give a nursing department and its health care organization a place of superiority in the marketplace. The nursing department needs to capitalize on those strengths that will produce better-than-average results in serving the consumer. This might be superior clinical expertise, outstanding outreach, or extraordinary patient teaching. It might be innovative approaches and distinctive nursing products. Care must be taken to assure that areas of strength are consistent with what the consumer is willing to purchase. In the final analysis, judgment about the superiority of nursing's services resides in the experience of the user, not in the intentions of the provider. A familiar example of positioning for success is military strategy in which the aim is to gain strategic advantage by capturing land, by eliminating the enemy, or by minimizing the ability of the enemy to wage war. In business, the aim is to gain strategic advantage by increasing market share. There is one marketplace. If one organization gains market share, another loses it. The degree to which the nursing department's strategy for patient care is consistent with what consumers recognize as excellent or superior parallels developing a dominant market share. This is precisely what is meant by competitive advantage. It follows that the nursing department's most important decision is identifying specific areas of excellence (niche) that the department will develop or refine to exceed the competition.

In strategic management, Igor Ansoff is noted to be one of the most important early thinkers. Combining the five concepts discussed previously with the thinking of Ansoff (1984), strategic management here is defined as *a systematic process of futuristic decision making which positions a nursing department to its environment in ways which assure its continued success and secure it from surprise as much as possible.* Ansoff emphasizes the need to anticipate the element of surprise because it is that aspect of the future that organizations are the least prepared to handle.

On a practical level, strategic management revolves around seven basic questions:

1. What business is the nursing department in? What consumer group does it want to serve? What are their needs? What are its technologies for meeting those needs?
2. What is the most appropriate set of ends—ie, mission, objectives, goals—to pursue in order to achieve the desired future?

3. What unique competencies does the nursing department have that favorably distinguish it from other competitors in the eyes of the consumer that will yield the greatest success at the least cost?
4. In what segment of the marketplace does the nursing department wish to compete?
5. What strategy should the nursing department select to achieve internal and external advantage?
6. How can the nursing department's internal functions, structure, and processes be redesigned to assure implementation of the strategy?
7. How can large-scale organizational change be managed?

When these seven questions are answered favorably and systematically, the ongoing process of strategy formulation and strategy implementation will be successful and the desired future will most likely emerge.

The model in Figure 4–2 illustrates the entire strategic management process. In it, the two major components are strategy formulation and strategy implementation. In strategy formulation, both the forces in the environment and the capabilities within the nursing department to respond to those forces are assessed. This latter activity is one of the primary distinctions of strategic management from strategic planning. The next step is to decide the ends (mission, objectives, standards, policies, procedures) that are a logical extension of the assessment. Knowing the ends, the means are then developed. Strategy is an important component of the means to the desired future. In strategy implementation, appropriate structures, processes, and controls are developed to assure achievement of the ends. Each of the steps of both strategy formulation and strategy implementation are presented in the next section on methodology.

METHODOLOGY FOR STRATEGIC PLANNING

To manage strategically, one must create a strategic organization. This includes: clear lines of responsibility; a broad, flat and lean structure; and, organization-wide participation. With this framework, the steps can be implemented.

The sequence of steps required for effective strategic management is neither simple nor straightforward. Experience has shown that applying the steps in an orderly fashion presents a supreme challenge. The nine chief challenges presented below are each discussed separately:

1. Motivating people to plan
2. Creating time for planning
3. Encouraging strategic thinking
4. Correctly interpreting the environment and its signals
5. Uncovering the unique competencies within the nursing department that will yield the best competitive advantage
6. Defining a relevant set of services that consumers will be willing to purchase
7. Formulating the right strategy
8. Fitting strategy to reality
9. Making appropriate use of people and the culture

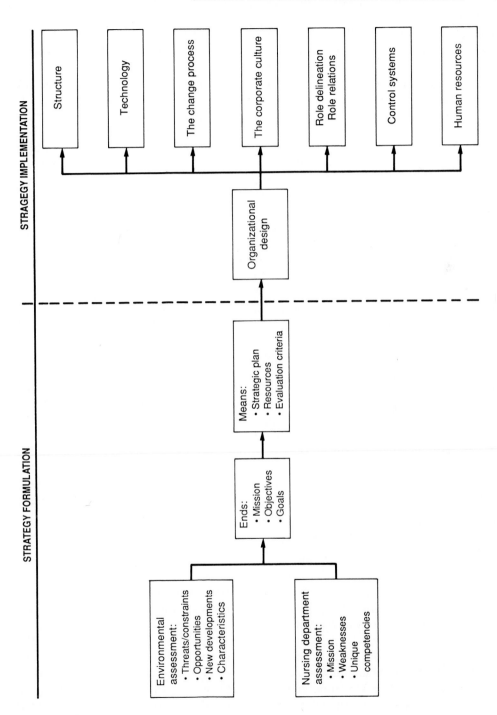

Figure 4–2. Strategic Management Process

Motivating People to Plan

Ackoff asserts that planners fall into four categories, depending on their orientation to time. The *reactive* planner prefers the past and has the desire to recreate a previous state of operation. The *inactive* planner prefers the present and resists change. The *preactive* planner believes that conditions are deteriorating rapidly and thus seeks to implement plans for the future rapidly. The *proactive* planner does not prefer the past, the present nor what is envisioned in the future. This planner prefers to create a desired future and invent ways to bring it about (Ackoff, 1972). It is often helpful to introduce the planning process with this concept as a means of motivating participants. This concept also tends to help participants to believe that being proactive can make a difference.

Creating Time for Planning

The day-to-day demands of operations as well as events occurring within the culture are prominent detractors from time to plan. A useful solution to this is to establish specific times and write them on all participants' calendars. The idea here is that activities for which participants set specific times and dates tend to be carried out. The potential for success with strategic planning meetings also is increased by creating an agenda that identifies an exact beginning and ending time. Nursing department members are busy and operate with limited time. Notifying them of the exact time frame affords them the opportunity to schedule other equally important activities. Interruptions should be kept to a minimum. Planning time also is conserved by emphasizing positive ideas rather than by discussing problems exclusively. This, in turn, inspires excitement about the future as opposed to the negative climate created by the discussion of only problems. It should be noted that with problem-centered planning, participants tend to formulate plans which state only what they do not want in the future. Eliminating what one does not want does nothing to assure the attainment of what one does want. Finally, when planning meetings have a negative, problem-oriented tone, participants become less interested in creating time for future meetings.

Encouraging Strategic Thinking

Health care delivery systems, of which nursing is one, are dominated by professionals. Professionals are socialized into an ideal model of service delivery. This can be translated into the difference between decisions made on the basis of theory and past practice. The opposite of this continuum are the demands created by environmental forces (eg, patients, market trends, reimbursement policies). Thinking strategically requires an appreciation for the demands of market forces as well as professional competencies. It means aligning professionally identified consumer needs with consumer wants. Consumers assume that providers can meet their needs. Beyond that, what consumers and, thus the marketplace, judge service delivery on is the degree to which that service is consistent with what the consumers want. This is often a difficult concept for professionals to embrace because it is interpreted as a compromise of their professional principles. The packaging of professional competencies to best match market requirements can yield enormous payoffs in consumer loyalty. Thinking in this direction must begin at the nurse executive level and filter throughout the nursing department. This thinking needs to be shared by the nurse executive on rounds and at any other opportunity to communicate philosophy.

Correctly Interpreting the Environment and Its Signals

One aspect of strategic management is that it can reduce the element of surprise. Surprise, if it is negative in nature, creates the need for quick reaction. The haste of such a reaction can waste resource utilization and reduce coordination of effort. In many instances, there are early warnings that dramatic change is impending, often called weak signals, which may go undetected. A critique of most chaotic administrative events will usually reveal that there were subtle warnings early on. The ability to interpret these subtle warnings develops with experience and conscious effort. While the approach to strategic management discussed here does not advocate a belief that one can predict and prepare for future events, it is strongly suggested that the nurse executive needs to develop a high level of skill in correctly interpreting events in the environment. Often, more change can be created in the nursing department by events in the environment than by events within the department. So, it is important to be alert to emerging events. Interpreting these events means going beyond a description of them to an explanation of them. Description answers the questions who, what, when, where, how, how much? Explanation answers the question why? Until one can adequately explain why events are occurring, one is apt to focus on the wrong aspects of the event and thus react inappropriately.

Uncovering the Unique Competencies Within the Nursing Department That Will Yield the Best Competitive Advantage

Every nursing department has unique skills and expertise. This uniqueness arises from at least two sources. On the one hand, it is created by the historical methods of delivering nursing care, from the unique capabilities of members of the department and from particular preferences of those members. On the other hand, it is created by the special demands and preferences of the consumers served by the nursing department, including patients, physicians, payors, the community at large and the containing organization. It is important that the nursing leader analyze the uniqueness that the department possesses and organize it in innovative ways that distinguish its services from those of the competition. The competitive advantage can often be created by doing the little things that count. Some examples include bilingual patient teaching or support groups led by former patients who are well aware of the needs of present patients. Other examples are discharge preparation teams that consist of members of each service used by the patient during treatment, business services as well as clinical services. In many nursing departments, these types of unique arrangements are already in place because the members already possess the required skill set. In other nursing departments, these unique arrangements must be consciously developed. The important point is that consumers, members of the nursing department, and the competition are all sources to decide the nursing department's unique and innovative approaches to service. Once discovered, these approaches must be capitalized on.

Defining a Relevant Set of Services That Consumers Will Be Willing to Purchase

With the advent of the prospective payment method of reimbursement of health care, competition for the health care dollar became a reality. A health care provider competes on the basis of price, quality of care, and service. Nursing is central to each of these mechanisms for competition. The price of care is based on the cost of delivering it. Nursing represents the largest single component of human resources in the delivery of care and nursing figures prominently in the quality of care. Both price and quality have been relatively easy to associate with nursing in the past. Relating service to nursing is less easy to demonstrate. This is probably because of beliefs related to professionalism. Nurses receive their professional socialization around a set of ideals which require that the nurse use a body of scientific knowledge to determine the needs, the care plan, and courses of action to convert a patient from an ill state to a well state. Nurses are taught to involve the patient in the planning of care but, in reality, the nurse typically maintains the dominant role in the treatment process.

Consumerism seems to be on the opposite end of a continuum from professionalism. Professionalism places the patient in a vertical relationship to the nurse; consumerism, a horizontal relationship. In that horizontal relationship, the patient becomes a consumer who has purchasing power and who can decide the type of service desired. There are clearly levels of consumer ability to decide. If nursing is to function in a competitive mode, it must approach the organization of its services with an appreciation of the consumer's contribution to the definition of those services. In the current competitive health care environment, the relevance of nursing's services is defined, in large measure, by their ''goodness of fit'' with the preferences of consumers. Ultimately, the best set of services will arise out of a combination of professionalism *and* consumerism, not professionalism *or* consumerism.

Consumerism encompasses consumers' wants as well as their needs. In all arenas of life, we as consumers purchase goods and services for two types of reasons—the intrinsic or extrinsic value that those goods or services add to our life. Intrinsic value fulfills our needs; extrinsic value satisfies our wants. Consumers' wants determine a particular type of lifestyle. In addition to meeting health care needs, nursing can package many of its services to address the lifestyle of consumers. Today's consumer seeks a lifestyle that includes being well informed, enjoying increased leisure time, communicating by electronic media, having access to services which simplify or eliminate basic chores, and the ability to exhibit choice, among other requirements. The challenge for nursing is to acknowledge consumer desires and address them because the services that address these desires are the services most remembered by the consumer. Some ideas for marketing nursing's expertise to consumers might include: (1) videotapes that highlight the array of nursing services available during the course of treatment; (2) discharge plans via electronic or auditory media; (3) self-directed health education; (4) nursing products from which the consumer can choose; and (5) self-directed nursing plans of care. These are not only services that the consumer has a high probability of being willing to purchase; they are also services that will distinguish nursing from other professions and make nursing memorable.

Formulating the Right Strategy

Whereas there is a strategy that is right for every nursing department, there is no one best strategy that can be prescribed for every nursing department. Strategy is entirely dependent on the environmental conditions confronting the particular nursing department and on the strengths within the department. Decisions that contribute to formulating the right strategy emerge from the answers to these questions:

- Do we choose to offer the same nursing services as competitors? In what quantity and variety?
- Do we choose to serve the same consumer groups as competitors? In what quantity and variety?
- Do we choose to offer an improved generation of nursing services which are innovative in content and/or form?
- What will be our overall approach to competitors:
  a. Frontal attack—going head-to-head with every service and every consumer group
  b. Flank attack—indirectly competing with select services and consumer groups
  c. Encirclement—providing greater numbers of services and pursuing a greater variety of consumer segments
  d. Bypass—providing the next generation of services or pursuing a different geographic segment of consumers
  e. Guerilla—building superior services to quickly overwhelm the competition and then retreat (Fahey, 1989)

Each strategy can be successful or unsuccessful, depending on the particular ends desired by a nursing department as well as its appropriateness. The "goodness of fit" or "rightness" of a strategy can be judged by its ability to galvanize all of the nursing department's potential for superior performance and concentrate that performance in ways that attract a major lion's share of consumers to the organization. The central task of formulating strategy consists of defining how one will gain or sustain competitive advantage. This requires asking fundamental questions, such as the ones above, and devoting adequate attention to finding their answers.

Fitting Strategy to Reality

Both the level of resources in the nursing department and conditions in the environment combine to determine how realistic a strategy will be. It is simple to craft an elegant statement of strategy. The question is, Will its implementation attract consumer groups as well as enhance the delivery system in the long run? For example, all nursing departments value the objective of being the leading provider. To achieve that objective, one strategy might be to exceed other providers in the variety of nursing services and the number of patients and physicians served in selected target services such as cardiovascular nursing or trauma care. Another strategy might be to offer the latest generation of care in obstetrical or rehabilitation nursing. When the realism of these strategies is considered, some difficult questions must be asked, namely:

- Are our resources adequate to seize opportunities that might be created by this strategy or to support the wants of consumers?
- Is this strategy the best one that can be selected to deploy our resources and win in the marketplace?
- Do consumers want and value our services in the form that we plan to offer them?
- Will this strategy and our services give us a commanding position in the mar-ketplace—eg, at least 30 percent market share?
- Will our services create a positive relationship between cost and price?
- Are our services intended to be specialty or commodity (commonly available) services? Which should they be? Can the selected type be afforded?
- Can we face the obligation to retreat if the strategy does not work?
- Are we inventing a new service that will be a popular fad only for a short time instead of making minor enhancements and marketing existing services, in which we have considerable strengths and which already favor for a long time?
- Can the consumer really use our services, now and in the future?

These and other questions help bring realism to strategy formulation. Entertaining them may not be pleasant but their answers, if good ones, will assure that realism prevails.

Making Appropriate Use of People and the Culture

To effectively implement strategy, a nurse executive needs a strong core group of staff and an appreciation of the organizational culture. The core group needs to include staff in all relevant positions. It is important to involve a wide variety of staff. Maximum utilization of staff can be achieved when expectations are clearly established, when participation is rewarded, and when recommendations are acted upon to the greatest extent possible. The culture of a setting is expressed in the prevailing philosophies, ideologies and aspirations of the nursing staff collectively. It is important to understand how these forces affect any move toward change. Using the culture appropriately is facilitated by the following actions (Albert, 1983).

1. Constantly survey and evaluate the strong beliefs, policies, and ideologies in the organization and in the nursing department. Beneficial ones should be separated from detrimental ones.
2. Determine the extent of the impact of negative values and plan how they will be managed so that readiness for change is uncovered.
3. Learn the aspirations which drive the beliefs and values of staff. Values determine the readiness and capacity for change. Aspirations reflect the staff's identification with future direction. It is important to know the different values and aspirations and to act accordingly. If the people and the culture are

known and used appropriately, endorsement and commitment to the strategy will follow. This is all important to the success of a strategy.

Each of the nine challenges discussed here are important to acknowledge as strategy is formulated and as preparation is made to implement the phases of strategic management.

Phases of the Strategic Planning Process

The strategic planning process involves eight major phases, each with their own series of steps. Following these steps enables the administrator to help the nursing department develop its preferred future.

Phase I—Before the Beginning

1. Review the organization's mission, objectives, and goals
2. Review nursing's mission, objectives, and goals
3. Clarify underlying assumptions of nursing leadership
4. Confront history and values operating in the nursing department

Phase II—Prepare for Strategic Planning

1. Outline the planning cycle
2. Plan promotional activities to be used
3. Design the strategic planning organizational structure
4. Describe the processes involved

Phase III—Analyze Information

1. Assess environmental variables
2. Assess the difference between nursing's goals and those of the organization
3. Assess the nursing department's strengths and weaknesses
4. Identify the nursing department's history of success
5. Assess the values and expectations of consumers

Phase IV—Ends Planning

1. Develop and revise statement of mission for nursing department
2. Develop objectives and goals
3. Develop idealized design of desired future

Phase V—Means Planning

1. Develop organizational structure for strategic planning
   a. Clearly delineate all roles to be included
   b. Clearly define the function of each role
   c. Describe how the roles will interact
   d. Conduct in-service to familiarize participants with their roles
2. Initiate activities of strategic planning

a. Generate participation of relevant individuals in formulating strategy
b. Develop plan to implement strategy through participation
    1. Determine meeting times, places, agenda, participants
    2. Write statement and description of strategy
    3. Identify actions required for successful implementation
    4. Delineate relevant positions, their functions, and their interactions
    5. Conduct in-services to assure understanding of plan
c. Develop standards, policies, and procedures to support implementation
d. Determine resource requirements for implementation

Phase VI—Controls

1. Develop measurable outcomes and evaluation criteria
2. Design control mechanisms (both reports and administrative actions)

Phase VII—Complete Written Strategic Plan

Phase VIII—Implement Strategic Plan

Phase I—Before the Beginning

A major and often overlooked obstacle to a successful strategy is the lack of a detailed description of the natural history of the present situation. This is described very well in the work of Sarason (1979). Before initiating the planning for new strategy, it is advisable for the nursing leadership to convene for a period of time (usually a day) to clarify the history and underlying assumptions toward change. This is important because the way the leaders view change and a strategy for the future is much more important than their skill in formulating and implementing it (Ackoff, 1972b). The previous structures, processes, and assumptions used in the nursing department explain the context from which new strategy emerges. They provide evidence of the strengths on which new strategy can build and weaknesses for which it must compensate. Three key aspects of history that warrant discussion in the group are: (1) the scope of nursing services previously offered; (2) the model for delivery of those services; and (3) resources available in the past.

Phase II—Prepare for Strategic Planning

Effective preparation includes laying out a schedule of activities and designing the structure and processes that will support strategic planning. This preparation yields several benefits. One, it allows participants to see the whole process which can reduce anxiety and resistance. Two, it reinforces the idea that planning is a process rather than an end in itself. Three, it provides an opportunity to anticipate risks and to offset them. Table 4–1 is an example of a full year of activities.

    The organizational structure designed for strategic planning is separate from the operations, organizational structure. There are two reasons for this. One, by its very nature, strategic management does not lend itself to an hierarchical structure. To plan strategy, communication must flow in all directions throughout the nursing depart-

TABLE 4-1. EXAMPLE OF STRATEGIC PLANNING CYCLE

Month	Strategic Management Activity	Operations Management Activity
January	Initial planning meetings[a]	Ongoing operations
February	Information analysis	Ongoing operations
March	Ends planning	Ongoing operations
April	Formulation of strategy	Ongoing operations
May	Means planning	Ongoing operations
June	Develop strategic plan	Ongoing operations
July	Convert strategic plan to operations plan	Initiate operations budget
August		Plan operations budget
September		Approve operations budget
October	Evaluate and revise strategic plan	Initiate new operations budget
November	Implement strategy	Implement strategy
December	Manage adaptation of culture to strategy	Manage adaptation of culture to strategy

[a]In the first meeting, the values and expectations of nurse leaders are discussed and history is confronted.

ment. Two, the focus of strategic planning is on the future. If the existing structure is used, there is the risk that future planning will be sacrificed for present moment issues and crises. The creation of a separate structure does not prevent the use of nursing operations staff from all levels. After all, planning is best done *by* the individuals affected, not *for* them. Figures 4–3, through 4–6 illustrate organizational structures which facilitate strategic management. Smaller organizations may choose to do strategic planning (see modified structures).

The second activity in preparation for strategic planning is designing an appropriate organizational structure. A frequently asked question is whether a separate structure for strategic planning should be created or if existing committees and roles should be used. The best decision, especially in a large organization, is to create a separate structure and to assign specific strategy-oriented roles to existing operations staff. There are two reasons for this. First, by its very nature, strategic planning does not easily lend itself to the hierarchical organizational structure used for daily operations. That is, horizontal collaboration, which is more akin to a matrix structure, is required. Also, the focus of strategic planning is on the future rather than on present moment, day-to-day issues. If strategic planning is not placed in a separate structure, there is a risk that future planning will be sacrificed for day-to-day issues and crises. Although a separate structure is created, it is essential that planning is done by operations staff from all levels of nursing rather than by corporate planning staff.

The organizational structure for strategic planning can be thought of on two levels: macro and micro. The macro level addresses the way the total process is organized. The micro level addresses the way individuals and committees function within the total structure. It is important to appoint individuals and committees who will participate throughout the entire process and not on an ad hoc basis. This assures that strategic planning will be understood as an ongoing process.

The macro level strategic management planning structure should involve staff

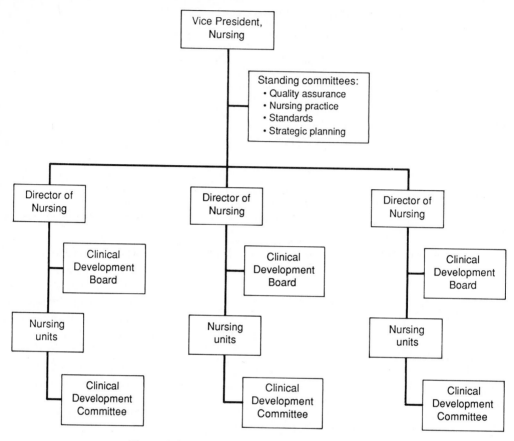

Figure 4-3. Macro Level of Strategic Management

from all levels of nursing. This involvement is manifested through appointments to the:

1. Nursing-wide strategic planning committee
2. Division level clinical development board
3. Unit level clinical development committee

The essential component of nursing's strategy is the strength of its internal competencies. Those competencies are continuously in the process of development, thus the name, clinical development, nursing-wide. At the nursing-wide level, strategy involves matching internal competencies with opportunities and threats in its environment. Each level committee is concerned with future direction. Each is interconnected and has overlapping membership. This creates a circular flow of information. In its entirety, this structure embodies important principles of interactive planning: participation, coordination and integration (Ackoff, 1972a).

The nursing-wide strategic planning committee is chaired by the nursing administrator and utilizes nursing staff membership as well as consultative input from con-

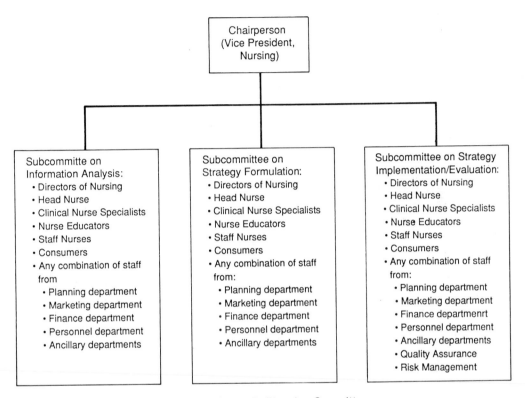

Figure 4-4. Strategic Planning Committee

sumers and other relevant departments, such as planning, marketing, finance, administration, personnel, ancillaries, and other. External staff involvement assures compatibility of the service level strategy with the overall organizational strategy. Consumer involvement assures compatibility with consumer demands. Participation from nursing staff increases acceptance of the strategic plan.

The charge of the strategic planning committee is to create the vision of future direction for the nursing department and to translate that vision into a realistic strategic plan. It performs this role through three subcommittees: information analysis, strategy formulation, and strategy implementation and evaluation. The information analysis subcommittee collects, analyzes, and interprets information about the environment and about nursing's unique competencies. Out of this arises an informed picture of challenges and capabilities. Information useful for this committee includes:

1. New providers and their impact on market share
2. New programs or services offered by competitors
3. Price changes by competitors

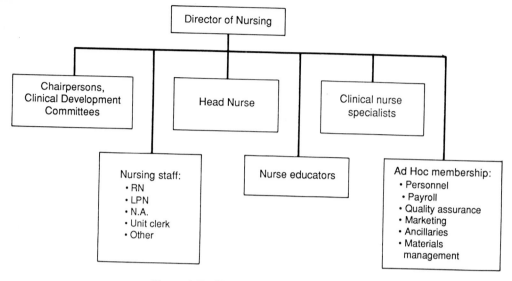

Figure 4-5. Clinical Development Boards

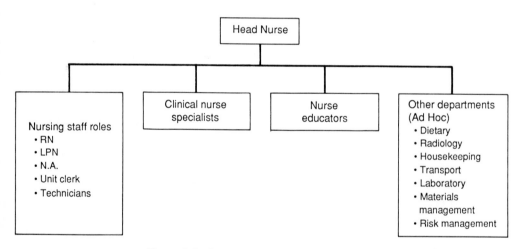

Figure 4-6. Clinical Development Committees

4. Reimbursement changes
5. Changes in payor mix
6. Changes in number and type of physicians, patients, payors
7. Changes in organizational strategy
8. Changes in regulations and laws
9. Bargaining power of consumers
10. Level of rivalry among competitors

11. Unique nursing programs, products, or services
12. Consumer satisfaction surveys
13. Cost of care
14. Human and other resource availability

The strategy formulation subcommittee takes the picture developed through information analysis and integrates it with the organization's strategic plan to create a service level strategy. They also develop the criteria for judging success of the strategy. The strategy implementation subcommittee develops a detailed work plan including resources required, programs, projects, standards, policies and procedures to support the strategy. They oversee the change process and evaluate the progress of the strategy.

Clinical development boards are established for each nursing division or for the most relevant cluster of nursing units that serve consumers with similar needs. These boards may access expertise from other departments or consumers at any point in their planning process. They consist of members from nursing administration, clinical nursing and nursing education. A clinical director of nursing (or mid-level manager) chairs this board. The board chair, as well as a select group of the board's members, also sit on the nursing-wide strategic planning committee. Each board's charge is to establish future objectives and goals, consistent with the overall direction of the nursing department. Its members transmit ideas to the nursing-wide strategic planning committee and participate in its activities.

The clinical development committee for each nursing unit performs the role of setting the direction for each unit, consistent with the division's direction. The members meet to discuss strengths of their patient care delivery methods, the quality of work life, and suggestions for new programs and emerging needs of consumers. Decisions which affect only one unit can be implemented without delay. Decisions which have the potential for affecting more than one unit are referred to the clinical development board for final decision. The same sequence of concurrence and approval occurs between division boards and the nursing-wide planning committee.

Phase III—Analyze Information

The most critical challenge facing the nurse executive in strategic management is to recognize important environmental developments and trends. The problem is usually not the trends themselves but the failure to recognize them and their potential impact on operations. This can be prevented if appropriate information is collected and analyzed.

Important factors to uncover about trends are why they exist, how they evolved, the degree of change the trends bring, the interrelationship among trends, and the trends that are most influential upon the nursing department. (See Figure 4–1 for areas of the environment that should be investigated for trends outside the organization.) Inside the organization, the focus of the analysis may be on such areas as employee attitudes, changes in leadership and availability of technology.

Factors in the nursing department itself that are important to understand include the variety and number of nursing services offered, the quality of care, and the image of nursing innovations. These factors should be viewed through the patient's eyes.

They determine both the relevance of services and the success of a strategy. To effectively plan strategy, all of these factors must be understood through rigorous information analysis.

Phase IV—Ends Planning

A strategy can be meaningful only if it fits with the framework of the nursing department's vision of a desired future. That vision is illustrated by the ends pursued. These are three levels of ends: mission, objectives, and goals, in decreasing order. Mission is a concise statement of who and what the nursing department aspires to be. An example is:

> The Universal Hospital Department of Nursing exists to improve the quality of life of citizens by offering a variety of health and illness-related services. The consumers toward whom efforts are directed are patients/families, physicians, the hospital and nurses themselves. We are committed to providing services that are free of error and outstanding in the value they add to the lives of consumers. We seek to be the single, most frequently accessed source of nursing services in this region.

The second level of ends are objectives. Objectives are slightly less abstract than the mission statement. The third level of ends are goals. The major difference between objectives and goals is the level of specificity and time relatedness of goals. That is, goals reflect measurable outcomes that can be achieved in a known time period. Criteria for selecting objectives and goals are:

1. Compatibility with mission
2. Specifically stated
3. Suggestive of the strategy
4. Representative of a balance between strengths and weaknesses in the nursing department
5. Cognizant of the threats and opportunities in the environment

The example below illustrates how objectives and goals may be stated.

- Objective: To enhance nurse retention through improved nurse:patient ratio
- Goal: To maintain the prescribed nurse:patient ratio for at least ninety percent (90%) of the nursing staff for the 180-day period, beginning January 1 and ending June 30.

Phase V—Means Planning

There are five generic strategies that nursing can follow in formulating its strategy:

1. Differentiation of services. The most feasible way to do this is to refine many of nursing's activities into specialty products that are delivered to consumers as complete packages. Some examples of specialty nursing products are a nursery hotline for parents, a hospital adaptation service to help patients and families adapt to the hospital, or a self-care lifestyling service to help con-

sumer's modify their lifestyle. The value of such differentiation of services is that it distinguishes a nursing department from its competitors.

2. Favorable cost structure. This is achieved through alterations in the amount or expense of resources for the delivery of services. The idea is to offer superior services at a lower cost than the competition.
3. Innovation. Nursing can excel in innovation by introducing models of service delivery that fundamentally change the way services are delivered.
4. Growth. Nursing can offer such excellent care and service that the volume of patients increases dramatically, thereby increasing the organization's market share. Since there is conceivably one market, this means that the organization would attract market share away from competitors.
5. Joint Venture. Nursing can create an alliance with other providers that leads to a competitive advantage or preeminence in the marketplace.

Let us suppose that the strategy selected is high differentiation and low cost. An example of a program to implement this strategy might be value-added nursing products. Projects consistent with this program might be a clinical development center, a client hotline, or self-care lifestyling.

The supporting structure for strategies consists of programs, projects, standards of care, policies and procedures. Programs are action plans which can be implemented through small projects. Standards, policies and procedures are specific types of guidelines that spell out how the strategy is to be implemented.

There are both professional and regulatory standards that must be considered when formulating strategy. Familiar examples are those enforced by the Joint Commission on Accreditation of Healthcare Organizations or by Medicare. Standards create legal obligations to perform; therefore, no strategy should be formulated that violates required standards.

Formulating and implementing strategy is both an art and a science. The art is in assembling the right people and resources to implement the strategy. These "right" people are those who believe in the strategy and have the appropriate values and skills. The "right" resources are workable new models of nursing practice and new rules of operation. The science is in acquiring appropriate information and using it properly.

Resource requirements for implementing a strategy should be considered at the time that the strategy is formulated. No matter how well-designed the strategy is, it cannot survive a serious lack of resources. It is advisable to fully cost out the total resource requirements for the entire term of the strategy, taking into consideration inflation and changes in personnel costs. If the financial expertise for this is not in nursing, the cost accountant or a staff member from financial planning usually will be willing to provide these services. The resources to be considered are human resources, technology, facilities, supplies, equipment, purchased services, and leases. The most feasible way to describe the resource requirements is by preparing a budget for each applicable fiscal year. Resource deficits should be avoided because this raises hopes of staff and subsequently lowers them, creating disappointment and loss of hope and trust. One of the most valuable resources often overlooked is time. Time estimates should be developed for each activity.

When various processes and structures have been described as supports to the structure, they often remain inactive until actual responsibilities are assigned. Many strategies fail for lack of momentum, once initiated. Therefore, particular attention should be paid to sequentially bringing all task forces and new staff to fill new roles and implement new programs and projects on line once the strategy and the resources for it have been approved.

Phase VI—Controls

Prior to implementation of the strategy, the nurse executive and the implementation team will need to assure that all aspects of the planning have been completed and that all matters related to the success of the strategy have been considered. A general checklist and measurable outcomes are useful to keep the work on schedule and to ensure success.

General Checklist

1. The strategy is appropriate and credible.
   a. It is focused on the right consumer and it targets the right changes in the organization.
   b. It has substance as well as form.
   c. The reorganization can realistically execute it.
   d. There are adequate types and numbers of resources available to execute the strategy.
2. Nursing operations is prepared to execute the strategy.
   a. The nursing care process is organized.
   b. The nursing care process is efficient.
   c. There is internal capability to continuously refine the strategy as deviations occur.
   d. There are sufficient, required elements of the operations in place including:
      • Leadership
      • Core management group competence
      • Information systems
      • Direct care staff
   e. A sufficient information system is in place to support operations and management.
   f. Human resource planing has been linked to the strategic plan.
   g. An appropriate organizational structure has been developed and roles are properly delineated.
   h. The processes necessary to coordinate and integrate patient care are in place and working well.
   i. Adequate relevant educational programs are in place for patients and staff, and others (eg stakeholders) affected by proposed changes.
3. The culture of nursing and the organization endorses the strategy.
4. A workable incentive plan is in place to reward implementation of the strategy.
5. A positive relationship exists between nursing and its stakeholders (physicians,

other intra-organizational departments, relevant organizations, patients and families).
6. Nursing's image is strong enough to support credibility of the strategy.
7. Scenarios of possible internal and external constraints have been anticipated and responsive actions developed.
8. The sequence of required activities for the strategy is accompanied by an implementation and control plan which specifies:
   a. Nature of the task to be carried out
   b. Relevant goal or objective
   c. Who is responsible for carrying it out
   d. Steps to be taken
   e. Who is responsible for each step
   f. Timing of each step
   g. Money allocated to each step, if any
   h. Critical assumptions on which the schedule is based
   i. Expected performance and when it is expected
   j. Assumptions on which the expectation is based
9. The strategy has been approved by appropriate officials
10. Morale and job satisfaction of staff have been checked out and repaired, if indicated

Measurable Outcomes. Specific outcome measures are determined prior to implementation. Results then can be used to demonstrate success of the strategy such as:

1. Value-added quality of care targets
   a. Increased patient/family knowledge, physician knowledge, other stakeholder knowledge
   b. Increased nursing products that satisfy consumer wants
   c. Increased intensity of patient contact which exceeds requirements
   d. Increased number of points of consumer contact by nursing
   e. Increased number of relevant employee skills
2. Error rate targets
   a. Decreased infections from previous level
   b. Decreased medication errors from previous level
   c. Decreased falls and other accidents from previous level
   d. Decrease in other sentinel events from previous level
3. Client volume targets
   a. Increased number of patient and physician visits
   b. Increased referrals from clients or physicians
4. Human resource targets
   a. Decreased turnover rate
   b. Decreased vacancy rate
   c. Decreased absenteeism
5. Value-added financial targets
   a. Revenues minus expenses, divided by number of employees, shows improved trend

   b. Positive trend in full-time equivalents per adjusted occurrence of patient contact
   c. Decrease in cost per unit of service
   d. Increase in profits resulting from new programs or new ideas
6. Market share indicators
   a. Targeted increase in market share
   b. Improved patient satisfaction

Simple, relevant, usable information systems can be created to reflect each of these parameters at appropriate intervals. It is preferable to create a logical order in the results reporting and to report as many parameters as possible on one form. The data processing department or management engineering can help design report forms. Any nursing department individual who is proficient with electronic spread sheets and graphics software can report results graphically, which is an invaluable asset when communicating outcomes.

Phase VII—Complete Written Strategic Plan
Each of the previous six phases culminates in the development of a written strategic plan. An outline is presented below.

Contents of the Strategic Plan
1. Executive summary
   a. Salient points
   b. Recommendations in capsule
2. Background
   a. Brief history of where nursing department has been
   b. Assumptions of the past
   c. Description of nursing department
      1. Size and scope of services
      2. Types of services offered
3. Environment
   a. Political and regulatory developments
   b. Social forces
   c. Economic trends
   d. Changing technology
   e. Competitor behavior
   f. Marketplace
   g. Demographic trends
   h. Employment trends
   i. Results of recent market surveys
   j. Factors in the containing organization
   k. Industry trends
4. General appraisal
   a. Context of the background and environment
   b. Projections for the future

    c. Emphasis on key questions that form basis for the strategy and plan of action

    d. Departmental strengths and weaknesses

    e. Requirements and history of success

5. Mission, objectives, and goals
6. Strategy
    a. General assumptions
    b. Options for addressing significant consumer needs
    c. Statement of selected options, with rationale
7. Programs and projects relevant to the strategy
8. Forecast
    a. Outcomes expected from the programs and projects
    b. Volume of patients served
    c. Expected revenue
9. Functional plans
    a. Personnel
    b. Finance
    c. Education
    d. Marketing
10. Resource requirements
    a. Cost of functional plans
    b. Cost of programs and projects
    c. Total combined resource required
    d. Scarce resources
    e. Human resources required
11. Financial analysis
    a. Income statement
    b. Balance sheet
12. Realism
    a. Test assumptions for realism
    b. Known uncertainties
13. Recommendations

Phase VIII—Implement Strategic Plan

Implementing strategy is a process of creating and managing large-scale organizational change. By its very nature, implementation creates change by revaluation rather than by evaluation. For this reason, the process requires extraordinary skill in anticipating and responding effectively to unanticipated events. The central point of strategic management is to minimize the element of surprise. It is important, therefore, to implement strategy in a way that is consistent with the goals of keeping surprise to a minimum.

    The important prerequisites for effective implementation are:

1. Gain nursing executive committee approval of strategic plan.
2. Translate strategic plan into operations plan and budget.

3. Include resource requirements for operations plan in annual operations and capital budget planning.
4. Gain approval of nursing operations budget and capital budget.
5. Allocate resources for operations plan.
6. Adapt operations plan to level of resources allocation.
7. Communicate operations plan throughout the nursing department and containing organization.
8. Modify the following as indicated:
    a. Mission, objectives, goals
    b. Policies and procedures
    c. Standards of care
    d. Educational offerings for all levels of staff
    e. Budgeting system
    f. Productivity monitoring programs
    g. Staffing standards, strength, mix
    h. Position control
    i. Efficiency report
    j. Risk management program
    k. Cost containment program
    l. Wage/benefits package
    m. Consumer relations program
    n. Technology assessment and acquisition
    o. Level and type of technology
    p. Type and/or availability of support services
    q. Revenue operating program
    r. Recruitment/retention programs
    s. Marketing program
    t. Organizational structure
    u. Role descriptions
    v. Patient flow
    w. Work methods
    x. Personnel policies
    y. Performance appraisal system
    z. Incentive/reward system
        (1) Model of nursing care
        (2) Image enhancement program
        (3) Codes of conduct
        (4) Quality assurance program
        (5) JCAHO/regulatory compliance
        (6) Information systems
        (7) Staff development (clinical, educational, management/leadership strategic thinking)
        (8) Interdepartmental procedures
        (9) Communication networks
        (10) Incentive/reward systems

        (11) Strategic planning system
        (12) Disciplinary procedures
        (13) Safety of nursing practice environment
        (14) Team building

9. Develop a schedule of implementation activities.
   a. Define the activity
   b. Make individual assignments
   c. Establish target dates
   d. Include an orientation program for key participants
   e. Conduct promotion activities
10. Generate consensus on schedule of implementation activities at all levels of nursing and with key stakeholders through a series of meetings.
11. Publish a finalized schedule of implementation activities throughout nursing and the containing organization.
12. Finalize evaluation control and incentive mechanisms.
13. Hold orientation sessions on evaluation, control mechanisms and implementation activities
14. Begin implementation of strategy.
15. Operationalize the strategy.
16. Elicit feedback and evaluate response by the culture.
17. Initiate internal consultation to reinforce implementation.
18. Initiate evaluation and control mechanisms.
19. Communicate interim results throughout the nursing department and the containing organization on an on-going basis.
20. Utilize feedback on results to:
    a. Determine success of strategy
    b. Make adjustments in:
       (1) Strategy
       (2) Timing of implementation
       (3) Resources
       (4) Evaluation and control mechanisms
       (5) Operating procedures
       (6) Information systems
       (7) Policies, programs
    c. Influence the culture
    d. Plan for the future
21. Reward high performers in accordance with incentive program.

The most successful implementation of strategy is accompanied by an effective combination of leadership, culture, organization, people, communication, and reward systems (Ackoff, 1972c). The leadership required to implement strategy begins with the top nurse executive and extends throughout nursing management. There is *no* substitute for the personal involvement of the nursing leadership. This personal involvement extends to letting the force of their personalities and commitment energize the organization. The leader must have strong interpersonal skills that can resolve conflicts and ease tensions as the discomforts of change arise. The leader must personify the nursing department's mission. Finally, the leader must be charismatic enough to inspire people, motivate them, and generate commitment.

The culture of the organization can either be a facilitator or inhibitor of effective implementation of strategy. It consists of the values and aspirations of the organizational members as a collective group. Not only is the culture within nursing important but the culture within the containing organization also is important. It is essential that the implementation plan take into consideration the prevailing philosophy, values, and aspirations. As was earlier stated, values are different from aspirations. Values point out the readiness of the group for change. Aspirations reflect the group's alignment with the strategic direction being taken. If these are not known, difficulties can be encountered during implementation, such as undue resistance, sabotage, or a compromise of overall results achieved. When culture is viewed as the security blanket that maintains stability of activities, those who are implementing strategy will be able to be sensitive to the human tendency to want to maintain the status quo while steering the group toward new vistas.

The structure and the decision flow process of the organization is important to strategy implementation. In order to achieve the outcomes desired, the organizational structure often must be altered. The effective organizational structure identifies the correct roles and appropriate individuals to occupy those roles. Also, the roles must relate to each other properly. Since decision making is the principal output of management, the decision-flow process also must be worked out beforehand. Often sound decisions can fail to get the proper action for lack of communication of them.

Those who are accountable for implementation of the strategy are essential to its success. They must be well informed about the who, what, when, where, how, and why of the strategy implementation. The most well-formulated strategy can go off course during implementation if those who are to implement it do not understand the spirit as well as the mechanics of it. To assure this, the strategic plan is translated into an operations plan and each section should have an action plan. The development of written plans is to be emphasized because of the obvious fallacies of word-of-mouth communications. To achieve the outcomes desired, people at all levels of the organization must be motivated and must have the ability to carry out its mechanics and to manage the change process. Therefore, the focus should be on recruiting and developing competent people and on the performance of individuals as well as work groups. People are the primary medium for successfully implementating strategy and achieving desired results.

Communication is one of the most powerful tools for assuring success in the implementation of strategy. It can be used to gain the understanding and support by stakeholders. It can be used to shape the culture in the desired direction. It can be used to resolve conflicts. Communication should move in all directions *to* staff responsible for implementation and *from* them. Information systems should be designed to reflect progress toward achieving goals. These information systems should not only be well-developed but they should be communicated effectively in order to publicize results.

Reward systems are one mechanism for mobilizing individuals toward successfully implementing a strategy. There needs to be very clear definition of the system of rewards and they should be attached to performance. The rewards may be financial and nonfinancial, including pay for performance, promotions, opportunities for career development, recognition, autonomy, and for greater involvement in decision making. The means of involving individuals should be designed so that the affected individuals can feel that their actions will directly affect the achievement of the desired goals. The basis of the reward system should be mutual goal setting by the managers and their direct reports and an objective performance should precede the distribution of rewards and should be directly related to specific goals. Finally, rewards should be commensurate with the level of contribution to the success of the strategy.

In addition to selecting, motivating, and rewarding a core group of managers, the nurse executive will want to take advantage of opportunities to involve a wide variety of staff in implementing the strategy. Such involvement can shorten the time required for implementation if the new direction is fully embraced. When committees are formed, it is important to manage them well by attending to fundamental decisions such as membership, breadth of representation, their charge, and the manner in which recommendations will be processed, once received by the nurse executive.

In an overall sense, implementating the strategy is an exciting opportunity to use the maximum creativity in managing the change process. A vision is set. The leadership works through the culture, the organization, the people, and the systems to impose change on an existing operation. Because of the powerful forces of resistance to change and the distractions involved in daily operations, those who implement change must utilize significant expertise in continuous goal setting, in performance and outcome measurement, and in gaining the cooperation of others. In the end, it is not sufficient to have people who *can* implement the strategy, it is necessary to have people who *want* to implement the strategy (Morse & Martin 1983).

SUMMARY

Strategic management is presented here as one of the three major responsibilities of a nurse executive. Operations, culture, and strategy must be of equal importance in the activities of the nurse executive. Representative guidelines, structures, and tools are suggested for use in strategic management. None of these tools is as important as the way individuals in the nursing department think about formulating and implementing a sound strategy for the future. That is, strategic thinking is more important than strategic techniques. What is needed is a way of thinking about the future of a nursing department which leads to a sound strategy for the future. That strategy emerges from a proper matching of the environmental forces, of consumer wants and of the unique competencies within the department. Strategic management presents equal challenges of managing operations and the culture. Ultimately, strategic management is a process that enables a nursing department to perform excellently in a strategically important area and thus achieve superiority in the market place.

REFERENCES

Ackoff RL. *A Concept of Corporate Planning,* New York: John Wiley & Sons, 1972a, 52–65

Ackoff RL. *Creating the Corporate Future,* New York: John Wiley & Sons, 1972b, 65–74

Ackoff RL. *Redesigning the Future,* New York: John Wiley & Sons, 1972c, 8

Albert KJ. *The Strategic Management Handbook,* New York: McGraw-Hill Book Company, 1983

Ansoff I. *Implanting Strategic Management,* Englewood Cliffs, NJ, Prentice/Hall, 1984

Drucker P. *Management: Tasks, Responsibilities, Practices.* New York: Harper & Row Publishers, 1974, 125

Fahey L. *The Strategic Planning Reader,* Englewood Cliffs, NJ, Prentice Hall, 1989

Morse EW, Martin KG. *Motivating the organization to implement change.* In: Albert KJ, *The Strategic Management Handbook.* New York, McGraw Hill Book Company, 1983, 171

Sarason SB. *The Creation of Settings and the Future Societies,* San Francisco, Jossey Bass, Inc, 1979

CHAPTER 5

Organizational Culture: Analysis of the Concept

Marjorie V. Batey*

ORGANIZATIONAL CULTURE

A central function of nursing administration is to develop and maintain environments that enable clinical nursing to be practiced professionally. Practitioners and students of nursing administration are challenged to understand theoretical perspectives by which health care organizations can be analyzed and to consider the implications of those perspectives for enabling or deterring nursing administration's central function. Previous chapters present selected theories and theoretical perspectives of complex organizations with particular emphasis on health care and nursing administration. The study of culture provides an additional perspective for organizational analysis (Bolman & Deal, 1984).

Organizational culture, with its roots in the perspectives of anthropology and

*The author wishes to acknowledge Noel J. Chrisman, Ph.D., for his participation in dialogues toward the clarification of culture in the context of organizations.

sociology, is rich in diverse meanings that can enhance an administrator's under-standing of the workplaces of nurses. The initial task of this chapter is to group those diverse perspectives of organizational culture according to two contrasting themes prevalent in current literature in order to elaborate on differences in meanings attrib-uted to the concept and to illustrate approaches to their study. Next, integration ver-sus differentiation of culture of an organization is examined. The former denotes a high level of internal consistency and consensus of culture throughout an organiza-tion suggesting that the organization is a single culture. The latter, in contrast, recog-nizes that inconsistency and limited consensus may exist between and among differ-ent organizational subunits, suggesting that multiple subcultures exist within the same organization (Martin & Meyerson, 1988; Young, 1989). The final task in the chapter is to address selected administrative problems—change, innovation, problem solving—from the viewpoints presented about organizational culture.

ANALYSIS OF THE CONCEPT

As a concept derived from anthropology and sociology, culture is a force that exists in all human groups that possess a history of interaction. The premise of culture is that people who share a past, who interact with relative frequency and who share a destiny, develop a system of beliefs that underlies their continuing interactions. Cul-ture is the basis for present behavior and contributes to continuity toward the future. In the words of Kluckhohn and Kelly (1945), ''culture is an historically created system of explicit and implicit designs for living, which tends to be shared by all or specially designated members of a group at a specified point in time'' page 66.

Over the past decade there has been a proliferation of literature in the organiza-tional sciences in which culture, previously used for societal analysis, has been exam-ined within and across organizations (Deal & Kennedy, 1982; Louis, 1985; Morgan, 1986; Pettigrew, 1979, Saffold, 1988; Sathe, 1983; Schein, 1985; Schein, 1990; Smircich & Calas, 1987; Wilkins & Ouchi, 1983). More recently organizational culture has be-gun to appear in the nursing literature (del Bueno & Vincent, 1986; Fine, 1989; John-son, 1987; Ray, 1989; Van Ess Coeling & Wilcox, 1988). While there is consensus that culture is a viable concept for understanding organizations, there are many different viewpoints on such questions as what it is, how it is manifested, its functions, how it might be studied, and in what ways its understanding may serve administrative practitioners and scholars in complex organizations. Answers to these questions are influenced by the disciplinary and theoretical perspective from which each author has derived his or her orientation to the concept.

One perspective is not necessarily more useful or valid than another. Rather, heightened awareness that the theoretical perspective underlying usage of a concept impacts the way one interprets situations and, concurrently, closes off alternative interpretations. Theories in use give shape to one's reality by directing what, within a situation, will be heeded or ignored (Bolman & Deal, 1984). Furthermore, when an applied discipline, such as nursing administration, borrows a concept that has its roots in other disciplines, the borrower needs to consider the full perspective and its underlying assumptions about the concept in the original field. Failure to do so can contribute to distorted interpretations (Meek, 1988; Martin & Meyerson, 1988).

LINKING ORGANIZATIONAL CULTURE

The study of organizational culture requires the linkage of two distinctly different concepts, those of organization and of culture. Historically, culture has been a concept central to the study of total societies (eg, clans or tribes that were remote from contacts with other societies) for purposes of understanding their patterns of human relationships. By attending to overt manifestations of relations as shown by uses of behavior, language, stories and myths, rituals, symbols and artifacts, an observer could discern directly the consistencies or regularities that comprise the society's explicit culture.

At the covert level, however, is a society's implicit culture that is not discernable through direct sight or hearing. Instead, the patterning of its content meanings is derived from the regularities depicted through the explicit culture. This level of culture comprises the underlying beliefs, values, and assumptions of a people that are largely out of awareness, that are taken for granted by the culture members, and yet which direct their "design for living" (Kluckhohn & Kelly, 1945; Bate, 1984). Beliefs, values and assumptions are shared by the culture members and are based on past learned ways of approaching problems of living. This implicit culture "frees individuals from having to make deliberate choices from among hosts of possibilities" (Thompson, 1967, p 102). Implicit culture is transmitted to new members through a process of socialization (Bate, 1984; Schein, 1985, 1990).

When culture is studied in a remote society in which the boundaries of the society are relatively fixed and interaction outside those boundaries is limited at most, the extent to which beliefs, values, and assumptions are shared, is not a central concern. Rather attention is paid to patterns across all human experiences—work, play, family—of the society's members. When the unit of analysis has boundaries that are continuously permeable, the probability of the unit having different subcultures, that is, less integration and greater differentiation, increases. This also is true for contemporary open societies, such as nations, or for subunits of those societies, such as organizations.

The second concept, organization, is the means used in contemporary society for uniting individuals and groups for collective action on some relatively circumscribed concern of the larger society. Attention in this chapter is on work organizations involved in some aspect of health care services (eg, hospitals, community health agencies, home health facilities). Continuing members of such organizations are its employees who fulfill the work segment of their lives in the organization but who leave the organization for other aspects of their lives. Outside the organization, members may or may not engage in interactions with one another but indeed do engage in interactions with persons (family, friends) who are not continuing members of the same organization. Furthermore, continuing members of an organization are drawn from different segments of the larger society, such as different social strata, occupations, and educational experiences. Within the work organization, interaction among members ranges from highly intense and continuing, eg, among nurses in an intensive care unit) to no contacts at all (eg, between ICU staff and outpatient rehabilitation unit staff). These variations heighten the potential for development of subcultures within an organization resulting in differences in the degree of integration and differentiation among the different parts of an organization.

THEMES IN ORGANIZATIONAL CULTURE

The rise of interest in the study of organizational culture, as reflected by the rapidly growing body of literature on the topic, seems to stem from at least three different forces. While it is beyond the scope of this chapter to examine those forces in detail, citing them places the themes in context.

First is the continuing search by organizational scientists for concepts to enhance both *understanding and explanation of organizations.* Study of organizational literature reveals a tendency to embrace each newly proposed explanation of organizational behavior only to reject it for a subsequent and seemingly more complete explanation. Such a tendency is noted throughout time beginning with scientific management, moving to systems analysis and structure and, more recently, embracing strategic management (Schein, 1990; Smircich & Calas, 1987). Is organizational culture but yet another succession of theoretical constructs? The promise held for this construct is in its potential for depicting ''variations in patterns of organizational behavior . . . (and for explaining) levels of stability in group and organizational behavior'' (Schein, 1990, p 110).

A second force underlying the organizational culture literature has arisen from the *changing external environments of organizations,* particularly in reference to national and global economic constraints (Turner, 1986) and a changing work ethic (Cummings & Srivastva, 1977; Harris, 1985). It is suggested that some organizations are more effective than others in dealing with these external environmental conditions and that their effectiveness is rooted in their internal culture (Deal & Kennedy, 1982; Ouchi, 1981; Peters & Waterman, 1982). Study, through comparative analysis, is directed toward identifying what effective organizations hold in common and how they differ from those less effective. The study of the exemplary magnet hospitals illustrates this comparative approach in the nursing literature (McClure, Poulin, Sovie & Wandelt, 1983).

Finally, in recent years there has been some shifting in research paradigms used to study phenomena of interest in the social sciences and in nursing. While survey and analytic research of the more positivist tradition continues very much in evidence, there now is a greater appreciation than in the past for the validity of social inquiry from an interpretive frame of reference such as ethnoscience or social interactionism (Turner, 1986; Schein, 1990; Smircich & Calas, 1987). Organizational culture studies using one or the other of these paradigms are based on different assumptions and, thus, can be expected to yield different findings. For example, researchers using a survey with structured questions, assumes that the questions reflect salient aspects of the concept, and, thus, that the concepts measured can be quantified within or across organizations. The interpretive paradigm, by contrast, assumes that an expanded understanding of culture is needed. Thereby, its methods call for descriptions of daily life experiences of the organizational members from their perspectives and as enacted by them. Of course, combinations of these contrasting paradigms can yield highly insightful results.

CULTURE OF AN ORGANIZATION

The two broad themes into which the organizational culture literature can be classified have been driven in part by differing assumptions that underlie theoretical perspectives about the concepts. One theme is that culture is a property or variable of an organization. As a variable, culture contributes to the explanation of problems addressed through organizational analysis. Therefore, culture can be managed, controlled, and manipulated in such ways as to vary the degree of organizational effectiveness along a range of criteria, including change and innovation, performance and productivity, creating commitment to the organization and recruitment and selection of personnel (Harris, 1985; Louis, 1983, 1985; Siehl, 1985. Trice & Beyer, 1984; Schall, 1983; Wilkens & Dyer, 1988; Harris, 1985; Pettigrew, 1979; Wiener, 1988).

Assumptions underlying the theme of culture as property of an organization follow closely with the biological and mechanistic metaphors of organizations in the functionalist and the structural functionalist perspectives of anthropology and sociology. This literature includes comparative management across different organizations in which culture is treated as a variable external to the organization and corporate culture is treated as a variable internal to the organization (Meek, 1988, Smircich & Calas, 1987).

As an internal variable, corporate culture is both a product and a property of an organization. Products are produced through particular designs of interaction in an organization such as rituals, legends, and ceremonies that serve as means to achieve shared values and beliefs among the organizational members (Smircich, 1983).

The sparse organizational culture literature in nursing is based mainly on the theme of culture as a property or variable of an organization. One example of comparative analysis is a survey study of the effect of shared values on job satisfaction and perceived productivity in nurses (Kramer & Hafner, 1989) in which the investigators found no relationship. Such results are consistent with Schein's (1990) view that work culture may be too abstract a concept to be measured by survey techniques, at least with our current state of knowledge about it. (Note: Kramer and Hafner used the term ''shared values,'' not culture, in their study; perhaps rather than culture, they were intending to study organizational climate, a more visible manifestation of an organization's environment.)

Other nursing literature has drawn selectively from the corporate culture perspective to illustrate how administration might bring about a desired change through alterations of specific intraorganizational variables thought to represent culture. Johnson (1987), for example, implied that the development and use of self governance through participative management in a nursing department would correct an "unhealthy culture." Perhaps that is so, but caution must be taken in interpretation. Successful transition from a traditional hierarchical organization with centralized decision making to a more egalitarian one entails considerable shifting of interlocking assumptions (implicit culture) throughout the organization.

The corporate culture literature has received considerable criticism suggesting that it conveys a management bias (Meek, 1988; Young, 1989) and, through its emphasis on manipulation and control of culture, that it will be no more effective for understanding organizations than was the earlier human relations approach to management. Turner (1986) criticized management by describing an "honest grappler" and a "pop culture magician." The former is the scientist who recognizes that there is a cultural dimension to organizations and is grappling with the complexities of studying and describing it. The "pop culture magicians," he asserted, draw only selectively from the culture literature and offer quick ways to diagnose and transform the culture through manipulation of its explicit representations such as symbols, myths, and artifacts.

These comments convey caution to administrators who are searching for management tools. Indeed, the more obvious, explicit manifestations of culture may encourage selected change in the short term; however, the implicit elements of culture—the engrained beliefs and assumptions—are relatively enduring. While these are capable of being changed over time, they are not amenable to manipulation and control and they are not subject to change in the short term.

ORGANIZATION AS CULTURE

The second theme of the organizational culture literature considers organizations as culture (Bolman & Deal, 1984; Morgan, 1986). Culture of an organization is its "expressive, ideational and symbolic processes" (Smircich & Calas, 1987, p 233). It is the socially constructed realities of the organizational members. Meanings, symbols, cognitions, and beliefs are constructed by the members and attributed by them. In turn they come to be learned (assimilated) by new members through continuing experiences as work life unfolds. Thus, the analyst of organizational culture asks "how individuals interpret and understand their experience and how these interpretations and understandings relate to action" (Smircich, 1983). These interpretations and understandings, thereby, are viewed as mobilizers of ways organizational members behave and interact within their primary work groups and across work groups.

Meanings are not necessarily shared by all members of the organization but rather different understandings and interpretations can exist across groups within an organization. Thus, study of culture in this perspective is not directed primarily or solely to the organizational leaders; instead, it seeks to account for and to understand diversity of cultural meanings across broad spectrums of organizational members. This perspective focuses on *understanding* (as contrasted to explanation) organizational culture through analysis of the symbolic processes enacted (Turner, 1986). It is based on the interpretive orientations of ethnoscience, phenomenology, and social interactionism as these are developed in sociology and anthropology and, to an increasing extent, in communication theory.

ORGANIZATIONAL PRACTICES, ARTIFACTS, AND CONTENT THEMES

Studies of organizational culture include one or more of three classes of data: *organizational practices, artifacts,* and *content themes.* Practices and artifacts represent explicit culture; content themes tend to overlap both implicit and explicit culture.

Organizational practices can be either formal or informal. Formal practices describe dimensions of organizational structure, including policies and activities occurring within organizations that prescribe or restrict behavior of organizational members (Dalton et al, 1980). These include organizational charts which depict how members are arranged in hierarchy and status, job descriptions, and policy and content of performance appraisal which depict expectations of members, and criteria for retention, promotion, pay and other resource distributions among members (Martin & Meyerson, 1988). Caution must be taken not to infer that culture and structure are necessarily the same thing (Meek, 1988). However, formal practices usually are components of structure that are guided by implicit assumptions about the nature of people and of work. Thus, examination of those practices can contribute to understanding the culture of an organization (Martin & Meyerson, 1988). Informal practices include means used by organizational members for acquiring access to resources not formally available, personal exercise of power such as informal opinion leaders, and communication norms or other non formalized expressions for "how we do things around here."

Artifacts is a general term that subsumes a range of verbal and physical symbols. These include stories and myths that convey "how we got to be who and what we are," rituals and ceremonies used for various symbolic purposes (eg, annual holiday lunch for nursing department), verbal or visual forms of humor (eg, cartoons on conference room bulletin board), and special language that sets boundaries between members (as pronoun usage of we and they) or that distinguishes members from nonmembers (eg, use of technical language or jargon among members which has little to no meaning to nonmembers).

Content themes are direct expressions by organizational members of what members say (espouse) are their beliefs, values, and assumptions, as well as inferences about beliefs, values, and assumptions drawn from interpreting practices, artifacts and members' direct expressions (Martin & Meyerson, 1988). When drawing content themes from what members express, both Schein (1985) and Martin and Meyerson (1988) emphasize the importance of distinguishing between that which is only espoused, and that which is actually used (Argyris & Schon, 1978). Espoused values and beliefs might be expressed only for some external public or may depict a desired condition yet bear little relation to what actually occurs in the organization. Schein's (1985) analysis of levels of culture placed values and beliefs at a higher level of awareness than assumptions. Assumptions, by contrast, are the most deeply ingrained aspects of culture, the least readily changed, and the essentially taken for granted views of how things are. Bate (1984) referred to this content as internalized social constructs, suggesting that they are deeply ingrained and not available for direct observation or to be readily changed and that their content is built and learned through interactions of group members.

A second example of content themes is the time dimension which illustrates variability across groups. What is the time sense within and between work groups? Is it oriented to the past (we've always done it this way), the present (tasks must be performed on time), or the future (what are we striving toward)? How does time sense vary from clinicians to middle managers to senior executives? To what extent is time viewed from a discrete (clock time) or a relative perspective? Time as a reference of content themes implies diverse administrative tasks including planning for and implementing change, understanding and managing intergroup conflict and incorporating new recruits to the nursing department from host cultures that hold different time orientations.

CONSISTENCY AND CONSENSUS

While the problems addressed by organizations or their subunits are considered universal, the assumptions guiding how they are approached, when coupled with the more explicit behaviors and artifacts, can reveal differing degrees of consistency and consensus. Martin and Meyerson (1988) developed three types of consistency: action, symbolic, and content. *Action consistency* exists when content themes are consistent with an organization's formal and informal practices and/or its artifacts and their uses. *Symbolic consistency* exists when there is congruence between artifacts and formal and informal practices. *Content consistency* refers to congruence among content themes.

Consensus includes the extent to which meanings are shared across organizational members. Consensus can be examined, for example, from the perspectives of the total organization, senior executives only, across departments, or across occupational groups. The extent to which there is consistency among the meanings generated from the three classes of culture (practices, artifacts, content themes) and that there is consensus among organizational members on these data reveal the extent to which a given organization has an integrated or a differentiated culture (Martin & Meyerson, 1988).

The two broad themes of organizational culture presented contain different perspectives about the extent to which it should be viewed from an *integrated* or a *differentiated* frame of reference. These contrasting views impact ways that organizational problems such as change, conflict, and ambiguity are addressed by practitioners and students of administration. The *integration* perspective implies that an organization has a single culture in which there is a high level of consistency and consensus on culture throughout an organization. It is most congruent with the theme of culture as a variable or property of an organization as presented in the comparative and the corporate culture literature. The *differentiation* perspective recognizes and allows for variation of culture across organizational subunits (eg, subcultures).

The term "strong culture" is used to imply a high level of integration and congruence of values and beliefs throughout an organization. Those with strong and healthy cultures are more effective in dealing with problems of external adaptation and survival as well as with problems of internal integration than are weak or unhealthy cultures (Schein, 1985; Deal & Kennedy, 1982; Peters & Waterman, 1982). Proponents of this view assert that, to the extent that an organization's culture is judged as weak, it is the responsibility of management to diagnose its limitations and to take measures, through use of symbolic means of rituals, artifacts and the like, to strengthen the culture.

Organizations that manifest a high degree of consistency and consensus among practices, artifacts, values and beliefs, and assumptions throughout the organization often are characterized as having a strong or healthy culture (Ouchi, 1982; Deal & Kennedy, 1982; Schein, 1985). The logical alternative of that argument is that weak or unhealthy cultures exist under conditions of differentiation. However, note that a strong culture does not necessarily mean a healthy culture, ie, one in which the members and their ideas can flourish internally and one that enables the organization to meet the problems of external adaptation and survival. A highly integrated culture could be quite repressive and nonadaptive!

In like manner, a differentiated organizational culture is not necessarily either weak or unhealthy. Rather, members of different subunits may have evolved different solutions influenced by the central focus of their work. A hospital operating room's cultural beliefs about humanity's dominance over nature can be expected to differ from the cultural beliefs of the ambulatory rehabilitation staff of the same hospital (Chrisman, 1990). At the same time, assumptions identified in the two units of the same hospital may reveal little if any variation in beliefs about the nature of human relationships. Thus, culture varies within an organization and across subunits depending on the issue.

Differentiation also may describe an organization that is in transition. Fine (1989) cautioned that organizational transition "requires that those wishing to progress to other organizational arrangements must let go of the past, disengage from the former patterns, and move into a 'twilight zone' in which thoughts and actions are geared toward new situations not yet fully defined" page 573. That past includes deeply held assumptions. The pace with which subunits are able to achieve disengagement and move out of the "twilight zone" and into the new organizational conditions can be expected to vary. Thus, during the transitional period, differentiation of organizational culture can be expected to exist. Hill (1989) described a nursing department transition when it adopted shared governance, nursing case management, nurse group practice, and a salary model rather than the past hourly wage model of compensation. These all reflect core assumptions about how nurses and their work are viewed and how it is compensated relative to achieving the business goals of the organization.

Differentiation of culture among organizational subunits does not necessarily mean that culture conflict exists; it means simply that there is variability. The form that the variability takes and the extent to which it serves what the organization needs to accomplish internally, as well as the organization's external adaptation and survival, must enter into judgment of the health or weakness of an organization's culture.

ADMINISTRATIVE IMPLICATIONS

Statements regarding the central function of nursing administration—to develop and maintain environments that enable the professional practice of clinical nursing to be enacted itself reflects a set of interlocking assumptions concerning the universal problems in administration. They convey values about the nature of nurses' work and of the people who conduct that work (content themes). They imply that a professional level of clinical practice is a particular form of nurses' work that is not simply prescribed and directed by others. It is discretionary work that involves self-directed processing of a wide range of information in order to reach and to implement decisions on clients' behalf (Cummings & Srivastva, 1977) and its objectives entail collaborative practice and colleagial relations between nurses and physicians (Brozavich & Shortell, 1984) and among nurses. Furthermore, the statement implies that the contexts and environments in which nurses' work occurs have an influence on the conduct and effective fulfillment of the work and that administrative practice, rather than being focused on the traditional elements of control and manipulation to achieve ends, is directed, at least in part, to enabling and mentoring functions.

Currently, however, there is not a meaningful body of research literature that addresses organizational culture in health care organizations, in a profession composed predominantly of women, or in departments of nursing. As a consequence, analysis of the concept has revealed many questions to which only speculative responses can be offered. Yet, the analysis does illustrate that culture is a viable dimension for studying organizations and its understanding is crucial to the practice of nursing administration. Further research is needed, however, to develop paradigms of the interplay among the universal problems and assumptions about organizations and within and between units in health care organizations.

REFERENCES

Argyris C, Schon DA. *Organizational Learning*. Reading, MA, Addison-Wesley, 1978

Bate P. The impact of organizational culture on approaches to organizational problem-solving. *Organization Studies*. 5:1, 43–1984

Bolman LG, Deal TE. *Modern Approaches to Understanding and Managing Organizations*, San Francisco, Jossey-Bass Publishers, 1984

Brozavich JP, Shortell SM. (1984). How to create more humane and productive health care environments. *Health Care Management Review*. Fall, 43, 1984

Chrisman NJ. Cultural shock in the operating room: Cultural analysis in transcultural nursing. *Journal of Transcultural Nursing*. 1:2, 33, 1990

Cummings TG, Srivastva S. *Management of Work*. San Diego, CA, University Associates, 1977

Dalton DR, Todor WD, Spendolini MJ, Fielding GJ, Porter LW. Organization structure and performance. *Academy of Management Review*. 5:1, 49, 1980

Deal TE, Kennedy AA. *Corporate Culture*, Reading, MA, Addison-Wesley, 1982

del Bueno DJ, Vincent PM. Organizational culture: How important is it? *Journal of Nursing Administration*. 16:10, 15, 1986

Fine RB. From the transition stage to the transformed organization. In: Henry B, Arndt C, DiVincenti M, Marriner-Tomey A, eds. *Dimensions of Nursing Administration*. Boston, Blackwell Scientific Publications, 1989, 573–581.

Harris PR. *Management in Transition*. San Francisco, Jossey-Bass Publishers, 1985

Hill BM. The McAuley experience with changing compensation within the context of a professional nursing practice culture. *Nursing Administration Quarterly*. 14:1, 788, 1989

Johnson LM. Self governance: Treatment for an unhealthy nursing culture. *Health Progress*. 68:4, 41, 1987

Kluckhohn C, Kelly WH. The concept of culture. In: Linton R, ed. *The Science of Man in World Crisis*. New York, Columbia University Press, 1945

Kluckhohn FR. (1953). Dominant and variant value orientations. In: Brink PJ, ed. *Transcultural Nursing: A Book of Readings*, Englewood Cliffs, NJ, Prentice Hall, 1976, (orig 1953) 63–81.

Kramer M, Hafner LP. Shared values: Impact on staff nurse job satisfaction and perceived productivity. *Nursing Research*. 38:3, 172, 1989

Louis MR. Organizations as culture-bearing milieux. In: Pondy LR, Frost PJ, Morgan G, Dandridge TC, eds. *Organization Symbolism*. Greenwich, Conn: JAI Press, 1983, 39–54

Louis MR. An investigator's guide to workplace culture. In: Frost PJ, Moore LF, Louis MR, Lundberg CC, Martin J, eds. *Organizational Culture*. Beverly Hills, CA, Sage Publications, 1985, 73–93

Martin J, Meyerson D. Organizational cultures and the denial, channeling and acknowledgment of ambiguity. In: Pondy LR, Boland RJ Jr, Thomas H, eds. *Managing Ambiguity and Change*. New York, John Wiley & Sons Ltd, 1988, 93–125

McClure ML, Poulin MA, Sovie MD, Wandelt MA. *Magnet Hospitals: Attraction and Retention of Professional Nurses*, Kansas City, American Nurses' Association, 1983

Meek VL. Organizational culture: Origins and weaknesses. *Organization Studies*. 9:4, 453, 1988

Morgan G. *Images of Organizations*. Beverly Hills, CA, Sage Publications, 1986

Ouchi WG. *Theory Z: How American Business Can Meet the Japanese Challenge*. Reading, MA, Addison-Wesley, 1981

Peters TJ, Waterman RH. *In Search of Excellence*, New York: Warner Books, 1982

Pettigrew AM. On studying organizational culture. *Administrative Science Quarterly*. 24, 570, 1979

Ray MA. The theory of bureaucratic caring for nursing practice in the organizational culture. *Nursing Administration Quarterly*. 13:2, 31, 1989

Saffold GS. Culture traits, strength, and organizational performance: Moving beyond ''strong'' culture. *Academy of Management Review*. 13:4, 546, 1988

Sathe V. Implications of corporate culture: A manager's guide to action. *Organizational Dynamics*. 12:2, 5, 1983

Schall MS. A communication-rules approach to organizational culture. *Administrative Science Quarterly*. 28, 557, 1983

Schein EH. *Organizational Culture and Leadership*. San Francisco, Jossey-Bass Publishers, 1985

Schein EH. Culture as an environmental context for careers. In: Steers RM, Porter LW, eds. *Motivation and Work Behavior*, 4th ed. New York: McGraw-Hill, 1987, 348–359

Schein EH. Organizational culture. *American Psychologist*. 45:2, 109, 1990

Schneider SC, Shrivastava P. Basic assumptions themes in organizations. *Human Relations*. 41:7, 493, 1988

Siehl C. After the founder: An opportunity to manage culture. In: Frost PJ, Moore LF, Lewis

MR, Lundberg CC, Martin J, eds. *Organizational Culture*. Beverly Hills, CA, Sage Publications, 1985, 125–140

Smircich L. Concepts of culture and organizational analysis. *Administrative Science Quarterly*. 28:3, 339, 1983

Smircich L, Calas MB. Organizational culture: A critical assessment. In: Jablin FM, Porter LL, eds. *Handbook of Organizational Communication*. Beverly Hills, CA, Sage Publications, 1987, 228–263

Thompson JD. *Organizations in Action*. New York, McGraw-Hill Book Company, 1967

Trice HM, Beyer JM. Studying organizational cultures through rites and ceremonials. *Academy of Management Review*. 9:4, 653, 1984

Turner BA. Sociological aspects of organizational symbolism. *Organization Studies*. 7:2, 101, 1986

Van Ess Coeling H, Wilcox JR. Understanding organizational culture: A key to management decision-making. *Journal of Nursing Administration*. 18:11, 16, 1988

Wiener Y. Forms of value systems: A focus on organizational effectiveness and cultural change and maintenance. *Academy of Management Review*. 13:4, 534, 1988

Wilkins AL, Dyer WG Jr. Toward culturally sensitive theories of culture change. *Academy of Management Review*. 13:4, 522, 1988

Wilkins AL, Ouchi W. Efficient cultures: Exploring the relationship between culture and organizational performance. *Administrative Science Quarterly*. 28, 468, 1983

Young E. On the naming of the rose: Interests and multiple meanings as elements of organizational culture. *Organization Studies*. 10:2, 187, 1989

CHAPTER 6

Organizational Effectiveness and Productivity Enhancement

Sandra R. Edwardson
Raymond A. Noe

Key Concept List

Effectiveness criteria
Organization life cycle
Systems model
Constituency
Production systems
Flow networks
Productivity

WHAT IS ORGANIZATIONAL EFFECTIVENESS?

Is there one correct way to assess the effectiveness of organizations? Is there a formula for determining whether an organization is effective? The answer to both of these questions is "no." There is not one universally acceptable definition of organizational effectiveness. Effectiveness differs depending on the types of criteria or measures of effectiveness the organization believes are valid measures of success. Because each organization exists for a different reason (consider the differences between a health care organization and a manufacturing organization), it is unlikely that there will ever be a "universal" measure of effectiveness.

The classic literature on organizational effectiveness illustrates the differences in how it is defined. Cummings (1977) believes that organizational effectiveness is determined by the extent to which employees feel that the organization is helpful in meeting their needs. Etzioni (1964) emphasizes goal attainment as the critical factor in organizational effectiveness. Yuchtman and Seashore (1967) emphasize that organizations need to attain resources from the environment in order to be successful. Georgopoulos and Tannenbaum (1957) and Pfeffer (1977) believe that in order for organizations to be effective they must successfully deal with resource demands and incompatibilities that result from the competing goals and objectives of departments as well as individual employees. Conflict must be minimized in order for the organization to remain productive and flexible enough to deal with changing environmental demands.

HOW IS ORGANIZATIONAL EFFECTIVENESS MEASURED?

In reviewing the organizational effectiveness literature, Campbell (1979) found a wide variety of criteria being used as shown in Table 6-1. These criteria can be divided into five major effectiveness categories: attendance, productivity, attitudes, strategy, and management (see Table 6-1). *Attendance criteria* suggest that effectiveness is the extent to which the employer gains employees' commitment to retain membership in the organization and to come to work on time. *Productivity criteria* relate to the quantity or volume of the product or service provided by the organization. This includes a comparison of performance versus cost (efficiency), amount of revenue or return on investment (profitability), and the quality of product or service as evaluated by clients and customers. *Attitudinal criteria* relate to employees' feelings and beliefs regarding the organization, the job, colleagues, and management. *Strategic criteria* such as growth, stability, and evaluation of external constituencies are important indicators of the extent to which the organization is maintaining its direction, achieving its objectives, and satisfying individuals with a vested interest in the organization including shareholders, suppliers and vendors, customers, and the larger community. Finally, *management criteria* are used to indicate the effective use of interpersonal and technical skills by managers which is critical for developing and supporting employees' performance efforts.

As is readily apparent from Table 6-1, it would be impossible for any organization to simultaneously maximize all effectiveness criteria or to limit effectiveness evaluation based on only one criteria. Therefore, organizations are forced to choose multiple effectiveness criteria based on organizational goals or strategies, the expectations of internal or external groups, and environmental influences.

TABLE 6-1. MEASURES OF ORGANIZATIONAL EFFECTIVENESS

Category	Criteria
Attendance	Absenteeism Voluntary terminations
Productivity	Efficiency Profitability Quality Value of human resources
Attitudes	Job satisfaction Motivation Morale Stability Evaluation by external constituencies
Strategic behavior	Planning and goal setting Flexibility/adaptation Readiness Utilization of environment Growth
Management behavior	Internalization of organizational goals Role and norm congruence Participation and shared influence Achievement emphasis Control Interpersonal skills Task skills Information management Training and development emphasis Conflict and cohesion

TRADITIONAL EFFECTIVENESS MODELS

The effectiveness models discussed in this section are considered traditional because historically they have been included in any discussion of organizational effectiveness. These two models include the goal approach and the systems approach.

The Goal Approach to Organizational Effectiveness

According to the goal model, organizational success is determined by the extent to which the organization meets its goals. Goals can be thought of as future states or conditions that contribute to the fulfillment of the organization's mission. Goals usually specify a desired outcome that the organization seeks to achieve. Goals can include productivity, efficiency, or outcomes related to employee satisfaction. For example, one goal of a public health agency could be ensuring that all children in the county receive their DPT vaccinations during the appropriate developmental period.

Because of the complexity of defining success and the number of important internal and external constituencies that must be satisfied, organizations usually have multiple goals. For example, a health care organization may simultaneously have goals related to patient care and satisfaction, productivity (number of procedures of a given quality performed for a surgical unit), and efficiency (illnesses treated with minimum inpatient costs).

Although goals may serve to direct and maintain the behavior of organizational units and employees toward the achievement of some common outcomes, there are some dangers in using goals as a way of assessing organizational effectiveness. First, goals may conflict with each other resulting in confusion for employees and departments regarding work priorities and reduced levels of employee and customer satisfaction. For example, until recently, health care providers have not been concerned with profit maximization as a key indicator of organizational effectiveness and survival. Increases in labor, insurance, and technology costs and competition for patient care have dictated, however, that efficiency and productivity goals are now necessary. Subsequently many hospitals must re-evaluate the length of hospital stay for many procedures. Although not endangering patient recovery, reduced length of hospital stays has caused the consumer to voice more dissatisfaction concerning patient care because they expect that recovery occurs best in the hospital. As a result, hospitals must balance productivity and efficiency goals with patient care goals (including post discharge planning) in order to ensure that patient care is not compromised.

Another problem with the goal approach to organizational effectiveness is that publicly stated goals may not be related to actual organizational objectives. Organizational goals can serve as a facade for legitimizing unit goals and the career ambitions of employees. Also, the operational goals at any time may vary depending on the politically dominant coalition. Organizational effectiveness will differ depending on the source of information used to identify organizational goals.

A final problem with the goal approach is that many times it is difficult to measure if goals have been attained. For example, AIDS research may have no immediate payoff but the cumulative effects of this research can help eradicate the disease.

The Systems Model of Organizational Effectiveness

The systems model views the organization as comparable to a biological system in which organizations are seen as a set of interdependent parts which together form a whole organization (Thompson, 1967). Because the organization is interdependent with the larger environment, survival of the organization depends on coordination between different internal systems and reactions to environmental disturbances.

According to Kast and Rosenzweig (1985) internal systems include the following:

- Goals and values subsystem: Related to the culture and philosophy of the organization
- Psychosocial subsystem: Related to interpersonal dynamics and attitudes
- Technical subsystem: Related to knowledge, techniques, facilities, and equipment
- Structural subsystem: Related to tasks, information flow, procedures, and rules
- Managerial subsystem: Related to managerial behavior such as goal setting, planning, organizing, implementing, and controlling

The systems model assumes that the organization is an open system that must acquire and use energy or inputs, transform these inputs into a product, and exchange this product with the environment in order to acquire additional resources or inputs needed for product development. The environment provides feedback to the organization regarding the extent to which its ''products'' or outputs are meeting its needs. For example, as shown in Figure 6–1, institutional inputs include its professional and administrative staff, equipment, supplies, patients, and working capital. For patients, the process consists of diagnosis, care and treatment, with the ultimate output being wellness, comfort, and satisfaction with the services rendered. If the larger environment is not satisfied, (eg, state and federal standards for patient care met, a return on investment for owners resulting from efficient treatment and medical

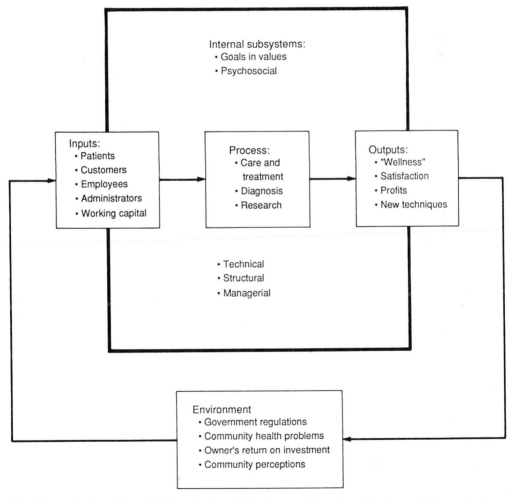

Figure 6-1. Systems Model of Organizational Effectiveness *(Based on Thompson JD.* Organizations in Action. *New York, McGraw-Hill, 1967)*

reimbursement, community health problems reduced) then it is likely that the institution will not receive sufficient inputs (money, patients, attraction of top-notch professionals) to survive.

The systems approach to organizational effectiveness emphasizes that the ultimate survival of the organization depends on its ability to meet environmental demands and balance internal subsystems. Administrators must review current changes in federal and state health care policies, community health care needs, and the characteristics of the customer population in order to provide services or "processes" to environmental needs and ensure adequate fiscal resources necessary for continued survival.

INTEGRATIVE EFFECTIVENESS APPROACHES

Integrative effectiveness approaches are based on the premise that organizations have multiple outcomes with which they must be concerned. In these approaches, multiple indicators or criteria are proposed to assess organizational effectiveness. These models include the *time-dimension model, constituency approach, competing values approach*, and *contradiction model*.

The Time-Dimension Model

Gibson, Ivancevich, and Donnelly (1988) point out that organizational effectiveness must account for the dimension of time. They argue that the ultimate or long-run criterion of organizational effectiveness is survival, ie, the degree to which the organization sustains itself in the environment. According to Cameron and Whetten (1981) organizations develop, mature, and decline according to how well they deal with environmental circumstances. If an organization is believed to be part of a larger system, over time the organization must acquire, process, and return resources to the environment in order to survive.

Different types of criteria are relevant depending on the maturity of the organization (see Fig. 6–2). In the infant stage or start-up stage of an organization, three types of criteria are important: production, efficiency, and satisfaction. Effectiveness is measured by the extent to which the organization produces the quantity and quality of output demanded by the environment (production criteria), makes good use of resources (efficiency criteria), and satisfies the needs of employees and customers (satisfaction criteria). Organizations that perform poorly in terms of productivity, efficiency, and satisfaction criteria will experience decline and eventual "death."

Once an organization has established itself by producing products in an efficient manner that satisfies customers and clients and allows employees to fulfill their work needs, the "adolescent" organization becomes concerned with responding to changes in the environment (adaptiveness criteria) and investing resources in a way to develop products and skills of its human resources (development criteria). Increasing attention is devoted to activities that attempt to sustain and formalize the organization's recipe for success. This includes goal setting, socializing new employees to fit the organization's culture, and information management. Research and development

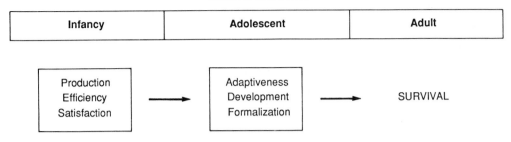

Figure 6-2. Time-Dimension Model of Organizational Effectiveness *(Based on Gibson, JL, Ivancevich, JM, and Donnelly, JH.* Organizations: Behavior, Structure, Process. *Plano, TX: Business Publications, 1988)*

activities attempt to ensure that the organization can adapt to changing client needs and incorporate new technologies and resources to yield a better product. It is also important that time and money be devoted to training and development activities in order to ensure that employees have the knowledge, skills, abilities, and motivational levels necessary to cope with changes in technology and new processes designed to produce a better product in a more efficient manner.

For example, survival of a health maintenance organization (HMO) initially depends on the extent to which health care services meet patient needs and are administered in an efficient manner. Once satisfactory enrollment levels are attained, HMOs must be concerned with addressing the changing needs of the patient population and using new technologies for treatment purposes. The increasing attention being paid to "wellness" by the general public demands that HMOs be prepared to conduct cholesterol screening, provide nutrition counseling, and discuss stress management techniques as part of routine physical examinations. HMOs that do not attempt to change the lifestyle of members at risk for cardiovascular disease and increase client awareness of the benefits of a healthy lifestyle will find themselves performing costly procedures that may have been avoided.

Constituency Approach
The constituency approach to organizational effectiveness considers the extent to which organizational stakeholders are satisfied. A constituency or stakeholder is any group within or outside the organization that has a vested interest in the organization's performance.

Table 6-2 presents some important constituencies and their effectiveness criteria. Common constituencies include owners, employees, customers, creditors, the community, suppliers, and the government. Each constituency likely has a different perspective regarding effectiveness. For example, customers (patients) will likely judge the effectiveness of the hospital or health maintenance organization on the degree to which they feel that their diagnosis was correct, services were performed in a timely and competent manner, and the treatment they received resulted in a return to good

TABLE 6-2. IMPORTANT CONSTITUENCIES AND THEIR CRITERIA OF EFFECTIVENESS

Constituency	Effectiveness Criteria
Patients/customers	Quality of care
	Treatment outcome
Employees/union	Pay, working conditions
Owners	Return on investment
Creditors	Debt payment
Suppliers	Demand for services
Government	Adherence to local, state, and federal standards
Community	Contribution to community activities and projects
	Continued employment of community members
Environment	Lack of pollution and minimal use of nonreplenishable resources

health. However, creditors such as vendor and suppliers of equipment and medications will judge effectiveness on the basis of the timeliness of debt payments. Shareholders will be most concerned with maximizing their return on investment.

The constituency approach highlights the difficulty in trying to identify one overall measure of organizational effectiveness. Organizational survival ultimately depends on how well the organization meets the demands of different constituencies, demands that are sometimes in conflict. It is critical for the organization to identify relevant constituencies and evaluate the importance of meeting the demands of any one constituency. This evaluation should be completed by referring to the organization's strategic goals which outline how much attention should be paid to meeting the demands of each constituency. In most health care organizations, the primary constituents are the patients. Correct treatment and patient comfort and satisfaction is the number one indicator of effectiveness. A second important indicator of effectiveness may be the extent to which the facility supports the community. It is unlikely, however, that community needs will ever take priority over patient care needs.

Given the current shortage of qualified nurses, nurse satisfaction is important for retention of nurses (employee constituency). Attitude surveys and other information gathering techniques should be used to obtain a perspective of current nursing staff needs and satisfaction with salary and benefits, working conditions, and opportunities to participate in development activities.

Competing Values Approach

Quinn and Rohrbaugh (1983) have developed a "competing-values" approach to organizational effectiveness. The competing values approach identifies two characteristics of organizations that are believed to be incongruent with one another. These two dimensions include the *focus* of the organization and the organizational *structure*. Focus refers to whether dominant values reflect issues that are internal to the organization, such as concern for employee satisfaction, morale, and efficiency of production. Organizational structure concerns include the degree to which the organization is concerned with stability or flexibility. An organization concerned with stability values characteristics of a mechanistic organization such as autocratic, top-down management control. An organization concerned with flexibility, an organic organization, values change and the ability to adapt to environmental changes.

In Figure 6–3 the competing values model is presented. Four possible models of organizational effectiveness are possible based on the value dimensions of structure and focus. An effectiveness model that values external focus and flexible structure is concerned with growth and resource acquisition. In the open systems model (shown in Quadrant I), effectiveness is determined by the extent to which the organization establishes a satisfactory relationship with its environment in order to acquire the necessary resources and increase its share of the market. The rational goal model (see Quadrant III) emphasizes structural control and an external focus. Organizational effectiveness is determined by the extent to which the organization is productive, profitable, and efficient. Management activity, such as goal setting and action planning, are likely to be valued in organizations with this view of effectiveness because these activities facilitate profitability and control. The internal process model (see Quadrant IV) emphasizes internal focus and structural control. Effectiveness is determined by the extent to which the organization can maintain its current status and market position. Information management and efficient communications are valued because they are mechanisms through which the organization can maintain itself in an orderly manner.

The human relations model (see Quadrant II) is concerned with maximizing the return on investment in human resources. This model incorporates the values of an internal focus and a flexible structure. According to this model, organizations that strive for effectiveness are interested in providing employees with motivating work experiences, promoting cooperation among work units, and usually have quite ad-

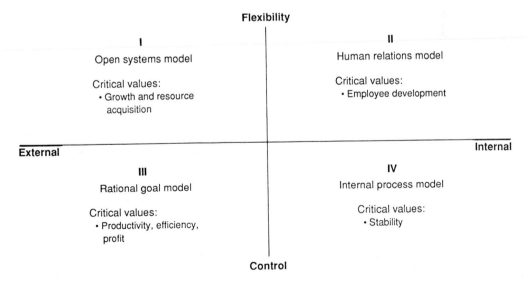

Figure 6–3. The Competing Values Approach *(Adapted from Quinn, RE and Rohrbaugh, J. A spatial model of effectiveness criteria: Toward a competing values approach to organizational analysis.* Management Science. *29, 363–377, 1983)*

vanced training and development systems. In the human relations model, employee development and satisfaction are more important than environmental demands.

The competing values approach makes an important contribution to our understanding of organizational effectiveness because it emphasizes the importance that organization values have in determining effectiveness criteria. Organizational values are the basic values and beliefs of the organization; they form the organization culture (Deal & Kennedy, 1982). (See Chapter 5 for a comprehensive examination of corporate culture.) Values provide a direction for the daily activities of the organization. In order to be successful according to this effectiveness model, organizations must determine their values, ensure that these values are communicated to all employees, and then use these values as their own effectiveness criteria.

Deal and Kennedy (1982) suggest that successful organizations place a great deal of importance on communicating values to employees and monitoring the values system by designing their appraisal measures around the value structure. If an organization is concerned with growth and resource acquisition, the organization must develop and use effectiveness indicators, such as client focus groups and marketing surveys, in order to examine whether customer and client needs are currently being met and identify new needs that could be satisfied by new product development or marketing strategies.

The competing values approach also emphasizes that effectiveness is a multifaceted concept with sometimes contradictory criteria. Management must consider the tradeoffs among the criteria and the value structure they represent in determining how to judge whether the organization is effective. Ultimately, the effectiveness criteria chosen communicates the values of the organization to its employees, the community, and customers and clients.

Contradiction Model

Hall (1987) argues that there are many contradictions inherent in organizational effectiveness. He suggests there are four contradictions which make it difficult to attempt to categorize an organization as effective or ineffective. These contradictions are *environmental constraints, goals, constituents,* and *time.* First, organizations face multiple and conflicting environmental constraints such as government regulations and constraints resulting from vendor and supplier demands for modified resources or new products. Constraints also arise from bargaining with competitors over market share. The organization is forced to negotiate with the environment, recognize and prioritize its dealings with competition, and attempt to predict the consequences of the chosen strategy for dealing with these constraints.

A second contradiction is the reality that the organization faces in dealing with multiple and conflicting goals. If an institutions's goals are profit-making and high return on investment and growth, it must deal with the conflict between return on investment to shareholders and investment in the development of new health care markets.

Third, organizations have multiple and conflicting external and internal constituencies. Unintentionally, organizations may take actions that damage relationships with their constituencies. Pollutants can damage the immediate community; unsafe products can cause death and injury to customers; and equipment failures can lead to misdiagnosis and incorrect treatments. In order to satisfy the demands of one constituency, the welfare of another constituency may be sacrificed. For example, employees may be displaced from their jobs in order to meet creditors' demands. Also, short staffing may occur in order to admit patients to satisfy physicians and to maintain hospital income. This likely has an adverse effect on the motivation and morale of the nursing staff.

Finally, all organizations have multiple and conflicting time frames. The life cycle stage of the organization dictates which goals should be met in order to be judged an effective organization. Productivity and profitability may be relevant effectiveness criteria for a newly founded organization while development and adaptability take on increasing importance as the organization becomes "mature" and hopes to meet changing environmental demands and survive.

According to the contradiction model, organizations need to control those constraints that they perceive to be central to the organization's mission and strategy in order to be effective. Organizations may acquire suppliers in order to reduce problems with fluctuating resource costs. To reduce the variance in health care costs, many organizations negotiate with health maintenance organizations to provide services at a specified cost level. Organizations may also attempt to manipulate the environment by lobbying for legislation that can have a positive impact on their business. For example, the pharmaceutical industry was successful up until a few years ago in protecting itself from competition by getting physicians to permit the industry to advertise drugs by their brand names rather than their generic names (Hirsch 1975).

The key contribution of the contradiction model to our understanding of organizational effectiveness is the emphasis it places on the reality of trying to identify a common set of effectiveness criteria. Any effectiveness measure must take into account the extent to which the organization is successful in dealing with the competing interests of groups in its environment and competing internal goals. Also, the relevance of any effectiveness criteria is going to depend on whether the organization is in its infancy (where productivity and efficiency are key) or in its mature phase (where development and adaptability are important).

PRODUCTION SYSTEMS

Now that the possible models for evaluating organizational effectiveness have been presented, an examination of production systems and how they can improve effectiveness follows.

Production—Concepts, Analysis, and Control

Most health care professionals do not think of the clinical process as a production process. Nor do they think of themselves as practicing within a production system. Nevertheless, it is instructive to examine production systems as a model for understanding the work of health care providers.

Hopeman (1976) describes a production system as a framework of activities within which an organization creates value by converting inputs into outputs (products or services) through a series of processes. The products and services are also inspected (evaluated for quality) and, in most nonservice industries, stored until needed.

Production systems, like other systems, have subsystems. In health care, subsystems tend to be defined according to major organizational activities such as the nursing or pharmacy subsystems. In addition, parallel support systems, such as management information systems are used to support the core subsystems (Hopeman, 1976). (This conceptualization of productions systems is similar to the Kast and Rosenzweig (1985) technical and structural subsystems.)

Besides the production function, organizations typically have two other basic functions which are marketing and finance. The marketing function includes making forecasts of future levels of demand and obtaining other pertinent data such as client feedback, expectations regarding amenities, technical quality of services, and new services. The finance function involves gathering budgetary information, analyzing investments, accumulating working capital, and gathering information on the general condition of the organization (Hopeman, 1976).

Health Care As A Production System

In general, there are two basic types of production systems—continuous and intermittent. The most familiar examples of continuous production systems are mass production assembly-line manufacturing industries. These systems are characterized by a very uniform, fixed-path production process that permits a high level of specialization of labor, special purpose machines and procedures, and economies of scale (Hopeman, 1976).

Few of the functions of a health care facility fit into the continuous production category. Rather, the delivery of health care services is more like a tailor's shop than a suit factory. Because each patient presents unique combinations of strengths, symptoms, and problems, the care and treatment plan is customized for each individual. Intermittent production systems are unable to achieve the economies of scale, uniformity of process, and predictability of work flow possible in continuous systems. Effectiveness in intermittent production systems is measured in terms of flexibility of both processes and workers.

The intermittent nature of the production process in health care is a major source of its production problems. In order to be effective, production systems must be able to plan, analyze, and control the operation or process of care. This requires that patients are scheduled rationally and routed through the various phases of the care process so that elements of care and treatment are sequenced in optimal order. While such scheduling and routing is theoretically quite simple, the fact is that patients appear for care at unexpected times and the course of illness and responses to treatment are often sufficiently unpredictable to require frequent revisions of the plan of care. This lack of predictability requires flexibility in the overall design of the production process with special attention to rapid turnaround time on work orders (See Overton, Schneck, & Hazlett (1977) for a discussion of how uncertainty, instability and variability have been found to differentially affect the organization of nursing units.)

Another major source of problems in production systems is design of the physical facility: its location and layout and its ability to handle patients, equipment, and supplies. In establishing a new health care facility, a site should be selected in relation to patient and physician markets, labor and materials supplies, and regulatory entities. Because most major health care facilities do not have the luxury of relocating, these same factors become the environmental givens with which the organization must grapple in designing its production system.

ORGANIZING A PRODUCTION SYSTEM

Organizing a production system requires development of a structural framework for the enterprise and definitions of administrative and operative relationships.

Types of Production Systems Organizations

Production system organizations tend to fall into one or more of the following types: *functional, location, customer, product, process,* and *project* organizations (Hopeman, 1976). (see Chapter 7.) Most hospitals combine functional and process systems for most of their work using project organization for ad hoc activities. Since the introduction of prospective payment systems, intense interest has developed in product management.

Functional systems are organized in divisions or units according to the specialized activities performed. An advantage of functional organizations is that workers with specialized knowledge and experience are assigned to do only their own specialized functions, theoretically improving their efficiency and effectiveness.

Organizing according to *process* involves dividing responsibilities by the processes involved. The nursing department, for example, is responsible for one distinct process in the overall production process. Organizing according to process permits greater coordination of the major units of production and greater continuity of process.

Project organization is generally selected for time limited special projects. Individuals are drawn from several functional or process departments to lend their expertise in completing the project at hand. Project management is frequently used for activities such as facility planning and construction.

Product organization is widely used in manufacturing but is a new entrant into methods for organizing health care. In the food industry, for example, a single company may organize itself along product lines, such as breakfast cereal, cake mix, entree, and drink mix. Product management allows each division to have control over the entire production process for products that have similar input and process requirements and seek to address a specific market.

In health care, product or service lines have been defined by *diagnosis related groups* (DRG) or by major clinical programs such as cardiovascular or neurological services. The manager responsible for the service line identifies and coordinates all of the services from the relevant functional and process units required by patients using its services (Bruhn & Howes, 1986). Responsibility for the entire set of services gives the manager an opportunity to understand costs, respond quickly to organization and environmental changes and remain competitive (Hesterly & Robinson, 1988).

Organizational Principles and Effectiveness of Production Systems

Regardless of the type of production system selected by an organization, basic management principles guide the details of the process of organizing. The principle of span of control suggests that organizations should be designed so that each supervisor is responsible for the number of workers and activities consistent with the complexity of the job, characteristics of the supervisor, and nature of the relationships. To be effective, each supervisor should have responsibilities that are narrow enough for effective supervision but broad enough to reduce cost, decrease communication problems and reduce red tape that accompany many levels within an organizational hierarchy (Hopeman, 1976).

Similarly, centralization and decentralization principles can guide the manager in improving organizational effectiveness. Fayol (1949) observed that, while centralization belongs to the natural order of things, the degree of centralization is dependent on the nature of the enterprise. Delegation and decentralization can lead to increased decision making authority for lower level managers. This not only reduces delays in reaching decisions, but also makes decisions more responsive to the specific concerns of the work unit. Too much decentralization, however, also can be problematic. Control mechanisms must be sufficient to assure coordination of activities among work units and accountability for overall organizational goals (Schermerhorn, 1986). Also, lower-level employees often must develop appropriate skills for newly acquired decision making responsibilities.

The use of horizontal or vertical integration methods also affects organizational effectiveness. In some situations, horizontal integration, in which one type of activity is performed in many locations, leads to greatest effectiveness. Examples include chain discount stores, chain restaurants, and hospital corporations with multiple autonomous or semi-autonomous hospitals.

In other cases, vertical integration, in which a firm performs many levels of activity from acquiring inputs to selling the finished product to the consumer, results in greater effectiveness (refer to Chapters 7 and 19). Health care organizations with a high degree of vertical integration could control primary care clinics, emergency rooms, acute care facilities, home care, long-term care, and pharmacies as well as data processing, supply acquisition, laundry, and food services. Those with a low degree of vertical integration would concentrate on only one or two of those markets. From nursing's perspective, a highly integrated production system includes responsibility for patients from the preadmission period through post discharge follow up rather than just during the acute care or home care portion of an episode of illness.

Horizontal integration permits greater responsiveness to local needs and allows the organization to take advantage of differences in local wage rates and supply costs. Vertical integration, on the other hand, allows an organization to control all relevant suppliers and subsystems, thereby reducing the possibility that inputs and distribution mechanisms will fail to meet standards and schedules. The chief advantage of the integrated system is that it allows the organization to ''capture'' the patient. For example, patients cared for by a hospital affiliated clinic or home care facility are more likely to be admitted to that hospital should the need arise.

Depending on the size of the operation and the level of analysis, both horizontal and vertical integration principles can be applicable. For example, a very large and highly integrated health care corporation may also have a system of semi-autonomous hospitals, clinics and nursing homes.

A final factor that can affect organizational effectiveness is the availability and use of information. It is no exaggeration to say that information is the chief integrating device in health care delivery systems. The plethora of paper and electronic communication devices in health care facilities is testimony to that. But to enhance organizational effectiveness, information needs to be both timely and pertinent. As illustrated in Chapters 9 and 21, when information is delayed, inaccurate, or irrelevant, the work of both managers and clinicians is delayed and is likely to be of inferior quality. One of the greatest potential advantages of the product line management strategy, for example, is that it increases the likelihood that at least one individual has a picture of the total care and treatment process. But highly integrated information systems also present problems. For example, computerization of information systems improves an organization's ability to centralize decision making and control. This may conflict with the ability to reap the benefits of decentralized decision making. Therefore, the effects of centralization and decentralization of information handling should be carefully weighed in relation to autonomy of the work units.

CONCEPT OF FLOW NETWORKS

In the organizational effectiveness literature, a flow network is defined as the series of steps in the production process from entrance of inputs from the environment through the flow of outputs back to the environment (see Chapter 19). In designing a production system, it is useful to divide an organization's work into several flow networks, each focusing on a set of like inputs, such as materials (patients), personnel, money, and other tangible resources (eg, equipment, supplies, facilities) (Hopeman, 1976).

The goal of an organization seeking to improve its productivity is often to accelerate the rate of work to achieve high levels of efficiency at low costs per unit (eg low costs per patient day). The worst fear of staff nurses is that productivity monitoring is nothing more than an excuse to reduce the number of nurses or increase workload in some other way.

In health care, as in other industries, this emphasis on efficiency often directly conflicts with quality goals. Demands to reduce health care costs are currently accompanied with demands to prove the effectiveness or quality of the service as well. Therefore, there is an increasing emphasis on incorporating feedback loops into production systems in order to monitor the inputs, the process of care, and quality of outcomes achieved. Effective organizations then compare this information with predetermined standards and effectiveness goals and make appropriate adjustments in the production process.

There are two flow networks in health care organizations that have a major impact on their effectiveness. The patient flow network describes the system for organizing the care and treatment of patients. The personnel flow network outlines the process of acquiring and maintaining the organization's employees. Both flow networks derive from the systems model of organization effectiveness.

Patient Flow Network

A generalized patient flow network for the process of providing nursing care in organizations is represented in Figure 6-4. It shows that the inputs include personnel, equipment, supplies, and capital. These inputs are combined in a wide variety of ways to form a patient care delivery system which has as its outputs patient days, hours of care, procedures and/or patient visits, depending on the type of service. Familiar patient care delivery systems include functional, team and primary nursing systems, each of which divides up the process of care and the tasks to be accomplished according to its unique philosophy and conceptual model of the nursing care process. More recently, nursing organizations have been making efforts to incorporate the processes of other departments into analysis and planning of the patient flow network for nursing care resulting in nursing participation and leadership in patient flow systems such as product line management and case management. (See Mayer, Madden, & Lawrenz, (1990), *Patient Care Delivery Models,* for a description of several options in organizing the patient flow network for nursing care.)

Care delivery systems are differentiated by their approach to decision making. How decisions are made in any care delivery system depends on the nature of the decision. Those care processes in which decisions are routine and similar lend themselves to development of standardized policies and procedures. Examples include admission and discharge routines, vital signs monitoring, patient classification systems, medically delegated procedures and treatments, and problem specific patient

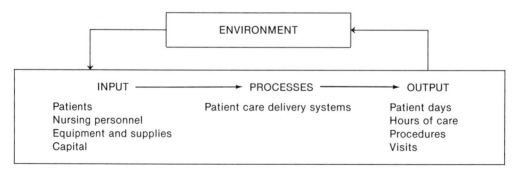

Figure 6-4. Patient Flow Network for Nursing Care *(Adapted from Jelinek RC & Dennis LC. A review and evaluation of nursing productivity. DHEW Publication No. HRA 77-15. Washington, DC: US Government Printing Office, 1976)*

education programs. Other decisions are nonroutine and nonrepetitive and must be custom tailored to a given situation. Planning care for patients with complex and interacting health problems requires use of judgment, experience, intuition, rules of thumb and specialized models (Hopeman, 1976). Knowledge about the type of decisions required to provide care for different patient populations is crucial knowledge for the design of care delivery models. It implies that a single care delivery model is unlikely to be optimal for caring for all patient populations and that a single large facility may find it necessary to use more than one model or several variations of a single model.

To guide the administrator in selecting an optimal patient flow model, several decision-making models may be employed. Physical models of a nursing unit may assist decision makers to visualize the way a unit's geography helps or hinders the care process and lead to innovative solutions to care delivery problems.

Traditionally, business organizations have used mathematical models such as break even and regression analysis for summarizing large amounts of complex information into a few key values. Break even analysis is especially useful in making decisions about whether or not to add a new service and at what level the service should be offered (Suver & Neumann, 1981). Regression analysis is particularly useful for making forecasts of demands for service. Health planning departments regularly use regression modeling to predict the number of patient days or visits a facility can expect to have in a forthcoming time period. Some patient classification systems also use regression modeling to improve the accuracy of forecasts of staffing requirements (Edwardson, Bahr & Serote, 1990; Giovannetti & Johnson, 1990).

A final decision-making model is the schematic model, a model that is more abstract than the physical model but less abstract than the mathematical. Examples include Gantt and Program Evaluation and Review Technique (PERT) charts used to schedule events. A schematic model currently receiving a great deal of attention in nursing is critical path analysis, a form of PERT charting (Warner & Holloway, 1978). A critical path is the optimum sequence of care and treatment activities that assures that the patient's care needs are met while at the same time ensuring that the patient gets appropriate and cost-effective care within a system of services (ANA, 1988).

Critical path analysis is one of the key components of the case management model used at New England Medical Center Hospitals. Critical paths are the abbreviated schematic models of case management plans developed for major patient groups. The case management plans or standards of care are detailed descriptions of the nursing diagnoses, clinical outcomes, intermediate goals, and nursing and medical interventions that facilitate movement toward each goal. The emphasis is on achieving goals within the DRG-allotted length of stay (Zander, 1988, 1990). Linkages to the environment through preadmission and discharge planning and control are other important ingredients of a useful critical path analysis.

Critical path analyses will have the biggest payoff for the organization if all of an organization's departments are included. But critical path analysis also can be used to analyze only one service (eg, nursing) and to explicate types of services needed and the optimum timing of services to meet patient care requirements.

Personnel Flow Network

A second flow network, crucial for achieving effectiveness in nursing care organizations, is the personnel flow network. The quality and performance of employees of service organizations, such as health care facilities, are crucial for organizational effectiveness because the actions of employees (services) is the product of the organization. What consumers know about an organization is their interaction with its employees. The quality of the care received is inextricably linked to the process of providing the care.

Figure 6–5 presents the personnel flow network, highlighting the steps involved in identifying personnel needs, recruiting, inducting, motivating, and terminating employees. Psychological research has aided our understanding of how elements of the personnel flow network affect the organization's effectiveness in converting its inputs into outputs. The extensive body of work related to work withdrawal behaviors such as absenteeism and turnover, for example, offers suggestions for the manager in maintaining effectiveness and organizational commitment (see Breaugh and Decker (1988) for more information). The personnel flow network is discussed in greater detail in the productivity section to follow.

Evaluating and Improving Production Systems in Nursing

Use of open systems concepts as a framework for analysis focuses on the means for attaining goals rather than on the goals themselves (Miles, 1980). In open systems, performance measures or effectiveness criteria are used as clues to the organization's ability to maintain its position and meet new opportunities and threats.

Productivity is one performance measure used to evaluate organizational effectiveness of great interest to nursing administrators. Productivity analysis is most often done within a systems framework with current conceptions attempting to integrate goal attainment or outcome indicators. Productivity measures can heighten awareness, provide the basis for tracking trends, serve as planning tools, and permit one facility to compare itself with others.

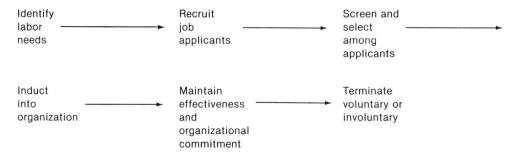

Figure 6–5. Personnel Flow Network

WHAT IS NURSING PRODUCTIVITY?

Productivity is often defined as an output/input ratio. The larger the ratio, the more productive the organization is believed to be because it gets relatively more output from each dollar invested. Most observers of health care are uncomfortable with such a definition, however, unless the quality of the output is specified. Jelinek and Dennis (1976) were among the first to recognize this need when they defined nursing productivity as follows:

> The concept of productivity encompasses both the effectiveness of nursing care, which relates to its quality and appropriateness, and the efficiency of care, which is production of nursing output with minimal resource waste. (p 3)

In other words, a more appropriate definition of productivity for health care services is the ratio of quality-adjusted output (or outcomes) per input expended.

Defining and measuring the inputs and outputs (outcomes of the health care process) is also difficult, however. Figure 6–4 shows the inputs of the patient flow network to include personnel, supplies and equipment, and capital. Some would also include patients' health problems (the "raw material" of the health care process) as inputs. Quantifying inputs presents difficulties. Supplies, equipment, capital, and, to some extent, personnel can be valued on a monetary scale. But the efficiency and effectiveness of nurses within occupational levels and job categories is known to vary widely and to affect the overall productivity of a nursing unit. While clinical ladder systems have been developed to tap these differences, a widely accepted evaluation method has yet to be found.

Quantifying patient input is especially difficult. Efforts to refine measures of patient inputs have been a byproduct of defining hospital output. Hospital output is most often defined as patient days. Recently researchers and policy makers have concluded that patient days are inadequate since they are not homogeneous entities. Of major concern is that fact that one patient day may require the use of many more resources than another. For that reason, methods for standardizing patient input have been developed to be more specific about the type of patient days. Examples include various case-mix or "patient classification" methods such as diagnosis related groups (DRGs).

Most elusive of all is the definition and measurement of quality-adjusted output or outcomes. Quality or effectiveness of a health care output refers to the safety, appropriateness, and excellence of care and to changes in health status, improved patient outcomes, and patient satisfaction (AMSI, 1980). In other fields, quality of outputs is more readily evaluated. A typist's productivity, for example, can be evaluated in terms of errorless pages typed per hour. While avoiding errors is certainly a necessary requirement for quality nursing care, it is hardly sufficient. Furthermore, definitions of errors are likely to vary depending on one's standards of practice and scientific knowledge.

Definitional and measurement problems in productivity evaluation derive from the fact that much of what nurses and health care facilities do is knowledge work. By definition the results of knowledge work often are not known for some time and the immediate result "is largely intangible, reflecting in part the unstructured, creative aspects of knowledge work . . . and exercise [of] substantial judgment and discretion in performing non-repetitive tasks" (Packer, 1985, p 161). As a result, measures of output and outcome often have a high level of subjectivity.

METHODS OF MEASURING NURSING PRODUCTIVITY

The preceding discussion suggests some problems in current methods of measuring nursing productivity. For example, the most common measures—nursing hours and salary costs per patient day—are of little value unless we know something about the quality of those patient days. Therefore, efforts are needed to standardize patient days to make them more homogeneous with respect to patient type and level of outcome. Examples include the number of resources required per patient day of specific types by categorizing patient days into DRGs or other medical or nursing diagnostic groupings. If the groupings are adjusted for severity, the validity of comparisons of nursing hours and nursing salary costs per patient day is improved (Edwardson, 1988).

Numerous costing studies reported in the nursing literature have shown that the DRG may not be sufficiently homogeneous to serve as a useful nursing input adjustment (Riley & Schaefers, 1985; Sovie, Tarcinale, Vanputee & Stunden, 1985; Vanderzee & Glusko, 1984). Study after study has shown that the nursing care requirements of patients in many DRGs vary widely. Many suspect this is due to differences in severity of illness, which suggests that severity-adjusted DRGs might be a good measure. But whether or not DRGs or severity-adjusted DRGs are an optimum output measure when evaluating nursing productivity, DRGs will remain a highly relevant output as long as DRGs are the basis of reimbursement.

Another commonly used productivity measure in nursing is to compare the hours of care required to provide care (as measured by a patient classification system) with the hours of care actually provided. This is one of the best day to day budget monitors available to nursing managers. But unless certain assumptions are made about required hours of care, it is more appropriately called a utilization rather than a productivity indicator. The required/actual ratio can only evaluate productivity as quality adjusted output per input if the nursing service assumes or has demonstrated that the required number of nursing hours can provide the quantity and quality of care that the organization wishes to provide. In other words, using employee utilization ratios to judge productivity is based on the assumption that the standard hours of care used by the patient classification system to calculate required nurse hours provide the desired level of service. If the organization has measured and is satisfied that the target level of staffing produces an acceptable quantity and quality of care, it may be an appropriate substitute for a direct measurement of productivity. The fact that many organizations expect the actual number of employees used to be less than the targeted level suggests that either the standards used to establish the target are too high or the organization is willing to compromise its standards (Edwardson, 1988).

H. L. Mencken once remarked that for every complex problem there is a simple answer, and it's wrong. The temptation exists to focus on easily countable indicators of efficiency and effectiveness rather than on indicators more important to core values and long-term viability. While some may concentrate on attaining certain goals (goal attainment model of organizational effectiveness), others will insist on knowing the relative importance of those goals in relation to the organization's mission (competing values model).

APPROACHES TO IMPROVING PERSONNEL PRODUCTIVITY

Because personnel costs are, by far, the most expensive inputs into nursing care, methods for improving personnel productivity receive considerable attention. The simplest approach is to reduce the costs of all input factors by reducing the size or skill mix of the staff. As Mencken cautioned, although it is simple, this approach is often wrong if a careful evaluation of the consequences for the quantity and quality of services is ignored.

Patient Classification

In order to make decisions to improve efficiency without reducing quality, the workload of the staff must first be measured. Patient classification systems used for nurse staffing are the most frequently used work measurement methods. Patient classification is the grouping of patients into a predetermined number of separate and identifiable groups which are homogeneous with respect to their nursing care requirements.

There are several types of patient classification systems. *Prototype systems* use broad descriptions of the characteristics of a typical patient and patients are classified according to which prototype statement best describes the patient. *Factor evaluation systems* uses sets of critical indicators, for which patients are rated independently. These critical indicators are then combined to provide an overall rating. *Tasking systems* employ lists of most of the activities required for a patient. The time values associated with each activity are added to produce a total care time requirement (Giovannetti & Burkhalter, 1988).

Regardless of the type of patient classification system in use, maintaining its validity and reliability is essential if the information is to contribute to organizational effectiveness. Systems vary in the ease with which reliability and validity can be maintained. Furthermore, system maintenance is not a particularly rewarding activity and for that reason requires concerted effort to see that ongoing monitoring occurs.

Assuming that the patient classification system is kept valid, it has several uses. The most common uses are to predict workload for subsequent shifts and to use cumulative workload information to develop and monitor budgets. Both of these applications can enhance the organization's efficiency and can contribute to its effectiveness by ensuring that resources are distributed according to need. In addition, some facilities use patient classification information to charge for nursing costs or to negoti-ate payment rates with third parties.

Use of Human Relations Principles

It is often assumed that the productivity of a nursing unit is an additive function of the productivity of individual nurses. This conflicts with another widely held as-sumption that the work of a group is more than the sum of the work of individual members. Furthermore, to focus only on the productivity of individuals fails to recog-nize that an individual's productivity in a complex organization is, in many ways, dependent on the performance of others.

Therefore, a reasonable alternative is to focus on individual performance with the understanding that performance is not synonymous with productivity. Then the individual nurse's performance can be seen as one contributing factor to a unit's pro-ductivity. This provides the logical basis for most productivity enhancing inter-ventions using human resource management and human motivation theories and techniques (Ilgen & Klein, 1988). (A discussion of these theories and methods can be found in Sullivan and Decker, 1992; Guzzo, 1988; and Berlinger, Glick and Rodgers, 1988. Also see Edwardson's (1988) discussion of productivity.)

SUMMARY

This chapter describes efforts to define and identify organizational effectiveness within the framework of various models. Attendance, productivity, attitudes, strate-gic behaviors, and management behavior are suggested criteria used to evaluate effec-tiveness. Since an organization cannot meet all criteria simultaneously, it is forced to choose effectiveness criteria based on organizational goals, expectations of its mem-bers, and environmental influences. Integrative effectiveness approaches include the time-dimension model, constituency approach, cometing values approach, and con-tradiction model. Effectiveness can be enhanced by improving the organization's pro-duction system which can be organized by function, location, customer, product, process, or project. Flow networks control the production process and, in health care, both the patient flow network and personnel flow network can be used to improve organizational effectiveness. Nursing productivity is difficult to measure because most indicators of productivity utilize quantitative measures (eg, nursing hours, sal-ary costs per patient days) without accounting for quality. Using a valid patient classi-fication system and recognizing the cumulative effects of individual nurses' produc-tivity assists the administrator in measuring and improving productivity.

REFERENCES

American Nurses Association (ANA). *Nursing Case Management*. Kansas City, MO, ANA, 1988
Applied Management Sciences, Inc. (AMSI). *Productivity and Health: Hospital Productivity—A Synopsis of the Literature* (DHHS publication no. HRA 80-14028). Washington, DC, United States Government Printing Office, 1980

Berlinger LR, Glick WH, Rodgers RC. (1988). Job enrichment and performance improvement. In: Campbell JP, Campbell RJ, Associates (eds.), *Productivity in Organizations: New Perspectives from Industrial and Organizational Psychology,* San Francisco: Jossey-Bass, 1988, 219–254

Breaugh JA, Decker PJ. Controlling absenteeism and turnover. In: Sullivan EJ, Decker PJ, eds. *Effective Management in Nursing,* (pp. 387–410). Menlo Park, CA, Addison-Wesley, 1988

Bruhn PS, Howes DH. Service line management: New opportunities for nursing executives. *Journal of Nursing Administration.* 16:6, 13, 1986

Cameron KS, Whetten DA. Perceptions of organizational effectiveness over organizational life cycles. *Administrative Science Quarterly.* 26, 524, 1981

Campbell JP. On the nature of organizational effectiveness. In: Goodman PS, Dennings JM, eds. *New Perspectives on Organizational Effectiveness.* San Francisco: Jossey-Bass, 1979, 36–39

Cummings LL. Emergence of the instrumental organization. In: Goodman PS, Pennings JM, eds. *New Perspectives in Organizational Effectiveness.* San Francisco: Jossey-Bass, 1977, 56–62

Daft RL. *Organization Theory and Design,* 3rd ed. St. Paul, MN, West, 1989

Deal TD, Kennedy AA. *Corporate Cultures: The Rites and Rituals of Corporate Life.* Reading, MA, Addison-Wesley, 1982

Edwardson SR. Productivity. In: Sullivan EJ, Decker PJ, eds. *Effective Management in Nursing.* Menlo Park, CA, Addison-Wesley, 1988

Edwardson SR, Bahr J, Serote M. Patient classification and management information systems as adjuncts to patient care delivery. In: Myer GG, Madden MJ, Lawrenz E, eds. *Patient Care Delivery Models.* Rockville, MD, Aspen, 1990, 293–313

Etzioni A. *Modern Organizations.* Englewood Cliffs, NJ, Prentice-Hall, 1964

Fayol H. *General and Industrial Administration.* New York: Pitman, 1949

Georgopoulos B, Tannenbaum AS. A study of organizational effectiveness. *American Sociological Review,* 22:534–540, 1957

Gibson JL, Ivancevich JM, Donnelly JH. (1988). *Organizations: Behavior, Structure, Process.* Plano, TX: Business Publications, 1988

Giovannetti P, Burkhalter B. *Test and monitor patient classification systems.* Minneapolis, MN, Health Management Systems, 1988

Giovannetti P, Johnson JM. A new generation patient classification system for nursing. *Journal of Nursing Administration.* 20:5, 33, 1990

Guzzo RA. (1988). Productivity research: Reviewing psychological and economic perspectives. In: Campbell JP, Campbell RJ, Associates, eds. *Productivity in Organizations: New Perspectives from Industrial and Organizational Psychology.* San Francisco: Jossey-Bass, 1988, 63–81

Hall RH. *Structures, Processes and Outcomes.* Englewood Cliffs, NJ, Prentice-Hall, 1987

Hesterly SC, Robinson M. Nursing in a service line organization. *Journal of Nursing Administration.* 18:11, 32, 1988

Hirsch PM. Organizational effectiveness and the institutional environment. *Administrative Science Quarterly.* 20, 327, 1975

Hopeman RJ. *Production: Concepts, Analysis, Control.* Columbus, OH, Charles E Merrill, 1976

Ilgen DR, Klein HJ. Individual motivation and performance: Cognitive influences on effort and choice. In: Campbell JP, Campbell RJ, Associates, eds. *Productivity in Organizations: New Perspectives from Industrial and Organizational Psychology.* San Francisco, Jossey-Bass, 1988, 143–176

Jelinek RC, Dennis LC. *A review and evaluation of nursing productivity.* DHEW Publication No. HRA 77–15. Washington, DC, US Government Printing Office, 1976

Kast FE, Rosenzweig. *Organization and Management: A Systems and Contingency Approach,* 4th ed. New York: McGraw-Hill, 1985

Mayer GG, Madden MJ, Lawrenz E. *Patient Care Delivery Models.* Rockville, MD, Aspen, 1990

Miles RH. *Macro Organizational Behavior.* Santa Monica, CA, Goodyear, 1980

Overton P, Schneck R, Hazlett CB. An empirical study of the technology of nursing subunits. *Administrative Science Quarterly.* 22, 203, 1977

Packer MB. Productivity analysis using subjective output measures: A perceptual mapping approach for "knowledge work" organizations. In: Dogramaci A, Adam, NR, eds. *Managerial Issues in Productivity Analysis.* Boston, Kluwer-Nijhoff, 1985, 161–181

Pfeffer J. Power and resource allocation in organizations. In Staw BM, Salancik GR, eds. *New Directions in Organizational Behavior.* Chicago: St Clair Press, 1977, 235–266

Riley W, Schaefers V. Costing nursing services. *Nursing Management.* 4, 40, 1985

Schermerhorn JR. *Management for Productivity.* New York, John Wiley & Sons, 1986

Sovie MD, Tarcinale MA, Vanputee AW, Stunden AE. Amalgam of nursing acuity, DRGs and costs. *Nursing Management.* 16:3, 22, 1985

Sullivan EJ, Decker PJ. *Effective Management in Nursing,* 3rd ed. Menlo Park, CA, Addison-Wesley, 1992

Suver JD, Neumann BR. *Management Accounting for Health Care Organizations.* Oak Brook, IL: Hospital Financial Management Association, 1981

Thompson JD. *Organizations in Action.* New York: McGraw-Hill, 1967

Vanderzee H, Glusko G. DRGs, variable pricing, and budgeting for nursing services. *Journal of Nursing Administration.* 14:5, 11, 1984

Warner DM, Holloway DC. *Decision Making and Control for Health Administration: The Management of Quantitative Analysis.* Ann Arbor, MI, Health Administration Press, 1978

Yuchtman E, Seashore SE. A systems resource approach to organizational effectiveness. *American Sociological Review.* 32, 891, 1967

Zander K. Nursing case management: Strategic management of cost and quality outcomes. *Journal of Nursing Administration.* 18:5, 23, 1988

Zander K. Managed care and nursing case management. In: Mayer GG, Madden MJ, Lawrenz E, eds. *Patient Care Delivery Models,* Rockville, MD, Aspen, 1990, 37–61

Organizing the Organization

CHAPTER 7

Organizational Structure and Environment

James P. Cooney
Philip J. Decker
Sandra M. Handley

> ## Key Concept List
>
> Organizational structure
> Dimensions of organizational structure
> Bureaucracy
> Health care organizational structures
> Organizational environment

Organizational structure is the framework through which resources, authority and responsibility are allocated to meet organizational goals and objectives. Environment is the atmosphere in which the structure functions. There are two types of environment within which all institutions must function: the environment external to the institution which includes the forces of society, politics, economics, and geography; and the internal environment of the institution which includes the organizational culture (Daft, 1988). (Organizational culture is discussed in Chapter 5.)

Both structure and environment can be the causes of and the cures for the nurse executive's problem of providing individualized and flexible nursing care in a highly structured, inflexible and impersonal environment. The effective nurse executive must identify which variables are resolvable and which are not, at least within the scope of current authority and responsibility. The effective executive will not battle every problem but will prioritize targets by their resolvability. Understanding the relationship between structure, environment, and individual productivity is essential for the nurse executive.

Daft and Steers (1986) discuss two dimensions of organizations: *contextual* and *structural.* Contextual dimensions are basic organizational properties that are stable over time and characterize the entire organization and its environment. They represent the important contingencies under which the organization operates and, therefore, contextual dimensions control organizational design. Structural dimensions are tailored to the organizations's contextual dimensions. Structural dimensions are the internal characteristics of the organization or the organizational design. Both contextual and structural dimensions are important in understanding organizations and improving their design. Contextual dimensions constitute the basic factors from which organizational function emerges, the ''givens'' in which structural dimensions must be developed. Structural dimensions are the building blocks which define the organizational shape and form.

CONTEXTUAL DIMENSIONS OF ORGANIZATIONS

According to Daft and Steers (1986), the three contextual dimensions of an organization are: size, organizational technology, and environment. *Size* is the magnitude of the organization and is typically measured by the number of employees. Other measures of size include the number of divisions and financial variables such as total sales and amount of assets.

Organizational technology is the production process used in the organization; it is sometimes termed core technology. Technology includes individuals' actions, knowledge and machines. In a service industry, people directly change organizational inputs into organizational outputs. In a health care organization, the machinery, knowledge, and action of health care workers are used to improve the health status of their clients. Technology varies from simple and routine to highly sophisticated processes. *Environment* includes all elements outside the boundaries of the organization. The environment contains several important elements of concern to the health care organization—for example, competitors, government regulators, suppliers, clients, family, the community, and general economic conditions. The environmental context varies from stable to rapidly changing or uncertain.

STRUCTURAL DIMENSIONS OF ORGANIZATIONS

Daft and Steers (1986) also identified six structural dimensions of organizations: formalization, complexity, span of control, centralization, professionalism, and personnel configuration. *Formalization* is the existence of written rules (policies) and procedures. In health care settings, these cover topics ranging from protecting clinical personnel from infectious disease to providing services to the medically indigent.

Complexity is the magnitude of subdivision of an organization into comparatively homogeneous parts or departments. Health care examples include the number of medical subspecialty units resulting from the scope of institutional clinical services, and a hierarchy of client care units such as intensive care, acute care, and self-care. *Span of control* is the number of subordinates managed by a single manager; for example, the number of staff nurses reporting to a nurse manager. *Centralization* involves the distance from top management that authority for decision making rests—for example, the authority to hire or fire personnel. *Professionalism* describes the distribution of educational levels among the work force such as the number of staff for which specialized education and/or training is needed to qualify for their positions. Professionalism is high when employees require long periods of training or when advanced degrees are required for entry to practice in the health care setting.

Personnel configuration is the comparative size of the work force distributed among professional, clerical, and administrative units. This is usually measured by ratios. The administrative ratio is the ratio of employees devoted to top administration to all employees. The clerical ratio indicates the clerical support needed to maintain the formal documentation and communication within the organization. The professional staff ratio indicates the amount of specialized technical staff used in the organization. An overall indirect/direct ratio may be used to show organizational efficiency regarding the percentage of employees engaged in direct production or service activities versus the percentage engaged in support activities.

INTERACTIONS BETWEEN CONTEXTUAL AND STRUCTURAL DIMENSIONS

There are interactions between contextual and structural dimensions. For example, organizational size, a contextual dimension, affects employee professionalism, a structural dimension. This is particularly true with professionals such as nurses. Increased organizational size is associated with greater conflict between bureaucratic and professional factions. Increasing size and bureaucracy occur as an organization produces a greater division of labor and more rules, both of which cause conflict between the organization and the autonomous employee. A large health care organization with a strong division of labor employs professionals such as physicians, nurses, and allied health personnel; however, sometimes the division goes too far and tasks are reduced to their smallest component. Division of tasks and the resulting routinization of the work may not utilize professional skills appropriately.

Financial pressures also force job components from one professional group to another, such as from physicians to nurses, or from nurses to ancillary personnel. Reassigning tasks from one group to another may cause conflict. Also, a seemingly routine task may require judgment or a higher knowledge level that the less educated group does not possess. The organizational response to conflict is often to increase formalization to standardize group behavior; however, highly trained professionals resent close supervision. Thus, the mixing of the professional norms and bureaucratic rules results in increased conflict. This is common in health care organizations.

Mintzberg (1979) distinguishes the *machine bureaucracy* from the *professional bureaucracy*. A machine bureaucracy is a mechanized system with high formalization and specialization. Employees in the production core usually are not professionalized. Yet, in a professional bureaucracy, the production core is composed of professionals. Hospitals, universities and consulting firms are examples of professional organizations. These organizations must be smaller, with fewer rules, and more employee autonomy. It appears that health care organizations are moving from machine to professional bureaucracy. This will be an overriding issue in the future reorganization of health care organizations.

The structural dimensions of organizations will closely parallel characteristics of the classic bureaucracy discussed in the subsequent section. These dimensions both independently and interdependently affect organizational performance. As opposed to contextual dimensions, structural elements are within control of management both initially and throughout the life of the organization. This difference in managerial control of structural over contextual elements means that the executive can most directly affect the structural dimensions. Contextual dimensions are much more difficult to affect directly.

FORM AND FUNCTION

In architecture, physical form follows or emerges from function. A warehouse or automobile assembly line each have its own unique physical shape or arrangement of people, resources, authority, and responsibly. Both physical and conceptual form must logically emerge from and support the functions of an organization.

The dictum of form follows function is applicable in health care in both a physical and conceptual sense. A health care organization's structure evolves from the goals of the organization and the functions which govern and accomplish the goals. All health care organizations have certain common functions (eg, patient care) which define the general shape or form of the organizational structure. Organizational structure therefore is critical to organizational performance—the effectiveness of the organization.

Technically, freedom exists in health care, as in most industries, for organizational form to follow function. In reality, however, health care organizations have limited their options in terms of the function- structure-effectiveness relationship. Until prospective payment systems were implemented in 1984, most health care institutions lived in a certain, static environment and had little reason to seek the innovation in shaping health care organizations that most are now seeking. Consequently, until very recently, hospitals often retained archaic structural forms and the major concern was the degree of bureaucratization. Reflecting on the multiple components required to manage the many services of a health care organization effectively underscores the necessity for subsystems and departmentalism. The necessity for using bureaucratic structure and form into the twenty-first century is not apparent, however. Consequently, we discuss classic bureaucratic organizational structure and then modern structures.

CHARACTERISTICS OF BUREAUCRACIES

The relationship of health services to bureaucratic structure is emphasized by Max Weber (1947) who was a manager of hospital services in Germany, and first labeled, defined, and analyzed bureaucratic structures. Many of his examples are drawn from the health care environment. Weber was one of the first authors who wrote about organizations. He conceptually described the following characteristics of bureaucracies in an attempt to show how modern (circa 1879) organizations should be developed. Following are concepts and their explanations of classic bureaucratic organizational structures.

Division of Labor

Each organizational member should have a clearly defined task and scope of authority and responsibility. No other individual in the structure will have the same domain of effort. Members will not interfere with the work assigned to another individual. This characteristic is perhaps the most basic as it sets forth the rationale for evolution of the individual "bureaus" or departments within the larger structure and functional structure (the most common structure of hospitals).

Nursing service is an excellent example of division of labor. Within the larger nursing service department there are multiple nursing units performing similar functions; yet each has a clearly defined clinical domain such as medicine, surgery, or pediatrics. Nursing units and their personnel do not interfere with the work effort of other units.

Hierarchy of Authority

Each labor division is supervised by a higher level of authority to ensure effective individual performance and consistency with organizational goals. A pyramid of authority results. In a typical nursing service department, the nursing unit is the smallest organizational unit within the department. The members of the unit are normally arranged in a superior–subordinate pattern; that is, those with greater delegated authority are higher on the supervisory ladder. Each unit is grouped with similar units into a larger organizational/supervisory unit. Such clusters continue to occur until the office of ultimate authority is reached—the nursing administrator. As nursing requires more autonomous decision making, this rigid bureaucratic hierarchy will be less successful; its rigidity and authoritarianism can overpower the autonomy and critical thinking needed by professional nurses in their daily practice.

The skills most critical for advancing up the supervisory ladder are managerial skills. This presents problems in an organizational structure developed to centralize clinical or technical skill. The skills that make a good clinician do not assure high skill as a manager. Yet, in management, there is less need for clinical nursing skills and more need for management skills.

System of Rules

A system of rules is developed and maintained to ensure each department performs predictably. In a health care organization, many services or components of services function continuously. Predictability of performance must occur uniformly throughout the organization because of the number of subsystems involved, the continual change in personnel, and the organizational distance of the individual from the ultimate authority.

Predictability of performance cannot be guaranteed under oral agreements. Expectations can be transmitted verbally and compliance can be observed but this will not guarantee predictable performance. Monitoring and evaluation of performance are necessary to maintain a consistent system of rules. The bureaucratic concept promotes standardization and predictability but does not allow for independent clinical judgments. As a result, conflict can ensue.

System of Records

Systematic records are established to provide continuity of action, an ''organizational memory,'' and a baseline for organizational evaluation. The two clearest examples of records systems in health care are the client's chart and the accounting records of the organization. The chart provides continuity of action among clinical personnel involved in client care. Many clinicians do not communicate with each other directly so the chart becomes the means of communication. Accounting records provide a true organizational memory and a critical mechanism through which to manage financial aspects of the organization.

Promotion on the Basis of Technical Competence

Qualification based on performance is required for both initial appointment and promotion. As previously noted, promotion on technical competence presents problems in a health care organization. Technical skills are a requisite for upward mobility but managerial skills are more important. This skill transference is not theoretically tolerated within the bureaucratic model. Health care organizations have attempted to develop career ladders that promote nurses without moving them away from patient care which is their area of expertise and source of gratification. Many clinical specialist roles have been usurped into management roles due to current economic constraints.

Impersonality of Relationships

To ensure fair and equitable service, impersonal relationships between client and employee and employee and employer are required in bureaucracies. This characteristic requires managerial ability to walk a thin line between equity among clients or personnel and effectively meeting individual needs. This perhaps is the heart of the managerial conflict within the bureaucracy of health care service.

Implications of Bureaucratic Theory

Many health care organizations can be fairly characterized as bureaucracies. However, the ''goodness of fit'' of health care to the concept is not strong because inherent characteristics of bureaucracy work against the effective delivery of health care. The often urgent nature of the health care service requiring so-called obedience with alacrity may be at odds with the rules required in bureaucracy.

Beside problems with the bureaucratic concept, there are inherent characteristics of many health care organizations that further complicate use of the pure bureaucratic model. The broad spectrum of professional skills required for the diversity of health care services complicates hierarchial decision making and increases interdepartmental confusion and conflict. Also, the large numbers of employees continuously required mandates supervision and yet such supervision may preclude a reasonable span of control and professionalism given the nature of clinical work. In addition, the continuous nature of nursing expands the service spectrum and the supervisory hierarchy often into an irrational organizational structure. Requiring predictable performance with a labor intensive work force such as nursing can result in failure of one or both outcomes; at other times they can be mutually exclusive.

Classical organizational theory suggests that a bureaucracy is necessary in large organizations. The bureaucratic form was developed to help organizations grow larger and more efficient. Rules, division of labor, and written records help management control the organization and increase its effectiveness. Bureaucratic structure provides control and coordination of large systems but bureaucratic characteristics are associated with slower responses to external change. Bureaucracy provides security for individuals and protects employees from capricious supervisory behaviors.

In modern society the term bureaucracy has a negative connotation and connotes having too many rules, too much paperwork, too many routine tasks and of being too rigid and inflexible. Employee behavior doesn't meet client needs but rather the needs of the bureaucracy. In bureaucracies, employees are often treated in an impersonal manner and they may feel constrained by rules and procedures. Jobs may become unchallenging, however, and employees may suffer job dissatisfaction and alienation. This form has many disadvantages in the twentieth and twenty-first century, especially in service industries.

Deciding which structure promotes highest efficiency and performance is often a matter of fit. Small organizations perform better with less bureaucracy, while large organizations perform better with more bureaucratic structure. Poor fit between bureaucratic structure and organizational size has been demonstrated in recent years in the acquisition of smaller companies and hospitals by larger, more bureaucratic corporations. The larger organization imposes its bureaucratic characteristics on the small firm resulting in significant problems and decreased efficiency in the smaller firm.

The optimal organizational structure integrates organizational goals, size, technology, and environment. Structural reorganization often results from changes in one or more of these four factors. When organizational structure is aligned with organizational needs, it is imperceptible. When structure is not aligned with organizational needs, organizational response to environmental change is diminished; delayed, overlooked, or low quality decisions are made; conflict results; and decreased organizational performance occurs. Organizational structure is an important tool through which managers can increase organizational efficiency. Thoughtful reorganization should not be avoided.

MODERN ORGANIZATIONAL STRUCTURES

Daft and Steers (1986) have discussed thoroughly the different structures found in modern organizations. Following is a summary of their examination of organizations.

Basically, all organizations fall within one of the four structures described and most health care institutions are functionally departmentalized. Furthermore, one can discuss the degree of bureaucracy in each structural form. Yet, bureaucracy ''fits'' best with the functional form and tends to lessen the effectiveness of the more complex forms. The environment of the organization also plays a part in the degree of bureaucracy and is discussed separately. Consequently, one has a complex contingency model where structure, environment and degree of bureaucracy may determine organizational or subsystem effectiveness independently of managerial skill or effort. We have discussed bureaucracy; let us now discuss organizational structure.

Functional Structure

In functional structures, employees are grouped in departments by task, with similar tasks in the same group, similar groups in the same department, and similar departments report to the same manager (see Fig 7–1). In a functional structure, all nursing tasks are under nursing service and the same is true of other functional areas. Functional structure is sometimes called a centralized structure because the decisions are made at the top of the organization and implemented down the pyramid. The functional structure tends to centralize decision making because the functions converge at the top of the organization.

The functional structure works best in small to medium-sized organizations with few products. Functional structure is used where technology is routine and where primary interdependence is between people within functions. Also, it works best when the environment is stable since activities are separated by functions. Difficult coordination across functions and slow response time, which are the disadvantages of functional structures, are not as critical in small stable environments. Functional structure also works best when the organizational goals require internal efficiency, high quality service, and technical specialization, such as in health care organizations.

Functional organizations use scarce resources efficiently because common tasks are grouped together for economy of scale. Employees are pooled by skill and no duplication of personnel or resources occurs. Functional structure simplifies training since employees in a department perform similar activities. Career progression is easier and promotion can be based on functional skill development. Employees identify with the department and work to excel in the functional activities. Decisions are centralized (see Table 7–1).

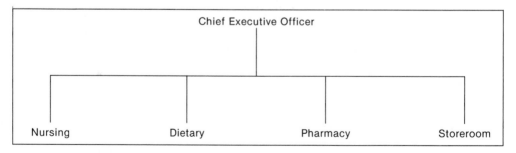

Figure 7–1. Functional Structure

TABLE 7–1. CONTEXT, STRENGTHS, AND WEAKNESSES FOR FUNCTIONAL DEPARTMENTATION

When to Use
1. Stable, certain environment
2. Small-medium size
3. Routine technology, interdependence within functions
4. Goals of efficiency, technical quality

Strengths
1. Efficient use of resources
2. In-depth skill development
3. Career progress based on functional expertise
4. Central decisions and direction
5. Excellent coordination within functions

Weaknesses
1. Poor coordination across functions
2. Decisions pile on top
3. Slow response, little innovation
4. Responsibility for performance difficult to pinpoint
5. Limited general management training

Source: Adapted from Robert Duncan, "What Is the Right Organization Structure?: Decision Tree Analysis Provides the Answer," *Organizational Dynamics*, Winter, 1979 (New York: AMACOM, a division of American Management Association, 1979), p. 429.

The functional structure has several weaknesses. Coordination across functions is poor; employees identify themselves with functions and are reluctant to cooperate with other departments. Decisions also can pile up at the top and overload senior managers who may be less informed regarding day to day operations. Responses to the external environment that require cross-function coordination are slow. The responsibility for performance is often difficult to analyze. The contribution of each department to meeting organizational goals may not be identified. General management training is limited because most employees move up the organization within functional departments. Most health care organizations meet many but not all of the criteria for a functional structure; most, however, have such a structure.

Self-contained Unit Structure

Self-contained unit structures also are called product line structures, and in nursing, service line structure. A self-contained unit structure means that all functions needed to produce a product or service are grouped together in an autonomous division. In functional structures, structure is departmentalized by resource or task; in a self-contained unit, it is structured by output (see Fig 7–2). Most large organizations contain some self-contained units. A large health care organization that acquires a smaller clinic may operate it as a self-contained unit. In order to be a true self-contained unit structure, however, *all units must be so organized*. The self-contained unit structure is decentralized and the units can be based on product, service, geographical mainte-nance, location, or type of customer.

Self-contained unit structure is preferred in situations where a functional struc-

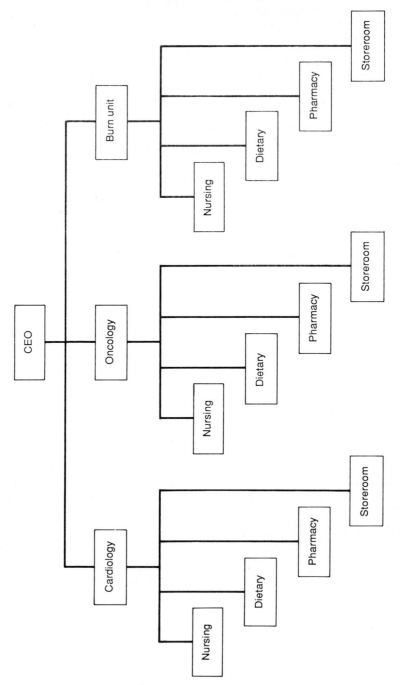

Figure 7-2. Self-contained Unit Structure

ture is inappropriate. The organization must be large and complex so it can be subdivided into divisions with responsibilities for specific services, markets, geographical areas, or products. Large organizations can assign the same activity to several self-contained units. Furthermore, the product structure is more amenable to change because all functions involved in a product or service are located in that division. Consequently, the self-contained unit structure is extremely appropriate when environmental uncertainty is high and the organization requires frequent adaptation and innovation to its environment (see Table 7–2).

One of the strengths of the self-contained unit structure is its potential for rapid change in unstable environments since each division is relatively small and product-focused and therefore, more flexible. Independent divisions can change to meet individual markets. Since each division is specialized and outputs can be tailored, high client satisfaction can be achieved. Also, customers know which division to contact to resolve problems. High coordination across functions occurs and employees identify with the unit and compromise or collaborate with other unit functions to meet unit goals and reduce conflict. Service goals receive priority under this organizational structure because employees see the product line as the primary source of their organization. The goals of production or client satisfaction, therefore, take priority.

Self-contained unit structures have several weaknesses relevant to health care. The major weakness is duplication of resources such as dietary, radiology, personnel, and nursing in each service line unit. Self-contained units do not provide good technical training and specialization because of the small size and range of the functional area. It is difficult to coordinate across product lines in a self-contained unit structure; divisions operate independently and often compete. In a typically functionally or-

**TABLE 7–2. CONTEXT, STRENGTHS, AND WEAKNESSES
FOR SELF-CONTAINED UNIT STRUCTURE**

When to Use
1. Unstable, uncertain environment
2. Large size
3. Technological interdependencies between functions
4. Goals of product specialization, innovation

Strengths
1. Fast change in an unstable environment
2. Client focus and satisfaction
3. High coordination between functions
4. Responsibility and control for multiple products
5. Develops general managers
6. Product goal emphasis

Weaknesses
1. Duplication of resources
2. Less technical specialization and expertise
3. Poor coordination across product lines
4. Less top management control

Source: Adapted from Robert Duncan, "What Is the Right Organization Structure?: Decision Tree Analysis Provides the Answer," *Organizational Dynamics,* Winter, 1979 (New York: AMACOM, a division of American Management Association, 1979), p. 429.

ganized hospital, each service line (which was independent and autonomous) has its own nursing staff and competes with other service lines with their nursing staff. Finally, since the organization is decentralized, top managers often feel they have lost control and the ability to influence the organization's direction. Central management acts more as a holding company or corporate consulting firm.

Hybrid Structure

When an organization grows, it typically organizes some self-contained units, although not all, and the result is a hybrid organization. Such an organization has functional departments that are centralized and product divisions that are decentralized (see Fig 7–3).

The strengths of the hybrid structure are that it provides simultaneous coordination within product divisions while maintaining the quality of each function, greater alignment between corporate and division goals, and the organization can adapt to the environment and still maintain efficiency. The organization can obtain economy of scale by centralization, and adaptability and innovation within functions by making them self-contained.

Hybrid structures have two basic weaknesses. One is the conflict between top administration and divisions. Top administrators typically do not have line authority over functional divisions, yet they must coordinate and influence their activities. Second, managers often resent administrators' intrusions. The buildup of large corporate staffs to oversee divisions and provide functional coordination across divisions puts increasing pressure on the product units. See Table 7–3 for uses, strengths and weaknesses of hybrid structures.

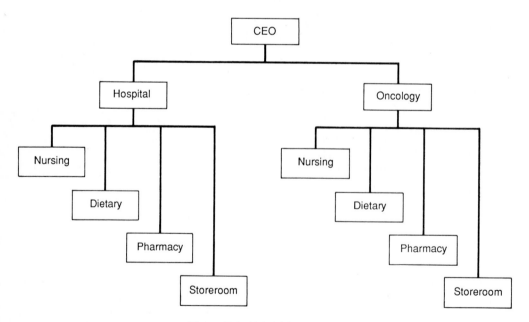

Figure 7–3. Hybrid Structure

TABLE 7-3. CONTEXT, STRENGTHS, AND WEAKNESSES FOR HYBRID STRUCTURES

When to Use
1. Unstable environment, especially in customer/competitor sectors
2. Large size
3. Technological interdependencies with both functions and product lines
4. Goals of product specialization and adaptation, plus efficiency in some functions

Strengths
1. Provides coordination within and between product divisions
2. Alignment between corporate and division goals
3. Helps organization attain adaptability in some departments and efficiency in others

Weaknesses
1. Conflict between corporation and divisions
2. Administrative overhead

Source: Adapted from Robert Duncan, "What Is the Right Organization Structure?: Decision Tree Analysis Provides the Answer," *Organizational Dynamics*, Winter, 1979 (New York: AMACOM, a division of American Management Association, 1979), p. 429.

Matrix Structures

The matrix organization is the most unique structure and is rare because of its complexity. When organizations find that neither functional, product line, or hybrid structures work, they often organize into a matrix. The unique aspect of a matrix is that both product and functional structures are implemented simultaneously (see Fig 7-4). Rather then separate functional and product structures, this structure overlaps both.

In a matrix structure, separate executives are responsible for each side of the matrix. One is responsible for functional tasks; the other for products or services. Within the matrix, departments and their heads report to both the functional and the product manager. They may receive conflicting demands from the matrix managers and often must resolve the conflict themselves. These two-boss department heads must be willing to work together and negotiate to solve problems. Matrices tend to exist where there are strong outside pressures for a dual organizational focus on product and function.

The matrix is appropriate in an environment that is highly uncertain, changes frequently, but also requires organizational expertise. It is typically seen in large organizations with extensive resources. (This may be a factor in its rarity in health care organizations.) The matrix also is seen in organizations with nonroutine technologies and high interdependence within and between functions.

The matrix structure enables an organization to meet demands from two sectors in its environment, especially product and functional demands. It provides for flexible use of resources within the organization. These resources can be allocated across several product lines. The structure adapts to environmental change and provides opportunities for the development of general management skills.

One of the major weaknesses of the matrix structure is the dual authority which can be frustrating and confusing for departmental managers and employees. The dual lines of authority can lead to interpersonal as well as role conflict. Excellent interpersonal skills are required for the managers involved. The implementation of a matrix

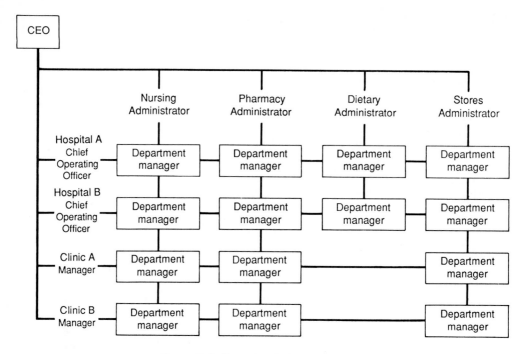

Figure 7–4. Example of Matrix Structure

structure usually requires human relations training in confrontation and conflict resolution skills. The matrix is time consuming because frequent meetings are required to resolve problems and conflicts and will not work unless participants can see the big organizational picture over their own functional area. Finally, if a matrix is implemented and the dual pressures do not continue, the side of the matrix more closely aligned with organizational objectives becomes more dominant. See Table 7–4 for the uses, strengths, and weaknesses of the matrix structure.

When complex structures such as hybrid or matrix structures are implemented, the organization must include integrating mechanisms in the organizational structure. Integrating structures are those that enhance coordination across departmental boundaries. These may not be apparent on the organizational chart, but they include information systems both written and computerized, planning meetings, schedules, liaison roles, ad hoc task forces, and permanent task forces for interdepartmental coordination. Especially useful is an integrating position, a full-time person or department to integrate activities of departments.

STRUCTURES UNIQUE TO HEALTH CARE

The organizational structure of the typical health care organization differs from both the straight bureaucratic model of Weber (1947) and the modern organizational structures of the very large, complex product-producing organizations as described. The

TABLE 7-4. CONTEXT, STRENGTHS, AND WEAKNESSES OF MATRIX STRUCTURE

When to Use
1. Very uncertain, shifting environment
2. Medium-large size
3. Nonroutine technology, high interdependence
4. Dual goals of product and functional specialization

Strengths
1. Can manage dual demands from environment
2. Flexible, efficient use of scarce resources
3. Adaptation and innovation
4. Development of functional and general management skills

Weaknesses
1. Dual authority cause frustration and confusion
2. High conflict
3. Time consuming
4. Special training required
5. Difficult to maintain power balance

Source: Adapted from Robert Duncan, "What Is the Right Organization Structure?: Decision Tree Analysis Provides the Answer," *Organizational Dynamics,* Winter, 1979 (New York: AMACOM, a division of American Management Association, 1979), p. 429.

typical health care organizational structure is the result of historical isolation and the complex relationships that exist between the formal authority of the health care organization and the authority of the medical profession. Consequently, a health care organization frequently has parallel structures rather than one organizational structure. Typically, the medical staff is separate and autonomous from the organization.

This results in an organizational dilemma: two lines of authority. One line extends from the governing body to the chief executive officer (CEO) and then to the managerial structure; the other line extends from the governing body to the medical staff. These two intersect in departments such as nursing in which decision making includes both managerial and clinical elements. Health care organizations with a functional structure and separate medical governance are termed parallel structures (see Fig 7-5).

Another unique aspect of health care is the corporate structure. The corporate structure is a functional structure in which each manager has financial control and responsibility for an area. That area's survival depends on the manager's expertise with the budget. Organizations where directors have become vice-presidents have a corporate structure.

Many health care organizations are controlled by a governing body which sets objectives and policies to accomplish the organizational mission and also may determine the effectiveness of those policies. Boards are composed of a variety of members, some with expertise and some without. Most hospitals have a joint hospital committee which acts as liaison between hospital management and the governing body of the medical staff. This is sometimes called the triad of health care. This committee is usually small and tightly knit; it rarely includes nurses. It is not uncommon for the CEO to be a member of the board.

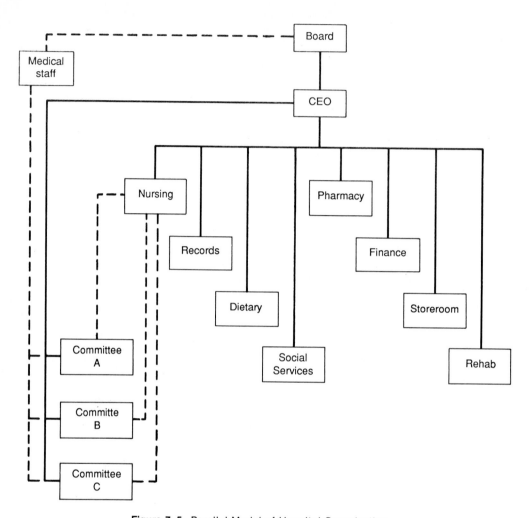

Figure 7-5. Parallel Model of Hospital Organization

Hospital organizations are changing because their environment is more fluid. A basic change is the increase in multi-institutional arrangements. Different types of arrangements include corporate ownership, cooperative services, consortiums, contract management, and consolidated multihospital cooperatives. These arrangements will radically change the face of health care over the next decades when, for the first time, health care will see large organizations control health provider units with different markets, geographical areas, and services. More business managers will be recruited to manage these entities.

Conceptually, the organizational structure of a health services institution results from an interplay between variables of a contextual nature (environment, size, and technology) and variables of a structural nature (complexity, decentralization, formalization), and its goal. Left to its own devices, the resulting structure often assumes the characteristics of a bureaucracy. Some of the theoretical aspects of a bureaucracy, however, are incompatible with effective delivery of health care services. Such incompatibility between the impersonality and inflexibility of bureaucracy and personal and flexible health care services presents a continual conflict to the nurse executive.

We have discussed all of the elements included in the basic contingency model explaining organizational effectiveness except the organization's environment. Most organizations are structured toward the product or service and goals pertaining to them. Yet, each organization exists in an environment which creates certain conditions, such as uncertainty, which interact with structure, degree of bureaucracy, and other contextual/structural variables.

ENVIRONMENT AND ITS IMPACT ON MANAGEMENT

Two types of environments affect an institution: external and internal. The former is generally beyond the control of management. The latter can be controlled to varying degrees by organizational management, however, the boundaries of such control are delineated by the authority of individual managers who can control areas they have the authority to change. External and internal environments both affect the functions and, correspondingly, the structure of an organization.

Organizational environment is vital to the success of an organization. Organizations are open systems; they must import resources and export outputs and services to the environment. To survive, the organization must interact with the environment efficiently. When environments are uncertain, the life of the organization is more difficult. Many environmental factors require difficult organizational responses, such as greater competition for employees, materials, and clients. Many structural features of organizations have developed to assist environmental adaptation and help them attempt to control their external environments.

The environment is divided into two parts, the task environment and the general environment (see Fig 7–6). The task environment includes the parts of an organization's external environment directly relevant to meeting organizational goals. The organization must respond or interact with these elements daily. In contrast, the general environment refers to those parts of the external environment that affect the organization indirectly or infrequently.

The task environment includes competitors, customers, work force and suppliers. Competitors are organizations in the same industry, customers are the clients the organization wants to attract, although clients also include physicians in most hospitals. The workforce includes current and potential employees. It also includes employee populations with a large supply of trained qualified personnel and those with a shortage of trained qualified personnel (such as nursing). The supplier sector includes organizations that supply raw materials and energy to the organization.

The general environment includes six sectors. The technological sector includes scientific and technological advances in industry and society. The government/political sector includes the legal system and laws concerning control, formation, and operation of organizations. The economic sector includes the economic health of the city,

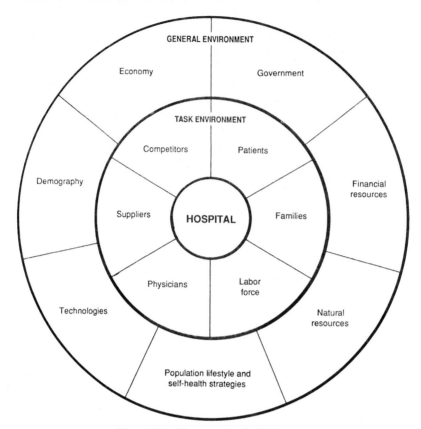

Figure 7-6. Elements in the Environment

county, region or country in which the organization operates. The cultural/demo-graphic sector includes the number, geographical distribution, and characteristics of the employee population. The financial sector pertains to the availability of money. The natural resources/geography sector includes the type, quantity and availability of natural resources and basic materials required for the organization.

EFFECT OF ENVIRONMENT ON NURSING SERVICE

The hallmark of the American health care system at its origins was "volunteerism." Each community developed its own response to the health problems of its citizens. While local needs may have been met, the local voluntary method provided no uni-formly common national access structure. In fact, a nonsystem emerged by virtue of its independent components. Today, local freedom to organize responses to health care problems has all but vanished. The erosion was gradual and in response to greater national controls and the inflation of health care costs as a proportion of the country's gross national product. Organizational structure and function are increasingly affected by external forces in the environment. Originally the health care contract was between the provider and the client. In the early 1930s a third party emerged and began to play a significant role in the contract; this third party originally was private health insurance, often "the Blues". In the 1960s, the federal government emerged as another third party. In the 1980s, due to the increasing cost of health care, business and industry emerged as a powerful fourth party in the relationship.

The service partnership began to expand in a series of tradeoffs. On one side were gains in quality and quantity of service for both the provider and the client. The other side was an increasing loss of autonomy. Today, third and fourth party payors increasingly control what occurs in health care settings. Such forces have an immediate effect on nursing departments and nurse executives.

Like "boxes within boxes" nursing services reside within a series of larger structures including those of the host institution and community. Nursing service obviously does not exist in a vacuum and is therefore subject to forces beyond the control of the nurse administrator. These forces must be understood to develop and maintain effective organizational response.

All organizations tend to feel uncertain about their environments, and consequently, health care organizations have become more cognizant of environments in the past decade. This uncertainty occurs because of three characteristics of an organization's environment: *change, complexity,* and *resource dependence.*

The speed of change is an increasing force on health care. Change is traumatic for an organization no matter how well planned. The degree of trauma can be controlled with management of and communication with the internal environment. However, despite such efforts, a significant element of uncertainty is introduced. Such uncertainty affects functions and organizational work units; personnel assignments are often restructured and reallocated to assure organizational survival in both economic and qualitative service terms. Greater stress is placed on management to adjust and function effectively.

An organization's environment may be simple or complex; complexity refers to the number of external elements and the degree of difference among these elements. Resource dependence occurs because all organizations must acquire and maintain external resources. The ability to acquire these resources depends on relationships with other organizations. Resource dependence is the relative power of the organization to obtain scarce resources from the environment or another organization.

All organizations must respond to environmental uncertainties by *internal change* or by *changing the external environment.* With internal change, the organization adapts its structure, patterns, or departments to the environment. Organizations can make a variety of internal changes in response to environment uncertainty. They can develop new departments or become more flexible. When organizations move toward increased flexibility, they become organic structures, a concept developed by Burns and Stalker (1961). These researchers found clear differences between organizational approaches that responded to changing external environments and those that did not and labeled them mechanistic or organic organizations (see Table 7–5). Mechanistic organizations have centralized control, extensive task specialization, and standardiza-

TABLE 7-5. COMPARISON OF MECHANISTIC AND ORGANIC SYSTEMS OF ORGANIZATION

Mechanistic	Organic
1. Tasks are highly fractionated and specialized: little regard paid to clarifying relationship between tasks and organizational objectives.	1. Tasks are more interdependent: emphasis on relevance of tasks and organizational objectives.
2. Tasks tend to remain rigidly defined unless altered formally by top management.	2. Tasks are continually adjusted and redefined through interaction of organizational members.
3. Specific role definition (rights, obligations, and technical methods prescribed for each member).	3. Generalized role definition (members accept general responsibility for task accomplishment beyond individual role definition).
4. Hierarchic structure of control, authority, and communication. Sanctions derive from employment contract between employee and organization.	4. Network structure of control, authority, and communication. Sanctions derive more from community of interest than from contractual relationship.
5. Communication is primarily vertical between superior and subordinate.	5. Communication is both vertical and horizontal, depending upon where needed information resides.
6. Communications primarily take form of instructions and decisions issued by superiors, of information and requests for decisions supplied by inferiors.	6. Communications primarily take the form of information and advice.
7. Insistence on loyalty to organization and obedience to superiors.	7. Commitment to organization's tasks and goals more highly valued than loyalty or obedience.

tion. Organic systems display decentralization, increased communication, and fewer rules. Mechanistic organizations are found in stable environments and organic organizations in dynamic environments.

Other responses to environmental uncertainty include boundary spanning roles or roles that coordinate the organization with other organizations. Boundary spanning roles look to the environment, protect core technology from external threat, and serve as gate keepers. Examples are market research analysts and nurse recruiters. In an organization with high differentiation (many departments doing different jobs), coordination across departments is difficult. So when differentiation is high, more coordination is needed. This coordination is defined as the quality of collaboration among departments to achieve unity of effort. Part of this integration takes place in planning, forecasting, budgeting, and other activities.

There are a number of means by which organizations attempt to change or control their environment. These include: (1) contractual arrangements, in which organizations develop legal contracts to ensure the predictable receipt of necessary resources; (2) coaptation, where organizations absorb individuals or organizations that threaten organizational goals; (3) advertising and public relations; (4) personnel exchanges such as sharing executives with organizational boards; (5) joint ventures; (6) political activity; (7) membership in trade associations; and, (8) mergers with other organizations.

Within health care organizations, there has never really been any environmental certainty. As a result both those who provide the professional technical services and those who manage are accustomed to dealing with individualized uncertainty. The recent change, however, is the removal of *institutional* certainty. The environment in which health care professionals function today is increasingly constrained by external forces. Change is frequent, rapid, and often incompatible with professional goals and sometimes, ethics. The manager must reduce the effect of such uncertainties to increase the ability of the work unit to function effectively. In a sense, that may be a definition of management: to function effectively in spite of problems.

SUMMARY

Despite all criticism, bureaucracies have a chameleonlike ability to change in order to survive problems and uncertain external environments. It is the ability for an organization to adapt, in a reciprocal manner, its goals, structure, size and environment that helps most survive. Each is unique and complex—and a significant conceptual problem for the nurse manager. Yet, the ability of the nurse manager to conceptualize this contingency and buffer staff from its forces is the most important element in assuring the efficiency of the core technology: patient care.

REFERENCES

Burns T, Stalker GM. *The Management of Innovations.* London, Tavistode Publishers Ltd, 1981

Daft, RL. *Management.* Chicago, Dryden Press, 1988

Daft RL, Steers RM. *Organizations.* Glenview, IL, Scott, Foresman & Company, 1988

Decker PJ, Rountree BH, Sullivan EJ. The nature of organizations in health care settings. In: Sullivan EJ,Decker PJ, eds. *Effective Management in Nursing,* 3nd ed. Redwood City, CA, Addison-Wesley, 1992

Herterley SC. Nursing in a service line organization. *Journal of Nursing Administration.* Nov 18:11, 32, 1988

Minzberg H. *The Structuring of Organizations.* Englewood Cliffs, NJ, Prentice-Hall, 1979

Weber M. *The Theory of Social and Economic Organizations,* trans by AM Henderson and T Parson. New York: Free Press, 1947

CHAPTER 8

Organizational Development and Change

Sandra M. Handley
James P. Cooney

Key Concept List

Organizational development
Change agents
Change processes
Process consultation
Quality of work life

In health care organizations, change is constant. Many forces encourage, promote, or mandate change. External forces, such as the federal government and third-party payors, and internal forces such as employee discontent, technological changes, and unions mandate organizational response to change. Organizations that successfully change and adapt are most effective.

Organizational development is concerned with designing and implementing organizational change in order to improve organizational functioning. This chapter provides an overview of current organizational development approaches and interventions and discusses their application to health care organizations and nursing.

THE PROCESS OF ORGANIZATIONAL DEVELOPMENT

Organizational development (OD) is based on two assumptions: An effective organization is able to solve its own problems; and an effective organization has both high productivity and high employee satisfaction (Harvey & Brown, 1988). The focus of OD is change that is planned and controlled by the organization. Such change can be directed, evaluated, and adjusted to maintain the change over time. Planned change differs from crisis driven changes, which are often unplanned, isolated, and thereby short-lived.

A theoretical perspective commonly used in planned change is the systems perspective of Kurt Lewin (1951) who suggests that change occurs in a system in a three-stage process: unfreezing, moving, and refreezing. Unfreezing occurs when the forces for change become stronger than the forces opposing change; these forces may be attitudes and/or external pressures. Unfreezing can occur by decreasing the opposing forces, increasing the change forces, or both. When the system is unfrozen, change can occur, and then the system "refreezes" into the changed version. Subsequent changes are repetitions of this process.

In operation, OD follows a nursing process-type format: assessment of the organization, identification or diagnosis of organizational problems, planned interventions, and evaluation of the interventions. Figure 8–1 illustrates the steps involved in the process.

THE CHANGE AGENT

An organizational development program may result in response to an identified problem within the organization such as decreased productivity, employee dissatisfaction, or the need for more current techniques. An OD program also may result from a change in management bringing a new vision to the organization. These can occur in the total organization or in one department such as nursing. The OD process is usually initiated by the chief executive of the organization or department in response to a problem or issue.

The initial step is to choose a change agent whose responsibility is to implement the program and manage the OD intervention. The change agent may be external or internal to the organization; each has advantages and disadvantages. An external change agent is an individual employed specifically to design and implement the

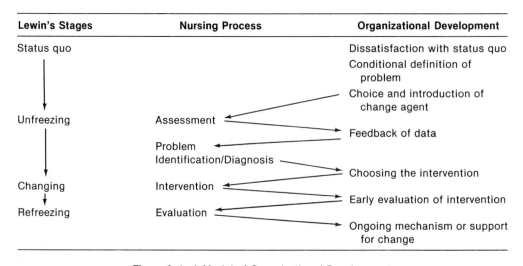

Figure 8-1. A Model of Organizational Development

OD program. The external change agent should be very experienced, objective, and unbiased concerning the organization. Since an early OD step is analysis of the organization, an external change agent may facilitate the assessment phase since an outsider may be more objective.

An internal change agent is an individual designated within the organization to manage the OD program. This may be an interim appointment. Some nursing organizations have a permanent position for such an individual (Hollefreund, Clark, & Wadsworth, 1986). The internal agent knows how the organization functions; however, this knowledge is biased by personal experiences. The internal change agent also has access to inside information and past experiences. Present concerns may affect the willingness of other employees to be honest and the change agent's ability to be objective.

An optimal compromise is a change agent team with both internal and external members. The internal member provides continuity and internal resources; the external member provides objectivity and authority. This collaboration expands the skills of the internal member and provides mutual support for both. When only one department is implementing change, an experienced change agent from another department may take the external role. Change agents vary on two dimensions: emphasis on productivity and emphasis on relationships. The optimal focus depends on the nature of the problem and the nature of the organization. An integrative style that includes both effectiveness and relationships is desirable, although difficult. Nurses in the change agent role can draw on their education and experiences which include both orientations; however, maintaining a balanced approach calls for experience.

ASSESSMENT

The first step in OD is to systematically assess the organization to describe current functioning and to define its problems and/or developmental needs. This begins with, but is not limited to, the problems initially defined by the program originator.

There are three assessment levels in an organization—the overall organization, the organization's subgroups or departments, and individual positions. Each level should be systematically assessed although the eventual intervention may focus on a particular level.

At the organizational level, assessment includes the organization's structure of departments, formal and informal departmental relationships, organizational resources in both personnel and finances, and the utilization of resources. Departmental assessment includes the group design, norms, member relationships, how the department is embedded in the organization, subgroups and their relationships, and the informal norms for those groups. Positions are assessed for the design and assessment of the group, its norms, and functioning. Positions can also be evaluated for skill variety, task identity and significance, autonomy, and feedback of results.

Since assessment is the first stage of the total process, the change agent has multiple goals for the assessment stage: (1) to obtain valid information concerning organizational functioning; (2) to develop a collaborative relationship with the organization;

and (3) to set the stage for constructive change. Four methods of assessment are commonly used—either singly or in combination—questionnaires, interviews, observations, and data from secondary sources. Each method has strengths and weaknesses.

Questionnaires are efficient; data from standardized questionnaires can be compared to other organizations or groups. Fixed choice items such as yes–no or Likert-type scales are easily analyzed. Questionnaires are particularly useful for large organizations or departments. A disadvantage is that the predetermined questions and categories do not allow for qualitative or individual responses.

Interviews allow a wider range of questions and build rapport resulting in more individualized data. Using a structured interview format, groups can be interviewed allowing a cross section of the organization or an intact work group to participate. These interviews generally focus on individual perceptions of organizational functioning. Interviews are time consuming both in actual interview time and in analysis time and they are subject to interviewer biases. This can be decreased by using standardized interview formats.

Observations include participant observation, videotaping, one-way viewing, or the counting of behaviors. Observations involve fewer inherent biases although collecting and coding observed data are time consuming.

Data from secondary sources such as organizational records can also be used, particularly data concerning absenteeism or productivity. Records are objective and can be quantified; however the change agent is limited to the data already collected and must assume its accuracy. It is important to interview the record keepers for the context in which the records are kept to determine systematic biases in the data. Records also may be an adjunct or a starting point for other data collection techniques.

Subject selection concerns from whom to collect data, how many, and how to select them. In a small organization, it may be possible to collect data from everyone. In a large organization this may be impractical and the change agent needs a sampling technique. Random sampling where all employees have an equal chance of being interviewed is one technique. Stratified random sampling where subjects are randomly selected within categories such as position level or department is another. It is important to interview a broad enough sample to identify a full range of issues and information.

Choice of assessment technique and subject selection are made by the change agent considering the type of organizational problem and the type of organization. The change agent must be able to apply any of the techniques skillfully and knowledgeably.

DEFINING THE PROBLEM(S)

Defining the problem, or diagnosis, is a systematic approach to understanding and describing the present performance of the organization by using the data collected. The goal is to identify problems and areas for improvement. Problems in organizations are usually related to or evidenced by decreased productivity, interpersonal issues, or a combination of both. Diagnosis ideally should be a collaborative process involving members of the organization *and* the change agent. Frequently the initially identified problem is a symptom rather than the real problem—eg, absenteeism may be defined as the problem when it is actually a symptom of employee dissatisfaction.

A common potential change agent error at this stage is premature diagnosis, making a diagnosis based on inadequate or biased information. This can occur when the change agent does not collect data from enough individuals or enough segments of the organization, when the initial problem definition is accepted at face value rather than examined more closely, or when the change agent has a particular theoretical orientation in which all problems are fitted. Since the intervention will be clearly based on the diagnosis, an inaccurate diagnosis results in inappropriate interventions.

The change agent team can validate their perceptions with each other. As the diagnosis evolves it may be useful to gather more data to confirm the diagnosis. When varied data sources result in the same conclusion, that conclusion is strengthened and validated.

FEEDBACK OF THE ASSESSMENT DATA

Feedback of data is an important step both in obtaining organizational cooperation and in developing a collaborative relationship. Initial planning should include how the data will be presented and to whom.

Quantitative data from questionnaires can be displayed using total scores, item means, and distributions; visual displays such as graphs and charts are particularly effective. Group scores can be compared with other segments of the organization or comparable groups in other settings. Qualitative data from interviews can be summarized into themes with frequency of responses in each category and categories of responses displayed. Representative quotes are an effective technique to exemplify common responses.

ASSESSING THE CHANGE FORCES

As the assessment progresses, the change agent needs to identify the organizational forces for and against change. Dissatisfaction with the status quo varies. In general, increased dissatisfaction results in increased readiness for change. If dissatisfaction is low, the change agent may need to increase it by providing new information, new ideas, or comparisons with other organizations. This can occur during feedback. Strategies to create readiness for change include: (1) sensitizing the organization to the pressures for change; (2) revealing discrepancies between current and desired states; and (3) conveying a shared vision of improved organizational functioning. External factors such as competition or technology may also be forces for change. The greater and more numerous the change forces, the more potential for change exists.

Resistance to change is certain and usually related to fear of the unknown or a threat to security. Employees should know why the change is suggested and the expected benefits for the organization and for the individual. Strategies for overcoming resistance to change include: (1) maintaining empathy for resisters and gathering data about actual and anticipated problems; (2) consistently communicating about how change will affect employees personally; and (3) including representatives of all employees on planning task forces.

The change agent also needs to assess the organizational climate for change. Information about past organizational changes and their implementation and results will be helpful in developing a strategy. In an organization with few recent changes, any change will be more difficult and require more preparation. If the change involves new technology or techniques, the education or sophistication of the employees may require evaluation.

Another component of the climate concerns the level of trust among employees and between employees and management. A successful intervention should benefit employees individually as well as the organization. A climate of distrust will make any intervention more difficult and less likely to succeed.

CHOOSING AN INTERVENTION

The type of intervention chosen depends on the type of problem, the type of organization, and the values of the organization. The intervention should be consistent with these factors to increase its success and should be chosen collaboratively by representatives of the organization and the change agent.

Interventions can be categorized by their focus on productivity or employee satisfaction and the organizational level affected: individual, group, or total organization. Three types of intervention are discussed here: *process interventions, technostructural interventions,* and *human resource management interventions.* While the intervention types are discussed separately, in practice, combinations of techniques are frequently used.

Process interventions focus on people in organizations and their interactions regarding communication, decision making, leadership, and group dynamics. Improving these interactions should result in both increased productivity and employee satisfaction. Process interventions at the individual or group level include sensitivity groups, process consultation, third-party interventions, and team building. Process interventions at the organizational level include survey feedback and normative approaches. These interventions focus on employee satisfaction and effective interactions at the group or organizational level.

Technostructural interventions focus on the structure of the organization and designing the structure to promote productivity and employee satisfaction. These interventions include organizational design and coordination, formal structure interventions, quality of work life programs, and work design interventions.

Human resource management interventions are aimed at managing employees in a manner that results in employee satisfaction and increased productivity. Interventions include goal setting, reward systems, career development, and stress management. These interventions are aimed primarily at the individual or small groups.

EVALUATION

Evaluation of the OD intervention occurs both during the intervention and at its completion. The evaluation during the intervention focuses on whether the specified intervention is actually occurring and whether it is occurring with sufficient strength. Problems may be related to insufficient preparation of organizational personnel or an unintended change in emphasis during implementation. Either issue, if discovered early enough, can be remedied by information or education.

Ongoing evaluation also attempts to determine the outcome of the intervention, whether the intervention appears to be meeting its goals. Again, if the outcome does not appear effective, it may be necessary to refocus the intervention or increase its strength. Persistent lack of positive outcome may call for a re-evaluation of the problem definition. Again, the earlier this discovery is made, the more effectively it can be addressed.

Evaluation at the end of the OD intervention focuses on whether the intervention met its goals and what mechanism is needed to maintain the change. This mechanism can be internal, where someone in the organization who is given responsibility for monitoring the changes made, or external, such as a periodic refresher workshop outside the organization.

The appropriate tools for evaluation are determined by the particular problem and intervention. The same types of data collected for assessment also may be collected and used for evaluation (questionnaires, interviews, observations, secondary sources). If an assessment instrument is appropriate for evaluation, pre- and post-intervention data can be compared. Since organizational problems usually concern employee satisfaction or productivity, these dimensions are important for evaluation. Multiple outcome measures along both dimensions are preferable when possible (see Chapter 29 on research).

ORGANIZATIONAL DEVELOPMENT INTERVENTIONS

These OD interventions involve the actual change that takes place after the organization is "unfrozen" and ready for change. An organizational problem may call for a combination of types of intervention.

Group Process Interventions

These interventions apply knowledge about group process to particular groups and situations. The goal is for individuals to learn about their behavior in a group and how that behavior contributes to the group's behavior in both the task and process aspects of the group—that is, the group aspects of getting the task done and the group processes involved. The overall goal is to increase the effectiveness of the individual's functioning in groups. Since most organizational and nursing functions occur in group settings, this knowledge should increase individual effectiveness in work groups.

Sensitivity groups. Sensitivity groups, or T-groups, are a process intervention focused on experientially teaching individuals about their interaction with other people in groups. This technique is most effective with groups of relative strangers. Sensitivity exercises with intact work groups have not been as effective in part because work groups have ongoing interpersonal processes that interfere with the focus on group process.

Organizational goals are more clearly met when the group focuses on tasks related to the work setting, for example, when a nurse manager group focuses on understanding their leadership style and its effect on others. While some sensitivity exercises are used in group teaching, the total sensitivity experience is rare in health care settings and replaced by other process interventions.

Process consultation. This intervention uses sensitivity group techniques with intact work groups. The goal is for the work group to understand its particular group processes. Frequently the change agent observes a group meeting and gives feedback. Particular group issues include roles and functions of group members, problem-solving processes, decision-making processes, group norms, and leadership. After identifying problematic interactions, interventions include teaching alternative communication techniques and helping the group differentiate issues that maintain the group process (process issues) from issues related to the actual work of the group (content issues). An effective group needs techniques for both process and content. The goal is to identify and teach the group techniques to increase its effectiveness. Although widely used, the effectiveness of this intervention in increasing work productivity has not been clearly shown (Schein, 1987; Kaplan, 1979).

Third-party intervention. This technique is used with interpersonal conflict that interferes with productivity between two or more persons within an organization. Dialogue with the involved parties and the change agent is used. Initially what triggered the conflict is identified and avoided, then limits are set on the conflict by rules for interactions between parties, and, lastly, the change agent helps the parties cope with the consequences of the conflict (see Chapter 24 on Conflict). The change agent can suggest coping techniques, such as reducing dependence on relationship, ventilating to friends, or other support. Resolution of the basic issues is desirable, if possible. The change agent's role is to remain neutral and unbiased, define problems with the individuals, help identify and clarify issues, and give feedback (Walton, 1987).

Team building. This popular intervention is used to build work groups and to improve teamwork and productivity. Team building is similar to process consultation but more tightly focused on the tasks and problem-solving abilities of the team. Team composition varies. Common examples are ad hoc groups focused on a particular issue, nurse-manager groups, and groups with a common manager, such as a nursing unit. Any group that needs to work together to accomplish a task is a candidate for team building. The first team task is to establish goals, clarify its purpose, and identify strengths and weaknesses. This may be done through an assessment tool or through participant observation by the change agent. Team building activities then focus on interventions to increase team effectiveness. Offsite meetings encourage the continuity necessary to complete team tasks. The team should develop processes for evaluating and maintaining its effectiveness. Research has been mixed on the results of team building (Dyer, 1987; Woodman & Sherman, 1980).

ORGANIZATIONAL PROCESS INTERVENTIONS

Group process can also be targeted to the total organization where the aim is improving communication, problem solving, and leadership for the entire organization or a major subsystem. Approaches for total organizations are variations of previously discussed techniques.

Survey Feedback

This intervention is part of the initial OD assessment and feedback process, however, it can also be an independent intervention when the additional step of problem solving and action planning is added. The data collected may be on attitudes or productivity. The total organization or involved department should be surveyed to increase the database and each employee's commitment to the process.

Usually feedback begins with top management. Each department gets feedback relevant to itself. When groups or departments are interdependent, it is important to share data between groups and to examine mutual issues. Ambiguity of purpose, distrust within the organization, and unwillingness to discuss particular topics decrease the effectiveness of survey feedback. The primary impact of survey feedback appears to be on attitudes. Survey feedback alone may not change behavior, but it can be a useful first step to further interventions (Cummings & Huse, 1989).

Organizational Confrontation

This process technique is useful in situations where the organization is under stress or there is a gap between management and the remainder of the organization. The process mobilizes problem-solving resources by identifying problems, setting priorities, and working on pressing problems. This all occurs in group settings. First, involved personnel are divided into small groups for an hour or more to identify problems; then the total group reconvenes and the small groups report. A master problem list is developed and arranged into categories. New small groups are formed to rank problems, suggest a plan, and again report back to the total group. This technique mobilizes the group and shares responsibility for the solutions. Organizational follow through is necessary to sustain the momentum. Periodic follow up on the status of the issues and solutions is crucial.

Intergroup Relations

This intervention uses group process techniques to resolve conflicts between departments, particularly interdependent departments. Both groups meet together, then each group separately makes a list of its attributes and the attributes of the other group. Then the two groups reconvene to compare lists. The separate groups then meet again to discuss discrepancies between the lists and why they exist. The groups again share their ideas concerning discrepancies and discuss a plan for reducing those discrepancies. The change agent should help the group decide on whether to focus on changing attitudes or behavior. The deciding factor should be the nature of the conflict itself.

Normative Approaches

Normative approaches, unlike most OD interventions, have predetermined outcomes. They are preplanned programs designed to promote or bring about particular types of organizational change that have been identified by the program developers. Two frequently used normative approaches are Likert's System 4 Management (Likert, 1967) and Grid Organization Development (Blake & Mouton, 1964). These approaches do not individualize the intervention to a particular organization; rather they are based on research and beliefs regarding organizational effectiveness. Their availability as preplanned programs allow an organization a clearer idea of the program they are purchasing.

Likert's System 4 Management. This format promotes a participative management approach with high levels of member involvement in decisions and goals. The system is designed around work groups, each of which is involved in goal setting, and decision making. Continuity across the organization is promoted by having group leaders at one level as group members at the next level so they are cognizant of current policies and organizational goals.

The beginning step of System 4 is questionnaire responses that develop a management profile of the organization and compares the organization to the optimal System 4. These data are shared with work groups using survey feedback techniques. Groups look at the difference between the current organization and the ideal and action plans are developed within the groups to move the organization toward the ideal. Likert suggests it takes 2 to 3 years for results to be seen. Some organizations have achieved success with the program; however, current research indicates the system may not be optimal in all organizations (Likert, 1967; Mosley, 1987).

Grid Organization Development. This program was developed by Blake and Mouton (1964) and is concerned with managerial style. According to the theory, the major barriers to organizational excellence are barriers to planning and communication which are symptoms of faulty management. The managerial grid assesses managers on two dimensions, productivity and interpersonal orientation (see Fig 8–2). An individual grid with both dimensions is developed for each manager. The 9,9 position, highest on productivity *and* interpersonal orientation is desirable; this manager strives to meet the needs of the organization and of the individual simultaneously.

The program begins with top management who are trained and then take each consecutive level through the training. This is followed by team and intergroup development activities. Next is the development of an ideal organizational model and plans for its implementation. Grid programs have been developed for a variety of profes-

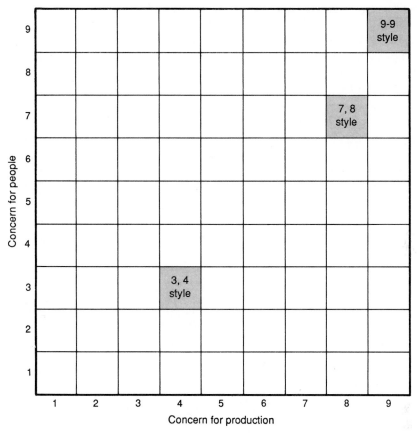

Figure 8-2. An Illustration of the Grid.

sions including nursing. Existing research has been mixed concerning results of use of the managerial grid (Blake & Mouton, 1976).

TECHNOSTRUCTURAL INTERVENTIONS

Technostructural interventions are OD interventions that examine the technology and structure of the organization, the division of labor into departments and coordination of the departments. These technostructural interventions are aimed at the organization level.

Organizational Design and Coordination

Lawrence and Lorsch (1969) developed a conceptual framework for organizational design and coordination (also termed differentiation and integration) from research on organizations. This framework examines organizations whose organizational design includes departments. Their research indicated that departments should be designed and coordinated according to the degree of environmental uncertainty facing the department.

Due to a somewhat different external environment, each department's design should fit their specific environment. In an uncertain environment, the department needs to be flexible. If the environment is certain or stable, the department should be more formal and inflexible. When the environments of departments are similar, the departmental designs are similar and simplify coordination.

The amount of coordination required is related to the degree of departmental interdependence; greater interdependence among departments requires greater coordination. Increased design differences among departments also requires greater coordination. When the need for coordination is high, integrating mechanisms, such as liaison positions or cross-departmental task forces, are needed. This is significant to health care organizations where departments differ greatly in design and have high interdependence signifying a need for greater coordination. Within a nursing department, subdepartmental designs are very similar and interdependence is lower, necessitating less effort in coordination.

A recent addition to the theory includes two new dimensions: *information complexity* and *resource scarcity.* An increase in information complexity produces a need for design flexibility. Resource scarcity, either human or capital, requires more efficiency and coordination. An organization needs an organizational design which incorporates both flexibility and coordination (Lawrence & Dyer, 1983).

The first stage in applying the theory is an assessment of the organizational design, coordination, environmental uncertainty, and departmental interdependence. Interventions may include survey feedback, education regarding the model, changes in departmental design and coordination, and changes in the relationship with the environment. Initial research has supported this framework; however, longer follow up is needed. Other research has suggested that pure service organizations may need less structure and formalization and a different structure than product-oriented organizations (Mills & Margulies, 1980).

Formal Structure Interventions

This type of intervention involves examining and changing the structure of an organization. The structure is the means by which organizational tasks are assigned to work groups and how those groups are coordinated. The organizational chart is the clearest representation of the structure. Structure should be designed with four organizational characteristics in mind: environment, size, technology, and goals of the organization. Several types of formal structures exist: traditional or hierarchical, self-contained, hybrid and matrix which were described in Chapter 7.

Collateral structures are permanent supplemental structures. Their goal is to work on specific issues or ongoing problems that the main structure does not have the format or expertise to resolve, usually these are issues that require a wide range of skills or knowledge. Ethics committees are collateral structures developed to address specific ethical issues in health care organizations and to make recommendations. In some organizations they are responsible for making decision. Quality circles are a type of collateral structure used for problems solving in work settings. Collateral structures may use more creative problem-solving techniques, such as workshops and retreats and may address a particular issue in greater depth and breadth. Ad hoc committees or task forces have the potential to become collateral structures if their purpose becomes permanent or of increased significance to the main structure.

Formal structure interventions focus on determining the optimal structure to meet organizational goals. When the optimal structure differs from the current structure, change is necessary. Because it affects the total functioning of the organization, structural change should be carefully prepared, presented, and thoughtfully instituted. To merely revise the organizational chart does not constitute structural change; the organizational chart represents relationships which must be restructured themselves. When structural changes are made without appropriate organizational preparation, members attempt to continue old structural patterns within the new structure and either subvert the change or introduce confusion.

A distinction needs to be made between organizational structure and the nursing care delivery structure, the difference between how the organization is structured and how nursing care is delivered. These two structures are correlated; a hierarchical organizational structure encourages hierarchical nursing care systems such as functional nursing. In both structures authority is centralized. Many newer nursing care systems are decentralized. This is consistent with the increasing need for decision making at the bedside. Such systems increase nursing autonomy and satisfaction and client satisfaction. However, the organizational structure must be philosophically consistent with the type of care delivery for the systems to be compatible.

Nurses are frequently more concerned with the nursing care structure than the organizational structure, but it is important to recognize their interrelationship. To provide a more decentralized, professional form of nursing care delivery an organization needs structure to provide support for such a change. If not, structural change may be a prerequisite to nursing care system changes.

Quality of Work Life Interventions (QWL)

The QWL interventions are aimed at increasing productivity and employee satisfaction by changing the work environment to promote and increase employee participation in work-related problems and decisions. Many of these interventions were initially developed in union-sponsored programs. Implementing QWL requires an organization that is reasonably flexible with little active competition among employees and between employees and management. QWL applications discussed here are cooperative projects, high-involvement organizations quality circles, and flexible work hours.

Union-management cooperative projects and high-involvement organizations.
These are business innovations. The first is a project in which union and management jointly decide workplace issues. Usually a joint union management committee (a collateral structure) oversees the project. External change agents may provide third-party facilitation, guidance, and evaluation of the project. While positive attitudes are increased, there are little data to suggest increased productivity. High-involvement organizations are usually small and developed around QWL principles. Characteristi-

cally they have horizontal structures, a high level of employee decision making, and all aspects of the physical and organizational structure are oriented toward increased employee involvement. This format seems to work best with interdependent technologies, small organizations where quality is particularly important. Little research currently exists regarding this format although high productivity has been reported (Lawler, 1982).

Quality Circles (QC). Quality circles, a popular QWL intervention, have been successful in Japan. In QC, small groups of employees meet to work on issues and problems directly related to their work and aimed at increasing productivity. Typically, a circle has 3 to 15 coworkers who have volunteered for the project. Circles are organized around particular work groups and multiple circles usually exist. These groups meet weekly to discuss issues related to their work and methods to increasing productivity. Some QC programs first train workers in problem solving and group process since these are crucial to success of the program. The circle leader, generally the area supervisor, guides the meetings and a group facilitator from outside the department directs the group process. A facilitator may work with several circles.

The circle follows the problem-solving process from defining a specific problem of mutual concern to implementing the selected solution. The process is based on the total group reaching consensus on one aspect of an issue before it progresses to the next. This process can be time consuming; however, circle members become individually committed to the results.

Support from management is crucial as the group needs the latitude to make decisions and implement solutions. For QC to be effective, group members must see the impact of their work. The management climate must be flexible enough to allow and encourage this process. Critics of QC have suggested that the participative Japanese management style is related to its success and may not translate as well into a different culture and management philosophy. Also research has not supported an increase in productivity related to QC (Ledford, Lawler & Mohrman, 1988; Mohr & Mohr, 1983).

Flexible work hours. Also termed flex-time, flexible work hours is another QWL approach. The employee can determine, within certain parameters, actual working hours. In one common application, all employees are present during predetermined core hours and may set their own arrival and departure to meet their contracted number of hours. This solution has practical implications for rush hours but it also allows an employee to arrange work hours consistent with other responsibilities. This is particularly meaningful in professions where employees must integrate their work schedules with child care or care of other family members.

Individually chosen work hours are unusual in nursing. The need to ensure adequate coverage has been at odds with flexible hours. Twelve-hour shifts have become popular solutions to personnel shortages and employee desires for increased off duty time. Nursing hours that overlap shift change are now common and developing work shifts to coincide with school hours has increased the number of employees in some organizations. The nursing shortage may encourage creative work-time solutions to retain and recruit nurses. Flex-time in business has led to improved attitudes and productivity (Cummings & Molloy, 1977).

Work Design Interventions

Work design interventions focus on designing jobs and work groups that increase employee satisfaction and productivity. Work design interventions may be included with QWL and/or other technostructural interventions. Work design is concerned with the compatibility between the technical dimensions of the job and the personal dimensions of the employee. Technical dimensions are the degree of technical interdependence or cooperation with other employees required in the job and technical uncertainty or unpredictability in the job. Personal dimensions are the employee's social, interpersonal, or growth needs or needs for challenge. Positions with high interdependence and employees with high social needs fit well with work groups. Positions with a high uncertainty and employees with high growth needs fit enriched jobs (Hackman & Oldham, 1980).

Four work designs are described using both the technical and personal dimensions: *traditional jobs, traditional work groups, enriched jobs,* and *self-regulated work groups* (see Fig 8–3). The latter two are often the focus of work design interventions.

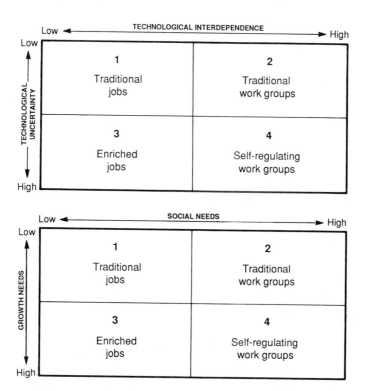

Figure 8–3. Work Designs Optimizing Technology (*Reproduced by permission of the publisher from T. Cummings, "Designing Work for Productivity and Quality of Work Life,"* Outlook 6 (1982): 39)

Traditional jobs and traditional work groups. Traditional jobs are low in both technical uncertainty and interdependence and fit employees low in social and growth needs. Few nursing positions are traditional due to the high technical interdependence in nursing.

In traditional work groups the work itself is routine (low technical uncertainty) but higher on technical interdependence due to related tasks. This work design fits employees with high social and low growth needs. Team nursing contains many elements of the traditional work group. The work is technically interdependent and occurs in settings with low technical uncertainty where patient care is somewhat predictable. Team nursing fits nurses with high social needs.

Enriched jobs. These jobs are specifically designed to include the five core job dimensions found by Hackman and Oldham (1980) to contribute to employee satisfaction, motivation, and retention. These core dimensions create critical psychological states that lead to personal and work outcomes (see Fig 8–4). The core dimensions are skill variety, task identity, task significance, autonomy, and feedback. The *Job Diagnostic Survey* (JDS) measures these core dimensions as perceived by the employee and indicates which dimensions should be enriched. Jobs can be enriched by forming

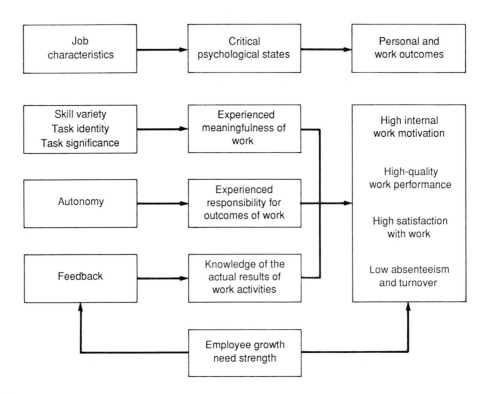

Figure 8-4. Work Designs Optimizing Personal Needs (*Reproduced by permission of the publisher from Cummings, ''Designing Work for Productivity and Quality of Work Life,'' p. 40)*

natural work units, combining tasks, establishing client relationships, decentralizing authority, and opening feedback channels.

Primary nursing and case management are examples of enrichment in nursing; the nurse has greater autonomy and greater accountability in these systems. Such nursing care systems may best fit nurses with high growth needs. Overall, more information is needed on how the growth needs of nurses relate to specific systems. Joiner and van Servellen (1984) report hospital nursing is enriched compared to other professions.

Self-regulated or autonomous work groups. In these work groups, employees with interrelated tasks form a relatively autonomous group. The optimal setting is one in which technical interdependence and uncertainty are high and optimal employees are high on social needs and growth needs. One example is the interdisciplinary team commonly found in community mental health centers. Some models of case management also fit this profile (Zarder, 1988, Kaener et al 1989).

HUMAN RESOURCE MANAGEMENT INTERVENTIONS

Human resource management is dealing effectively with the human resources of the organization. This is particularly significant when resources are limited as in nursing. Specific interventions discussed here include *goal setting, reward systems, career development,* and *programs to decrease organizational stress.* These interventions are focused on the individual and on promoting optimal performance and development within the organization. Many of these interventions can be implemented through revision of existing procedures.

Goal Setting

This technique allows employees and managers to identify and monitor specific goals for the employee. Clear goals focus and energize work behavior. Successful goal setting requires determining the difficulty and specificity of the goal, receiving specific feedback from the manager regularly and active employee participation in goal setting. Goals should be difficult enough to encourage performance but not unattainable and should be specific enough to focus behavior.

Goal setting begins with an assessment of the position, identifying the specific goals, feedback, and managerial support. Periodic review and revision of goals provides an important feedback loop. Research on goal setting suggests positive results in productivity and is focused on identifying the situations and individuals for whom goal setting is most effective (Latham & Locke, 1979). Goal setting can easily become a component of regular evaluation.

A specific type of goal setting is *management by objective* (MBO). In MBO, the employee and manager collectively analyze and set the employees work goals within the framework of organizational goals. These goals are identified specifically and include criteria for evaluation. Personal and career goals of the employee are also addressed within the context of the organization.

Keys to MBO effectiveness are the climate of the total organization, how MBO is implemented, and the degree of input from the employee. A major drawback occurs when the employee perceives the goals as imposed rather than collaboratively chosen. Research has been mixed partially due to the variety of implementations (Wickens, 1968). Health care organizations and nursing departments have experimented with MBO approaches; their tendency has been to integrate MBO within the total evaluation system (Pollok, 1983).

Reward Systems

Intrinsic and extrinsic rewards are necessary for both employee satisfaction and performance. The QWL interventions are examples of intrinsic rewards. Pay and promotions are extrinsic rewards. To be effective, the reward should be sufficient to satisfy basic needs, consistent with competing organizations, distributed fairly, and consistent with the values of the employee (Lawler, 1977).

Pay. Pay is an important reward. Many organizations have a skill-based plan where pay increases as the employee learns new job skills or elements of work. In nursing, the new nurse graduate's salary increases with licensure and then with appropriate performance until the individual reaches the top of the pay scale within that grade. This element of "topping out" represents the problem with skill-based pay. When the employee reaches the top of the position scale, the employee must change positions or organizations to increase salary. The topping out phenomenon contributes to salary compression, which is the small difference between initial and final career salaries in nursing.

When the supply of staff nurses is adequate, health care organizations do little to reward nurse longevity. This contributes to a lack of organizational loyalty and a mobile work force in nursing. The nursing shortage and the cost of orienting new employees encourages re-examination of this policy. In some organiztions, new salary levels have been added and other internal rewards, such as career ladders, and flexible work shifts are also possible.

All-salaried work force. In this system, all levels of employees in an organization are salaried. Frequently this system is combined with other work design interventions. These plans are popular because their implementation in industry frequently allows some independent scheduling of work time and treats employees in a more professional fashion.

Gain-sharing. This format allows employees to share the gain from improvements in the organization, particularly gains made through participative management and employee feedback. Problem-solving techniques are solicited. If selected and used, the gains made are shared. In health care, gain sharing is largely unexplored because of the complexity of health care expenses and the lack of participative management. Health care organizations have experimented with bonus payments when an employee recruits another employee. In nursing, such programs have had an unprofessional flavor.

Career Development Interventions

These interventions are at the interface between the personal needs of the employee and the human resource needs of the organization. There are benefits for both the individual and the organization in career development, particularly if the organization can utilize the increased career skills. Two career development formats exist: internal formats where the employee makes a career within the organization and moves upward with appropriate gains in knowledge or skills specific to that organization; and external formats where the employee gains skills and knowledge outside the organization through training or education programs. External programs transfer better between organizations and have benefits for the employee. Internal programs provide a means to develop a needed employee and are of benefit to the organization. Particular groups who may benefit from career planning include women, career initiates, and employees in midcareer. These groups tend to be at points where career planning is important and motivating.

Career planning is the setting of career objectives. Several methods for accomplishing career planning exist. One method involves communicating career opportunities and resources within the organization by job posting and bulletin board information. Making self-development materials available is another. Career counseling, either by external counselors or properly trained managers, is a more formal route. Such counseling can be incorporated into individual goal setting. Another option is an assessment program. This can identify talent for the organization, help employees to recognize their particular talents, and focus on career goals consistent with those talents.

A *career stage* schema was developed by Super (1957) and modified by Hall (1976) that identifies four stages of career development: (1) *exploration;* (2) *establishment;* (3) *maintenance;* and (4) *disengagement.* Each involves specific career concerns. These stages can be addressed through organizational programs.

Exploration lasts from one's first serious position until approximately age 25. The individual has chosen a career, received the appropriate education and entered a first career position, usually as a graduate or staff nurse. This first nursing position can strongly effect future experiences (Schein, 1987). The position needs to challenge but not overwhelm. Organized learning experiences and feedback are essential. The nurse should be encouraged to assess personal strengths and weaknesses. Appropriate organizational programs are realistic job previews to decrease reality shock, nursing internships, and ongoing performance feedback and counseling.

The *establishment* stage involves becoming established in a career, usually when aged 25 to 45. This stage may involve advanced training or specialization, or a graduate degree in a clinical specialty. Optimally, the nurse makes a commitment to the profession and prepares for a long-term responsible position appropriate to one's abilities. Promotions to managerial roles occur during this stage. For many women this stage involves determining a balance between career and family roles since these years are also primary childbearing and childrearing years. Organizations can facilitate this stage by providing challenging and visible assignments, providing sponsorship or mentoring, and encouraging realistic career goals through career development programs. Organizational commitment may occur during this stage, so employees need information on internal career paths. Flex-time programs encourage integration of work and family as does onsite day care.

During the *maintenance* stage, approximately aged 45 to 60, the individual's primary concern becomes maintaining the career gains that have been made. This employee has a broader perspective on a career and the organization. Mentoring others is characteristic of this stage. Workshops that develop counseling or mentoring skills are appropriate. In-service programs ensure that these employees are current on newer techniques and skills. Plateauing or becoming stagnant are organizational concerns for maintenance stage employees. Lateral transfers or job enrichment that develops new skills and challenges may be helpful.

The *disengagement* stage occurs as the employee prepares to retire. The employee is concerned with planning a meaningful retirement and passing on knowledge to the organization. Consultation roles maintain contact with the organization or profession. Professional organizations also are a means to stay involved. Organizational responses during this period can include retirement planning and phased retirement.

Exceptions to the age-related career stages may occur in people who enter nursing in midlife, as second careers, or following military service. These nontraditional populations are becoming more prevalent today. They may be out of age sequence regarding career stages or they may bring with them experiences and knowledge that move them rapidly through the career stages.

Career ladders are an organizational career mechanism that identifies a particular set of nursing skills and rewards their attainment. Career ladders vary in extent and can be internal or external although internal programs are more common. Career ladder criteria are set within institutions. A nurse meeting the next level criteria can be promoted within grades. Larger organizations are more able to provide the range of experiences necessary for advancement. One problem with the internal or organization based career ladder is that achieving a particular spot on the ladder may not have transferable meaning in another organization. External career ladders involve workshop participation or pursuit of courses or particular degrees assisted by the organization. Certification is an example of a credential that is transferable to other organizations and locations.

Stress Management

An area of organizational concern that frequently falls under organizational development is the management of job related stress. The two types of stress are organizational and personal. While a correlation exists between the two, organizational stresses are the primary concern for the nurse executive. Stress can be loosely defined as the reaction of individuals to the environment. It can be managed in several ways by increasing awareness of stress and its causes, by modifying those causes, and by increasing the capacity to cope.

Stress is inherent in life and work with a certain amount of stress necessary for optimal functioning. This amount varies individually. Some work environments are more stressful than others. Certainly, intensive care units have particular elements of stress but nursing in general is considered a stressful profession. Common organizational stressors for nurses are role conflict or conflict between how a nurse and nursing executive view the work, role ambiguity, or defining appropriate work activities. Diagnostic interventions include identifying organizational and personal stressors through the use of scales that measure both stressors (Holmes & Rahe, 1967) and the physiological effects of stress. Some health care organizations hold periodic health fairs where employees can be tested and receive a health profile that indicates (generally) the amount of stress in both personal and professional lives. Health care organizations are in a good position to do this and to encourage nurses and other employees to practice the good health habits they teach.

Organizational interventions can include role clarification with managers, either individually or in group settings. An environment that encourages supportive relationships among employees may decrease stress as social support mediates the effects of stress. Exercise facilities also allow employees to work off stress effects and improve general health.

ORGANIZATIONAL DEVELOPMENT (OD) IN HEALTH CARE

Health care is one of the last frontiers for organizational development. While OD programs have been developed and instituted in some areas, generally it has made little impact on health care organizations. An organization that is well-managed and organized does not need OD. Health care organizations are neither well-managed nor well-organized for their tasks today. Many health care managers do not have a background in management principles and are not sufficiently familiar with management theories to implement them. Therefore, OD does not occur in spite of the need for it.

Organizational development is not needed when the mission of the organization is clear. While health care organizations may have understood their mission in the past, today they are being pressured by outside forces and economic considerations to reconsider that mission in more concrete (and frequently less humanitarian) terms. In organizations where the mission is not congruent with reality, the resulting schizophrenic environment is not conducive to OD.

All this suggests a need for change in approach in health care organizations. The basic elements of mission, organization, and managerial competence need to be assessed as a preliminary step and if inadequate structures and knowledge bases exist, interventions should be begin there. In nursing, the move toward the combined MBA/MSN degree or the masters in nursing with a strong business track indicates recognition that a strong business background is needed.

SUMMARY

The process of organizational development and types of interventions follows a problem-solving format similar to the nursing process that includes systematic assessment of the organization, definition of the problem(s), interventions, and evaluation. Assessment may utilize questionnaires, interviews, observations and data from secondary sources. Feedback of the data to the organization itself is the next step. Interventions are chosen in collaboration with the organization and consider the nature of the organization.

The person responsible for the OD intervention is the change agent. The change agent may come from outside the organization, outside the department, or inside the organization. A combination of internal and external agents on a team is optimal. The change agent must be impartial to any particular segment of the organization.

Interventions can be at the individual, group, or organizational level depending on the identified problems of the organization. There are three types of interventions: process, technostructural, and human resource management.

Process interventions are aimed at the group or organizational level. The goal is to examine group dynamics. Technostructural interventions are aimed at designing the structure and technology of the organization for optimal employee satisfaction and productivity. Human resource management interventions involve increasing employee satisfaction with resulting increased productivity. These interventions are aimed at the individual or small groups.

Organizational development in health care has been limited by the lack of basic organizational structures in health care settings and the absence of managers with experience in organizational development.

REFERENCES

Blake R, Mouton J. *The Managerial Grid*. Houston, Gulf, 1964

Blake R, Mouton J. *Organizational Change by Design*. Austin, TX, Scientific Methods, 1976

Cummings TG, Huse EF. *Organization Development and Change*, 4th ed. St. Paul, MN, West, 1988

Cummings TG, Molloy E. *Improving Productivity and the Quality of Work Life*. New York, Praeger, 1977

Daft RL, Steers RM. *Organizations: A Micro/Macro Approach*. Glenview, IL, Scott, Foresman, 1986

Dyer W. *Team Building: Issues and Alternatives*, 2nd ed. Reading, MA, Addison-Wesley, 1987

Hackman J, Oldham G. *Work Redesign*. Reading, MA, Addison-Wesley, 1980

Harvey DF, Brown DR, (1988). *An Experiential Approach to Organizational Development*, 3rd ed. NY: Prentice-Hall, 1988

Holmes TH, Rahe RH. The social readjustment rating scale. *Journal of Psychosomatic Research*. 11, 1967

Kaplan R. The conspicuous absence of evidence that process consultation enhances task performance. *Journal of Applied Behavioral Science*. 15: 346, 1979

Koerner JG, Bunkers LB, Nelson B, Santema K. Implementing differentiated practice. *Journal of Nursing Administration*. 13:2, 13, 1989

Latham G, Locke E, (1979). Goal setting: a motivational technique that works. *Organizational Dynamics, 8,* 68–80

Lawler E III. Reward systems. In Hackman J, and Suttle J, eds. *Improving Life at Work*. Santa Monica, CA, Goodyear, 1977, 163–226

Lawler E III. Increasing worker involvement to enhance organizational effectiveness. In: Goodman P, ed. *Change in Organizations.* San Francisco, Jossey-Bass, 1982

Ledford G Jr, Lawler E III, Morhman S. The quality circle and its variations. In: Campbell JP, Campbell JR, eds. *Enhancing Productivity, New Perspectives from Industrial and Organizational Psychology.* San Francisco, Jossey-Bass, 1988, 225–294

Lawrence P, Dyer D. *Renewing American Industry.* New York, Free Press, 1983

Lawrence P, Lorsch J. *Developing Organizations: Diagnosis and Action.* Reading, MA, Addison-Wesley, 1969

Lewin K. *Field Theory in Social Science.* New York, Harper & Row, 1951

Likert R. *The Human Organization.* New York, McGraw-Hill, 1967

Mills PK, Margulies N. Toward a core typology of service organizations. *Academy of Management Review.* 5:255, 1980

Mohr WL, Mohr H. *Quality Circles.* Reading, MA, Addison-Wesley, 1983

Mosley D. System four revisited: Some new insights. *Organizational Developmental Journal.* 5: 19, 1987

Pollok CS. Adapting management by objectives to nursing. *Nursing Clinics of North America.* 18:3, 484, 1983

Schein E. *Process Consultation Volume II: Lessons for Managers and Consultants.* Reading, MA, Addison-Wesley, 1987

Super DE. *The Psychology of Careers.* NY, Harper & Row, 1957

Walton R. *Managing Conflict: Interpersonal Dialogue and Third-Party Roles.* 2nd ed. Reading, MA, Addison-Wesley, 1987

Wickens J. Management by objective: an appraisal. *Journal of Management Studies.* 5, 365, 1968

Woodman R, Sherwood J. The role of team development in organizational effectiveness: a critical review. *Psychological Bulletin.* 88, 166, 1980

CHAPTER 9

Communication Systems

Karen Kelly Schutzenhofer
Sandra R. Shelley
Sharon L. Pontious

Key Concept List

Assertiveness
Communication
Computers as communication tools
for nurse executives
Effects of computerization on nursing
Strategic communications

COMMUNICATION PROCESSES

The success or failure of every human interaction is a result of the effectiveness of communication. For nurses executives, communication skills are essential to the organizational effectiveness of a contemporary nursing department (Farley, 1989). As noted by Wolf (1986), ''Effective communications are the bricks in the road to corporate excellence'' (p 26).

The Nature of Communication
Communication is more than just an exchange of words or ideas or the giving of information. Physiological, cognitive, and effective abilities are all used in any interac-

tion. A message is shaped by the communication skills, attitudes, values, and knowledge base of the sender and then filtered by the communication skills, attitudes, values, and knowledge base of the receiver. The feedback from the receiver is then shaped and filtered and the process of communication continues. This process of effective communication and its applications for nurse executives provide the focus of this chapter.

Channels of Communication

In any organization the formal channels of communication are defined in the organizational chart. Within these formal channels, downward communication uses letters and memos; large and small group meetings, including dyads; phone calls; manuals and handbooks; newsletters and other written and electronic documents. Channels of formal upward communication include suggestion systems, grievance procedures, and attitude surveys, as well a variety of personal interactions, particularly small group and dyadic interactions.

Informal channels of communication, which move horizontally, vertically and diagonally, transcend the official channels of communication. They are often verbal, more direct and more effective than the official channels, and may be viewed as the means by which work really gets accomplished in an organization.

Nurse executives focus much of their communication efforts along formal channels with policies, procedures, and administrative expectations and actions which are transmitted formally from executives to the various levels of managers and then to the nursing and support staffs. The effectiveness of formal channels needs to be considered by the executive to ensure that all personnel, especially off-shift and part-time employees, understand the upward and downward flow of information. Equally important to the nurse executive, and sometimes even more critical to one's effectiveness, is the lateral and diagonal flow of information to and from other departments outside nursing. Successful communication with executive peers and various levels of managers outside nursing is essential to the overall success of the nurse executive.

Modes of Communication

In any organization written communication is a primary mode of communication. Nurse executives, whether using paper and pen or computerized communication systems, generate a range of written communication including correspondence, memos, reports, performance evaluations, budgets, proposals, policies, procedures, and job descriptions. The effectiveness and clarity of these written communications, from a single paragraph memo to lengthy proposals, are enhanced by simplicity and brevity.

Oral communication is, of course, the most commonly used mode of communication and, in many ways, the most complex. Oral communication includes both verbal and nonverbal aspects. Verbal communication refers to the spoken words in an interaction between two or more people. Nonverbal communication includes the body language and gestures that accompany verbal messages; the personal space, or spatial relationship, of the persons communicating; the paralanguage of a message, including tone, pitch, pace, and voice quality; and personal attributes, such as grooming, clothing, hair style, and cultural qualities.

A verbal message always has a nonverbal component; congruence between these two aspects of a message is essential for the effectiveness of the verbal aspect. When there is conflict between the verbal and nonverbal aspects of a message, the nonverbal will be perceived as more powerful. Nonverbal communication is so powerful that it exists in the absence of a verbal message. Consider a busload of commuters at the end of the day. Without speaking a word, the riders relay powerful messages about their work and how their days were spent in their posture, facial expressions, and personal appearance.

Communication Skills

Verbal skills. Verbal skills enable the sender to shape a message so that the message received by the listener is the message intended by the sender. Verbal skills, including the selection of language appropriate to the intended audience, enable nurse executives to present their messages clearly and succinctly and, in turn, enable them to assist others in the effective expression of their ideas. Two basic rules of effective verbal skills are (1) avoid jargon and (2) don't use a big word when a smaller, more common word will do the job.

Nonverbal skills. Nonverbal skills include the presentation of self to the receiver. The credibility and persuasiveness of the speaker is as much determined by image as by expertise and authority. Gestures, posture, facial expression, clothing, and grooming all communicate powerful messages before the speaker utters a word. As a predominately female group, nurse executives must deal with the same dilemmas faced by other female executives regarding wardrobe and grooming. To appear too feminine may send the wrong messages about one's competence; to appear unfeminine may indicate a repudiation of one's peer group of women.

Gestures, posture, and facial expressions can emphasize a verbal message or send a powerful opposing message. Dramatic, sweeping hand movements may undermine the impact of verbal content. A smile may accentuate good news or confuse the receiver when the message is bad news.

Eye contact is an important nonverbal skill. While eye contact is avoided in some cultures, our cultural norms call for frequent eye contact during interactions. The mutual glance indicates a readiness to communicate. One must be particularly aware of the eye contact used in an interaction. Frequent eye contact, especially when accompanied by frequent smiles, may be viewed by the opposite sex as interest beyond the bounds of a professional relationship.

Spatial relationships, or body space, communicate powerful messages. Most social and business interactions occur within a social zone of approximately 4 to 12 feet distance. Social interactions are more likely to involve a distance of 4 to 6 feet, while business interactions are more likely to occur with the participants 10 to 12 feet apart. Business interactions that occur within a personal zone of 1.5 to 4 feet may indicate an attempt by one participant to intimidate the other.

The effectiveness of verbal communication is not only determined by what words are spoken but also by the way those words are spoken. Pace, rhythm, volume, and enunciation all affect the spoken word. The selective use of silence and pauses can contribute much to a verbal message. Verbal messages punctuated with frequent non-fluencies, like *uh, er,* or *um,* can greatly detract from an otherwise well constructed message.

One needs to be especially aware of the tone and pitch of his or her voice. Stereotypes of vocal qualities may work to the disadvantage of women, especially those with very high or very husky voices. A raise in pitch during an emotionally charged interaction can also decrease the effectiveness of the spoken word.

Issues of status can influence communication. Distortions can occur because of perceived status barriers, such as titles, location and layout of an office, or other factors that may seem as hurdles by persons of lower status in the organization. A nurse executives's secretary may screen calls for appointments primarily for the efficient use of the executive's time; a staff nurse may perceive this as purely an effort to prevent direct communication with the staff.

Active listening. Listening is the receptive communication skill that includes physiological, cognitive, and affective processes. It differs from hearing, a purely physiological process. Active listening requires that one focus on both the verbal and non-verbal messages of the sender. Nursing has historically emphasized the need to develop these listening skills among clinicians; executives also need to use these same skills in daily interactions. Sullivan (1988) offers these principles of active listening:

1. Find a place to talk with a minimum of distractions or interruptions.
2. Sit or stand so that you can look directly at the other person.
3. Listen to words but pay closest attention to nonverbal clues.
4. Ask questions to develop points further.
5. Be empathic—try to put yourself in the other's place.
6. Obtain feedback for your impressions of the other's thoughts or feelings.
7. Acknowledge positive contributions of the other.
8. Respond to the other's message and meaning.
9. Be patient. (p 164)

These principles demonstrate the interdependence of listening skills with verbal and nonverbal communication skills.

Assertiveness skills. Assertive communication is a communication style that acknowledges and deals with existing conflict, acknowledges other people as equals, and includes a direct statement of feelings. Assertive communication protects one's own rights in a situation, while respecting the rights of others; enhances self-esteem and esteem for others; and supports a sense of trust. Assertiveness is often confused with aggressiveness. Aggressive communication, in contrast, creates or escalates conflict; disregards the feelings and rights of others; allows no room for compromise; and is a selfish means of expression. Historically, many of nursing's professional woes can be traced to a legacy of passive communication (Ashley, 1977), seasoned at times with a hint of passive aggressiveness. Passive communication is characterized by avoiding conflict even at a great cost to one's self-esteem; creating self-anger, accepting the infringement of one's own rights; and allowing others to ignore one's needs and feelings.

Assertive communication allows one to exercise power in a constructive manner. Learning to communicate powerfully is an important step. Nurse executives, who are predominately female, must communicate frequently with people in positions of power within health care organizations, powerful people who are predominately male. These interactions can reflect the same stereotypes and problems seen in other female–male relationships. Assertive communication transcends gender differences.

Chenevert (1988) identifies four levels of assertiveness: *remedial, basic, advanced,* and *beyond assertiveness.* We reach our highest level of communication effectiveness at beyond assertiveness. Those who function beyond assertiveness evidence high self-esteem and esteem for others, valuing their time and talents. They feel comfortable saying "no" but take delight in saying "yes!" They are able to take personal and professional risks and do not consider "power" a dirty word. In seeing the big picture long beyond tomorrow, they are able to move from leadership to fellowship. They recognize their own interdependence, while achieving a strong internal locus of control. They communicate support of others and others seek their support.

Principles of Communication

As noted earlier, communication is more than just giving information. There must be interaction, which includes feedback, between two or more people for communication. For the executive, giving information to subordinates becomes communication only when there is feedback from the subordinate that confirms that the message has been received.

Clarity of a message is the responsibility of the sender. The modes and skills of communication previously noted are offered to nurse executives as means for ensuring the clarity of a message. The vision of the nurse executive cannot be operationalized by staff unless communication is clear and effective. It is not the responsibility of the staff to read the mind of the executive. The message must be made clear to be well understood.

Sometime during our earliest nursing experiences, we learned to use simple and exact language to ensure that our messages were understood by patients, their families, and our colleagues. Nurse executives, while no longer directly responsible for patient care, are still responsible for using language that clearly communicates their messages to the various constituencies with whom they interact.

As noted above, communication occurs only when the sender's message elicits feedback from the receiver. Feedback can prevent many misunderstandings. The executive must encourage feedback. The executive must seek feedback from those reluctant to provide feedback, accept and evaluate feedback that is unpleasant or uncomplimentary, and respond to feedback constructively.

A speaker must be credible. Celebrity spokespersons for consumer products are often chosen because they lend credibility to advertising. For nurse executives to function as effective communicators, they must be perceived by others as competent, trustworthy, and reliable professionals. As noted earlier, credibility and persuasiveness are influenced by expertise, authority, and image. It is impossible to persuade others to carry out one's vision for nursing without a high level of credibility.

An important principle of assertive communication is to acknowledge others and their contributions. While such acknowledgment is easily given when there is harmony and cooperation, during conflict much greater effort is required to acknowledge the efforts, ideas, and values of others.

Children play a game of "telephone" where a message is whispered from one player to another until it is repeated to the child who started the game. Everyone laughs at the distorted message at the end. This simple childhood game is evidence that direct channels of communication are the most effective. When numerous people have to interpret and pass on a message, the chances for distortion intensify. Direct communication offers greater opportunity for feedback. Although not always feasible, and sometimes not always desirable, face-to-face interaction offers the greatest opportunity for immediate feedback and the advantage of greater use and interpretation of nonverbal communication skills.

Barriers to Effective Communication

The verbal and nonverbal communication skills and the principles of communication previously noted are tools to help the nurse executive avoid some common barriers to effective communication. Communication problems arise when we only hear the words but do not listen fully to the messages of others. Information can be manipulated or filtered so that only part of a message is passed on or the original message is obscured, thus impairing the sender's credibility. Value judgements and status issues become obstacles to effective communication when we fail to acknowledge assertively the equality of others. Clarity of message is lost when we fail to use simple and exact language and, instead, lapse into jargon or become involved in semantic differences which sidetrack from the issue at hand. In response to time pressures, it may seem expedient to skip some levels in the formal channels of communication in order to bring a project to fruition; this may eventually undermine the success of the project because those who were skipped over later fail to support the project.

Communication is a complex process that involves far more than the imparting of information. Effective communication requires the nurse executive to use verbal and nonverbal skills to convey messages and to employ active listening skills to obtain feedback to complete the cycle of communication. The skills and principles offered in this chapter provide no magic formula for effective communication but are simply tools to be used wisely.

PRACTICAL APPLICATIONS OF COMMUNICATION SKILLS

Emphasis on Verbal Skills

Much of the nurse executive's verbal communication occurs in dyads and other small groups. Henry and LeClair (1987) cite research that indicates that three quarters of the nurse executive's day is spent talking with others. Three specific types of common one-to-one interactions are coaching, discipline, and performance appraisals.

Through coaching the nurse executives tries to eliminate or decrease a performance problem in an employee. Coaching also serves a motivational function by encouraging the employee to perform more effectively. Effective coaching may prevent a performance problem from becoming so serious that it becomes an issue for discipline. Discipline is used when a rule or policy is breached, especially a violation that puts patient safety at risk, violates confidentiality rights, or reduces the quality of patient care. Performance appraisal is a behavioral evaluation, which reviews past performance with a view toward future expectations. Each of these types of interactions calls for stating problems (or strengths) in clear, behavioral terms, precise definition of the nurse executive's expectations, and a mutually agreed plan for follow-up. The reader is referred to Chapters 13 and 16 and to Breaugh (1992) for more specific information on these kinds of communications.

Small groups. Small group interaction offers nurse executives the opportunity to share their ideas, goals, and expectations with others, with the added advantage of immediate feedback. Small groups may demonstrate greater problem solving and creative abilities than the same individuals working alone. Nurse executives can use small groups to empower nursing colleagues to work together as a collaborative, professional group rather than simply an aggregate of individuals. Committees, councils, and task forces are examples of small groups. Through these groups the executive can communicate content, facts, aspirations, goals, and visions, and teach interpersonal skills through example. Small groups provide an excellent medium for teaching one's colleagues new ideas, skills and attitudes. The support, cohesion, and trust that characterize effective small groups create an excellent environment for learning.

There is often much opportunity to manipulate the environment to support small group effectiveness. Creating an environment that supports communication for a dyad or other small groups follows the same principles. Arrange seating to ensure good eye contact and to achieve appropriate spatial relationships. Close doors and redirect phone calls to minimize distractions. Hold the interaction on your own ''turf'' when control is an issue; move to a neutral site to avoid control issues.

Exit interviews. Exit interviews may be part of the formal system of communication within a department. They may be handled by the executive, a staff person, the human resources department, or an outside organization. The validity of the data obtained may be strengthened by having a neutral party, ideally someone from outside the organization, conduct the interview, especially with employees who are involuntarily terminated or leave voluntarily under hostile conditions. The interview is directed at determining the exact reason for the employee's resignation, identifying problem areas in the department that require corrective actions, and promoting good relations with departing employees. The interview may be an opportunity to retain a valued employee if the cause of dissatisfaction can be identified and addressed. The interviewer needs to maintain a relaxed atmosphere, use open-ended questions that encourage employees to share their perceptions, experiences, and feelings, and clarify any statements made by employees that are incomplete or unclear. Valued employees who resign should leave the interview knowing that they are welcome to return to the institution in the future. The interview should be kept to a maximum of 15 to 30 minutes. This offers sufficient time to collect the desired data without seeming to impose on departing employees.

Speeches. Speeches and other presentations test the skills of even the most effective communicator. Nurse executives generally will speak publicly to inform and to persuade. When preparing for presentations, have your goals clearly in mind. If you are an invited speaker, make sure you fully understand the expectations of those who have issued the invitation. What is the precise topic you are to address? Who is the audience and what do they expect? What are the time limits? Will audiovisual support be available? May you prepare handouts to distribute? Should you bring copies or will they copy the handout for the group? Effective communication promotes your credibility and strengthens the effectiveness of your presentation. For the novice speaker, public speaking courses are available through various organizations, including local community colleges.

Following are some suggestions to help with public speaking skills. Focus on communicating the content of the presentation. Nonverbal skills support the effectiveness of the content. Smile when appropriate and make eye contact with selected members of the audience. Demonstrate a lively tone of voice. Make sure the speed of the presentation and the pitch of your voice is appropriate. Use hand gestures to emphasize words. Some presentations are enhanced when the speaker moves into the audience. Adapt material to the audience. Attend to the nonverbal messages they are sending and make revisions in the content using examples to clarify or less detail if appropriate. Once you begin your presentation stop worrying about how you look and sound and how the audience perceives you. Think confidently and you will become confident.

Grapevines. Grapevines were previously identified as an informal channel of communication. The grapevine cannot be ignored by the nurse executive; it exists and always will. Despite some distortions and inaccuracies, the grapevine is on target as much as 75 percent of the time (Aldag & Stearns, 1987; Gibson et al, 1988). Strengthening the formal systems of communication in the department will reduce the role of the grapevine. However, the grapevine can meet departmental needs for the quick dissemination of information that the formal system cannot or will not accommodate (Aldag & Stearns, 1987; Gibson et al, 1988).

Role modeling. Role modeling by nurse executives represents both the verbal and nonverbal practical application of communications. Bandura (1971), the author of social learning theory, posits that most direct learning occurs by observing the behavior of others. One means of strengthening communications within departments is for nurse executives to model effective communication skills to their subordinates, who in turn model their behavior after the executive, and then role model their communication skills to their own subordinates. This role modeling can occur in dyadic, small group, or large group interactions. The effect can be contagious throughout a department.

Emphasizing Practical Nonverbal Communication Skills

As noted earlier, the most effective written communication is succinct. For any written communication, clarity, simplicity, and brevity are essential. Keep paragraphs short, simple, and focused on a single topic. Use charts, graphs, and other illustrations to clarify content, not as a substitute. Use active, nor passive verbs (eg, *"The nursing executive team prepared the report,"* not *"The report was prepared by . . . ."*). Use personal pronouns carefully, avoiding sexist language (Davis & Newstrom, 1985; Hanser & Avadian, 1989).

Memos. Schutz, Decker, and Sullivan (1992) offer five characteristics nurse executives should consider when writing a memo. The *subject* should be clearly identified. What are you really writing about? The *purpose* of the document is well-defined: Why are you writing? Could a telephone conversation or face-to-face interaction handle the situation as effectively? What *format* will the written communication take? Will this be a memo (less formal) or a letter (more formal)? Is this a concept paper to stimulate discussion or a proposal for an action to be taken? Will this document include many details or will it just convey a brief piece of information? Who is the *audience* of this document? The intended audience will influence form, vocabulary, length, and other characteristics of this written message. Finally, what *voice* will be used in the document? The role or tone taken by the writer is influenced by the document's degree of formality, the intended audience, the content, the timing and current departmental/organizational climate, the purpose of the document, and the format used. Even a budget sends powerful messages, in this case, about the allocation of resources for the nursing department, reflecting its value and status in the organization.

Policies, standards of care, performance standards. Policies, standards of care, and performance standards are formal, written communications that convey powerful messages about the nursing department. These documents must be written clearly so that they are meaningful to even the least experienced staff nurses. They must incorporate the current and collective thinking of the department and of the nursing profession, including the state's nursing practice act. Such documents must also reflect the policies and collective thinking of the organization. Systems must be identified for the development, distribution and revision of these documents. Policies, standards of care, and performance standards are not only written documents but they should be the driving forces in the day-to-day activities of the department. Nurse executives must develop formal systems that ensure easy access to, thorough understanding of, and adherence to these written communications. This requires effective communication with the various levels of nursing management and the nursing staff.

Newsletters and bulletin boards. Newsletters and bulletin boards commonly are used communication tools in any organization. Information on new policies and procedures, continuing education programs, new career opportunities, and new programs and employees are frequently communicated through these systems. Clarity and brevity are as essential for these systems as they are for formal documents. Bulletin boards loaded with outdated brochures and fliers are common sites on many nursing units. Systems for bulletin board posting and review can keep the content current and attractive. Newsletters offer an opportunity to involve many people within the department in production and distribution.

Surveys. Organizational surveys are another common communication tool in most nursing departments. Surveys are valuable administrative tools for planning, establishing and evaluating an environment conducive to quality patient care. Various organizational surveys may cover anything from staff development interests and needs to cafeteria food, from job satisfaction to attitudes about the nursing executive team. Data from these surveys may be used for strategic planning, specific program planning, budgeting, performance appraisals and other purposes. In any survey, questions of validity and reliability must asked. The reader should consult a research text for further information on the development and implementation of valid and reliable surveys. Discussion of the methods of organizational surveys is found later in this chapter.

ORGANIZATIONAL COMMUNICATION

Just as communication skills are important for personal effectiveness, fluent organizational communication is vital to both the success of individual people within the organization and the organization itself. Central to achieving success in this arena is strategic communication—employing appropriate communication strategy to the specific circumstances present in the work environment to obtain the maximum outcome. The contemporary emphasis on leadership puts rejuvenated interest in communication processes within organizations.

Conrad (1985) describes the three functions of communication within organizations as: command, relational, and ambiguity management. In organizations, the *command* function involves both directions and feedback. Organizations must give their members information on the work to be done, how it should be done, and subsequently, how it was done. The command function of communication is essential to coordinating the interdependent actions of people involved in producing the commodities, services, or information of the organization.

Organizations, like cultural or social groups, are comprised of complex interpersonal *relationships.* Most cultural or social situations involve a certain degree of voluntary participation. In contrast, employees are involved in ''imposed'' relationships, dictated by the structure of the organization. Work relationships often lack the customary bonds of commitment and permanence inherent in social relationships. However, individuals in work relationships must have a common understanding about each others' actions and motivations, so that cooperation toward work objectives can be achieved. Communication is the catalyst by which work relationships are formed and the sustaining force by which they are maintained. Work relationships have a strong bearing on employee perceptions of the work to be done and actual performance of that work.

On a daily basis, members of organizations must make choices concerning the interests of self, relationships, and the organization. If the expectations and consequences for making those choices are clear, there is little difficulty; if not, a certain degree of *ambiguity* results. This ambiguity can be compounded by disrupted rules and norms resulting from organizational changes. Employees use communication to reduce or manage the ambiguity. They can use communication to create a common understanding of the different circumstances that present themselves in organizations (ambiguity reduction). In addition they can use communication to share their coping strategies for dealing with organizational uncertainty (ambiguity management).

One school of thought on organizational decision making emphasizes the rational nature of organizations: organizations are comprised of people; people are rational beings; decision making is done by people; thus, organizational decision making must be rational. In the process of maturation, we are socialized to believe mature adults do not make impulsive decisions. Rather, they use a logical process, involving deliberate consideration of multiple factors related to carefully set goals. This process of individual rationality is often used to describe an organization's decision-making process.

Certain organizational scientists believe that in reality, however, that most organizations appear to act rationally some of the time, and irrationally at other times. Consequently, organizational rationality is more a myth that describes how organizational decisions *ought* to be made, rather than what really occurs. Yet, organizations still must make decisions in order to be productive. Bem's (1972) theory of ''self-perception'' suggests that people make decisions, and often act upon them, before constructing logical explanations to support their choices. Conrad (1985) believes that ''organizational decisions are made, and once they are made, the participants begin to construct, share, and publicize a rational explanation and justification'' (p 155).

Processes

A common understanding about information is that the use of it is power, that is, you can't use information you don't have. Access to communication in organizations often is linked to sources of power and authority. Since communication is the dominant modality for transmitting information, it too is closely associated with organizational influence. Thus, an understanding of how communication flows in organizations is necessary for developing one's sphere of influence. It was previously suggested that communication patterns have an influence on employee productivity and satisfaction. Thus, the ability to comprehend and manipulate communication flow is often a determinant of success in organizations.

In most structured institutions, formal communication flows in a vertical direction—from the top down, or from the bottom up. Endorsed communication channels closely follow the reporting lines in an organization. It is no surprise that formal power gradients follow the same lines on the organizational chart.

Both downward and upward communication serve specific purposes in an organization, as discussed elsewhere in this chapter. Downward communication, provides subordinates with specific information about the work to be done, and their role in performing that work. Another aspect of downward communication is the transmission of information about rewards and punishments associated with organizational compliance. The success of a reward and punishment system depends on effective communication. First, there must be a set of clearly communicated rules and norms that subordinates understand to be relevant, objective, fair, and supported by an appropriate reward and punishment system. They also must know that the rewards and punishments were fairly and equitably distributed in the past, and will continue to be in the future. Finally, employees' experience with the reward and punishment system should be consistent with their own self image.

Upward communication usually involves specialty or technical information related to job tasks. It plays an important role in the feedback aspect of communication. Individuals higher up in the bureaucracy depend on those closest to the work product for information on job related processes and problems.

Several inherent obstacles in organizational hierarchies increase information distortion. Some are structural in nature. In most organizations, information flows between several bureaucratic layers from its origin to its destination. These multiple communication links cause information to be interpreted differently as it passes from one point to another. In addition, the large size of many bureaucratic hierarchies prevent messages from reaching their destination at the appropriate time and with maximum efficiency. Information is further distorted as people assimilate it to their work roles. The more indoctrinated employees are in their specific work culture and the more accustomed they become to their individual job tasks, the less they are able to interpret messages accurately which are foreign to their own tasks, or to empathize with situations outside of their particular environment.

Other distortions of vertical communications relate to interpersonal phenomena. Organizational echelons convey differences in power and status that contribute to an "us versus them" attitude. This mind set can foster mistrust among people in different organizational levels, which often results in communication barriers. Subordinates who feel their chances for advancement may be hurt by sharing certain information also may inhibit information flow. Some supervisors consciously or unconsciously discourage communication through their words and actions. And finally, the organization itself may have overt or covert norms that stifle information sharing.

Distorted communication contributes to ambiguity and, thus, can be the source of conflict in organizations. Although conflict is an inevitable phenomenon, it must be recognized and managed to prevent deleterious outcomes. Employees react to conflict in different ways based on the particular expression of conflict and their unique orientation to it. Knowing how employees react to conflict can help individuals structure situations so the appropriate communication strategies can be utilized to manage the conflict (see Chapter 24 for more information on conflict management).

NEGOTIATING

This history of nursing and the stereotypes of nurses demonstrate a legacy of compliant, passive behavior (Ashley, 1977). The tendency of nurses to try to be all things to all people has created an expectation that nurses will never say no and has left many nurses with few skills in negotiating. Steves (1985) points out that nurse executives must learn not only when and how to negotiate, but also when not to negotiate. As previously noted, assertive communication will prevent nurse executives from negotiating away their authority. Using communications skills in situations that call for negotiation allows executives to deal effectively with their own power and others in various positions of power.

Approaches to Negotiating

In positional bargaining, opposing positions are taken on an issue and each side tries to come to a resolution that fulfills its own interests. In a "hard" position (playing "hard ball"), participants become adversaries, with each side demanding concessions from the other, while digging in to their own positions. In this contest of wills, pressure is applied until one side makes concessions. Much time is wasted and distrust builds between the sides as people, as well as problems, are critically attacked. In a "soft" position, participants remain friendly and try to reach agreement through mutual concessions without criticism of people or problems. Soft negotiators are willing to concede to a one-sided resolution of the problem, emphasizing a need to reach agreement over reaching a satisfactory resolution.

Fisher and Ury (1983) offer principled negotiation as an alternative to the approaches noted above. In *principled negotiations,* the participants are problem solvers, not adversaries. The approach separates people and personalities from the problem at hand. The interests of both parties are served, but positions are not taken irrevocably. As part of the problem-solving process, a variety of options for action are generated before a decision is made. The outcome of the negotiations is based on some objective standard (eg, market value of a service or commodity, expert opinion, custom, professional standards or law). The principled approach avoids ego damage and enables people to work together on a problem without taking opposing sides. The opposing sides are able to share perceptions of the situation and examine ownership of the problems. Assertive communication skills and active listening are used with facility.

Principled negotiation avoids the "dug in" positions assumed in hard negotiating that often obscure the basic interests of the involved parties related to the problem at hand. Blaming is avoided when interests are shared instead of positions being held.

Negotiation Problems

There are times when the other party will not budge from a position. Avoid attacking the other party's position; it will only create defensiveness and lock you into a untenable position. Explore the other party's position: What are the interests of the other party? Are there any common interests? Invite a critique of your ideas before it is offered with hostility. Ask open-ended questions and offer plenty of "think time." Clarify and restate the other party's position; this could lead to brainstorming. Some people will use dirty tricks when negotiating, ploys that are designed to deceive. Often just recognizing the tactic eliminates it; raise the question explicitly.

MEASURING ATTITUDES

Organizational Surveys

As noted earlier in this chapter, organizational surveys are a common event for nurse executives. Surveys are conducted to measure employee attitudes about and reactions to organizational policies, events, practices, programs and structures (Dunham & Smith, 1979). Surveys may include all employees within an organization or may be limited to a particular department. Organizational surveys are used to analyze known problems; identify potential problems; evaluate current policies and practices; assess organizational change; and to collect data for the development of interventions to decrease turnover, absence and tardiness and to increase organizational effectiveness, including identification of staff development needs.

Using a survey requires far more than the distribution of a questionnaire. Some stimulus triggers the need for most survey programs, even if the stimulus is a date on the calendar in the case of regularly scheduled surveys. Recognizing the need for a survey should lead to a careful review of current organizational (or departmental) documents, including philosophies, missions, and goal statements. Key people in administrative and in staff positions need to be included in the initial discussions of the need for a survey. The focus and the intended outcomes of the survey need to be clearly identified. The timing of the survey is important. If a crisis triggers the survey, the process is less likely to be systematically implemented than if the survey is part of a regularly scheduled assessment program. This emphasizes the need for a well developed assessment plan within any organization.

The purpose of the survey will guide the selection of the type of survey chosen. The characteristics of the target group also will help determine the survey format. The communication skills of the target group, for example, will influence selection of the survey. If the survey is being conducted to assess needs or opinions, a sample of the target group will be adequate. If the outcomes of the survey will result in some change process, the entire target group needs to be included to support the process of planned change. If the survey will focus on professional employees, sophisticated questionnaires can be used with greater confidence in the data then if employees with limited reading and writing skills are included.

Surveys can be conducted through observation, interviews, or questionnaires. Observation can measure both formal and informal interactions. Data collection is heavily influenced by the skill of the observer and validity and reliability of the instrument used. When more than one observer is used, interrater reliability (the consistency of observations) can strengthen or weaken the quality of the data. Observation also is very costly.

Interviews allow for indepth exploration of a topic and for the clarification of responses. Consistency of data from one survey to the next depends on the skills of interviewer or interviewers (interrater reliability) and on the quality of interview schedule. Interview surveys also can become very costly when large numbers of employees are included.

Written surveys offer the consistency of a single, uniform experience for all those surveyed. Anonymity is another advantage of written surveys. Written surveys generally take less time to complete than if the same questions were asked by an interviewer.

Surveys can be designed to address an organization's specific needs at the moment. However, such self-designed surveys raise questions about the validity and reliability of the instruments. Self-designed surveys need to be pilot tested and revised, with this process repeated, if necessary. Standardized questionnaires may be more valid and reliable but may also be less exact in meeting the organization's need. Whatever kind of survey is selected, professional assistance is likely to be needed to address survey construction and distribution, psychometric issues, ethical concerns, and data interpretation. Such assistance may come from in-house experts or from external consultants.

Once a survey instrument is selected, the method of administration must be decided. Observations may be conducted by persons from within the organization or by external consultants. Interviews may be conducted by the same personnel. Written surveys can be mailed to the employees' homes, distributed with paychecks, distributed by managers or other appointed persons, or completed at a meeting. Anonymity of responses is best guaranteed by surveys mailed to the home and returned by mail to a third party outside the organization.

Data analysis can be a complex and costly process. Computer answer sheets can be scanned for written surveys if forced choice answers were given (eg, yes-no, scales of 1 to 5). Open-ended response items, interviews and observational data may only be suitable as handwritten responses, which must be categorized and tabulated by hand. These data usually require content analysis for valid interpretation, with categories emerging from the responses without using predetermined classifications. These rich data may provide more valuable information, but the analysis is time consuming.

Once data analysis is completed and the data have been interpreted meaningfully, it is essential to provide feedback to employees. Written reports or either large- or small-group meetings may be used. Findings should be presented with the most favorable findings identified first, the mixed findings next, and the negative responses last. The report also must include those planned actions to be taken in response to the survey and what actions indicated by the survey will not be taken because of economic, time, or other constraints. This feedback needs to be provided in a timely fashion and with opportunity for employee feedback.

Job Satisfaction Measures

Organizational surveys commonly focus on job satisfaction. During nursing shortages, job satisfaction surveys of nurses occur with much greater frequency as organizations try to position themselves favorably in a tight nursing market. Factors generally examined in job satisfaction surveys include the work itself (intrinsic interest, variety, opportunity for learning, difficulty, creativity, amount of responsibility and authority, opportunity for success, control/autonomy, scheduling); pay (amount, equity, method of payment); promotions (opportunities for advancement, fairness); communication; recognition; benefits; working conditions; quality of supervision; management and administration (Farley, 1989; Locke, 1983).

Job satisfaction measures are used prospectively to retain valued employees as part of ongoing organizational planning. Such surveys can also be triggered by increased employee turnover, tardiness and absenteeism, other productivity problems, and the threat of unionization. A variety of measures are used in industry: self-report rating scales, observations, action tendency scales, and interviews. The Job Description Index (Smith, Kendall, & Hulin, 1969) is commonly used in nursing (Roedel & Nystrom, 1988). This 72-item scale is a modified adjective checklist that measures satisfaction with pay, promotion, co-workers, supervision, and the quality of work. The scale takes 10 to 15 minutes to complete, is backed by extensive normative data, and reports acceptable reliability and validity.

The nursing literature reveals an increasing body of research on job satisfaction among nurses. Many studies use general measures of job satisfaction; some measures of nursing-specific job satisfaction are emerging. McCloskey and McCain (1987) have developed a 33-item Likert-type Reward/Satisfaction Scale with items categorized as safety rewards, social rewards, or psychological rewards. Extensive validity and reliability data have yet to be established.

Organizational Climate

Organizational climate is an individual's perception of an organization's environment. Climate is influenced by the structure of the organization, including the chains of command and channels of communication, role structures and the status system. However, structure variables are characteristically measured by objective data, such as organizational charts, job descriptions, and committee structures, while climate is a perceptual, personal phenomenon. Climate is a measure of how people feel within the organization (Thomas, Ward, Chorba, & Kumiega, 1990). Measures of organizational climate may examine an individual's perception of work autonomy; the degree of structure imposed on a position; reward structure; consideration and support from management and peers; and orientation to development, progressiveness, and risk taking. Measures may also include objective data such as tardiness, absence and vacancy and turnover rates. Perceptions are shaped by the attitudes, values, and beliefs of the individual and, in turn, influence the individual's performance within the organization.

Climate is not the same as organizational culture, the commonly shared attitudes, values, and behaviors within an organization. Climate is an individual's *perception* of the organization. When there is fit between corporate culture and the individual's perceived climate, the performance and motivation of the individual is much more positive than when culture and climate sharply conflict (Thomas et al, 1990). (See Chapter 5 for more on culture.)

COMPUTERS AND COMMUNICATION

Computer systems have been used to manage and support information and communications in health care organizations for over thirty years. Initially, these systems were used primarily for financial, business, and medical information processing (Bailey, 1988). Nursing passively observed these developments while writing extensively about the possible benefits of computer applications to management activities since 1970. Nurses did not actively seek to use nor empirically validate the worth of using computers to assist them in the actual provision of nursing care until recently (Bailey, 1988; Staggers, 1988). Only in the last few years has nursing truly realized the "frightening potential" of computers and related computer information systems "for determining the course of nurses' clinical practice and, subsequently, influencing the development of nursing's body of knowledge" (Graves & Corcoran, 1988, p 168). Nursing executives must be prepared for direct involvement in the selection, use, and design of computerized health care systems in order for nursing to assume its place as the leader in the health care delivery industry—in controlling the flow of systematized patient information and nursing personnel information.

Many terms, abbreviations, and information systems are used when describing computers and associated programs used by nurses. Information is the collection and organization of data so that inferences and decisions can be made and appropriate actions taken. A system is "the combination and interaction of computer hardware, software and data with the accompanying input and output mechanisms" (Cox, Harsanyi, & Dean, 1987, p 154). Thus, an information system (IS) is an automated or computerized collection and organization of data (accumulated from throughout the institution and across departments) so that inferences or appropriate actions can be taken to meet a set of organizational goals.

The initials IS used before denotes the base of the system or the main user of the system. For example, **HIS** (hospital information system) is a computer information system used in several hospital departments. A typical HIS includes computerized admission, bed assignment, supply and diet orders, laboratory and radiology test requests and results, and patient billing. MIS stands either for a medical or management information system. A medical information system is designed for physician use. A management information system is used primarily by executives and is designed to facilitate the managerial functions of the institution. MIS functions usually include patient classification, personnel data base, staff scheduling, quality assurance, budgeting, staffing projections, institutional statistical data and a variety of reports on institutional issues. NIS, nursing information system, denotes a computer system primarily for the practice of nursing with computerized nursing documentation as well as care planning and reports on nursing care of patients. NIS usually includes nursing orders, nursing histories and assessments, care plans, documentation of nursing care, and patient reports for change of shifts. It can also include computer-assisted instruction modules for nursing orientation and inservice, capabilities for retrieval of literature to support patient care, and clinical decision support from an expert decision support system (Graves & Corcoran, 1988; Kiley et al, 1983). In an *expert decision system*, content experts develop programs to determine the best intervention to use for particular patient problems. Patient care information system, *(PCIS)* describes a large integrated system that incorporates management, hospital, medical, and nursing information systems in such a way that each component can "talk" to the other. One piece of information inputted in one area automatically is copied into every other appropriate one. Conceptually, the PCIS computer system can manage all information relating directly or indirectly to the care of patients by interdisciplinary personnel of an institution.

Nursing Information Systems

A primary application of computers in patient care is to monitor patients' conditions. Computers continually monitor the progress of the patient and alert the nurse either on the monitor or by sounding an alarm when a significant change occurs. Today an integrated NIS assists nurses to care for patients from admission through discharge. With an NIS compatible with the hospital's PCIS, information entered by the nurse while caring for the patient is automatically communicated for administrative functions including patient classification, patient billing, quality assurance checks and personnel management.

An integrated PCIS assists in the collection, organization, and analysis of patient information from first contact through discharge. Initially, the historical information is gathered (via either direct input by the patient or admission staff or by automatic transmission from other information systems). Patient assessment data (immediately entered at the bedside by health care personnel), lab and x-ray data, and continuous monitoring data (eg, vital signs, fluid intake and urinary output, cardiac and renal functions) is continually updated, organized, analyzed, and interpreted. The computer immediately alerts caregivers to any undesirable trends or patient changes, suggests therapeutic actions and/or implements preprogrammed closed-loop therapy (van Bemmel, 1987), and protects against medication or treatment errors. Dates, times and personnel identification occurs with each entry which facilitates quality assurance, personnel evaluations, and enhances risk management.

Advantages of an NIS integrated in a PCIS include: decreased time for charting, ordering of tests or supplies, scheduling, and transporting patients to various departments; increased precision, completeness, and accuracy of nursing records; improved identification of life-threatening changes in patient's conditions; and increased authority, responsibility, and accountability for nurses in the care of patients (Cox et al, 1987; Sullivan & Decker, 1992; van Bemmel, 1987). The biggest advantage is the amount of time saved on indirect patient care activities, thus using budgeted time for more effective direct patient care. Time-management studies demonstrate that computerization can save 70 percent of the time a nurse spends on information handling, with the average nurse currently spending 30 percent of the day dealing with information (Barry & Gibbons, 1990). Others have demonstrated time savings ranging from 13 minutes per patient per shift (Viers, 1983) to 20 to 25 minutes per patient per shift (Soontit, 1987), with a considerable saving in overtime pay. Many nurse executives recognize an NISs potential for retention of nurses but no empirical data have been yet reported.

Management of Information

Computers were initially used to manage the voluminous information hospitals stored about patients, with billing and materials management among first areas to be computerized. Next, hospital and nursing executives used computers for management purposes such as statistical reports, patient classification, staffing, budget, and quality assurance.

Computerized Schedules

Nurse executives can use the computer to forecast how many and what mix of nursing personnel will be needed for the next shift on each unit and to modify the preplanned schedule as necessary. Many computerized staffing systems collect information on each staff member, such as desired shifts, days off, vacation or flex time, abilities and specialization, and then automatically compile these data to derive staffing schedules based either on actual or forecasted patient acuities. These schedules can be provided to nursing staff one or more months ahead of time. Advantages of such scheduling include more effective and flexible use of staff with the appropriate mix of nursing personnel with resulting cost effectiveness through reduced overtime, increased patient satisfaction, and increased staff satisfaction with increased retention (Bergmann & Johnson, 1988; Cox et al, 1987; Gallagher, 1987). In addition, computerized staffing decreases scheduling time for the nurse executive, thus allowing more time for personnel management activities.

Automatic Audits

Computer systems which integrate an automated nursing documentation system with the patient classification and staffing systems also enable executives to audit the quality and quantity of nursing care provided by nurses to one or more types of patients. Administration can determine which category of patients is provided with the most cost effective nursing care and which is requiring more nursing care than that for which the hospital is reimbursed. Actions regarding any unacceptable care or patient reimbursement problems can then be identified and corrected.

Graphics

Graphics packages allow the executive to assemble a variety of information quickly and present it concisely with significant relationships identified pictorially for immediate understanding, especially for those outside nursing. Computer graphic use clarifies information and speeds one's comprehension so reports are more useful and helpful.

Budgets

Executives frequently use computers to develop budgets, evaluate productivity, forecast needs, and make quantitative decisions about personnel and their activities. Computers can quickly sort and then compute appropriate statistical results; they are ideal assistants for these projects. Even without the availability of HIS or PCIS, the nurse executive can use one of the various spreadsheet programs to solve ''what if'' problems to help make the best decisions.

New Technology

New computer technology will have a major impact on the future of nursing in all health care settings. One of the greatest challenges to nursing is to develop stringent definitions of nursing diagnoses and intervention using one or two nursing theories so that computers can relate data in such a way that the user can extract needed elements into meaningful information about nursing assessments, actions, and patient observations. Werley, Devine and Zorn (1988) have begun developing a Nursing Minimum Data Set (NMDS). This data set will allow for collection, analysis, and comparison of nursing data locally, nationally, and internationally ultimately to strengthen the base of nursing science. Development of a coordinated computerized system using one data set is strongly supported by the third recommendation for utilization of nursing resources developed by the Secretary's Commission on Nursing (1988):

> The federal government should sponsor further research and encourage health care delivery organizations to develop and use automated information systems and other new labor-saving technologies as a means of better supporting nurses and other health professionals. These systems and technologies should be applicable and cost-effective across all practice settings (p VI).

Implications of New Technology for Nurse Executives

Nurse executives and managers need skills in computer use, statistics, and cost data. The executive needs to make decisions concerning personnel requirements and retention of staff based on evaluation data generated by automated nursing information systems (McCormick & McQueen, 1988). In addition, nurse executives have to decide who and for what purpose particular nursing personnel have access to various components of the computerized patient and personnel data bases. To the extent that information is power, restricted access is both resisted and resented. Yet nurse executives must ensure patients' and nurses' rights to privacy and confidentiality (Romano, 1987).

Since computers are changing nursing roles and responsibilities, nurses need to become familiar and comfortable with using computers to control the information flow about patients. New roles and skills for nurses are in demand for the future. All nurses prepared at the basic educational levels must be able to assume the role of information specialist, understanding the basics of what, when, where, how, and why of computer technology. Graduate level nurses need to be prepared to become system specialists, with a background in needs evaluation, research methodology, systems theory, nursing theory, implementation strategies, economic and business theory, hardware and software application, evaluation strategies, and organizational and sociological theories (Cox et al, 1987). The system specialist assists in the design of computerized information systems and teaches other nurses how to use them.

SUMMARY

Effective communication is an essential skill for nurse executives. One's effectiveness within the nursing department and within the organization as a whole is enhanced and supported by communication skills. Effective communication does not just happen: It is deliberate and strategic. The appropriate channel, mode, and skills all contribute to the effectiveness of communication, both in the sending and the reception of messages. Relationships in the work setting depend on the effectiveness of communication.

The introduction of computer systems in nursing has been a slow process. However, the growth of these systems are influencing the delivery of nursing care and the administration of the departments which provide that care. Nurse executives who have not yet developed facility in using computer systems will soon find themselves desperately in need of this new area of communication skills.

REFERENCES

Aldag RJ, Stearns TM. *Management.* Cincinnati: South-Western Publishing, 1987

Ashley JA. *Hospitals, Paternalism, and the Role of the Nurse.* New York, Teachers College Press, 1977

Bailey DR. Computer applications in nursing: A prototypical model for planning nursing care. *Computers in Nursing.* 6, 199, 1988

Ball MJ, Snelbecker B, Schechter D. Nurses' perceptions concerning computer uses before and after a computer literacy lecture. *Computers in Nursing.* 3, 1985

Bandura A. *Social Learning Theory.* Morristown, NJ, General Learning Press, 1971

Barry CT, Gibbons LK. Information systems and technology: Barriers and challenges to implementation. *Journal of Nursing Administration.* 20:2, 40, 1990

Bem D. *Beliefs, Attitudes and Human Affairs.* Belmont, CA, Brooks-Cole, 1972

Bergmann C, Johnson J. Managing staffing with a personal computer, Part I. *Nursing Management.* 19:7, 28, 1988

Breaugh JA. Performance appraisal. In: Sullivan EJ, Decker PJ, eds. *Effective Management in Nursing,* 3rd ed. Menlo Park CA, Addison-Wesley, 1992

Chenevert M. *Special Techniques in Assertiveness Training: STAT,* 3rd ed. St. Louis, CV Mosby, 1988

Conrad C. *Strategies for Organizational Communication.* Fort Worth, TX, Holt, Rinehart and Winston, 1985

Cox, HC, Harsanyi B, Dean LC. *Computers and Nursing: Application to Practice, Education and Research.* Norwalk, CN, Appleton and Lange, 1987

Davis K, Newstrom JW. *Human behavior at work: Organizational behavior,* 7th ed. New York: McGraw-Hill, 1985

Dunham RB, Smith FJ. *Organizational Surveys: An Internal Assessment of Organizational Health.* Glenview, IL, Scott, Foresman, 1979

Farley MJ. Assessing communication in organizations. *Journal of Nursing Administration.* 19:12, 27, 1989

Fisher, R, Ury W. *Getting to Yes: Negotiating Without Giving In.* New York, Penguin Books, 1983

Gallagher JR. Developing a powerful and acceptable nurse staffing system. *Nursing Management.* 18:3, 45, 1978

Gibson JL, Ivancevich JM, Donnelly JH, Jr. *Organizations,* 6th ed. Plano, TX: Business Publications, 1988

Graves J, Corcoran S. Design of nursing information systems: Conceptual and practice elements. *Journal of Professional Nursing.* 4, 168, 1988

Hanser M, Avadian B. Improving your written communications. *Journal of Nursing Administration.* 19:12, 18, 1989

Henry B, LeClair H. Language, leadership, and power. *Journal of Nursing Administration.* 17:1, 19, 1987

Kiley M, Halloran EJ, Weston JL, Ozbolt JG, Werley, HH, Gordon M, Giovanetti P, Thompson JD, Simpson RL, Zielstorff RD, Fitzpatrick JJ, Davis HS, Cook M, Grier M. Computerized nursing information systems. *Nursing Management.* 14:7, 26, 1983

Locke EA. The nature and causes of job satisfaction. In: Dunnette MD, ed. *Handbook of Industrial and Organizational Psychology.* New York, John Wiley and Sons, 1983, 1297–1349

McCloskey JC, McCain BE. Satisfaction, commitment and professionalism of newly employed nurses. *Image: Journal of Nursing Scholarship.* 19, 20, 1987

McCormick K, McQueen L. New computer technology. In: Johnson M, McCloskey JA, eds. *Series on Nursing Administration, Vol 1.* Menlo Park, CA, Addison-Wesley, 1988, 59-69

Roedel RR, Nystrom PC. Nursing jobs and satisfaction. *Nursing Jobs and Satisfaction.* 19:2, 34, 1988

Romano C. Privacy, confidentiality, and security of computerized systems: The nursing responsibility. *Computers in Nursing.* 5, 99, 1987

Schutz C, Decker PJ, Sullivan EJ. *Nursing Management: An Experiential/Skill Building Workbook,* 3rd ed. Menlo Park, CA, Addison-Wesley, 1992

Secretary's Commission on Nursing. *Secretary's Commission on Nursing: Final Report.* Washington DC, US Department of Health and Human Services, 1988

Smith PC, Kendall LM, Hulin CL. *The Measurement of Satisfaction in Work and Retirement.* Chicago, Rand McNally, 1969

Soontit E. Installing the first operational bedside nursing computer system. *Nursing Management.* 18:7, 23, 1987

Staggers N. Using computers in nursing: Documented benefits and needed studies. *Computers in Nursing.* 6, 164, 1988

Stevens BJ. *The Nurse as Executive,* 3rd ed. Rockville, MD, Aspen Publications, 1985

Sullivan EJ. Communication skills. In: Sullivan EJ, Decker PJ, eds. *Effective Management in Nursing,* 2nd ed. Menlo Park, CA, Addison-Wesley, 1988

Sullivan EJ, Decker PJ, eds. *Effective Management in Nursing,* 3rd ed. Menlo Park, CA, Addison-Wesley, 1992

Thomas C, Ward M, Chorba C, Kumiega A. Measuring and interpreting organizational culture. *Journal of Nursing Administration.* 20:6, 17, 1990

Thomas K. Conflict and conflict management. In: Dunnette M, ed. *Handbook of Industrial and Organizational Psychology.* Chicago, Rand McNally, 1976

Van Bemmel JH. Computer assisted care in nursing: Computers at the bedside. *Computers in Nursing.* 5, 132, 1983

Viers VM. Introducing nurses to computer world. *Nursing Management.* 14, 24, 1983

Werley H, Devine EC, Zorn CR. Nursing needs its own minimum data set. *American Journal of Nursing.* 88, 1651, 1988

Wolf GA. Communication: Key contributor to effectiveness—A nurse executive responds. *Journal of Nursing Administration.* 16:9, 26, 1986

CHAPTER 10

Military Executive Nursing Systems

Clara L. Adams-Ender
Barbara Goodwin
Mary F. Hall
Sandra S. Lindelof
Margaret Armstrong
John M. Hudock
Patricia Porter
Claudia Bartz
Joanne M. Black

Key Concept List

Dual mission
Dual role
Planning, programming, and budgeting system (PPBS)
Closed system
Reserve component
Active component
Medical treatment facility (MTF)
Program Budget Advisory Committee (PBAC)
Self-management

The military nurse executive thrives in a paradoxical system. Civilians control the whole military system. Military health care providers train for mobilization and war. Staff turnover is continual, making training/retraining needs constant and substantial. Two strong and tradition-filled systems, the officer and noncommissioned officer systems, must co-exist. The system is saturated with politics but the executive has an equal and interdependent partnership with other executive staff due to the rank structure. While care of patients and families is paramount at each facility, the executive also is responsible for development of staff to benefit the whole system.

Military nursing shares many features with civilian nursing in regard to professional practice. Educational preparation; clinical specialization; staff development; continuing education; standards of practice, care, and performance; patient and family care activities; quality assurance and documentation; and nursing research are all areas that form a solid bond between the civilian and military nursing communities. Military nurses take the same licensure and certification examinations and are subject to the same accreditation review. In peacetime, military nurses care for patients whose illnesses or injuries are essentially the same as those found in civilian facilities. The workload and job-related stresses are no different than those in civilian nursing with staff shortages and threats to state of the art nursing practice being key dissatisfiers among military nurses. Leadership and management expertise are critical to the survival and progress of professional nursing in both the military and civilian health care sectors.

Nonetheless, major differences exist between civilian and military nursing because of differences in the mission and organization of the military health care system. In brief, military nursing is committed to a dual mission with each military nurse having a role as officer *and* professional nurse. The medical departments of the armed services have dual missions. The primary mission is to prepare for delivery of health care to military combatants in the event of mobilization for war in defense of the United States or its allies. At the same time, medical departments must provide peacetime health care to active military members and other beneficiaries.

Career military nurses are expected to cope with periodic relocation and changes of position as a normal part of professional development and military life. As more members of the Nurse Corps are married and have families, mobility may be somewhat decreased. Nurses who must reside in only one geographical area eventually may have to decide between family and military career obligations.

Military service requires a high degree of conformity, standardization and wartime readiness. Military nursing is infused with traditions, courtesies, and discipline. The vital role performed by 13,000 active duty military nurses demands flexibility, versatility and sacrifice in a health care delivery system made more complex by its dual mission.

It is paradoxical that within a structured military system under the control of the President, the Congress, and a civilian staff at the Department of Defense, military nurse officers experience autonomy, respect, and scope of authority that exceeds that of their civilian counterparts. Nurse autonomy does not preclude multidisciplinary turf battles; however, recognition of the dual mission and staff interdependence, especially during mobilization, may be factors in minimizing strife and disagreement among health care professionals.

Military nursing assignments vary from administration, clinical practice, research, or education in a modern medical center to the management and provision of combat casualty care in an austere land, sea, or air environment. Military nurses are prepared for this range of assignments through formal undergraduate and graduate nursing programs, internships or preceptorships, speciality nursing courses, speciality military courses, leadership courses, and professional military education programs.

Military nurses' entry to practice level is, for the most part, at the baccalaureate level. Each service makes exceptions to this policy to meet critical staffing requirements. Nurses who are new to military nursing often receive orientation to their role at the facility to which they are assigned. Each service has an internship and/or preceptorship program to prepare new nurses for the transition to practice and assumption of the officer role (see Fig 10-1).

The three military departments support graduate education, with the number of officers being sent for master's and doctoral degrees depending on validated position requirements, personnel availability, and budget constraints. Graduate education encompasses all nursing specialties to include clinical specialties, nursing and health care administration, informatics, and education.

Specialty nursing courses are provided by each service in response to clinical staffing requirements. Such courses include critical care, nurse practitioner, hyperbarics, perioperative, pediatric/neonatal, obstetric/gynecologic, psychiatric, renal dialysis and community health nursing. Courses for special environments include aeromedical and combat casualty nursing. Specialty military courses address topics including biological warfare and infectious disease, chemical casualties, medical effects of nuclear weapons, and training for nuclear hazards.

Leadership and management courses are designed to address levels of progression in the career development of nurse officers. Nurses assigned to intermediate, advanced and executive level management roles attend courses of the respective departments or courses offered by other federal or civilian institutions.

The senior levels of military education are integrated with officers from the respective medical department, the military department, Department of Defense, or the federal sector. Newly appointed officers attend an officer basic orientation course.

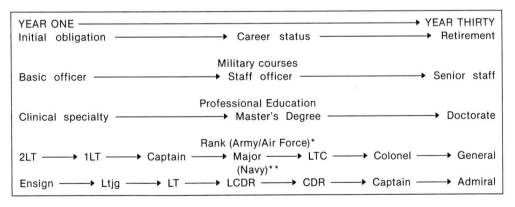

Figure 10-1. Career Progression in the Military Nurse Corps

*2LT, Second Lieutenant; 1LT, First Lieutenant; LTC, Lieutenant Colonel; General, Brigadier General.

**LTjg, Lieutenant Junior Grade; LCDR, Lieutenant Commander; CDR, Commander; Admiral, Rear Admiral.

Later, advanced officer, staff officer, and senior service courses are available. As the level of professional military education increases, the number of Nurse Corps officers attending each program decreases, emphasizing the selective preparation for senior leadership positions.

The military health care departments cooperate with two other major federal health delivery systems on matters of federal nursing policy. The United States Public Health Service, while a uniformed service having a considerable medical mission, is part of the Department of Health and Human Services rather than the Department of Defense. The Department of Veterans Affairs has a broad medical mission that is met by federal, nonuniformed employees of that department.

MILITARY HEALTH CARE SYSTEM

Department Of Defense Structure

The President of the United States is the Commander in Chief of all armed services (see Fig 10-2). The President, the administration, and the Congress collaborate to develop national policy which establishes the mission of the Department of Defense (DoD). The Department of Defense is under civilian control, with the Secretary of Defense having oversight responsibility. There are three military departments (Army, Navy, Air Force) and five military services. The Marine Corps is a service in the Department of the Navy. The Coast Guard is a service under the Department of Transportation, except when operating under the Department of the Navy during mobilization. Each military department is controlled by a civilian secretary. Each military service (Army, Navy, Air Force, Marine Corps and, during mobilization, Coast Guard) is managed by the senior military officer of that service.

The three military departments are assigned common functions, primary func-

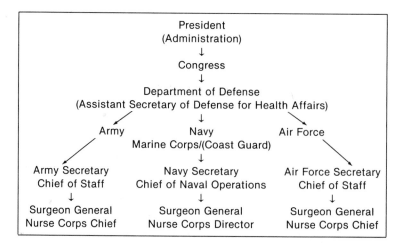

Figure 10-2. Organizational Chart (Simplified)

tions, and collateral functions. Common functions address maintenance of readiness and mutual assistance; primary functions focus on the department's speciality. For example, the Army provides land forces while the Navy/Marine Corps provides sea-going forces. Collateral functions address joint responsibilities, for example, the Air force provides air-to-air refueling in support of naval campaigns (Joint Chiefs of Staff, 1986).

The military health care system is part of the infrastructure supporting the overall mission of the military services. The Surgeons General of the Army and Air Force report to their respective Chiefs of Staff and the Surgeon General of the Navy reports to the Chief of Naval Operations. The Chiefs of Staff of the Army and Air Force, and the Chief of Naval Operations, report to their respective service secretaries. The Assistant Secretary of Defense for Health Affairs, appointed by the President, has responsibility for overall supervision of the health affairs of DoD and is principal staff assistant and advisor to the Secretary of Defense for all DoD health policies, programs, and activities (US Army, 1989–1990).

The Chief Nurse Executives (CNE) for the Army, Navy, and Air Force report to their respective Surgeon General. The CNE for the Army and Air Force is the Chief of the Nurse Corps. The CNE for the Navy is the Director of the Navy Nurse Corps. The CNEs occupy a unique position in nursing through their oversight of the policy and operations required to acquire, distribute, educate, and develop Nurse Corps officers. The basic goal of the CNEs is to ensure that quality nursing care is provided across a worldwide system. The CNE is a principal architect for medical force structural changes. The CNE is the proponent for all nurse recruitment and retention strategies.

Planning, Programming, and Budgeting System (PPBS)

Congress establishes the basic guidance for military policy. The President's budget, submitted yearly to Congress, includes a budget for the Department of Defense. The Congress holds hearings and negotiations which eventually result in authorization of military and other programs and appropriation of funds for those programs. Since the Congress is involved with the whole federal budget, DoD priorities are determined in the context of other priorities of the country.

When the budget process is on schedule, authorization and appropriation legislation distributes the resources to DoD programs including personnel, equipment, operations, maintenance, and research and development. If the authorization and appropriation process is not completed by the end of the fiscal year (September 30), a continuing resolution is required of Congress so that funding can continue at least at the previous year's levels.

The planning, programming, and budgeting system (PPBS) is the means by which the six-year defense program (SYDP) is established, maintained and revised (see Fig 10–3). The Department of Defense, the military departments, and the health care system within each department participate in a complex budget process to support the military mission. Checks and balances are applied to the budget process to ensure the balance of power in our country. The PPBS is a biennial process used to

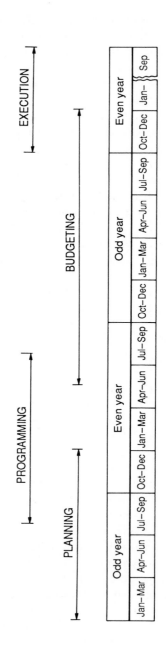

Figure 10-3. Planning, Programming, and Budgeting System (PPBS)

formulate the budget and to manage DoD resources throughout the budget cycle. The PPBS translates national military strategy into personnel and material.

The SYDP is the official document summarizing DoD programs. It is a detailed compilation of the total resources (forces, personnel, procurement, construction, research and development, and operation and maintenance dollars) programmed for DoD, divided into 11 major defense programs. For example, program 8 is training, medical, and other general personnel activities. This program is critical to the functioning of the medical departments of the military departments.

The planning process addresses three broad time periods: long-term planning focuses on 9 to 20 years in the future; midterm planning focuses on 2 to 9 years in the future; and near-term planning takes place for resource management during the next 2 years. As a result, three to four cycles of the budget will be in review simultaneously. Long-term and midterm planning are conducted within the DoD and are generally not subject to public review. However, near-term planning involves budget execution and is closely scrutinized by the Congress and, with the exception of classified programs, is available for public review. Figure 10–4 shows the DoD involvement in the Congressional budget process.

Programming is the second step in the PPBS cycle (see Fig. 10–5). Programming matches dollars available against the most critical needs and priorities. The military department secretaries propose changes, additions, and deletions to the SYDP. The result is the six-year program proposal from each department called the program objective memorandum (POM). The POM is reviewed for overall balance across the services in view of the national military strategy. The Office of the Secretary of Defense (OSD) and the Office of Management and Budget (OMB) review the departments' POMs and suggest alternatives to some proposals. Before the budgeting step can begin, the POM must be approved by the Secretary of Defense in a program decision memorandum (PDM).

Budgeting is the third step in the PPBS cycle. Budgeting involves refinement of detailed costs and development of the individual department budget estimate submission (BES) needed to accomplish the approved program. Following review and approval by OSD and OMB, the budget serves as input to the President's budget on which legislative action is taken. The President reviews the DoD budget, balances defense requirements with domestic and other national programs, and decides on program adjustments and funding levels. The DoD budget submitted to the Congress is structured according to major appropriation categories: military personnel; operations and maintenance; procurement; research, development, test and evaluation; military construction, family housing, and Army stock fund. All of the appropriation categories are applicable to the PPBS cycles of the medical departments of the military services.

The budget formulation cycle concludes after the President's budget request is sent to Congress and the SYDP is updated. The SYDP allows interface between the output oriented DoD and input oriented Congress. The budget is subject at any time, even after approval, to alterations resulting from administration changes, Congressional policy revisions, and DoD mission changes.

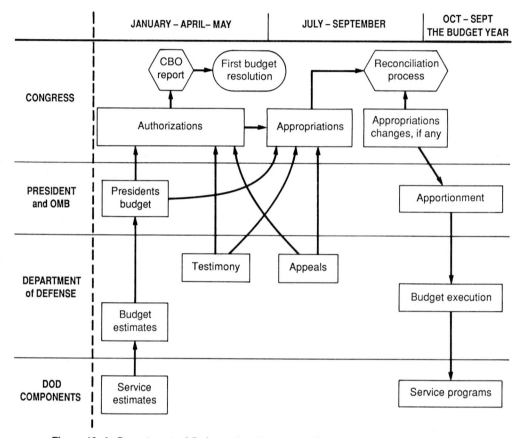

Figure 10-4. Department of Defense Involvement in Congressional Budget Process

The budget process is centralized at command and local levels until execution or allocation. For the military health care system, command level is similar to corporate headquarters and local level is comparable to the medical center or community hospital. The centralized process is extremely effective in providing equitable funding for the military services' ongoing health care operations. However, it lacks the immediacy required to respond quickly to unanticipated situations such as increased personnel requirements because of changed demands for health care services. As a result, individual military facilities may be somewhat slower than civilian health care facilities in accommodating surge demands for personnel resources. Budget appropriations for health care come from tax dollars. Consequently, every effort is made to ensure efficient and judicious use of these fiscal resources.

Military Health Care System Scope
The military health care system is extensive, consisting of more than 500 worldwide medical treatment facilities of varying sizes, including 168 hospitals. The beneficiary

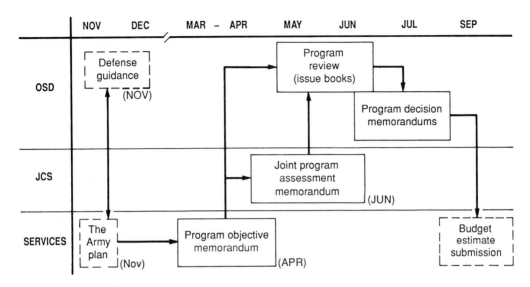

Figure 10-5. Department of Defense Programming

population totals 9.3 million people with approximately 2.2 million active duty personnel. The remainder are retirees and family members of active duty, retired, or deceased military personnel.

The system is closed in that it provides full-service, direct care services around the world to a defined population in specified treatment facilities. Beneficiaries of the military health care system can seek or be referred to civilian health care providers. The full-service aspect of the system means that the military nurse executive is responsible for ensuring that standards of nursing practice, care, and performance are met across all levels. In contrast, the civilian nurse administrator may be responsible for only one aspect of care such as home, long-term, or inpatient care.

Military medical treatment facilities are comprised of medical centers, community hospitals, clinics, and transportable facilities which offer all levels of modern health care to DoD beneficiaries. Transportable hospitals can be deployed for use in civilian disasters where fixed medical facilities are not available. The personnel required to staff these hospitals maintain their preparation while assigned in a fixed facility.

The military services have a reserve component which includes medical units. The reserve components are divided into Army, Navy, and Air Force reserve units and Army and Air National Guard units. Reserve units are organized by geographic region while Guard units are organized by state.

The Army, Navy, and Air Force Nurse Corps maintain a relatively stable number of nurses (about 13,000) on active duty as part of the DoD medical departments. The Navy provides health care for the Marine Corps. The active component is supplemented with nurses in the reserve components (about 25,900) whose mission is to mobilize and augment the active duty forces in a national emergency. In addition, a substantial complement of civilian nurses (about 4000) are federal employees, working in nonmilitary positions in DoD medical treatment facilities.

Skilled enlisted personnel are another enormous resource supporting patient care delivery. Enlisted personnel or paraprofessionals are trained in sequenced educational programs in individual department programs similar to civilian emergency medical technician, licensed practical nurse, and paramedic programs. Education and training continue on the job in clinical settings and in field settings such as aid stations in support of military training exercises. The constant theme of preparation for mobilization and wartime patient care scenarios differentiates military education from comparable civilian programs. About 63,000 active duty enlisted personnel provide support to nursing and patient care in all types of settings.

Medical Treatment Facility (MTF) Organization

The health care system of each military department is organized differently. The distribution of command and control functions depends on historical evolution of the system counterbalanced by requirements engendered by a complex, modern health care system.

For the Army and Air Force, a physician is usually the commander of a military medical treatment facility (MTF), with full responsibility and authority for the facility's operations. The Navy, since 1982, has utilized other health professionals including nurses in command. This Chief Executive Officer role would ordinarily be held by a nonphysician in civilian institutions. The authority of the MTF commander can be conceptualized as both management executive and professional clinician. Administrators on the executive staff bring managerial expertise and authority while nurses and physicians on the executive staff bring both managerial and professional expertise and authority. The military nurse executive participates in an equal and interdependent partnership with other executive staff members to achieve optimal patient care and administrative outcomes in the treatment facility.

Military nurse executives exercise power and influence to effectively advance professional nursing. The military services have an officer force (size) and rank structure; therefore equity, stability and respect are promoted among health care professionals. Since the visible rank adds power of position to existing professional power, military nurse executives may have more influence than civilian nurse executives within the treatment facility.

The budget process and expenditures at each military medical treatment facility are the responsibility of the commander. However, all members of the executive committee are responsible for the execution or allocation of their respective portion of the budget. The executive committee varies depending on the military service and on the size of facility within each service. The executive committee generally includes officers responsible for medical, nursing, and administrative services. All executive staff members act interdependently and rarely, if ever, independently, on budget matters. A Program Budget Advisory Committee (PBAC), comprised of health care executives, meets regularly at military medical treatment facilities to collectively negotiate and make decisions about resource priorities within each facility. The PBAC is the medical treatment facility's portion of the DoD PPBS cycle.

MILITARY NURSE EXECUTIVE DEVELOPMENT

The military nurse executive is a commissioned officer who serves in a variety of roles: chief or director of the corps, chief nurse, assistant chief, senior staff officer or facility commander. As a commissioned officer, the military nurse ''must be capable of providing leadership, management, and planning expertise as well as directing and coordinating the work of others'' (Secretary's Commission on Nursing, 1988). As a manager, the military nurse ''must have the organizational skills and flexibility to respond to the demands of military health care and be responsible for all aspects of nursing care in peacetime and in time of mobilization'' (Secretary's Commission on Nursing, 1988). The professional and career development of the military nurse executive is described in this section.

Self-Management Model

Professional and personal development as a military nurse executive is based on a self-management model. Self-management balances conceptual entities in preparation for the accomplishment of goals and objectives. These entities are necessary within the executive's realm of experience to ensure success and progress of nursing programs in complex health care organizations. The five entities which must be kept in balance are *philosophy, values, knowledge, relationships,* and *endurance* (see Fig 10–6).

Philosophy is the set of basic beliefs which underlie action. The military nurse executive must hold a multidimensional philosophy that, at a minimum, addresses leadership, management, nursing, nursing management, and military nursing. The executive must be able to clearly articulate these dimensions to anyone at any time.

Values are the things of importance to oneself and to others. A clear sense of values assists the military nurse executive in knowing what is of real importance and helps him or her to readily determine the values of subordinates, peers, and superiors. It also is important to acknowledge differences in values so that one can recon-

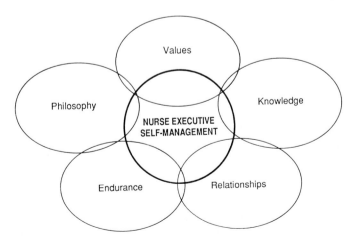

Figure 10–6. Self-Management Model

cile differences and resolve conflicts since the majority of conflicts in health care settings arise from conflicting values.

Knowledge is a fact or condition of knowing something with familiarity gained by way of experience or association. The responsibility and accountability for the judicious leadership and management of nursing personnel during war and peace make it imperative that the military nurse executive possess a depth and breadth of professional nursing knowledge in clinical practice, administration, research, and education. The daily pursuit of knowledge and understanding of complex and diverse topics assist the executive in placing events in their proper perspective within the military setting. The executive must seek knowledge constantly to remain current about professional nursing and the political, social, economic, and cultural issues on local, national, and international levels. The global implications of national security policy necessitate knowledge of the international scene. The deployment of a military force and its possible engagement in combat with subsequent requirements for health care services necessitates indepth knowledge of the military mission and the threat, as well as tactics and strategy.

Relationships are sustained through the rapport established and maintained with others. The closed nature of the military health care system makes it likely that the nurse executive will work with colleagues and collaborators in several settings including combat and contingency situations. Consequently, the executive must concentrate on developing relationships in which teamwork and comradery are fostered.

Endurance is a combination of stamina and persistence. The maintenance of both physical and mental stamina is of immense importance to the military nurse executive. Physical stamina is acquired through a program of deliberate and regular physical fitness and avoidance of substance and dietary excesses. Mental stamina is the maintenance of high mental acuity and alertness via reading and study.

The military nurse executive begins early professional and personal development in leadership by learning and practicing self-management. Self-management is the process whereby philosophy, values, knowledge, relationships and endurance are kept in balance and consciously emphasized in accomplishing goals and objectives.

Roles and Education

Professional development means a well-balanced combination of career area professional expertise, leadership, and management. Professional development synthesizes learning situations and experiences throughout the career, culminating in a nurse executive, educator, clinician, or researcher who balances vision with pragmatism.

Usually, the military nurse executive's first administrative role is that of individual unit manager. The next level in a medical treatment facility could be as a clinical service supervisor or clinical coordinator. Assignments as nurse executive in a medical treatment facility would follow. A chief nurse (CN) or director of nursing services (DNS) at a medical center would be a more senior nurse executive than the CN or DNS of a small community hospital. Military nurse executives might also move to staff jobs at major commands and department (Army, Navy, or Air Force) level organizations.

The military nursing system provides formal education for advanced and executive level management positions. The focus for advanced management development is management theory and practice as applied to middle management responsibilities. Problem-solving, interpersonal relationships, and communication skills for the nurse manager are emphasized. The focus for senior nurse executives is on corporate level decision making, interpersonal collaboration, and analysis of organizational dynamics and structure applicable to the administration of nursing services. Regulations and standards, medical readiness, quality assurance, and policy development and operationalization are integrated throughout learning situations. Professional development conferences, civilian education offerings, and graduate education programs are sources of this education.

MILITARY NURSE EXECUTIVE PRACTICE

Sources of Oversight

The military health care system functions under a framework of laws, directives, regulations, and policies. The military nurse executive is guided by civilian and military standards of health care. Civilian oversight of health care practices comes from the Congress, the Office of Personnel Management (OPM), and the General Accounting Office (GAO). Civilian oversight includes, but is not limited to, the Joint Commission on Accreditation of Healthcare Organizations (JCAHO), the Occupational Safety and Health Administration (OSHA), the Environmental Protection Agency (EPA), and the Center for Disease Control (CDC). As in the civilian community, standards from professional nursing organizations provide important direction for the executive. Military oversight comes from military department and Department of Defense levels and includes the service audit agencies and the Inspector General system. Figure 10–7 lists the civilian and military sources of oversight.

Civilian Oversight. Congress and the civilian elements within the DoD are responsible for broad policy and budget guidance that is eventually operationalized at each military medical treatment facility. The military nurse executive plans with the executive staff of the facility for distribution of financial resources. The OPM sets policy for hiring and performance evaluation of the civilian employees in the nurse executive's department. The GAO audits numerous programs and issues which are directly or indirectly related to the nurse executive's scope of responsibility. GAO audits are directed by the Congress in response to concerns about, for example, quality assurance, health care provider licensure, or medical care in clinics or civilian settings.

As in civilian health care facilities, the JCAHO accredits military health care facilities and provides benchmarks for military health care practice. The military nurse executive uses the JCAHO standards as a basis for the management of nursing services within the facility. Quality assurance programs developed in the facilities are also in keeping with JCAHO standards. These programs can provide ongoing and

```
┌─────────────────────────────────────────────────────────┐
│                    CIVILIAN OVERSIGHT                     │
│                                                          │
│                        Congress                          │
│            Office of Personnel Management                │
│               General Accounting Office                  │
│  Joint Commission for Accreditation of Healthcare Organizations │
│       Occupational Safety and Health Administration      │
│            Environmental Protection Agency               │
│               Center for Disease Control                 │
│             Professional Nursing Standards               │
│                                                          │
│                    MILITARY OVERSIGHT                    │
│                                                          │
│                 Service Audit Agencies                   │
│                   Inspector General                      │
│                      Regulations                         │
│                       Policies                           │
└─────────────────────────────────────────────────────────┘
```

Figure 10-7. Oversight Agencies for Military Nurse Executives

systematic evaluation of nursing care, staff professional development, and education and training programs.

The physical plants and grounds of military medical treatment facilities are subject to OSHA and EPA regulations. For example, radiographic and laboratory equipment must meet standards; building structure must conform to requirements in terms of space, fire prevention, and safety considerations; contaminated and dangerous wastes must be disposed of properly; and water and sewage systems must meet federal codes.

Military Oversight. The department audit agencies are similar to the GAO in that issues or problem areas identified in the health care system are tasked to these agencies for review. The audits may involve the nurse executive's department. The audits provide information about the department's health care system that could assist the nurse executive in establishing policies and overseeing development of standards and procedures of benefit to nursing practice.

The Department of Defense and Army, Navy, and Air Force Inspector General (IG) Systems are wide-ranging agencies charged with inquiring about and/or investigating matters of fraud, waste, abuse, compliance, and systemwide issues. The IG, serving as confidential advisor to the commander, can focus on a person, unit, or system. The nurse executive thus can anticipate interaction with the IG for personnel, patient care, or health care system issues, such as cost or efficiency of services. The IG is internal to DoD and has no disciplinary or punitive authority.

Military Personnel Management

The military nurse executive has responsibility for officers and enlisted personnel in facilities that range from small to large and fixed or mobile facilities, located around the world. Generally, the nurse executive's rank and experience are directly related to the magnitude of the responsibilities assumed. Corporate models for organization, professional development and clinical practice evolve from their adaptability across a large, heterogenous system. Military nurse executives in DoD hold 563 positions out of a total of 13,338 budgeted positions for the combined Army, Navy, and Air Force Nurse Corps. In a smaller facility, the executive's scope of responsibility may include officers from medical support services, such as pharmacy or respiratory therapy, and administration.

The military health care system provides little flexibility in personnel resources. Regardless of documented personnel requirements for overall mission performance, budgetary constraints determine numbers of personnel actually assigned. The military nurse executive distributes the personnel resources to meet mission requirements and to use them efficiently and effectively to achieve a desired level of productivity. Decisions to combine health care services, reduce operating beds or units, or limit patient admissions to certain units are based on data supplied by the nurse executive to the executive staff. The hospital commander has responsibility for the final decisions in these matters.

Officers. The military nurse executive manages most nurse officers in the facility. The constant turnover of officer staff due to reassignment, retirement, and release from active duty is a challenge in order to maintain consistently high standards and morale as new officers replace those who have been there two to four years. Replacements may or may not be available in time to have an orientation overlap with their predecessors. The nurse executive's effectiveness is tested by the constant turnover. Each executive expects to receive, and is expected to send to the next facility, officers with maximum education and clinical performance capability.

All military members are employed by the system and thus the process of hiring and firing does not rest with one executive. While the process of removing an employee from the system may be cumbersome at times, it does not threaten safe nursing practice. The nurse executive has the authority to remove unsafe or poor performers from clinical practice and to initiate the administrative or disciplinary process necessary to determine the member's employment status.

Three broad categories of nurse officers staff a medical treatment facility: first-term officers, nurse officers who have made the decision to remain beyond one term, and career or senior officers (see Fig 10–8). First-term officers come with varied expectations about nursing and about the military system. They originate from various geographical areas. Accession standards provide selection criteria for new officers in that their nursing education, nursing experience, character, and civilian employment history concerning malpractice and legal matters are reviewed closely prior to their selection for service. Personal health is evaluated and applicants must meet preset physical standards. The new officers are a more diversified group since age limits for recruitment have become more liberal. The military nurse executive sets expectations for the staff concerning the new officers in the facility. For example, orientation programs, preceptorship programs, and socialization to nursing and the military are all

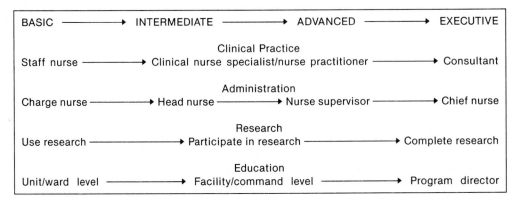

Figure 10–8. Professional Development for Nurse Executives

key elements for moving the new nurse officers toward the ability to provide quality professional nursing care. In addition, the fulfillment of the military nurse executive's expectations should set the groundwork for the newly accessed nurse's progression toward military career status.

The second category of nurse officers for whom the executive is responsible ranges from nurses who have made the decision to stay in the military beyond their first term to middle managers and a variety of clinical specialists, nurse practitioners, and junior staff officers. This group is evaluated by the nurse executive and identified for development as senior military leaders, preparation for senior staff roles at major commands, service departments or Department of Defense levels. The executive must set standards for the administrative and clinical senior staff who will, in turn, challenge the middle level officers to improve their professional nursing skills and knowledge, advance their military education and experiences, and successfully pursue civilian graduate education. While promotion in the early ranks is assured if the officer's record reflects good performance, promotion in the middle ranks becomes much more competitive and requires an outstanding record. In the Army and Air Force, these promotions are to Captain and Major; in the Navy the comparable grades would be Lieutenant and Lieutenant Commander. The officer will decide whether to make a firm commitment during these middle years, planning for a military career of 20 to 30 years.

The third category of nurse officers are the senior managers, clinicians, educators and researchers. These officers generally have graduate degrees in nursing or related fields; their military education is at the staff officer level. The military nurse executive works most closely with this core group, with the number of staff being determined by the mission of the facility. The executive works through this group to disseminate a personal philosophy of nursing that sets the stage for the philosophy, goals, and objectives that guide the work of the department of nursing.

The military nursing executive is assigned with some knowledge of the state of nursing in the facility and with variable knowledge about the staff in place and the anticipated, normal military staff turnover. The executive is challenged to pull the senior staff together into a cohesive, productive unit. The executive has the authority and responsibility to optimally configure the department within constraints of total numbers of officers authorized and assigned to the facility. The executive works with this senior group to accomplish personnel management changes, for example, centralization or decentralization. Senior staff members have made a career commitment to the military; nonetheless, the executive has the responsibility for stimulating their professional development and advancement within the system.

The military nurse executive represents the department of nursing staff to the rest of the military health care system. The constant challenges in facilities between peacetime health care and mobilization training for war, demand that the executive's beliefs and values concerning personnel management and professional development are based in the context of the military health care system as a whole.

Enlisted Personnel. The military nurse executive is responsible for enlisted personnel assigned to the health care facility or to a facility elsewhere (eg, clinics in remote locations). The military system always will have a mix of professional and paraprofessional staff, given the mobilization requirement of care ranging from the battlefield to the general hospital. In wartime, basic medics serve on the battlefield and paraprofessionals, with more specialized training (eg, licensed practical nurses), serve at first line treatment sites nearest the battlefield.

The assignment of enlisted personnel to medical treatment facilities is generally controlled by enlisted personnel management systems of the service branches. Enlisted personnel come with widely diverse ages, training, experience, and levels of motivation for the military system and for health care. The turnover rate is high among paraprofessionals after they complete their first enlistment of three or four years. Every military medical facility and health care setting is influenced by the substantial training needs of the enlisted personnel and by the loss of investment in training when they leave the service.

Enlisted personnel have to be able to provide care within the designated scope of practice for their specialty. They also must successfully complete progressive military training programs which are prerequisites to promotion and retention. In addition, when assigned to a medical treatment facility, enlisted personnel have numerous other tasks and duties which are critical to the facility but do not contribute directly to the patient care mission. When enlisted personnel are assigned to units that would be directly involved in combat (for example, an infantry battalion in the army) their health care duties are supervised by more senior paraprofessionals, physician's assistants, or by professional staff.

The noncommissioned officer (NCO) system is strong in all branches of the service; the hierarchy and the benchmarks for advancement are well-established. Consequently, the executive is expected to carefully balance the senior officer's role in enlisted nursing personnel management and evaluation with the NCO system's role. The demand for safe practice at all levels is paramount for the quality of health care delivered in the facility.

As with officers, enlisted personnel cannot be hired or fired per se. Administrative and disciplinary actions are the responsibility of officer or senior enlisted personnel. The nurse executive does have sufficient authority to relieve those with poor clinical performance through evaluation procedures.

Military Evaluations. Performance evaluation for military nurses and enlisted personnel is accomplished through Officer Evaluation Reports (OER) or Enlisted Evaluation Reports (EER). The Navy uses Officer Fitness Reports and Enlisted Performance Evaluations. Reports are prepared by specified individuals within the rated person's chain of command. The report documents the caliber of performance during the rating period and identifies potential for promotion and assignment to positions of higher responsibility.

As a management tool, evaluation performance data are used as a basis for various personnel actions such as retention and advancement in the military, school selection, specialty designation, and, for officers, command selection. The evaluation report is the single most important document in the career file of the military service member. Evaluation fairness is enhanced by having input from at least two raters. Service members have the option of appealing unsatisfactory reports through a process defined by service-specific regulations.

Civilian Personnel Management

The military medical departments also have civilian registered nurses and paraprofessional nurses. The military nurse executive ensures that all staff with responsibility for civilian personnel have the knowledge necessary to sustain this important component of the military health care system. Civilians new to nursing and the military system need orientation, preceptorship, and clinical guidance. Experienced civilian nurses warrant continuing education and clinical advancement and the effective military nursing executive ensures these processes. Civilian employees work in direct patient care and nursing management positions. Civilians also hold specialist roles such as nurse practitioners, nurse anesthetists, and occupational health nurses. While some contracting for agency nurses occurs, most civilians are federal employees and are part of the General Schedule (GS) Classification and Pay System.

Generally, civilians are a stable core of staff in a military MTF and thus are extremely valuable. Of the three services, the Army has the greatest number of civilian nursing employees. The Army depends on senior civilians to keep units and sections running smoothly, given the military turnover and constant need for education and training of nurses and enlisted and civilian paraprofessional personnel.

Classification. Civilian nursing positions are all classified according to the Classification Act of 1923. Position Classification Standards are published by the Civil Service Commission after extensive public research of occupations; detailed guidance is provided for evaluation and corresponding grade allocation. A pay grade, an occupational code, and a title are given by a personnel specialist during the classification process. Decisions on grade and code are made by comparing one or more position classification statements to the nursing tasks to be performed and responsibilities to be met on the job. Grades for nursing personnel are from GS-3 for nursing assistants to GS-12 for civilians in supervisory or senior staff roles.

Evaluation. Under the Civil Service Reform Act, all government agencies including health care facilities must have a system for timely and accurate appraisal of employee job performance. The appraisal results then are used as a basis for education and training, rewarding, promoting, retaining, reassigning, changing grade level, or removing employees. A formal performance rating is normally made annually. Major and critical job elements are identified and, together with performance standards, are communicated in writing to each employee at the beginning of the rating period. The job elements encompass all of the duties in the particular job. Five levels of performance ranging from exceptional to unacceptable are used to document employees' job performance. Yearly performance appraisals do not necessarily signal a pay raise or bonus. Several programs exist where monetary performance awards can be given. Salary increases would come with grade or step-within-grade promotions.

Promotions. The Federal Merit Promotion Program provides that promotions for civil service employees will be fair and that promotion practices will support the organization's effort to select and retain the best qualified employees. Opportunities for civilian advancement occur when new positions are established because of reorganization, when responsibilities are added to an existing job description, or when an employee vacates a position. Promotable employees meet qualification requirements and time-in-grade requirements while also being evaluated as fully successful in their performance appraisals. Promotions can be competitive or noncompetitive; the employee can be promoted within the career ladder that provides for successive upward promotion to an established full performance level or the employee's position may be reclassified at a higher grade level due to the addition of more complex duties and responsibilities.

SUMMARY

The dual role of military nurse executive as professional nurse and officer of substantial rank provides the challenge and rewards that make military nursing exciting and unique. The context for military nurse executives' professional practice includes both the military structure and professional nursing. The military health care system is part of the Department of Defense structure. Budget processes, scope of the system and medical treatment facility are all organized within this system. Civilian control of the Department of Defense and thus the three military departments must be recognized as the driving force behind organization and budget for military health care.

Military nurse executive development uses a self-management model for nursing executives to demonstrate the process of professional and personal development toward key positions in the Nurse Corps. Standards, both civilian and military, provide policy and direction to military nurse executives. A large part of the nurse executive's responsibility is personnel management emphasizing career professional development for military and civilian professional and paraprofessional staff.

REFERENCES

Army Command and Management: Theory and Practice. (1989–1990) US Army War College. Carlisle Barracks, PA, 24–30

Joint Chiefs of Staff (JCS) Publication 2. 1986, 2–1, 2–13

Secretary's Commission on Nursing. US Department of Health and Human Services, vol II, 1988, VI-A-6

Organizing HRM Systems

CHAPTER 11

Nursing and Employment Law

Helen Conners
Jim Guthrie

Key Concept List

Sources of law: Civil, Contract, Criminal, and Administrative Law
Liability, negligence, and malpractice
Incompetent practice
Equal Employment Law (Title VII)
Affirmative action
Age and usage discrimination
Employment-at-Will Law
Occupational Safety and Health Law

As the role of the professional nurse has expanded to include increased expertise, specialization, autonomy, and accountability, so has the number of malpractice lawsuits against nurses. The paternalistic attitudes of the past, where physicians and health care institutions assumed responsibility for the acts of their employees are no longer the norm. Although the doctrine of *respondeat superior* still exists, individuals also are being held accountable for their own negligent acts. Nurses and nurse executives must develop an increased understanding of the changing legal climate and of what their responsibilities are, as viewed by the public and the legal system (Luquire, 1989).

SOURCES OF LAW

Understanding sources of law and the various types of law assists in determining their impact on nursing practice. Each of the three branches of the government creates law, and these, in conjunction with the Constitution, form the basis of the judicial system of this country. The Constitution is the supreme law of the land. It defines the structure, power and limits of the government and guarantees people certain fundamental rights as individuals. The influences of the legislative, judicial and executive branches of the government are reflected in statutory law, common law, and administrative law (Northrop & Kelly, 1987).

Statutory Law

A statute is law enacted by the legislative branch of government. It is designed to declare, command, or prohibit something. State and federal governments have broad powers to legislate for the general welfare of the public. The federal government's explicit power is invested in it by the Constitution, whereas the states have broad inherent powers to act except where the Constitution reserves the power to the federal government. The state's power to govern is referred to as "police power." Generally, this term is defined as the power inherent in the state to legislate, within the limits of the state and federal constitutions, reasonable laws necessary to maintain the public order, health, safety, welfare, and morals (Northrop & Kelly, 1987). Licensure laws for health care providers, including nurses, are statutory law. These laws are designed to protect the welfare of the public from incompetent practitioners. Other statutory laws affecting nursing practice are: guardianship codes, statutes of limitation, informed consent, living will legislation, and protective and reporting laws.

Common Law

Common law is the law made as the result of a judge's decision as opposed to law created by the legislature. This type of law is derived from earlier decisions made by the court which are referred to as legal precedent. Common law establishes a custom or tradition by which other similar cases are judged. It is not absolute; earlier decisions can and frequently are overturned. As time and circumstances change, court decisions become obsolete and may require a different opinion.

Each state has its own body of common law related to the delivery of health care within that state. These laws must be known by health professionals as a basis for accountability, quality assurance, and risk management within their professional practice. As the number of malpractice suits involving nurses increases, the body of common law regulating nursing practice also increases. An awareness of this law will help nurses to function within their role boundaries and to advocate for nursing practice.

Administrative Law

According to statutes, administrative agencies are granted authority to enact rules and regulations that will carry out the specific intentions of the statutes. These regulations are adopted by the agencies according to a well-defined approval process. This type of law making allows the legislature to delegate to an administrative agency the authority to create rules and regulations governing a specific area of practice, using experts in that field. Legislators could not be expected to process the necessary knowledge and expertise to dictate such practice regulations. For example, state boards of nursing are authorized by nurse practice acts (statutory law) to write rules and regulations governing the practice of nursing. These rules and regulations are as binding as the statutory law itself. Nurses, especially nurse managers and executives, need to monitor these proposed rules and regulations because of their possible future effect on nursing practices.

Another example of administrative law is the opinion of the attorney general. Frequently, the attorney general is requested by an individual or an agency to give an opinion regarding the interpretation of a law. The response to this request is considered a form of administrative law. It is binding until a subsequent statute, regulation or court decision is made which contradicts the attorney general's opinion.

TYPES OF LAW

The two basic classifications of law are criminal and civil law. Criminal law deals with an individual's relationship to the state or society. It is an offense against the state and a breach against society. Civil law deals with the relationships between individuals. It is an infringement against an individual's rights. When an individual's rights are violated, the aggrieved person may seek restitution by filing a civil action suit. Civil law can be further classified to include tort law, contract law, and protecting and reporting laws. Criminal law is broken down to include misdemeanors and felonies.

Civil Law

Tort Law. Tort law is divided into two categories, unintentional and intentional. Negligence and malpractice (professional negligence) fall under the category of unintentional torts. Intentional torts consist of assault, battery, false imprisonment, invasion of privacy, disclosure of confidential information, libel, slander, misrepresentation and fraud, and defamation of character. The most common type of law affecting nursing practice is that of unintentional torts (malpractice). Malpractice will be discussed in detail later in this chapter.

Contract Law

A contract is a legally enforceable agreement or promise to do a certain thing. For example, an employment contract is an exchange of promises between two persons who are legally capable of making such an agreement. It consists of a promise by the employee to perform certain specified services during a specific time frame in return for a promise by the employer to give a certain monetary payment and other benefits. An employment contract should be in writing, stating the specific terms of the agreement. When the job is for a specific period of time, the employer cannot terminate the employee before that time ends unless the employer has just cause. Failing to report to work or stealing from an employer constitutes just cause. The employee, however, has more latitude to end the employment arrangement. Usually, the courts do not force employees to work for employers if they do not desire to do so. Reasonable notice is also a consideration in terminating an employer–employee contract. Written employment contracts usually are reserved for executive level employment (Hunt, 1988; Calloway, & Kota, 1989). Some states accept the doctrine of "employment at will," in which a contract, unless it is expressly written, will not be recognized and an employee may be terminated "at will." This concept is further discussed later.

Certain basic premises must exist for a contract to be legally binding: (1) the parties involved must be present in order for a contract to be legally binding; (2) an offer or promise must be made between the two parties; (3) the offer must be mutually understood and accepted; and (4) the parties agree that only lawful actions be performed in return for something of value. If any of these four elements is not present, the contract usually will not hold up against a legal challenge (Northrop & Kelly, 1987). It is important for nurse executives to become familiar with contract laws that impact their practice. For example, a breach of contract may exist when a private duty nurse terminates services provided to a patient without giving reasonable notice (Fiesta, 1988).

Protective and Reporting Laws. Protective and reporting statutes are designed to provide for the safety or rights of a specified class of individuals. For example, many states have enacted statutes which require mandatory reporting of suspected elder abuse. The same is true for child abuse. Other protective and reporting laws include: violation of the privacy act, age of consent statutes, privileged communication statute, abortion statute, good samaritan act, living will legislation, and mandatory reporting of incompetent practice.

Additional Civil Laws. Additional civil laws affecting employer and employee relationships will be discussed later in this chapter. Labor laws, which protect workers rights to bargain collectively and outlaw unfair labor practices, are discussed in Chapter 18.

Criminal Laws

A crime is an act of omission or commission which is punishable by the state. Crimes require a particular state of mind which is referred to as a criminal intent. The necessity to prove criminal intent is one of the criteria that distinguishes criminal acts from torts. Generally, torts do not require willfulness or specific intent. Intentional torts, as the name implies, are the exception.

Crimes are classified into two major categories: *misdemeanors* and *felonies*. Some jurisdictions define misdemeanors as acts punishable by fine and/or imprisonment in jail, and felonies as crimes punishable by death or imprisonment in the state penitentiary or prison. Others define the two according to length of imprisonment. Misdemeanors are crimes punishable by less than 6 months in prison or under $500 in assessed fines. Felonies constitute acts punishable by an amount above that specified for misdemeanors (Fiesta, 1988; Northrop & Kelly, 1987).

Homicide and manslaughter are examples of crimes. If a nurse intentionally kills a patient, the nurse may be prosecuted by the government for a crime. Euthanasia, involuntary manslaughter, rape, and elder or child abuse are examples of criminal offenses against nurses.

LIABILITY

As individuals, nurses are responsible and accountable for their own actions or inactions. This is referred to as *personal liability*. In addition, the law ascribes negligence to certain parties who may not be negligent themselves but whose negligence is implied because of association with the negligent person. This is called *vicarious liability* and is based on the legal principle of "respondeat superior" which means "let the master speak." This doctrine allows the courts to hold the employer responsible for the actions of the employee when performing services for the employer.

All too frequently, the nurse has a false sense of security concerning the doctrines of respondeat superior and vicarious liability. Employees sometimes believe that the institution's responsibility protects them from being sued as individuals; this is not the case. Patients have the right to sue both the employee and the institution when they have suffered injuries as a result of substandard care. Also, the employer has the right to sue the employee for damages it incurred as a result of the nurse's substandard care. This action is based on the principle of indemnification. This principle is applicable when: (a) the employer is held liable only because of the negligent actions of the employee and (b) the employer is assessed monetary damages because of the employee's negligence (Guido, 1988). This is why it is important for staff nurses to carry their own personal liability insurance.

Nurse managers frequently do not recognize their responsibility and liability for their acts of delegation and supervision of employees. Nurse managers must be cautioned to know the extent of their liability. Delegation and supervision are part of the nurse manager's job responsibilities and, therefore, they are held individually accountable for these actions. If the nurse manager makes an assignment to one known to be incompetent, liability on the part of the nurse manager could result. There is no liability for the nurse manager under the doctrine of respondeat superior because the nurse manager is not the employer. However, the employer could be held responsible under this doctrine for the nurse manager's actions as the institution would be for any employee. This concept is discussed further in the section on delegation and supervision.

Employers also are subject to corporate liability. Corporate liability holds the institution responsible for its own wrongful conduct. The health care institution has the responsibility of maintaining an environment that allows for quality health care for its consumers. Corporate liability issues include: the duty to hire, supervise, and maintain qualified, competent, and adequate staff; the duty to provide, inspect, repair, and maintain reasonably adequate equipment; and the duty to maintain safety in the physical environment. These duties are very broad and require that responsibilities for achievement be delegated to management even though the institution is ultimately responsible. Nursing administration assists the institution in fulfilling these duties. For example, hospitals usually have a mechanism in place for reporting incompetent, unethical, and illegal practices. If the nurse manager (or administrator) is aware of such practice but does not report it, the responsible administrators also are liable. Many states have statutory laws regarding mandatory reporting of legal and ethical issues (Luckenbill-Brett & Stuhler-Schlag, 1987). The individual nurse's or manager's legal duty is satisfied as long as they fulfill their duty to communicate issues within their job responsibilities.

NEGLIGENCE AND MALPRACTICE

Negligence. Negligence is defined as the failure of an individual to perform an act or not perform an act that a reasonably prudent person would or would not perform in a similar set of circumstances. *Malpractice* is professional negligence. It refers to any misconduct or lack of skill in carrying out professional responsibilities. In most states, expert testimony is required to prove professional negligence. Ordinary negligence does not usually require the testimony of an expert.

For malpractice to exist, four elements must be present: duty, breach of duty, causation, and injury. If any one of these elements cannot be proven by a preponderance of the evidence, then the judge or jury will hold in favor of the defendant.

Nurses, by virtue of their professional responsibilities, have the duty to provide the degree of nursing care that a reasonably prudent nurse with comparable education and training would provide in a similar set of circumstances. The more educated and the more specialized the nurse is, the higher the standard of care. Duty is breached when the nurse does not perform according to the professional standard of care.

The professional standard of care can be established by a variety of sources. Nurse practice acts of each state define the scope of nursing practice and the rules and regulations that guide the practice of nursing in that state. Over the years, nurse practice acts have changed to reflect the changing practice of nursing. The rapidly expanding role of the nurse has led many states to define nursing more generally allowing rules and regulations to guide practice and specify educational requirements. Several state boards of nursing have promulgated rules and regulations governing advanced and specialty practice, including nursing administration.

Other sources are used to determine practice standards. The American Nurses Association (ANA) and other specialty organizations have formulated and published standards for nursing practice. The overall framework for these standards is the nursing process. Standards that are formulated and published by a recognized authority are generally acknowledged as describing the minimal acceptable behavior for that specific area of practice (Cushing, 1988). The Standards for Nurse Administrators developed by ANA provide a framework for organizing and operating nursing services in a variety of health care settings. These standards are outlined in Table 11–1 (ANA Standards for Organized Nursing Services).

TABLE 11-1. STANDARDS FOR ORGANIZED NURSING SERVICES

Standard I

Organized nursing services have a philosophy and structure that ensure the delivery of effective nursing care.

Standard II

Organized nursing services are administered by qualified and competent nurse administrators.

Standard III

The nurse executive determines and administers the fiscal resources of organized nursing services. The nurse executive has an interactive role in the determination of the organization's fiscal resource requirements and their acquisition, allocation, and utilization.

Standard IV

Within organized nursing services, the nursing process is used as the framework for providing nursing care to recipients.

Standard V

An environment is created within organized nursing services that enhances nursing practice and facilitates the delivery of care by all nursing staff.

Standard VI

Organized nursing services have a quality assurance program.

Standard VII

Organized nursing services have policies to guide ethical decision making based on the code for nurses.

Standard VIII

Within organized nursing services, research in nursing, health, and nursing systems are facilitated; research findings are disseminated; and support is provided for integration of these findings into the delivery of nursing care and nursing administration.

Standard IX

Organized nursing services provide policies and practices that address equity and continuity of nursing services and recognize cultural, economic, and social differences among recipients served by the health care organization.

American Nurses Association. *Standards for organized Nursing Services and responsibilities of nurse administrators across all settings.* (NS-31 3.5M). Kansas City, MO, 1988

Accreditation standards, such as those established by the Joint Commission for Accreditation of Healthcare Organizations (JCAHO), assist in establishing the standards for health care facilities accredited by JCAHO. These accreditation standards address a variety of hospital, clinic, home health, and long-term care operation procedures including nursing services. In addition, federal and state accreditation standards or regulations for health care facilities can be used to establish the standard of care for those institutions governed by such standards.

Institutional policies, procedures and bylaws as well as job descriptions serve to establish internal standards of care. Violation of these standards can be held against one in a court of law. Failure to follow these directives demonstrates a breach of duty. These documents must be drafted with care and must be communicated to those employees responsible for their implementation. Following such rules, regulations, and policies does not necessarily mean that the defendant met the proper standard of care (Fiesta, 1988; Northrop & Kelly, 1987; Calloway & Kota, 1989).

Professional publications, textbooks, and journals provide another measure of determining the standard of care. These are used to prove facts in issue or to discredit the testimony of an expert witness (Cushing, 1988). Nurses need to be familiar with current literature in their area of practice to guide their practice.

The most important factor in establishing the standard of care in a malpractice case is the expert witness. When the nurse's alleged negligence involves professional skills, expert testimony is required by law to establish that the duty of care was breached, and that the defendant acted improperly. The purpose of the expert opinion is to explain to the judge or jury the intricacies of nursing practice as applied to a given situation.

Expert testimony is not required if the doctrine of *res ipsi loquitur* exists. Literally this phrase means "the thing speaks for itself." For this doctrine to apply three conditions must exist: (1) the injury must be the kind that would ordinarily not occur in the absence of negligence; (2) the injury must be in the exclusive control of the defendant; and (3) the plaintiff must not have voluntarily contributed to the injury in anyway (Fiesta, 1988). If these circumstances exist, then the nature of the injury is probably within the scope of jurors common knowledge and an expert witness may not be needed.

For malpractice to exist there must be a preponderance of evidence to demonstrate that the breach of duty was the direct or proximate cause of the injury which occurred. If there is not a connection between the breach of duty and the reported injury, or if there is no resulting harm, physical, financial or emotional, then malpractice does not exist and damages will not be awarded. Only when plaintiffs are able to prove that they suffered calculable harm directly related to the treatment rendered to them can they be economically enumerated in order to make them "whole" again.

COMMON CAUSES OF MALPRACTICE FOR NURSE ADMINISTRATORS

The nurse administrator has the legal responsibility to control the quality of nursing care rendered within the institution (Northrop & Kelly, 1988). This includes the responsibility of providing direction and programs that assure the development and productive performance of nursing personnel.

DELEGATION AND SUPERVISION

Nursing management encompasses supervising nursing care and the personnel who provide that care. The nurse manager is personally liable for the reasonable exercise of delegation and supervision activities. Failure to delegate and supervise within accepted standards of professional nursing may be viewed as malpractice. This does not absolve the individual nurse's responsibility, but extends the liability to the nurse manager. In addition, the health care institution or employer also can be held liable for the nurse manager's negligent acts committed within the scope of employment under the doctrine of respondeat superior. It is important to emphasize that nurse managers are not liable just because of supervisory status of their positions. They are liable only if they personally committed the negligent act or are negligent in their delegation and supervision of others. Since nurse managers usually are not the employer, the nurse manager cannot be held liable under the doctrine of respondeat superior. Also, if it can be proven that the nurse manager delegated appropriately and had no reason to believe that the assigned nurse was anything other than competent, then the nurse manager cannot be held personally liable in the case.

The nurse manager must be aware of the staff's knowledge, skills, and competencies when delegating tasks and must supervise appropriately. Unfortunately, because there are no clear-cut legal guidelines to describe adequate supervision, a common-sense approach is recommended. Nurse managers have a legal duty to ensure that the staff members reporting to them are performing in a manner consistent with the standard of practice. Knowingly allowing staff to function below the accepted standard of care increases one's personal liability as well as employer liability. If a nurse manager makes an assignment to a nurse who the manager knows is not competent to perform that assignment, the nurse manager can be liable if the patient is injured. The employer also will be held liable (Calloway & Kota, 1989).

Staffing

An unprecedented demand for nurses compounded with the increased technology has created staffing dilemmas for hospitals and other health care institutions. According to established standards, the institution must provide adequate staffing with qualified personnel (Calfee, 1987). The responsibility of the institution to maintain an adequate staffing level often falls on the shoulders of nurse managers and nurse executives. The institution that fails to retain the level of nursing personnel required to provide safe quality care may be held liable under the doctrine of corporate liability if an injury occurs and is shown to be related to "short staffing." On the other hand, if it can be shown that the injury resulted from the staff nurse's inappropriate actions, regardless of the staffing issue, the individual nurse can be held personally liable, and the employer also is liable under the doctrine of respondeat superior. Inadequate staff is no excuse for negligent acts.

The *Horton v Niagara Falls Memorial Medical Center* case is illustrative of inappropriate actions of a charge nurse. In this case a charge nurse on an understaffed unit was held liable for failure to communicate the situation to the supervisor when a confused patient was injured in a fall from a balcony. Construction workers reported to the charge nurse that the patient was on the balcony outside his room requesting a ladder. The charge nurse called the patient's wife and asked if she could come and sit with the patient. The wife stated that she would send her mother who was 10 minutes away from the hospital and requested that the charge nurse assign someone to watch the patient in the meantime. The charge nurse stated that this would not be possible because the unit was understaffed. The charge nurse provided no supervision nor did she notify the supervisor of the problem. During the 10-minute period before the patient's mother-in-law arrived, the patient jumped from the balcony and was injured. The court held the charge nurse liable for failure to properly supervise the patient and failure to communicate the staffing problem to the supervisor. The hospital was liable under the doctrine of respondeat superior. In ruling, the court noted that there were orderlies from other areas of the hospital as well as a registered nurse assigned to the charge nurse for orientation, who could have stayed temporarily with the patient. In addition the charge nurse allowed a nurse's aide to go to supper during this time (Calloway & Kota, 1989; Fiesta, 1990). Although understaffing may have been an issue in this case, it was not the cause of the negligence; poor judgment on the part of the charge nurse was the cause.

As always, it is the nurse manager's responsibility to maintain a reasonable standard of care on the nursing unit. If short staffing compromises that care, and you have done all in your power to alleviate the situation, then you must communicate your concerns to upper levels of management. Frequently, a short staffing problem needs to be addressed to top management levels. Upper management may choose to make business decisions regarding staffing which they must defend in the event of a malpractice suit. As long as the staff nurse and nurse manager acted reasonably under the circumstances the liability rests with the institution. If the institution is aware of short staffing and makes a business decision not to fill vacancies there is nothing the staff nurse or nurse manager can do about the problem. In addition, in some cases, if it can be demonstrated that management has taken appropriate actions to alleviate the staffing crisis, then they may not be held liable (Fiesta, 1990).

Staffing an institution is not as clear-cut as it may seem. Although the institution has some guidelines to follow, such as those mandated by the Joint Commission as well as federal and state regulatory bodies, these guidelines are broad and require a certain amount of judgment. Even though they specify minimum nurse patient ratios, adequate staffing mix of registered nurses to other personnel, and a statement that patient care assignments be made by a registered nurse based on assessed patient needs and qualifications of the staff, other factors involved in providing adequate staff are somewhat subjective and the responsibility of the institution. Acuity instruments are helpful in that they provide an objective measure of the number of staff needed; however, they do not take into consideration whether these staff are experienced or inexperienced. They also do not take into consideration whether adequate equipment is accessible, appropriate policies exist, and sufficient supervision is available, all of which would be helpful adjuncts during a staffing crunch (Fiesta, 1990).

Floating Staff

Health care employers have a legal duty to ensure that all areas of the hospital are adequately staffed. With fluctuating patient census, this often places the hospital in a position where floating nurses from one area of the hospital to another is the only way to balance the needs of the unit and the safety of the patients. This practice is commonplace in today's hospital; however, it does raise some concern on the part of the staff nurse and the institution. Floating nurses to unfamiliar areas, especially specialty areas, increases the chance of error and increases the nurses' anxiety levels. According to JCAHO criteria, assignments must be made in accordance with the qualifications of the nursing personnel. Floating a nurse to a completely unfamiliar area is in violation of this standard.

Floating hospital personnel is a necessary evil that in many instances cannot be avoided. Nurses have no legal ground to refuse to float unless it is previously specified in their contract, the institution has policies and procedures to the contrary, or the nurse is not competent to carry out a specific assignment. Nurses who refuse to float may face the possibility of discharge on the grounds of insubordination. Nurses must realize that they have a professional responsibility to serve in the best interest of the patient. The administrator must recognize that to achieve adequate staffing requires consideration of patient care requirements, staff expertise, unit geography, available support services, and patient care delivery systems. Open communication regarding staff limitations and concerns as well as creative problem solving can assist with alleviating some of the stress associated with floating (Calloway, 1986).

Temporary Personnel

The increased use of temporary personnel or agency nurses has caused some administrators to question their accountability for the actions of these individuals. In the past, nurses and other health professionals not employed by an institution were considered independent contractors. As such, the employer was not held liable for their actions. Recently, the courts have begun to refute this principle of no liability with the legal theories of ostensible agency or apparent authority. These principles apply when it is reasonable for a patient to believe that the health care provider is an employee of the institution. In other words, if it appears that the nurse is an employee of the institution, he or she may be considered an employee (Fiesta, 1990).

If the principles of ostensible agency or apparent authority apply, the employee may be placed in a position of vicarious liability for the agency nurse just as for its own staff nurse. For this reason, if the administrator believes that the agency nurse is incompetent, this must be communicated to the employer of the agency nurse. In addition, screening of the agency personnel must be done as carefully as it is for regular employees of the institution. A critical need for nurses is no justification for accepting incompetence. The use of agency personnel and float nurses requires a higher degree of supervision.

Equipment

When a patient is injured by a piece of equipment, the immediate issue is whether the injury was a result of a product defect or whether the injury was due to equipment misuse or lack of maintenance. Product liability cases often involve the manufacturer of the product, the institution, and the individual using the equipment. Generally, accountability follows control; therefore, those who have control of the solution to the problem will be held liable. Design or construction defects, a breach of warranty, or failure to provide adequate warnings are examples of manufacturers' liability issues (Cushing, 1988; Fiesta, 1989).

The health care institution, as a corporation, has a duty to make sure that equipment is available and in working order. It also is the institution's duty to provide adequate training to teach nursing personnel how to operate equipment and what to do in case of equipment failure. The institution must have policies governing the use and maintenance of equipment, especially complex equipment (Cushing, 1988). The institution relies on the staff nurse and nurse managers to assess equipment, ensure proper maintenance, and report faulty or malfunctioning equipment. Maintaining proper functioning of equipment also has been expanded to include ensuring that equipment is not contaminated and that hospital policy is followed when cleaning and storing equipment (Guido, 1988). Since accountability follows control, the staff nurse may be held individually accountable for improper use of properly functioning equipment. Frequently, nursing personnel fail to recognize equipment usage as part of their scope of responsibility.

Policies and Procedures

Policies and procedures are required by JCAHO for all accredited health care institutions. These documents serve to set standards for care and guide practices. They must be well delineated, clearly stated, and based on current and actual practice.

When the nurse is responsible for performing procedures that require judgments beyond the usual scope of nursing practice a standardized procedure or protocol is necessary. These procedures must be written and authorized by the institution. Routinely, the standardized protocol must specify: (1) the functions the nurse may perform under specific circumstances; (2) any requirements that must be followed in performing the function; (3) education, experience, and training requisites of the nurse performing the procedures; and (4) the method for evaluating competence of the nurse performing the practice (Walker, 1980).

RISK MANAGEMENT

Since the early 1970s health care organizations have recognized the importance of risk management programs. Although risk management was always a consideration, it was not formalized or required as it is today. In recent years, many states have enacted statutory risk management requirements with mandatory reporting mechanisms in an attempt to reduce the risk of malpractice lawsuits. In addition, the federal government and insurance companies have enacted safety laws and rules governing risk prevention.

The American Hospital Association (AHA), instrumental in the development of risk management programs, defines risk management as "the science for the identification, evaluation and treatment of the risk of financial loss" (Dankmyer & Groves, 1977). The goals of such a program are: (1) to assess areas in which claims can be prevented; and, (2) to identify, analyze, evaluate, and treat risk factors in order to reduce preventable injuries and minimize financial severity of claims. Many institutions now have established management committees to assess areas of real or potential risk and to develop programs to reduce the risk of malpractice. An important responsibility of this committee is to educate nursing staff regarding their legal accountability.

The key to successful functioning of a risk management program is a systematic reporting mechanism. An institutional policy and procedure shall define a reportable incident and delineate the proper reporting mechanism. The policy should be readily accessible and disseminated to other personnel involved in the reporting. Incident reports, the usual mechanism for identifying risks in the health care setting, can be a very valuable tool if designed and implemented correctly. Staff must be carefully instructed regarding completion of these reports. Although some states still hold that incident reports are not discoverable, under the attorney/client or insurer/insured privilege rule, this is not always the case. In recent years, health care records have come to be considered as ordinary business records and as such may be admissible as evidence in court. For this reason, the incident report itself, or reference to such a report, must not be part of the medical record, and it is wise that individuals writing the reports assume that it may be viewed by others in the event of a malpractice suit (Cushing, 1988).

Incompetent Practice

Boards of nursing are responsible to protect the public welfare. Reporting of incompetent practice is a necessary element. Many states report an increase in filing of complaints against practitioners since the inception of mandatory reporting statutes. The vast majority of the complaints and disciplinary actions are for alcohol and drug abuse or drug diversion (Calloway & Kota, 1989).

The scope of impairment due to substance abuse among health professionals is alarming. It is estimated that from 5 to 10 percent of health care professionals are impaired by alcohol or drugs (Creighton, 1988). In addition, 67 percent of the disciplinary cases coming before state boards of nursing are drug related (Sullivan, Bissell & Williams, 1988). One state reports the annual cost for disciplinary actions involving drugs is $300,000 (Hutchinson, 1986). Since licensure is granted upon meeting specific criteria, it can be revoked when legal standards are not met. Nurse executives cannot ignore the risk of allowing the impaired nurse to function within the institution or the profession (see Chapter 16). Enacting punitive policies without offering assistance to nurses whose practice is impaired by alcohol or drug abuse may result in a loss to the profession of a nurse who could return to practice with appropriate treatment. Knowledge of the disciplinary process and availability of employee treatment programs are vital components of the nurse executive's role.

Many states have instituted mandatory reporting of incompetent practice. The purpose of this statute is to safeguard the public welfare. Guidelines for reporting professional misconduct are available through the state board of nursing. Mandatory reporting is a complex process that involves both legal and ethical parameters.

Informed Consent

To provide treatment without the patient's consent, except in an emergency, could result in liability for unauthorized touching or battery. There are three basic requirements necessary for informed consent: *capacity, voluntariness,* and *information.*

Individual capacity to consent is determined by age and competence. Generally, one must be an adult in the technical and legal sense to consent to treatment. The legal age for adult status is established by state statute and varies among states. Based on state statute, minors may consent to certain types of treatment such as abortion and substance abuse treatment. Adults are considered competent when they can make choices and understand the consequences of their choices.

Individuals act voluntarily when they exercise freedom of choice without force, fraud, deceit, duress, or any other form of coercion.

The third element of informed consent is information. Information must be supplied to patients in a manner which is understandable to them. Lay terminology is preferred to professional terminology. The information must include:

1. An explanation of the treatment to be performed and the expected results
2. A description of risks and discomforts
3. Likely resulting benefits
4. A disclosure of possible alternatives
5. An offer to answer the patient's questions
6. A statement that the patient may withdraw consent at any time
7. The risk of no treatment

The legal responsibility to provide the necessary information for informed consent rests with the individual who will perform the treatment. When a nurse asks a patient to sign a consent form, the nurse is merely attesting to the fact that there is reason to believe that the patient is informed regarding the impending treatment, and witnessing the signature. If the nurse asks the patient to sign a consent knowing that the patient has had no prior explanation of the treatment, however, the consent is invalid and the nurse also may be liable if the patient sues.

Right to Refuse Treatment

Just as competent adults have the right to consent to treatment, they also have the right to refuse treatment. This refusal must be an informed refusal and patients must clearly understand the results of their actions. In addition, guardians of incompetent adults and children may have the right to refuse treatment for them dependent on prior expressed choices of the patient.

The right of competent adults to refuse treatment is guaranteed by the Constitution and has been tested in court with several landmark cases. In recent years, most states have adopted statutory laws to protect these rights and to protect the health care provider.

EQUAL EMPLOYMENT OPPORTUNITY

Equal employment opportunity (EEO) is influenced by constitutional amendment, legislation, executive orders, and judicial decisions emanating from federal, state, and local levels. The fifth and fourteenth amendments of the Constitution mandate due process and equal protection of the law, forming the basis for EEO. Employment practices in the public sector are sometimes challenged as being discriminatory under these amendments. An employment decision treating or classifying an employee differently may be "unconstitutional if it bears no rational or reasonable relation to a legitimate purpose" (Arvey & Faley, 1988, p 65).

Subsection 1981 of the Civil Rights Act of 1866 has been applied to workplace discrimination cases. This section guarantees individuals the same contractual rights as "white citizens." Although not generally applicable to sex discrimination, cases involving race and national origin have been actioned under this law (Levin-Epstein, 1987).

The most significant legislation affecting EEO today is the 1964 Civil Rights Act (CRA) as amended (43 Fed. Reg. 1978). The 1964 CRA contains several "titles" outlawing discrimination in different settings (eg, education, federally funded programs). Section 703(a) of Title VII makes it illegal for an employer:

1. To refuse to hire, discharge any individual, or otherwise to discriminate against any individual with respect to his compensation, terms, conditions, or privileges of employment because of the individual's race, color, religion, sex, or national origin
2. To limit, segregate, or classify employees or applicants for employment in any way which would deprive, or tend to deprive, any individual of employment opportunities or otherwise adversely affect his stature as an employee because of such individual's race, color, religion, sex, or national origin.

Essentially, Title VII of the 1964 CRA prohibits any employment decision based on race, color, religion, sex, or national origin (eg, selection, promotion, discipline, training, rewards). As amended by the Equal Opportunities Act of 1972, Title VII applies to private employers with 15 or more employees, state and local governments, labor unions, and employment agencies.

Enforcement of the Act

The federal agency which oversees the administration and enforcement of Title VII is the Equal Employment Opportunity Commission (EEOC). It was created by the 1964 CRA and received broadened powers in the 1972 Equal Employment Opportunities Act. The primary activity of the EEOC is processing complaints of employment discrimination. This consists of three phases: investigation, conciliation, and litigation. If a state civil rights agency exists, the case reverts to it for 120 days. Investigation by the EEOC focuses on determining whether or not the employer has violated Title VII. If the EEOC finds "probable cause," an attempt is made to reach an agreement (ie, a conciliation) between the EEOC, the complainant, and the employer. If conciliation fails, the EEOC may file suit against the employer in federal court or issue the complainant the right to sue.

The EEOC also promulgates written regulations that reflect its interpretation of Title VII and other laws under its auspices. These include the *Uniform Guidelines on Employee Selection Procedures* (1978), which relates to employers' staffing practices. They stipulate that organizations should determine if their staffing decisions could discriminate against protected groups and, if so, employers must establish procedures to eliminate unfair practices or justify them as being job related (ie, valid).

The *Uniform Guidelines* also require employers to maintain detailed documentation of staffing patterns. The courts have traditionally given the *Guidelines* the deference of law.

The EEOC also has produced *Guidelines on Discrimination Because of Sex* (1980), which cover sexual harassment. Because individuals can be harassed on the basis of their sex (a protected characteristic), sexual harassment is considered discriminatory under Title VII. As defined in these *Guidelines:*

> Unwelcome sexual advances, requests for sexual favors, and other verbal or physical conduct of a sexual nature constitute sexual harassment when (1) submission to such conduct is made either explicitly or implicitly a term or condition of an individual's employment; (2) submission to or rejection of such conduct by an individual is used as the basis for employment decisions affecting such individual; or (3) such conduct has the purpose or effect of unreasonably interfering with an individual's work performance or creating an intimidating, hostile, or offensive working environment.

The courts have generally agreed with the EEOC in defining sexual harassment quite broadly, as seen in the above definitions. The EEOC outlines proactive policies and practices for employers to implement both to sensitize employees to this problem and to prevent its occurrence. It is the duty of employers to prevent employees from sexually harassing other employees.

Disparate Treatment versus Disparate Impact. Two categories of employer discrimination have evolved for court decisions: disparate treatment and disparate impact. The *disparate treatment* basis for discrimination hinges on finding that an employer treats members of protected groups less favorably or differently than others due to their race, color, religion, sex, or national origin (Twomey, 1986). A disparate treatment basis for discrimination involves evidence indicating discriminatory intent on the part of the employer (Arvey & Faley, 1988). A *disparate impact* (sometimes referred to as adverse impact) claim of discrimination does not center on an employer's intentions. Instead, a finding of disparate impact would follow evidence showing that an employer's policy or practice adversely affects one of the protected classes of employees whether discrimination was intended or not (Castagners, 1988). The emphasis is on the *consequences* of employer practices.

Title VII Exemptions and Exceptions

There are a number of bases on which employers may seek exceptions to Title VII. Exceptions include the use of bona fide occupational qualifications (BFOQs) and bona fide seniority or merit systems. The BFOQ exception stipulates that it is lawful to make employment decisions on the basis of national origin, religion, and sex (but not race or color) if this is necessary for the normal operations of the enterprise. This exception is construed very narrowly by the courts. Examples which might qualify under this exception would be theater groups hiring actors on the basis of sex, or an organization which lobbies on behalf of citizens of a particular national origin hiring on this basis (Hunt, 1988). Employment decisions (eg, promotions, layoffs) based on bona fide seniority or merit systems are permissible under Title VII, regardless of the consequences to members of protected groups, (*Firefighters Local 1784 v Stotts*, 1984).

Another important exception is business necessity. To meet this standard, a challenged employment practice must be ''so essential to the safe and efficient operation of the business as to override any racial impact'' (*Robinson v Lorillard Co*, 1971). This was established in *Griggs v Duke Power Co* (1971), a case involving race discrimination where the US Supreme Court ruled that:

> The touchstone is business necessity. If an employment practice which operates to exclude Negroes cannot be shown to be related to job performance, the practice is prohibited (p 431).

Employers must show that decisions adversely affecting members of protected groups are demonstrably related to job performance.

EEO Courtroom Procedures: The Burden of Proof

Employment discrimination cases have an established sequence of events or procedures. First, the complainant bears the burden of establishing that there is prima facie (apparent) evidence of discriminatory behavior on the part of the employer. The burden of proof next shifts to the defendant (the employer) to defend its employment practice(s). If successful, the burden of proof then shifts back to the plaintiff to challenge the employer's defense. The US Supreme Court established the disparate *treatment* criteria for a prima facie claim of discrimination in *McDonnell Douglas Corp v Green* (1973). In this case, it was ruled that plaintiffs initially must show that: (1) they are a member of a group protected from discrimination under the law; (2) they applied and were qualified for a job opening with the defendant; (3) they were rejected; and, (4) subsequent to rejection, the position remained open to applicants of equal or fewer qualifications (Twomey, 1986). If the plaintiff meets these criteria, the employer then bears the burden of proving that there is a legitimate, nondiscriminatory reason for having rejected the plaintiff.

The *Griggs* case set forth the criteria necessary to establish a prima facie finding of discrimination based on a claim of disparate *impact*. Plaintiffs must show that an employer's general practices act to exclude members of their protected class. The US Supreme Court ruling in *Wards Cove Packing Co v Atonio* (1989) has made establishing a prima facie disparate impact finding more difficult. In addition to showing that employers' actions have had a deleterious effect on members of a protected class, this decision requires that plaintiffs also identify the specific employment practices that are discriminatory. If the prima facie criteria are met, employers may defend their practice(s) by showing that they meet the business necessity standard.

Age Discrimination in Employment Act of 1967 (ADEA)

This act made it unlawful for employers, unions, and employment agencies to discriminate against older men and women. As of 1986, the law prohibits discrimination against individuals over the age of 40. It is illegal for employers conducting more than $10,000 of business with the federal government to discriminate based on age. These prohibitions against age discrimination have the practical effect of making mandatory retirement a "thing of the past" (Arvey & Faley, 1988, p 59). The majority of ADEA discrimination suits are argued on a "disparate treatment" basis.

As with Title VII, there are a number of defenses that an employer may invoke. An employer has the legitimate right, for example, to use a reasonable factor other than age (RFOA), such as bona fide seniority or performance evaluation systems, in making termination or layoff decisions. Bona fide occupational qualifications (BFOQs) also are permissible exceptions under very limited circumstances. A legal defense arguing that age is a BFOQ due to the physical demands of a job would be tenuous (Levin-Epstein, 1987). BFOQ exceptions based upon age are more likely to be accepted in cases involving public safety (Ledvinka, 1982).

Vocational Rehabilitation Act of 1973

The Vocational Rehabilitation Act of 1973 prohibits discrimination against handicapped individuals solely on the basis of their handicap. In *Drennon v Philadelphia General Hospital* (1977), a job applicant with a history of epilepsy successfully sued the hospital employer when rejected for the job on the basis of this condition. The definition of "handicapped person" is fairly broad. A handicapped person is defined as one who: (1) has physical or mental impairment which adversely affects a major life activity; (2) has a history of such impairment; or, (3) is regarded as having such an impairment. In order to be protected under this Act a handicapped person must be able to perform "the essential functions of the job" with "reasonable accommodations" by the employer (Twomey, 1986, p 91). Thus, individuals who are recovering from alcohol or drug dependency may be entitled to protection under this law, provided that their addictions do not interfere with their ability to perform their jobs. State practice acts and board of nursing regulators designate criteria to assure employers that nurses recovering from additions are safe practitioners. Many states now define individuals afflicted with AIDS as handicapped (Levin-Epstein, 1987), and employers must consider these individuals as having legally protected handicapped status. As noted by Arvey and Faley (1988, p 65):

> In the case of employment, at least, *any* mental or physical restriction that substantially limits an individual's ability to gain employment, yet does not perceptively affect the individual's ability to *perform* the job is likely to be actionable under the Act.

AFFIRMATIVE ACTION

Although often discussed in tandem, a policy of affirmative action (AA) differs from a policy of equal employment opportunity. EEO is concerned with utilizing employment practices which *do not discriminate against or impair* the employment opportunities of members of protected groups. AA centers on the use of policies and practices *enhancing employment opportunities* of protected class members. The former policy advocates the use of practices which are "neutral" with regard to protected characteristics, while the latter policy specifically gives preferential treatment to members of protected groups.

AA and Title VII of the 1964 CRA

A strict interpretation of this law leads to the conclusion that preferential treatment for members of protected groups, to the detriment of the majority group (''reverse'' discrimination), is illegal (Ledvinka, 1982). *Weber v Kaiser Aluminum and Chemical Corp* (1979) set the conditions under which AA plans may be acceptable. Kaiser and its union included an affirmative action plan in their collective bargaining agreement. The plan called for 50 percent of openings for craft training programs to be set aside for black employees until racial parity with the local labor market was achieved. This resulted in black employees with less seniority being admitted ahead of their white counterparts. Kaiser was sued by one of the white employees (Weber) who was denied admittance in favor of blacks with less seniority. The US Supreme Court ultimately found in favor of Kaiser. The majority opinion focused on the intentions of the lawmakers who wrote and passed Title VII and the fact that Kaiser's AA plan was voluntarily agreed to by the employer and its union. The court did not want to vitiate the right of employers to voluntarily utilize practices designed to rectify a history or pattern of discrimination.

AA and the Vocational Rehabilitation Act of 1973

Section 503 of this Act mandates affirmative action measures for handicapped individuals on the part of federal contractors with contracts exceeding $2500. Employers meeting this criterion must make reasonable attempts to accommodate physically and mentally handicapped individuals who would otherwise be qualified for jobs. In addition, the US Labor Department has issued regulations pertaining to this act which require that contractors with 50 or more employees or doing more than $50,000 in contract business formulate written affirmative action programs which are to be available to employees and enforcing agencies.

AA and the Vietnam Era Veteran's Readjustment Act of 1974

This Act requires that employers with government contracts exceeding $10,000 take steps to enhance the employment opportunities (ie, hire and promote) of disabled veterans and other veterans of the Vietnam era.

Office of Federal Contract Compliance Programs (OFCCP)

The US Secretary of Labor is charged with overseeing the compliance of federal contractors. The Office of Federal Contract Compliance (OFCCP) was established by the Secretary of Labor for day-to-day administration and enforcement of E.O. 11246 and other EEO/AA laws and regulations pertaining to federal contractors. The OFCCP has issued Revised Order No. 4 detailing AA requirements for covered employers (Twomey, 1986).

WAGE DISCRIMINATION: EQUAL PAY ACT OF 1963

The Equal Pay Act (EPA) of 1963 makes it illegal to pay lower wages to employees of one sex when the jobs: (1) require equal skill (experience, training, education and ability); (2) require equal effort (mental or physical exertion); (3) are of equal responsibility (accountability); and (4) are performed under similar working conditions (physical surroundings and hazards).

Definition of Equal

The definition of "equal" has evolved through various court decisions. A 1970 court case, *Schultz v Wheaton Glass Company* (1970), involved a company which maintained two classifications for the same job, one male and one female. The employer paid the male job classification a 10 percent premium, based on its claim that the males performed additional tasks which justified the additional payment. Thus, the defendant claimed that the jobs were not equal. The plaintiff contended that these additional tasks were infrequently performed by men and that the jobs were, therefore, equal. The court ruled that the jobs were "substantially" equal, and the extra duties performed by the men did not justify paying the men additional compensation. This "substantially equal" criteria has now become the standard for assessing whether or not jobs are equal (Milkovich & Newman, 1990).

Factors Other Than Sex

Unequal pay for equal work may be justified under the EPA if wage differences are attributable to one of four defenses: *seniority, merit, incentive systems,* or a *factor other than sex.* Pay differences based on shift differentials, production incentive or bonus systems, performance or longevity raises, bona fide training programs, etc, will generally be found to be valid exceptions to the EPA (Levin-Epstein, 1987). If challenged, employers must show that wage differences across opposite sex employees holding "substantially similar" jobs are legitimated by business-related (eg, productivity, performance or profitability) differences.

WAGE DISCRIMINATION: TITLE VII AND THE COMPARABLE WORTH DOCTRINE

As noted earlier, Title VII prohibits workplace discrimination based on a number of characteristics, including sex. The 1963 EPA outlaws pay discrimination based on sex for jobs which are "substantially similar". Despite these laws, the weekly median earnings of women remains at about 70 percent of the weekly earnings of men. One reason for this disparity is the disproportionately large number of women working in a limited number of historically low paying occupations including nursing. Proponents of the "comparable worth doctrine" believe sex differences in earnings are attributable to societal discrimination in that women tend to be crowded into a limited number of occupations due to long-term gender socialization and stereotyping in education, hiring, and promotion practices. Furthermore, these occupations are under-compensated because they are dominated by women. Employers often maintain that wages are attributable to the market forces of supply and demand. Women earn less because they choose lower wage jobs that permit relatively easy entrance and exit and require relatively less training, and have working conditions which are not "onerous or dangerous" (Milkovich & Newman, 1990, p 467). Disparate treatment and disparate impact have been difficult to apply to issues of pay because of the legality of pay differences attributable to dissimilar work.

Dissimilar Jobs and Dissimilar Pay

In *County of Washington v Gunther* (1981), the US Supreme Court established the legitimacy of applying Title VII to pay discrimination cases involving "substantially different" jobs. In this case, four jail matrons claimed that their jobs were comparable to work performed by male guards. They were being paid at only about 70 percent of these jobs even though the defendant's own assessment of job worth indicated that the matrons' jobs should be paid at 95 percent of the male guards' jobs. Although settled out of court, this set the important precedent that pay discrimination charges for jobs of unequal content can be brought under Title VII.

Use of Market Pay Data

Comparable worth court cases invariably focus on what the "market" pays different occupations. A number of these cases have involved health care workers and nurses. In *Lemons v The City and County of Denver* (1980), the plaintiff nurse held that her female-dominated job class was illegally paid less than other (male dominated) jobs paid by her public employer (eg, tree trimmers, sign painters, tire servicers). Lemons argued that nurses' jobs required more education and skill than these other jobs and that pay rates for these "male jobs" were unduly influenced by the local labor market. Lemons maintained that market differences in pay reflected historical patterns of discrimination and using them as a basis for compensation decisions only perpetuated this discrimination. The court found in favor of the defendant, noting that Title VII was not intended as a basis for adjusting market disparities.

Briggs v City of Madison (1982) also involved nurses and market rates but focused on jobs which the court ruled to be substantially similar. In this case, comparing nurses ("female" job) and public health sanitarians ("male" job), the court found prima facie evidence of discrimination, although the jobs were similar (in terms of skill, effort, responsibility, and working conditions), the pay difference between the two jobs was great. By using market data, the employing organization (the city of Madison) was able to successfully defend its compensation practices. Madison was able to show that pay market differences compelled them to pay sanitarian workers a higher wage in order to attract and retain these workers.

Spaulding v University of Washington (1984) again affirmed the right of employers to use market rates in their pay decisions, despite their adverse impact on female dominated occupational groups. In *Spaulding*, the predominantly female faculty of the Department of Nursing claimed they were illegally underpaid relative to faculty in other departments. The court ruled that to hold employers responsible for market pay differences "would subject employers to liability for pay disparities with respect to which they have not, in any meaningful sense, made an independent business judgment.''

In sum,

> These court decisions imply that pay differentials between dissimilar jobs will not be prohibited under Title VII if the differences can be shown to be based on the content of the work, its value to the organization's objectives, and the employer's ability to attract and retain employees in competitive external labor markets (Milkovich & Newman, 1990, p 461).

EMPLOYMENT-AT-WILL AND WRONGFUL DISCHARGE

The employment relationship has been construed historically as being characterized as a ''free will'' relationship: Employees were free to take or leave a job at their pleasure, and employers were likewise free to hire, retain, or discharge employees for any reason, be it good, bad, or indifferent. But employers' rights to terminate employees have been steadily eroding. EEO laws affect an employer's ability to discharge members of protected groups. About 70 percent of the US working population are considered employees at-will (EAW); they do not have tenure, civil service, or labor contract agreements protecting them against (wrongful) termination. Federal legislation does not cover the EAW issue and state laws vary considerably. Evolving case law provides three exceptions to the broad doctrine of EAW: (1) public policy exceptions; (2) implied contract exceptions; and, (3) good faith and fair dealing exceptions.

Public Policy Exception
This involves cases where an employee is discharged in direct conflict with established public policy (Twomey, 1986). Examples include firing an employee for the following reasons: serving on a jury; failing to commit perjury on behalf of the employer in a trial; reporting an employers' illegal actions ''whistle blowing''; and filing a worker's compensation claim. The public policy exception to EAW tends to be interpreted fairly narrowly.

Implied Contract Exceptions
This exception to EAW involves situations considered to form an implied contract. The courts have generally treated employee handbooks, company policies, and oral statements as framing the employment relationship (ie, the ''contract'' between the employee and employer). For example, in *Toussaint v Blue Cross and Blue Shield* (1980), two managerial employees were told during the hiring interview that as long as they ''did the job,'' they would be able to maintain employment with BC/BS. Further, the company's personnel handbook stated that it was the company's policy to require ''good cause'' for discharge. The court held that such written and oral statements provided for an enforceable contract between employer and employee. In

Hillsman v Sutter Community Hospitals (1984), the plaintiff successfully argued that the employer discharged him without following company termination procedures.

Good Faith and Fair Dealing

This exception to EAW exists to prevent unfair or malicious terminations. It implies that there is a "covenant of good faith and fair dealing" in the employment "contract" such that the parties to the contract will not abuse, injure, or act unjustly toward one another. In *Fortune v National Cash Register* (1977), the plaintiff was discharged just prior to signing the final contract for a $5 million dollar sale for which he would have received a large commission. The court found that the employer had acted in bad faith toward the salesman and ordered reasonable compensation. To date, only three states have written statutes supporting EAW exceptions based on a theory of "good faith and fair dealing" (Koys, Briggs & Grenig, 1987).

Implications

Employers have responded to these developments by taking a number of steps. Organizations have reviewed company documents (eg, employee handbooks, recruiting brochures) to remove unwanted statements implying job security or other unintentional promises. Companies also are establishing and communicating policies to reinforce the right to discipline and discharge in light of poor performance or rule-breaking. Managers also are being trained to resist retaliating when employees report acts of a questionable ethical or legal nature. Finally, some employers are requiring employees to sign an agreement stipulating that they are truly "at-will" employees who may be discharged at the employer's discretion.

OCCUPATIONAL SAFETY AND HEALTH LAW

Responding to rapidly increasing incidences of occupational disease and worker injury and death, Congress passed the Occupational Safety and Health Act (OSHA) of 1970. This act created administrative bodies which have promulgated standards and procedures to enhance employee safety and health. With the exception of federal and state governmental employers, most other employing organizations are covered by the act. Health care institutions contain many threats to the health and safety of their employees including equipment, supplies, and diseases. The onslaught of the AIDS epidemic and increasing awareness of the dangers of hepatitis emphasize the risks to health care employees inherent in such employment.

Administration

The Occupational Safety and Health Administration (OSHA) is the primary federal agency for creating standards, conducting inspections, and engaging in enforcement activity. The National Institute of Occupational Safety and Health (NIOSH) is an occupational health and safety research center which recommends standards to OSHA and provides aid and assistance. The Occupational Safety and Health Review Commission (OSHRC) processes appeals made by employers following OSHA citations charging them with violations.

Standards

Standards involve the imposition of rules pertaining to safety procedures or hazardous materials. There is a fairly involved procedure which OSHA must follow to issue new permanent standards (Twomey, 1986). If the Secretary of Labor believes that workers are at risk, he or she has the option of bypassing these procedures to issue temporary (six month) emergency standards.

Individuals or employers may contest a new standard by filing a petition with the US Court of Appeals. The Secretary must then demonstrate that the standard addresses a factor posing a ''significant risk'' to worker health and safety.

Significant Risk and Feasibility

The significant risk standard is decided on a case-by-case basis. The court must be convinced that without the standard workers risk disease or injury. OSHA is not required to show a balancing of costs and benefits but is charged with the duty of adopting the most protective, yet ''feasible'' standard. The feasibility of standards historically has been very contentious.

Exemption from Standards

Variances are exemptions from standards granted to employers. Temporary variances are granted if organizations prove they are taking all steps necessary to protect employees and are moving in the direction of standard compliance. A permanent variance may be granted if worksite methods or procedures are at least as safe as those designated by OSHA standards.

General Duty Clauses

A clause in the OSHA Act stipulates that employers ''shall furnish to each employee employment and a place of employment which are free from recognized hazards that are causing or are likely to cause death or serious physical harm to the employee'' (Ledvinka, 1982, p 166). This covers disease and safety hazards which may arise outside of the OSHA standards. Employers are in violation of this cause if they fail to reduce or remove a recognizably serious hazard.

Protection from Retaliation

Workers are protected from retaliation resulting from exercising rights granted by the Act. *Whirlpool Corporation v Marshall* (1980) established the right of employees to refuse hazardous work. This is restricted to situations in which employees perceive a clear threat to their health or safety.

Record Keeping and Reporting

Employers having eight or more employees are required to maintain records of occupational injuries and illness. OSHA has specific definitions for each of these categories and requires the use of OSHA forms which must be available to OSHA compliance officers. Employers must also post these records to keep employees informed of the employer's safety and health record.

Inspections, Citations, and Penalties

OSHA has the authority to inspect every worksite which is covered by the Act. Situations involving death or serious injury are the highest inspection priority, followed by inspections prompted by employee complaints. High-risk industries also are singled out for inspection. Final priority is given to general worksite inspections, conducted on a random basis. Inspections are conducted by compliance officers and reported to OSHA area directors. Then a decision is made as to whether citations and/or penalties are in order.

State Programs

The Act encourages states to develop their own occupational safety and health programs. A number of states have instituted "right to know" laws guaranteeing workers the right to be informed of any hazardous substances in their workplace. Notification of the presence of hazardous substances to employees' physicians and local fire and public health officials also is sometimes required.

EMPLOYMENT ISSUES AND RIGHT TO PRIVACY

The right to privacy is the right to be free from unwarranted intrusion by others and the right to be left alone (Hunt, 1988). Both employers and employees have had privacy rights curtailed. Employers may be required to file EEO reports with government agencies and to report safety and health data. Employees' privacy often is diminished when employers elicit information while recruiting and hiring. The primary concern in workplace privacy is with this latter issue. The Privacy Act of 1974 outlines strict requirements for the handling of personnel data. A number of states have passed legislation giving employees the right to view their personnel files. Other states have laws limiting the rights of employers to test employees for the presence of the AIDS antibody, examine job applicant's criminal record, and search an employee's clothing or possessions.

Given the growing legislation and the upsurge in computerized data banks (sometimes referred to as human resource information systems or HRIS), companies are beginning to adopt employee privacy programs. These are often designed to:

> (1) restrict the types of employee data that can be kept to only those that are clearly job related, (2) provide for the periodic purging of outdated data, (3) provide a mechanism for promptly responding to employee inquiries about the data and for resolving disputes over data accuracy, (4) regularly provide printouts for employees containing much of the data the company keeps on them to permit instant correction, and (5) assure employees that personal information will be released outside the company only with their approval, except to verify employment or to comply with legitimate legal investigations (Heneman, Schwab, Fossum & Dyer, 1986, p 216).

In order to reduce exposure to tort liabilities, some companies are limiting the practice of giving references or recommendation letters. Employers have been sued for defamation of character and/or invasion of privacy for releasing information to outside agents, such as scores on tests of general intelligence (Hunt, 1988).

OTHER LAWS AFFECTING THE WORKPLACE

In addition to the laws affecting the workplace reviewed here, there are many others, including laws pertaining to labor relations and collective bargaining and the structure and administration of compensation and benefit programs. These are discussed in Chapter 18, Labor Relations, and Chapter 14, Budgeting and Compensation.

REFERENCES

ANA. *Standards for Organized Nursing Services* and responsibilities of administrators across all settings. Kansas City, MO, American Nurses' Association, 1988

Arvey RD. Faley RH. *Fairness in Selecting Employees*, 2nd ed. Reading, MA, Addison-Wesley, 1987

Brett JL, Schlag MS. Mandatory reporting: Legal and ethical issues. *JONA*. 17:12, 32, 1987

Briggs v City of Madison, 536 F. Supp. 435, 1982

Calfee BE. Understaffing. *Nursing Life*, 7:6, 25–29, 1987

Calloway SD. *Nursing and the Law*. Eau Clair, WI, Professional Education Systems, Inc, 1986

Calloway SD, Kota JM. *Legal Issues in Supervising Nurses*, 2nd ed. Eau Clair, WI, Professional Education Systems, Inc, 1989

Castagners JO. *Personnel Law Answer Book (1990 Supplement)*. Greenvale, NY, Panel Publishers, 1989

County of Washington v Gunther, 452 US 161, 25 FEP Cases 1521, 1981

Creighton H. Legal implications of the impaired nurse—Part I. *Nursing Management*. 19:1, 21, 1988

Cushing M. *Nursing Jurisprudence*. Norwalk, CT, Appleton & Lange, 1988

Dankmyer T, Groves J. Taking steps for safety's sake. *Hospitals*. 51:10, 60, 1977

Drennon v Philadelphia General Hospital, 14 FEP 1385, 1977

Fiesta J. *The Law and Liability: A Guide for Nurses*, 2nd ed. New York: John Wiley & Sons, 1988

Fiesta J. The nursing shortage: Whose liability problem? Part I. *Nursing Management*. 21:1, 24, 1990

Fiesta J. The nursing shortage: Whose liability problem? Part II. *Nursing Management*. 21:2, 22, 1990

Firefighters Local 1784 v Stotts, 467 US 561, 34 FEP Cases 1702, 1984

Fortune v National Cash Register Co, 373 Mass. 96, 264 NE 2d 1251, 1977

Griggs v Duke Power Co, 401 US 424, 3 FEP Cases 175, 1971

Guidelines on Discrimination Because of Sex, 45 FR 74676, 1980

Guido GW. *Legal issues in nursing: A source book for practice*. Norwalk, CT, Appleton & Lange, 1988

Heneman HG, Schwab DP, Fossum JA, Dyer LD. *Personnel/Human Resource Management*, 3rd ed. Homewood, IL, Irwin, 1986

Hillsman v Sutter Community Hospital, 153 CAL App 3d 743; 200 CAL Rptr. 605, 1984

Horton v Niagara Falls Memorial Medical Center, 380 NYS 2d 116 (NY 1976)

Hunt JW. *The Law of the Workplace*, 2nd ed. Washington, DC: Bureau of National Affairs, 1988

Hutchinson S. Chemically dependent nurses: The trajectory toward self-annihilation. *Nursing Research*. 35:4, 196, 1986

Koys DJ, Briggs S, Grenig J. State court disparity on employment-at-will. *Personnel Psychology*. 40, 565, 1987

Ledvinka J. *Federal Regulation of Personnel and Human Resource Management*. Boston, MA, Kent Publishing Co, 1982

Lemons v City and County of Denver, 620 F. 2nd 228, 1980

Levin-Epstein MD. *Primer of equal employment opportunity*, 4th ed. Washington, DC: Bureau of National Affairs, 1987

Luckenbill-Brett JL & Stuhler-Schlag MK. Mandatory Reporting. *Journal of Nursing Administration*, 17:12, 32–38, 1987

Luquire, R. Nursing Risk Management. *Nursing Management*, 20:10, 56–58, 1989

McDonnell Douglas Corp v Green, 411 US 792, 5 FEP Cases 965, 1973

Milkovich GT, Newman JM. *Compensation*, 3rd ed. Homewood, IL, BPI/Irwin, 1990

Northrop CE, Kelly ME. *Legal Issues in Nursing*. St. Louis, MO, CV Mosby, 1987

Robinson v P. Lorillard Co, 444 F2d 791, 3 FEP Cases 653, CA4, 1971

Schultz v Wheaton Glass Co, 421 F2nd 259, 9 FEP Cases 502, 1970

Spaulding v University of Washington, 35 FEP Cases 217, CA4, 1984

Sullivan EJ, Bissell L, Williams E. *Chemical Dependency in Nursing: The Deadly Diversion*. Menlo Park, CA, Addison-Wesley, 1988

Toussaint v Blue Cross and Blue Shield, 408 Mich. 579, 292 NW 2d 880, 1980

Twomey DP. *A Concise Guide to Employment Law: EEO & OSHA.* Cincinnati, OH, South-Western Publishing Co, 1986

Uniform Guidelines on Employee Selection Procedures, 43 Fed. Reg. 38290-315, 1978

Walker LJ. Nursing 1980: New Responsibilities, new liabilities. *Trial*. 16:12, 42, 1980

Wards Cove Packing Co v Atonio, NO. 87-1387, 1989

Weber v Kaiser Aluminum and Chemical Corp, 443 U.S. 193, 1979

Whirlpool Corporation v Marshall, US 1 445, 1980

CHAPTER 12

Staffing, Recruiting, and Selecting

Steven D. Norton
Susan Crissman

Steven D. Norton
Susan Crissman

Key Concept List

Equal Employment Law
Job analysis
Human resource planning
Recruiting
Validity and reliability of selection systems
Selection devices
Interviewing

This chapter addresses the critical process of bringing nursing staff into the organization and promoting them. Although nurse executives generally do not themselves hire staff nurses and other unit personnel, they select their own direct subordinates and have managerial responsibility for ensuring that adequate numbers of qualified nurses are employed by the hospital. Recruiting, selecting, and promoting are highly related to the other aspects of human resource management (HRM) (Chapter 13), including employment law (Chapters 11 and 18), performance appraisal, and compensation (Chapter 14). All three must be carried out in a fair and lawful manner. The organization's performance appraisal system should be based on performance factors similar to those used in hiring decisions. Of equal importance are compensation practices which must be fair if applicants are to accept job offers and current employees are to remain with the organization and accept promotions.

SELECTION AND EEO LAW

Hospitals have been affected by Equal Employment Opportunity Law as much as any American institution. They draw on minority applicant pools and employ large numbers of female employees. Employee selection procedures, whether formal such as paper-and-pencil tests or informal such as unstructured interviews, are subject to the *Uniform Guidelines on Employee Selection Procedures (Uniform Guidelines)* (EEOC, 1978). The *Uniform Guidelines* are the enforcement guidelines for Title VII of the Civil Rights Act of 1964, as discussed in Chapter 11, which prohibits discrimination on the basis of sex, race, religion, or national origin ("protected classes"). Other legislation prohibits discrimination on the basis of age (over 40 years), veteran status, or handicapped status.

HUMAN RESOURCE PLANNING

Ideally, human resource planning should direct recruiting and selecting so that an organization always has the required employees available. Most organizations carry out human resource planning but do it unsystematically. Figure 12–1 illustrates a planning process beginning with the establishment of organizational objectives for existing and new services.

Planning for an adequate nursing work force is difficult because nurses are in short supply and their work is highly specialized. Although human resource planning in nursing is difficult, it is highly cost-effective because recruiting is expensive. Furthermore, poor planning can lead to underutilization of expensive facilities if nurses are not available to staff them. There is typically a three-month lag from the time a nurse resigns until a replacement reports to work. This lag leads to using overtime or hiring expensive temporary nurses until the empty position is filled. Either alternative lowers morale and may increase turnover.

Efforts to improve retention also are cost-effective. Nursing turnover is quite high nationally, with the average cost to recruit a nurse approximately $20,000 (Droste, 1987). Analyzing reasons for turnover can help change management practices to reduce turnover of current employees and help to select employees who are more likely to remain with the hospital. Turnover analysis includes exit interviews and analysis of employment data.

Labor market information and recruiting practices of other area institutions are part of human resource planning. Advertisements from other institutions should be monitored and nurses who have applied to other hospitals can be asked tactfully about other institutions' recruiting methods. As specialty nurses leave the organization, it may be possible to avoid recruiting by retraining current employees and subsequently replacing them. For example, a surgical nurse might be interested in moving to coronary care. Effective use of training requires information on the abilities and interests of the current nursing work force as well as information on how appropriate training can be obtained.

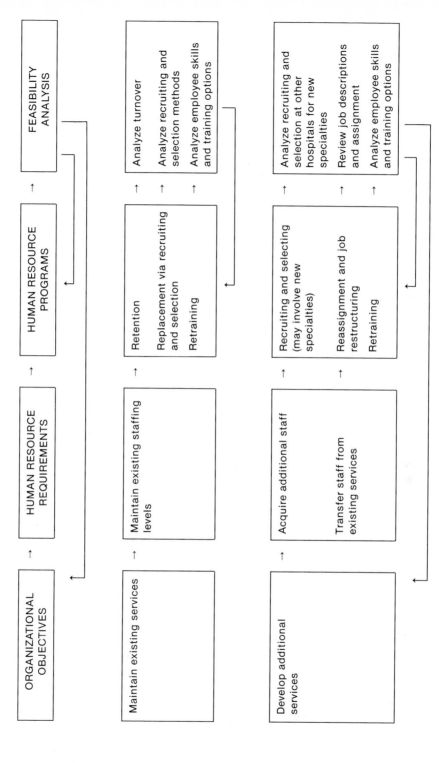

Figure 12–1. Human Resource Planning (Scarpello and Levinka. Personnel/Human Resource Management. PWS-KENT Publishing Company. Copyright 1988, p. 224)

DETERMINING DEMAND AND SUPPLY

Effective human resource planning requires that demand and supply be determined as accurately as possible. Federal documents, especially the Seventh Report of the Status of Health Personnel help to identify national and regional needs (USDHHS, 1990). Individual institutions can forecast their demands by using statistical methods or outside consultants. Forecasts incorporate plans for maintaining current services as well as developing additional services.

Forecasts depend on the accuracy of the hospital's personnel records. It is possible to use past data to demonstrate how useful this model could have been for past years. For example, the prediction of supply and demand for 1990 could have been based on the data available in late 1989 and can then be compared to actual supply and demand during 1990.

Net demand for nursing staff (turnover plus demand for additional nurses) depends on seasonal fluctuations in turnover and on demand for additional nurses. Seasonal turnover fluctuations will be relatively constant across specialties. For example, there is not likely to be a difference between the turnover rates of pediatric nurses and trauma center nurses depending on the season. On the other hand, the demand for additional nurses in these two specialties will vary because childhood illnesses are more prevalent in the winter and accidents are more prevalent in the summer (see Fig 12–2). Therefore, the emphasis should be on hiring additional trauma center nurses in the spring and additional pediatric nurses in the autumn. In addition to overstaffing in critical specialties, the institution may wish to seek nurses who are qualified in more than one specialty for more flexible staffing. Finally, an institution may adapt an approach to pay determination that is increasingly common in industry, paying employees according to the number of skills they possess, rather than their current position. The rationale is that more versatile employees are inherently more valuable

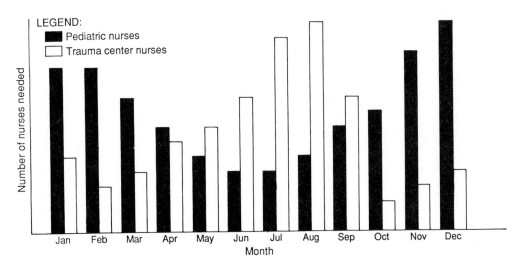

Figure 12-2. Example of Seasonal Fluctuation in Demand for Pediatric and Trauma Center Nurses

to the organization. For example, a hospital facing the situation illustrated by Figure 12–2 would be aided by hiring nurses who were competent in both trauma center and pediatric nursing.

Supply can be determined primarily by examining the annual graduations of local nursing schools. The number of nurses currently not working in practice is quite small but some who dropped out to have children might be recruited to return at least part time. It may be possible to recruit nurses from other locations but recruiting and relocating costs are high. Since such nurses also will not have local roots, turnover may be high. When possible, it is more cost-effective to be the "preferred employer" and let *other* institutions recruit nurses from other locations. An excellent resource on becoming the preferred employer is *Magnet Hospitals* by the American Academy of Nursing (ANA, 1983).

JOB ANALYSIS

Job analysis is the process of collecting information about the work performed and the worker characteristics required in a job. The first step in carrying out a job analysis is determining the use of the resulting information. Job analysis allows decisions regarding recruiting, selecting, training, appraising performance, compensating, and human resource planning to be made with systematic knowledge of individual jobs and of the relationship among jobs. Job analysis systems developed for this purpose are likely to be useful for most other personnel purposes, except compensation.

SCOPE OF THE JOB ANALYSIS PROCESS

Job analysis is about describing work. This must be done to create human resource management systems for selection, performance appraisal, and/or compensation. Work can be broken down into several component parts (US Department of Labor, 1972), as shown in Table 12–1. Staff nurses all carry out the same major tasks, including assessing, planning, intervening, and evaluating care, but in a variety of settings. Job analysis starts with a *job specialty,* which is a group of positions identical in almost all of its tasks. Pediatric nurse is an example of a job specialty. Individual nurses fill *positions* as pediatric nurses.

Many job elements of a nurse's position may also be performed by other personnel under certain circumstances. For example, a nurse assistant may bathe a routine postoperative patient, but a nurse would bathe a critically ill patient. Other elements are legally the purview only of the nurse, and may require specialized skills. Starting a preoperative intravenous infusion requires technical knowledge of IVs, knowledge of the patient's condition, fluid and electrolyte balance, as well as the emotional needs of the patient.

Job analysis begins with a detailed job description. Agreement should be reached by job holders and their supervisors regarding the job tasks or duties performed by the incumbent. The job description must include job specifications, such as experi-

TABLE 12–1. COMPONENTS OF WORK FOR A PEDIATRIC NURSE

Component	Example	Definition
JOB ELEMENTS ↓	Start IV	Smallest step of work activity
TASKS ↓	Pre-operative preparation	One or more elements of distinct activity leading to a result
POSITIONS ↓	Pediatric nurse, Sally Jones	Collection of tasks that constitute a single employee's assignment
SPECIALTY ↓	Pediatric nursing	Group of positions identical in almost all of their tasks
JOBS ↓	Staff Registered Nurse (R.N.)	Group of positions identical in their major tasks
OCCUPATIONS ↓	Nursing	Group of jobs found within or across organizations and based on common knowledge, skill, training, and type of work
JOB FAMILIES	Patient care	Jobs related in some important way

ence and education required. Jobs may be grouped into occupations and job families to achieve different purposes. For example, a performance appraisal system may be developed for the "patient care" job family, which could include nursing, occupational therapy, respiratory therapy, medical technicians, and so on. Salary studies may be done for the entire occupation of nursing. Selection methods usually are based on an analysis of jobs, occupations, and job families. For example, a structured selection interview for pediatric nurses might contain some questions unique to that position (How do you reduce a child's fear of the hospital?), some questions asked of all nurses (How do you deal with an MD who seems too rushed to listen to you?), and some asked of all patient care personnel (How do you deal with a patient's complaint about another employee?).

Rather than try to analyze every single job in the pool of jobs, those being analyzed should be representative of other jobs. For example, the job of a medical/surgical nurse is representative of other staff nursing jobs. Job demands would be very similar, except for specific technical knowledge. However, some jobs may be so critical to the success of the organization that they should be analyzed even if they are not representative. An example would be the nurse manager in charge of the trauma center. Finally, a very careful job analysis should be carried out for any job in which current selection methods have a high adverse impact against minority groups, as revealed by a study of how many minority applicants are hired.

PARTICIPANTS

Successful job analysis requires a partnership between the HRM department and the nurse managers responsible for the function in which the jobs are located. Most HRM departments are experienced in job analysis for wage and salary systems but may have less experience in job analysis for staffing systems. HRM and nurse management need to determine whether the job analysis should be carried out by HRM staff, a consulting firm, or HRM staff aided by a consulting firm. One of the direct subordinates of the chief nurse executive should be assigned to the project in order to provide managerial oversight. Needless to say, many nurses and nurse managers will provide input at various stages in the process.

Any HRM project will be the source of countless rumors. Open, honest communication is the best antidote. Information on the job analysis process and how it will be used should be widely distributed as soon as possible. Except for the details of tests and interview scoring protocols, no information needs to be confidential.

METHODS OF JOB ANALYSIS

Job analysis can be either task-oriented or worker-oriented, depending on the nature of the position and the use of the results. Task-oriented job analysis focuses on the results produced by the employee and tends to be very job specific. Worker-oriented job analysis focuses on the behaviors involved in job activities and tends to be less job specific. The latter is more common in nursing. An advantage of worker-oriented techniques is that the knowledges, skills, and abilities to be measured by the predictor can be addressed directly in job activities rather than being inferred from tasks. The three most common methods of job analysis are interviews, questionnaires, and direct observation.

The *job analysis interview* is a structured interview. Task statements are developed from responses to the interview which include: What action is performed? To whom or what is the action directed? What output is expected? What tools, equipment, aids, or processes are used? The interview is most useful in smaller organizations and in the early stages of developing a job analysis system.

The *job analysis questionnaire* is a printed questionnaire which is more standardized, less open to distortion, and less expensive than an interview. Incumbents are usually asked to rate the frequency and importance of tasks. A job analysis questionnaire is particularly useful in large organizations and in fine tuning a system developed through interviews.

Direct observation is most applicable when the important job elements are clearly observable. It is particularly useful in verifying the results of interviews or questionnaires rather than as a primary information source.

Other job analysis methods include technical conferences (a form of group interview), worker diaries, critical incident questionnaires, and work participation (the analyst actually performs the job).

Standard-oriented job analysis is a method of developing a selection system that meets the content validity requirements of EEOC regulations. The major steps are: (1) identifying major job duties; (2) rating their frequency and importance; and (3) identifying or developing measures which reflect those duties which are high in frequency and importance (Biddle, 1982).

When the goal is to learn about the differences among jobs and among incumbents, job analysis frequently begins with a structured interview with incumbents of representative positions. The results then are used to develop a job analysis question-naire that can be widely distributed. When the goal is to learn about the basic nature of the occupation, job analysis frequently begins with the collection of critical inci-dents (challenging skills). Benner (1984) applies the critical incident technique in nurs-ing (Table 12–2).

The best examples of job analysis for nursing specialties are those performed by national certification boards. A committee developed a large number of task state-ments that were then sent to a large sample of practicing nurses and nurse managers (Chase, 1988; Fox & Blue, 1988). The most important tasks were determined and the behaviors associated with those tasks identified. The focus was on behaviors that demonstrated a high level of proficiency just below the expert level.

RECRUITING

Recruiting is a process in which the needs of both the institution and the individual must be satisfied. The institution must satisfy its needs for nursing staff in order to survive. The individual must decide to work in an institution in general, and this hospital, in particular, rather than in a physician's office, nursing home, clinic, home care, schools, or industry. Satisfied employees are the best recruiters and dissatisfied employees will counteract the most sophisticated marketing campaign. However, re-lying on current employees as recruiters tends to perpetuate the current racial and ethnic mix. Outreach activities may be needed to ensure a proper mix of employees. Some hospitals pay a bonus to employees who recruit new employees, a sign-on

TABLE 12-2. INTERVIEW QUESTIONS FOR NURSE MANAGER POSITION RELATED TO BENNER'S (1984) DOMAINS OF NURSING PRACTICE

1. The helping role	What do you see as the primary issues in dealing with a pa-tient who may not recover?
2. The teaching-coaching func-tion	What are the primary issues in helping a patient and spouse cope with a chronic debilitating disease?
3. The diagnostic and patient-monitoring function	Suppose you had an inexperienced nurse caring for a newly diagnosed diabetic. What signs and symptoms would you encourage the nurse to be aware of?
4. Effective management of rap-idly changing situations	Have you ever been a supervisor in an intensive care unit or trauma center? Tell how you handled an unusually busy day? What would you do if a patient was in acute respira-tory distress and a physician was not readily available?
5. Administering and monitoring therapeutic interventions and regimens	What are the most common errors made by inexperienced nurses when they start IV therapy? How do you ensure the safe administration of medications over all three shifts?
6. Monitoring and ensuring the quality of health care prac-tices	How would you respond to a physician who wanted a patient to receive discharge instructions that you believed to dem-onstrate a lack of understanding of the patient's condition?
7. Organizational and work-role competencies	How would you deal with a staff nurse who is a chronic com-plainer? What methods have you utilized in the past so that all shifts are kept informed?

bonus to the new employees themselves, or a re-enlistment bonus to employees who remain. If the purpose of bonus is to attract long-term employees rather than to fill a temporary need, it may be desirable to withhold the bonus until the new employee remains with the hospital for a specified amount of time. See Table 12–3 for the advantages and disadvantages of these three types of bonuses.

MARKETING TO PROSPECTIVE EMPLOYEES

Recruiting is really marketing. You are selling your organization as an employer. Marketing involves analyzing a market, preparing the message, selecting the appropriate media, and analyzing the results.

1. *Analyze the market.* Market analysis has been discussed in determination of supply. In the context of marketing, the market also is analyzed to find the media most likely to reach the potential supply. For example, are there nurses who live close enough to commute but are not likely to read the local newspaper?
2. *Prepare the message.* One good way to prepare the message is to ask current staff what they like about working in the organization and then use these statements in advertisements. Other sources are marketing materials from other local institutions and interviews with staff members who have worked other places.
3. *Decide on the media.* Most advertisements for staff nurses are placed in the classified sections of local newspapers in order to attract nurses who are working for other employers or who are not currently in the work force. Advertisements in nursing journals may be effective in recruiting specialized nurses and nurse managers. Local radio stations may offer a low-cost method of reaching nurses whether or not they are actively in the job market. In order to ensure that they are reaching minority communities, organizations also should consider advertising in local newspapers and on radio stations that are focused on those communities.
4. *Analyze the results.* Applicants always should be asked why they decided to apply for a position. The results should be tracked by date of application so that the effect of advertising campaigns and other efforts can be tracked. It is

TABLE 12–3. ADVANTAGES AND DISADVANTAGES OF THREE TYPES OF BONUSES

Type of Bonus	Advantage	Disadvantage
Recruitment (given to employee who recruits)	Rewards current employees; attracts new hires	New hires may leave after a short period
Sign-on (given to new hires)	Attracts new hires	Irritates current employees
Re-enlistment (given after "x" period of service)	Rewards current employees; provides an equivalent to sign-on bonus	Does not "buy" anything unless employee would have left without the bonus; employees may leave immediately after bonus is earned

helpful to keep information on the application process, employee performance, and reason for leaving in separate files to simplify later analysis.

Methods of Recruiting

If done properly, visits to nursing schools are a very effective way of recruiting new graduates. Emphasize the schools where most of the nurses employed at your hospital received their education. If possible, recruiters should be graduates of the school they visit, should be high performers with good interpersonal skills, and should be trained in "selling" the organization. When visiting a local school, the recruiter primarily "sells," rather than screens applicants. On visits to geographically remote schools the recruiter may have to combine the two functions to avoid paying travel expenses for unqualified applicants.

Nursing students' positive clinical experiences in the institution are indirect ways of recruiting. Students are alert to both verbal and nonverbal clues about the working conditions and ambience of the institution. Nurses who have worked with students can directly recruit them as well. Establishing a professional environment conducive to nurses' practice can be an important factor in the institution's reputation among students as well as in the larger community.

Other recruiting sources include walk-ins, employment agencies, and internal recruiting. *Walk-ins* are applicants who present themselves to the HRM office without an appointment. They may have seen an advertisement or heard about the hospital from a friend. If possible, a nurse recruiter should be "on-call" during the normal business day to welcome walk-ins. Job openings should be routinely posted at *public employment agencies* as part of your affirmative action program. Positions should always be posted internally before being advertised to the public (except for special affirmative action efforts).

Effectiveness of Various Recruiting Methods

Recruiting methods can be evaluated in two ways: whether they generate candidates and whether the candidates become good employees. In a comprehensive survey, personnel specialists rated sources for recruiting various types of employees (Bureau of National Affairs, 1979). Professional and technical employees were recruited best by newspaper advertising, private employment agencies, and visits to colleges and universities, in that order. Walk-ins and employee referrals were less effective. Another study of recruitment methods found that applicants referred by current employees have more realistic expectations and thus lower turnover than those recruited through newspaper advertisements. Breaugh and Mann (1984) found that walk-ins have both lower turnover and higher performance, possibly because they were highly motivated to work in that particular organization.

The effectiveness of recruiting methods varies considerably, depending on the local labor market and competitors. Fortunately, the effectiveness of various methods is easy to evaluate by asking applicants how they found out about the vacancy. The effectiveness of recruiting minority employees can be evaluated immediately. It is necessary to note the methods of recruiting in the employees' personnel records and wait six months to a year to determine their tenure and performance. In general, nurses who stay at least 3 months are satisfied with the work environment and will stay for at least a year. Nurses who stay at least 3 years are settled in the community and are likely to stay for several more years.

SCREENING AND SELECTING

Hiring is a two-stage process: screening for basic qualifications and selecting those likely to perform acceptably. Screening verifies that the candidates have the appropriate nursing education and have passed (or are eligible to take) the state licensing examination. Unlike screening, selecting is a *measurement* process because it concerns the *level* of the applicant's performance on the job.

FUNDAMENTALS OF PERSONNEL MANAGEMENT

Measurement is the process of assigning numbers to objects in order to represent the quantity of some attribute. HRM measures (including selection interview ratings) will be more or less accurate depending on how well they measure what they are intended to measure (validity).

A *predictor* is a measure that can be taken at the time of selection and used to make a decision about selecting a candidate for a position such as nurse manager, based on an inference about subsequent job performance. A *criterion* measure measures outcomes or actual job performance.

Criterion measures should be relevant, unbiased, and adequate. A performance rating of a nurse manager by a supervisor would be *relevant* to the extent that importance aspects of job performance were rated. It would be *biased* to the extent that factors not related to performance influence the ratings. Such factors could include the race or sex of the nurse manager, departmental problems unrelated to performance, or the opinions of others. Rater training should reduce rating bias. If the nurse manager's job duties required technical, interpersonal, and managerial ability and one of these was absent from the performance rating system, the rating of a manager would not be an *adequate* measure of job performance.

When possible, criterion measures should be objective measures of performance, rather than ratings which depend on the supervisor's judgment of the effectiveness of the individual's performance. Criterion measures for nurse managers could include financial performance of the unit and patient satisfaction measures. Some measures, such as treatment outcomes, may be beyond the control of the nurse manager.

Every time a score is obtained for an individual on a measure, the obtained score has two parts, a *true* component and an *error* component. Reducing error in measurement is always important (Gatewood & Feild, 1990). Good test design and administration will minimize error score, leaving obtained score as close to true score as possible.

The effectiveness of a predictor depends on its reliability and its validity. *Validity* is the extent to which evidence supports inferences about the subject made from a measure. The statistic commonly used to describe validity in personnel measures is the correlation coefficient.

Table 12-4 illustrates the hypothetical results of interviewing 10 candidates for nurse manager by having two interviewers (A and B) rate their predicted performance as a nurse manager and then having their supervisor rate their actual performance (in three dimensions: technical, interpersonal and managerial) as nurse manager a year later. The scores in the two right columns (Interview Score and Job Performance Score) are overall measures obtained by summing the two interview scores and the three job performance ratings respectively.

Looking down the last two columns in Table 12-4, high scores on the interview seem to be associated with high job performance. The three nurse managers who are low in job performance were only marginal in the interview (see Fig 12-3). Of the five who are moderate in job performance, two were low in the interview and three were high. Both of the nurse managers who are high in job performance were high in the interview.

RELIABILITY

Reliability and validity are different aspects of measurement. Reliability is the extent to which a measure is repeatable. Even though a measure may be highly repeatable, it may not be valid. Height, for example, could be measured very reliably but would not be a valid predictor of ability as a nurse manager. Reliability usually is described by the correlation between two administrations of the same measure. For example, the blood samples of a group of subjects could be split in half and each half could be analyzed for sugar content using the same procedure. The correlation between the two samples would be the reliability of the procedure. The reliability of standardized paper-and-pencil tests is best determined through the use of alternate forms, two versions of the test that are equally difficult (yield the same average score). The two forms are given on succeeding days and half of the group receives each form first. In a variation called the split-half method, the two versions of the test are combined so that the even-numbers items are one version and the odd-numbered items are another version.

For a selection interview, the measurement of reliability is difficult with only one interviewer. Both the interviewer and the subject would be affected if the interview were to be repeated. Instead, two raters evaluate the candidate and their rating are correlated. As shown in Table 12-5, Interviewers A and B rated the 10 subjects. The correlation between these two ratings is 0.836 which is very good reliability. Careful training of interviewers and good interviewing conditions will increase reliability.

VALIDITY

Validity is the extent to which evidence supports inferences about the subject made from a measure. The three types of validity are criterion-related, content, and construct (see Fig 12-4).

TABLE 12-4. INTERVIEW RATINGS AND RATINGS OF JOB PERFORMANCE FOR TEN NURSE MANAGERS

	Interviewers		Job Performance			Sums	
Subject	A	B	Technical	Interpersonal	Managerial	Interview Score	Job Performance
1	6	6	5	6	6	12	17
2	7	7	7	6	5	14	18
3	8	7	8	6	7	15	21
4	9	8	10	10	10	17	30
5	7	7	6	7	8	14	21
6	6	6	7	7	8	12	22
7	7	8	8	9	7	15	24
8	5	6	6	7	5	11	18
9	9	10	8	8	7	19	23
10	8	8	10	10	8	16	28
Mean	7.2	7.3	7.5	7.6	7.1	14.5	22.2
Standard deviation	1.317	1.252	1.650	1.578	1.524	2.461	4.260

269

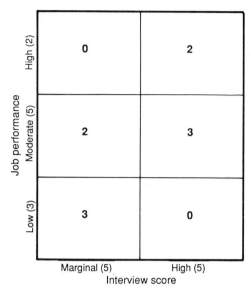

Figure 12-3. Relationship between Interview Score and Job Performance for 10 Nurse Managers

Criterion-related Validity

Criterion-related validity is the correlation between a predictor score and a criterion measure of job performance. Criterion-related validity requires a range of scores on the predictor measure. Rather than simply making a hire or not hire decision, it is necessary to rate the potential for success of successful candidates.

Table 12-5 shows the correlation between the interview ratings and three supervisory ratings: technical ability, interpersonal ability, and managerial ability. The overall validity of the interviewers' ratings for predicting job performance is the correlation between interview score and job performance (0.667). The correlation between the interview score and the three job performance factors (technical, interpersonal, managerial) are 0.725, 0.572, and 0.489, respectively. The correlation of Interviewer As ratings with job performance was 0.705, while Interviewer Bs ratings correlated at only 0.57. Thus, Interviewer A was a better predictor of future job performance than Interviewer B.

Content and Construct Validity

"Evidence of the validity of a test or other selection procedure by a content validity study should consist of data showing that the content of the selection procedure is representative of important aspects of performance on the job for which the candidates are to be evaluated." (*Uniform Guidelines*, §1607.5, B.) "Evidence of the validity of a test or other measure through a construct validity study should consist of data showing that the procedure measures the degree to which candidates have identifiable characteristics which have been determined to be important in successful performance in the job for which the candidates are to be evaluated." (*Uniform Guidelines*, §1607.5, B.) The difference between content and construct validity is that in the

TABLE 12–5. CORRELATIONS AMONG INTERVIEW RATINGS AND RATINGS OF JOB PERFORMANCE FOR 10 NURSE MANAGERS

| | Interviewers | | Job Performance | | | Sums | |
	A	B	Technical	Interpersonal	Managerial	Interview Score	Job Performance
A	—	0.836[b]	0.767[a]	0.524	0.598	0.960[b]	0.705[a]
B	0.836[b]	—	0.619	0.574	0.332	0.956[b]	0.570
Technical	0.767[b]	0.619	—	0.811[b]	0.641	0.725[a]	0.916[b]
Interpersonal	0.524	0.574	0.811[b]	—	0.666	0.572	0.922[b]
Managerial	0.598	0.332	0.641	0.666	—	0.489	0.852[b]
Interview Score	0.960[b]	0.956[b]	0.725	0.572	0.489	—	0.667[a]
Job Performance	0.705[a]	0.570	0.916[b]	0.922[b]	0.852[a]	0.667[a]	—

[a]$p < .05$; [b]$p < .01$

271

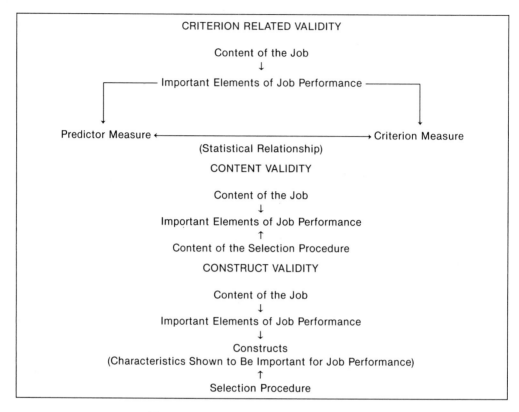

Figure 12-4. Models of Evidence for Validity

former, the content of the selection procedure is representative of important aspects of performance and in the latter, the procedure measures identifiable characteristics which have been determined to be important in successful performance.

Content validity is evident when important aspects of the job are reflected in the predictor or when the predictor is representative of the job content domain. For an interview to be a content valid predictor of the job of a nurse manager, questions have to be based on a job analysis of the nurse manager position. Table 12-2 contains interview questions that are related to Benner's (1984) domains of nursing practice.

Need to Demonstrate Validity

Conforming to EEO guidelines does not require that all selection practices be validated. It is only when practices have disparate impact on protected classes that an employer is required to validate the use of those practices. The "rule of thumb" is that the selection ratio for the protected group should be at least $\frac{4}{5}$ of the selection ratio for the majority group (*Uniform Guidelines*, §1607.5 B.). Suppose that 50 out of 100 white applicants are selected and only 20 out of 60 black applicants are selected.

The adverse impact ratio is calculated as: $\frac{20}{60} \div \frac{50}{100} = \frac{1}{3} \div \frac{1}{2} = \frac{2}{3}$. Since $\frac{2}{3}$ is less than $\frac{4}{5}$, the selection practice would have an adverse impact and the employer would need to defend its validity. It is both prudent and ethical to establish the validity of a selection practice before its use rather than waiting to determine whether or not it has adverse impact.

SELECTION METHODS

Applications

Applications serve several purposes: (1) They can be used to determine whether a candidate meets the basic job requirements; (2) they can be analyzed statistically, including a study to ensure that the scoring method does not discriminate against protected groups; and (3) they can be used to prepare for a selection interview. Gatewood and Feild (1990) suggest that the interviewer be provided only with basic information about the candidate's previous employment. Other information can be taken into account when the selection decision is made.

Almost every organization asks job candidates to complete an application form, even if the candidate has submitted a resume. The advantages of an application over a resume are: (1) It forces candidates to supply information, such as a career history with dates, that they may have omitted from their resume, and (2) it speeds up the screening process because the reader knows exactly where to find particular information. Every question asked *should* be job related and should not violate either the candidates' privacy or their civil rights. The key is to ask about the applicant's ability to meet the needs of the job, not about his or her personal life.

Data on applications are sometimes falsified or omitted. Candidates should be asked to sign a statement giving their permission to verify the information they have provided. They should be warned that they may be dismissed at a later date if the information is shown to be false. However, they should also be given the option as to whether their current employer is notified that they are seeking other employment.

Selection Interviews

The selection interview is the most commonly used selection procedure. The validity of the interview depends on how well it is planned and implemented. This section deals with planning the interview process, planning the interview itself, and implementing the interview.

Planning the Interview Process. Planning the interview is the responsibility of the interviewer, or lead interviewer in the case of a panel interview. (Be sure one of the interviewers is in charge!) The interviewer should review the applicant's job history and develop a set of questions to measure the skills identified in the job analysis. For the position of staff nurse or below, most of the questions may be standardized, so that the interviewer need only decide which of the candidate's previous positions is likely to be relevant to a particular question. For nurse manager, and above, the interviewer may have to adapt standardized questions or prepare new questions to measure how well the candidate is prepared for a particular skill. Like any first-level supervisory position, a nurse manager requires both technical skills and interpersonal skills. It is much easier to teach particular technical skills to a nurse manager candidate with good people skills than to teach people skills to a technically competent candidate.

An effective interviewer should:

1. Create an open communication atmosphere.
2. Deliver standardized questions consistently.
3. Avoid questions not related to the applicant's ability to do the job (see Fig 13–5, Sullivan & Decker, 1988, p 307).
4. Maintain control of the interview.
5. Be a good listener and note taker.
6. Keep the conversation flowing without leading the candidate.
7. Appropriately interpret nonverbal cues.
8. Ask good followup questions to evaluate the use of higher level cognitive skills during routine patient care (Adapted from Gatewood & Feild, 1990).

The interviewer should be very careful to avoid casual questions that might reveal the applicant's personal life, such as questions about finances, spouses, or children. Applicants who are members of a minority group should not be told that their status makes them particularly attractive candidates because such a statement implies that they are not as qualified as other candidates.

Planning includes: (a) training interviewers; (b) developing standard interview questions for each position; (c) screening candidates, including telephone interviews for out-of-town candidates; (d) determining who should interview a particular candidate, or type of candidate, and scheduling interviews; (e) comparing internal to external candidates; (f) follow up with successful and unsuccessful candidates; and (g) determining the role of the HRM department.

Training Interviewers. Interviewer training increases the validity of the interview process. Training should include learning questioning techniques, rating responses, practice using role playing and videotapes, and avoiding typical interview errors (eg, excessive talking by interviewer, inconsistent questions, overemphasizing first impression) (Gatewood & Feild, 1990).

Developing Standard Interview Questions. Based on job analysis, standard questions should be developed which are valid measures of each required skill and reflect the institution. For example, for a skill such as "monitoring and ensuring the quality of health care practices," an interview question could be "What would you do if a physician ordered 100 mg of Demerol IM for a child weighing 35 pounds?"

Determining Who Should Interview and Schedule. Candidates for nurse manager and nurse executive positions can be interviewed by subordinates, peers, supervisor, peers of the supervisor, and physicians. (Involvement of other department heads and physicians provides a realistic job preview and ownership in the selection decision.)

Interviews should be scheduled during relatively quiet periods in the interviewer's day. Interviewers should arrange for someone to handle all but the most critical emergencies so that the interview is not interrupted. For high level jobs, it may be cost-effective to have an initial interview with only a few interviewers and bring the best candidates in for a second visit with more extensive interviewing. A well-planned telephone interview is an important cost cutter for out-of-town candidates. If a large number of candidates are being interviewed, especially for entry level positions, it is appropriate to be vague about the length of the interviewing process. Unsuccessful candidates may be terminated early in the process.

Internal and External Candidates. When management level positions are being filled, external candidates frequently compete with those already in the organization. Although it may seem artificial, the best procedure is to treat the two types of candidates as much alike as possible. Interviews with internal candidates must be scheduled as carefully as for external candidates. If they are not successful, internal candidates will be very sensitive to any irregularities in the selection process. Feedback to unsuccessful internal candidates is particularly tricky since the organization shares some responsibility for their career development. It is easy to make a statement such as "All you need is a little more experience" that appears to the employee to be a promise of future promotion. An employee who wants to be a manager and is viewed by his or her current organization as having low potential (even with further experience) is likely to seek other employment. The best course of action is to give honest feedback so that the employees will either adjust their expectations or seek employment elsewhere. On the other hand, internal candidates do have a disadvantage in that both their strengths and weaknesses are known to the organization. Do not make the mistake of rejecting an internal candidate because of minor faults that would not be visible in an external candidate.

Follow up with Candidates. Follow-up issues include: Who does the follow up? When does feedback take place? What kinds of discussion is held with successful and unsuccessful candidates?

In most cases, the supervisor of the position being filled will do the follow up. Feedback may take place at the end of the interview day if the individual is clearly unqualified or mentions other open job offers. In most cases, feedback should take place after all candidates have been interviewed or at least within a day or two of the interview. In a lengthy interview process with many candidates, those who are still under consideration should be notified and told how long the entire process will last. The best candidates may be entertaining other offers and may want to know whether they are the highest rated among those candidates who already have been interviewed. Depending on the situation, the best candidates may be interviewed first or last in the process. If there is no need to interview every candidate, the best candidate may be interviewed first and the process discontinued if she or he accepts the position. If the plan is to interview every acceptable candidate, the best candidate may be interviewed last so that the job offer can be extended at the end of the interview process or shortly thereafter.

For successful candidates, the job offer discussion is the first step in their orientation to their new position. The supervisor should express pleasure with the candidate's acceptance of the job offer (if it is accepted at that time) or offer to answer questions if the candidate is undecided. Critical or unusual aspects of the position should be reviewed. If the candidate is going to reject the job offer, it is better to be able to offer it to the next most qualified candidate immediately. For unsuccessful candidates, particularly at the nurse manager level and above, the key question is how much feedback to give. One's natural inclination may be to give extensive feedback. Since giving reasons for not selecting an individual may open the organization to legal challenges, detailed feedback should only be given by a high-level official, with consultation from the HRM department. Subordinates and peers of the position should be told to not discuss the selection decision with unsuccessful candidates.

Role of the HRM Department

Depending on the organization, the role of the HRM department in the interviewing process may vary from managing the entire process to having no contact with candidates until after they have accepted a job offer. Large organizations will either have a nursing representative within the HRM department or a mini-HRM department within nursing. All too often, this arrangement depends on the quality of the relationship between nursing and the HRM department. Being able to control your own HRM department may be very tempting to the nurse executive. However, the nurse executive would have to become expert in HRM and remain current in that rapidly changing field. A better understanding of the HRM function and how nurse executives can collaborate with their HRM departments should be encouraged.

Improving the Selection Process

Suppose a hospital interviews 10 candidates a year for nurse manager and hires 7, a selection ratio of 60 percent. A cutoff of 14 on the interview score (see Table 12–4) is required in order to hire 7 candidates, which means that only about 71 percent of the candidates will be successful. There are three ways to improve the success rate.

1. Develop a more valid interview, which will lessen the number of false positives, candidates for whom success is falsely predicted.
2. Interview a larger number of candidates so that a higher cutoff can be used to select the top 7 candidates. Attracting a larger number of candidates might require only the one-time expense of more advertising or might require the continuing expense of offering higher salaries.
3. Increase the overall quality of the candidate pool by becoming the preferred employer. This option was discussed earlier.

The first alternative, developing a more valid interview, may be the least expensive, especially in a situation where about half of the candidates are hired. However, the validity of the interview in our example is already 0.667, which is quite high. A major improvement is unlikely. In the example given, the least expensive way to improve the selection process would be to decrease the selection ratio by increasing the number of applicants rather than attempting to increase the validity of the selection interview.

Evaluation of Education, Training, and Experience

Depending on the position, the *educational level* of candidates may range from an associate degree to a doctorate. *Training* is used to describe a learning experience that is shorter in duration and does not carry credit for a degree. Training may vary from informal on-the-job training to continuing education course that is identical to a course taught for credit. *Experience* may be thought of as continuing on-the-job training. A good senior nurse or nurse manager is constantly training subordinates. When training or experience are being evaluated, a primary issue will be whether basic skills or cognitive decision-making skills were gained.

Other Selection Measures

Paper-and-pencil tests can measure mental ability or personality traits. These tests which utilize only written material (rather than equipment) may be administered to more than one subject at a time. The responses may be multiple-choice, short answer, or essay. Such tests have the advantage of being objective, inexpensive, and quick. In general, all testing will be done by the HRM department.

Ability Tests. An ability test measures how much a person has learned about a knowledge domain or how well a person can carry out a task. Formal distinctions among tests of ability, aptitude, and achievement have not proven to be useful. The licensing examination is an ability test. Ability tests have proven less useful for predicting success as a manager, since employees who are below average in general ability tend to be screened out as candidates for management positions. Assessment centers, discussed later in this chapter, use work samples of the manager's job and can be very useful in selecting managers and executives.

Personality Measures. Personality inventories are multiple-choice measures of an applicant's personality characteristics, how the individual approaches and responds to life situations. Other personality measures may ask the applicant to complete sentences (eg, Most nurse managers are ____.) or to tell a story about a picture. If personality measures are used, the characteristics favored by the measure should be consistent with the climate in your hospital. Validating a personality test is difficult at best and should be done by an expert. Interest inventories compare the applicant's interests to those of thousands of subjects in a number of occupations. Their validity depends on the assumption that applicants are more likely to be successful in an occupation if their interests are similar to others in the occupation. Interest inventories have better empirical support than personality inventories but would be difficult to defend in an EEO lawsuit. In general, a personality inventories should be avoided.

Work Samples

Work samples and other performance tests are widely used in industry, particularly for jobs involving trade knowledge and manual skills. For example, a welder will be asked to perform a particularly tricky weld on scrap metal. Fortunately, there are no "scrap patients" in hospitals. However, work samples can be developed by preparing detailed questions to ask nurse candidates claiming competence in a particular specialty. More complex clinical simulations are possible with computer-aided instruction, interactive video, or role playing.

Assessment Centers

An assessment center is not a place but a process for selection, usually for a supervisory position. In an assessment center, candidates perform a series of exercises that have been specially developed to (1) reflect the demands of a position and (2) elicit behavior that can be observed and evaluated. Teams of trained assessors (usually supervisors of the target position) observe and evaluate the candidates. Assessment centers are useful when competence in a nonsupervisory position is necessary (eg, clinical nurses) but is not sufficient to demonstrate performance to be a supervisor (eg., nurse manager). Assessment centers especially are useful to the chief nurse executive for selecting the managers who report directly to the executive (Sullivan, Decker, & Hailstone, 1985). Simulations similar to those found in assessment centers can also be used to determine training needs in newly hired nurses.

Developing an assessment center begins with a job analysis to determine the important job tasks. Then, the tasks are combined into skill dimensions. The skill dimensions tend to be very similar for a wide variety of managerial jobs, with the exception of technical job knowledge. However, the time spent on job tasks is not wasted because the next step is developing exercises that incorporate the job tasks and measure the dimensions. Then assessor training materials are prepared and assessors are trained. Finally, candidates are screened and go through the assessment center. Many organizations allow any professional with adequate work experience to try the assessment center.

Dimensions measured in a typical assessment center include leadership, delegation and control, planning and organizing, sensitivity, problem analysis, verbal and written communication, performance under pressure, and technical knowledge. Typical assessment center exercises include a leaderless group discussion, an in-basket, a managerial case study, an employee counseling exercise, a personnel scheduling exercise, and a technical case study. Exercises must be pretested and are likely to be modified extensively as a result.

Assessment is a very demanding task carried out by teams of two or three assessors. It is *very* important to select the best managers as assessors rather than those who can be most easily spared. An assessor who is a weak manager will be a burden to teammates and is likely to be forced from the team. Assessor training typically lasts 2 or 3 days and includes a discussion of the material and a "mock" assessment center. Assessors usually find the training to be extremely relevant to their day-to-day duties as managers.

Assessment centers are highly effective, but expensive. If properly designed and administered, they are much more likely to be objective than other methods of comparing internal candidates to each other and to external candidates. In the long run, they are cost-effective because high performers are identified and because candidates who do poorly are more likely to accept the results than candidates who receive low evaluations in a typical promotion process.

An assessment center is a demanding process that requires high involvement on the part of hospital administrators, assessors, and candidates. However, it provides the best methodology for comparing internal and external candidates (a difficult task) and is usually seen as a valuable experience by both assessors and candidates. A complete discussion of the assessment center method is found in Thornton and Byham (1982).

CLINICAL LADDERS

Clinical ladders provide a means of recognizing and rewarding highly skilled nurses by providing an alternative to traditional promotion from patient care to supervision. In most hospitals, staff nurses who are highly competent must choose between continuing to work in direct patient care or increasing their status and pay by seeking advancement as a nurse manager. Clinical ladders offer an opportunity to remain involved in direct patient care. A nurse who has advanced on the clinical ladder typically provides highly skilled nursing care and acts as a coach and role model for less experienced nurses (Mackay et al, 1987).

The advantage of a clinical ladder is that it enables the institution to make the best use of nurses who may not be skilled, or interested, in managing. Nurses who desire to remain at the bedside can be recognized and rewarded for their expertise. Developing criteria for advancement and documenting the progress of each nurse is time consuming but very worthwhile for both the individual and the organization. Documenting the progress of nurses as they advance on the clinical ladder will be simpler and less subjective if objective factors such as educational level, years of experience, continuing education, and cross training are used in addition to evaluations of clinical skill.

REFERENCES

American Academy of Nursing. *Magnet Hospitals: Attraction and Retention of Professional Nurses.* Kansas City, MO, American Nurses Association, 1983

Benner P. *From Novice to Expert: Excellence and Power in Clinical Nursing Practice.* Menlo Park, CA, Addison Wesley, 1984

Biddle RE. *Guidelines Oriented Job Analysis.* Sacramento, CA, Biddle and Associates Inc, 1982

Breaugh JA, Mann B. Recruiting source effects: A test of two alternative explanations. *Journal of Occupational Psychology.* 57:261, 1984

Bureau of National Affairs. Recruiting Policies and Practice. Survey No. 126. *Personnel Policies Forum.* 1979

Chase JA. Certification and job analysis. *Orthopaedic Nursing.* 7:2, 26, 1988

Droste T. High price tag on nursing recruitment. *Hospitals.* 61 150, October 5, 1987

Fox V, Blue, Sister MR. Job analysis, national certification board: Perioperative Nursing Inc, document. *AORN Journal.* 47:5, 1256, 1988

Gatewood RD, Feild HS. *Human resource selection*. Chicago, Dryden, 1990

Mackay RW, Storey RG, Mcclean LC, Misick JD, Glube RH, and Pereira L. Job design: Matching jobs to staff nurses interests. *Nursing Management*. 18:4, 76, 1987

Scarpello VG, Ledvinka J. *Personnel-human resource management: An environmental approach*. Boston, PWS-Kent, 1988

Sullivan EJ, Decker PJ. *Effective Management in Nursing*. Menlo Park, CA, Addison Wesley, 1988

Sullivan EJ, Decker PJ, and Hailstone S. Assessment center technology: Selecting head nurses. *Journal of Nursing Administration*. 15:5, 13, 1985

Thorton G, Byham W. *Assessment Centers and Managerial Performance*. San Diego, CA, Academic Press, 1982

US Department of Health and Human Services. *Seventh Report to the President and Congress and the Status of Health Personnel*. (DHHS Pub. No. HRS-P-OD-90-1). Washington DC, US Government Printing Office, 1990

US Department of Labor. *Handbook for Analyzing Jobs*. US Training Employment Services, Manpower Administration. Washington DC, US Government Printing Office, 1972 (Updated Supplement, 1982)

US Equal Employment Opportunity Commission, US Civil Service Commission, US Department of Labor, US Department of Justice. Uniform guidelines on employee selection procedures. *Federal Register*. 43:38290, (August 25, 1978)

CHAPTER 13

Performance Appraisal Systems

Jeffrey S. Kane
H. John Bernardin
Kimberly F. Kane

Key Concept List

Performance appraisal
Job functions and outcomes
Internal staffing
Force reduction
Legal constraints on appraisal
Designing an appraisal system
Rating errors
Appraisal formats

Performance appraisal has long been regarded as one of the most troubling areas of human resource management. While over 95 percent of organizations use formal systems of appraisal, the majority express considerable dissatisfaction with it. This includes not only the raters and ratees themselves but those who administer the appraisal systems as well. The nursing profession is no exception to this general attitude toward appraisal. Nurses who are evaluated are generally unhappy with the process, those who do the evaluating would rather do just about anything else, and administrators are inundated with problems related to the process and actions taken as a consequence of appraisals (Bernardin & Abbott, 1985).

Several surveys have revealed widespread dissatisfaction in relatively large organizations (eg, *Fortune* 500 companies) which presumably have the resources to acquire the best appraisal technology available. In nursing, Cardy and Korodi (1990) found that 50 percent of the respondent nursing directors questioned the validity of evaluations and 75 percent believed that politics played a significant role in appraisal.

Appraisal in health care is more important today for several reasons. First, in today's cost-effective environment, hospitals must be certain that all personnel are working to the best of their ability. Second, hospital performance appraisal practices are now closely examined by regulatory bodies. The Joint Commission for Accreditation of Healthcare Organizations (JCAHO) requires hospitals to have "measurable standards" for the evaluation of nurse performance for purposes of accreditation. Third, performance appraisal is the most heavily litigated personnel practice today (Bernardin & Kane, 1991). Legal grounds for challenging appraisal systems are expanding, so litigation can be expected to increase. Fourth, there is increasing diversity in populations entering nursing. Ever greater proportions of new nurses will be members of minority groups and older workers. Unfairness and biases already present in appraisal systems may be magnified by differences between raters and ratees. Finally, in an effort to retain experienced nursing professionals, health care institutions need to remove performance appraisal as a source of dissatisfaction and bring it to a level acceptable to professionals. Health care organizations consequently will need to be increasingly scrupulous regarding fairness and objectivity in appraisal practices and personnel decisions (Ghorpade, 1988). Since appraisal may be used in the future as a method to increase productivity, organizations have more pressure to use it correctly.

Although a nurse's work performance depends on some combination of ability, effort, and opportunity, it is measured in terms of outcomes or results produced. Performance is defined as: The *record of outcomes produced on a specified job function during a specified period.* The nurse's job can be broken down into smaller components (ie, job functions) that do not overlap and that are specified at about the same level. For example, the extent to which the nurse complies with hospital and departmental policy. Performance then can be measured on each of these component job functions. Performance on the job as whole is equal to the sum (or average) of performance on these functions. The definition of performance refers to a set of outcomes produced during a certain period of time, and does not refer to traits or personal characteristics of the performer.

Outcomes are defined as goal attainment or nonattainment. These goals are tied to job functions as specified in nursing standards and policies. Performance is widely acknowledged to be the product of a stable factor (ie, ability) and variable factors (ie, effort, opportunity). It is not reasonable to dismiss variations in the outcome levels achieved. Variations in nurse performance across a performance period could be due to fluctuations in the effort invested in one's work and represent important information about how the nurse has performed.

USES OF PERFORMANCE APPRAISAL

Performance appraisals are used for four primary purposes:

1. Performance management
2. Internal staffing
3. Training needs analysis
4. Research and evaluation

Performance Management

Performance management is the systematic effort to identify performance deficits, to specify target levels for performance improvements, and to utilize incentives to motivate performers to the target levels. This includes all pay-for-performance programs such as merit pay and even bonus awards. Performance management programs may be focused at one or more of the following organizational levels:

- Individual performers
- Work groups or organizational subunits
- Organizationwide

Individually-focused programs use performance appraisal results to identify deficiencies in a person's job performance. Typically, arbitrary target levels for all substandard areas of performance should be set. In industry, computer programs are now available that start with a target level of overall performance and proceed to analyze the employee's appraisal scores to determine the easiest set of performance improvements in job functions necessary to raise overall performance to the target level. Merit pay raises, bonuses, or other incentives can be tied to the attainment of the target level.

Work-group or *organizational subunit-focused* programs essentially do the same things as those focused on individual performers, the only difference is that the performance of the work group or subunit is evaluated. In order to determine the collective performance of a work group or subunit, it is necessary to have an appraisal system with scores for different jobs that are directly comparable and thereby capable of being meaningfully averaged. Only when the numbers have the same meaning for all the jobs over which performance is to be averaged, will the average meaningfully reflect collective performance (eg, critical care nurses). If collective performance data are available, high and low performing work groups or subunits can be identified (eg, coronary versus surgical ICU nurses). High performing groups can be allocated higher pay increases and/or bonuses and low performing groups can be subjected to more detailed analysis to determine the causes of the performance deficits. Such deficiencies may be traceable to particular individuals, job titles, occupations, hierarchical levels, periods of time, or to unitwide phenomena. The source(s) of the problem can be identified and efforts directed to alleviate the problem during the subsequent appraisal period.

Organizational-focused approaches require performance measurements that are comparable, not only across all jobs in the organization, but also to measurements used in previous periods or other similar organizations. Comparisons over time are important to track the success of improvement efforts from one period of operation to the next or to spot undesirable trends. Appraisal results can pinpoint the units, work groups, or individuals that seem to be negatively affecting the organization's overall performance.

Internal Staffing

Once people have become employees of an organization they are subject to two basic types of selection decisions: *promotion* and *force reduction*.

Promotion. To the extent that promotions are viewed as serving staffing purposes exclusively (and not as rewards for past performance), the basis for selecting people for promotion is their predicted performance in the higher level job. Unfortunately, appraisal results have had limited usefulness in predicting performance at a higher level because they usually focus strictly on the functions of the present job. This means that appraisal results only have the potential to predict performance in the portion of higher level jobs that contain functions similar to those in the candidates current job. To the extent that the head nurse job entails distinct job functions from the staff nurse's job, the appraisal system involving only staff nurse functions is deficient for promotion. However, the performance appraisal system is useful as a developmental device.

Since conventional appraisal systems are limited in their ability to assist with promotion decisions, organizations often resort to written and oral examinations, interviews, and, more recently, assessment centers. It has long been recognized that a person's job performance is the best source of information about the typical levels of various abilities that a person exhibits. The problem, however, is in extracting the generalizable (and potentially predictive) information about typical ability levels from assessments of performance on job specific functions or projects.

Force reduction. This selection decision is the opposite of promotion not only in the response it produces among those "selected," but also in the degree to which it has traditionally relied on appraisal as the selection criterion. While in the unionized work force seniority is the principal basis for force reduction (ie, layoff) decisions, in the rest of the work force, performance is the key in such decisions. The federal government's current guidelines for "reduction in force" specify that equal weight be given to performance and length of employment. In many private sector organizations, performance is the basis used though nursing organizations typically use attrition.

In states that have laws that require terminations to be based on "just cause," force reduction decisions based on appraisal systems shown to be biased, unreliable, or inaccurate may not be defensible. Moreover, when force reductions are based on comparisons of appraisal scores, the organization must be prepared to defend the comparability of appraisal scores.

Training Needs Analysis

Performance appraisal also can be used to determine the training needs of an organization as a whole. Any organization has a limited budget for training and it must determine where it should spend the money to get the greatest return on its investment. Appraisals can be invaluable in this determination but once again, their usefulness depends on a method that allows direct comparisons of scores across all jobs. Assuming this degree of score comparability, the basic strategy would be to compute the following index for each job:

$$\text{Average decrement from maximum performance} \times \text{Average pay level of job incumbents} \times \text{Number of incumbents in job}$$

Jobs then are ranked by this index. Jobs with the highest levels on this index yield the highest returns for each increment of performance improvement produced by training.

Research and Evaluation

Evaluation is needed to verify whether personnel activities to enhance performance are effective. Examples occur in both employment selection and in training. Criterion-related validation studies of the tests used to select applicants for employment are needed to verify their use. These studies involve examining the extent to which people who score higher on the tests also perform more effectively on the job. Appraisals are the most commonly used measures of job performance in such studies (see Chapter 12 for a description of criterion-related validation studies).

Organizations should evaluate the effectiveness of their training programs more often than they actually do. Many evaluations simply consist of questionnaires asking participants how much they liked the program. Any meaningful evaluation of a training program should try to assess its effects on the job performance of participants. Appraisals can furnish the measures of job performance needed for this purpose.

LEGAL CONSTRAINTS ON APPRAISAL

Since performance provides the basis for many important personnel decisions (eg, pay, promotion, selection, termination), it is understandable that the basis for such decisions—performance appraisal—is the main target of legal disputes involving employee charges of unfairness and bias (Barrett & Kernan, 1987; Koys, Briggs, & Grenig, 1986). The legal grounds for challenging appraisal systems are increasing so it is reasonable to expect that legal activity involving performance appraisals will continue to increase.

There are several legal avenues a person may pursue to obtain relief from unfair or discriminatory personnel practices based on performance appraisals. While there are a myriad of federal, state, and local laws, the major sources of legal protection for complaints involving performance appraisal are Title VII of the Civil Rights Act (1964) and the Equal Employment Opportunity Act (1972); the Age in Discrimination in Employment Act (ADEA, 1967); and exceptions to the "employment-at-will" doctrine (see Chapter 11).

One recent case (*Watson v Fort Worth Bank & Trust*, 1988) involved promotions that were based on the subjective judgments of performance made by white supervisors. White applicants were selected instead of Watson (a minority female) for promotion to four supervisory positions. The US Supreme Court ultimately ruled that subjective evaluation criteria is subject to the same analytic scrutiny as "neutral" employment practices such as standardized tests or credentials.

Termination of an employee for poor performance is the most common reason for litigation under ADEA. Employers have lost numerous cases due to differences between the employee's formal record of performance and the employer's claims of poor performance. The formal performance records of the employee as well as the methods of appraisal used by the employer are a vital part of the employer's decision whether to settle out of court or to continue litigation. Experts in performance appraisal who have been expert witnesses report that personnel decisions based on performance appraisal systems with relevant ratings are much more defensible than those lacking these qualities (Bernardin & Kane, 1991). Employers are more likely to lose with only an undocumented system of evaluation although written records indicating satisfactory or exemplary employee performance (commonly due to lenient or inflated performance ratings) can be used to rebut an employer's argument of poor performance.

"Employment-at-will" refers to an employer's right to discharge an employee for any reason at any time. This common law doctrine exists in some states though many states recognize an "implied contract exception" that an employee will not be terminated if performance is satisfactory. A less widely recognized exception to the employment-at-will doctrine is an "implied covenant of good faith" which holds that all employees must be treated fairly and with good faith. The implication for performance appraisal is that terminations must be made for "just cause" based on documented performance deficits and a good faith effort to avoid unfair terminations.

Defensible Performance Appraisals

In view of the legal ramifications of personnel decisions based on indefensible performance appraisals, there are several recommendations for conducting fair appraisals and avoiding (or winning) litigation in nursing. These recommendations are based on case law and research on performance appraisal (eg, Barrett & Kernan, 1987).

1. Legally defensible appraisal *procedures*:
   - Personnel decisions should be based on a formal, standardized performance appraisal system.
   - Performance appraisal processes should be uniform for all nurses within a job group, and decisions based on those performance appraisals should not be effected by the race, sex, national origin, religion, or age of those who are rated.
   - Specific performance standards should be formally communicated to employees.

- Employees who are rated should be able to formally review the appraisal results. Further, there should be a formal appeal process for employees who wish to contest the rater judgments.
- Raters should be provided with written instructions on how to conduct appraisals properly to facilitate systematic, unbiased appraisals.
- Personnel decision makers should be informed of antidiscrimination laws and made aware of legal and illegal activity regarding decisions based on performance appraisals (Klimoski & London, 1974).

2. Legally defensible appraisal *content*:
- Performance appraisal content should be based on a job or task analysis of the nursing job (eg, Lang, 1988).
- Appraisals based on individual traits such as attitude, initiative, and dependability should be avoided (Feldman, 1986).
- Objective, verifiable performance data should be used whenever possible (ie, not rated performance) and constraints on employees performance which are beyond their control should be prevented from contaminating the appraisal to ensure that all employees within that job group have equal opportunities to achieve any given appraisal score.
- Specific job-related performance dimensions should be used rather than global measures or single overall measures of performance.

3. Legally defensible *documentation* of appraisal results:
- A thorough written record of evidence leading to termination decisions should be maintained (eg, performance appraisals and performance counseling to advise employees of performance deficits and assist poor performers to make improvements).
- Written documentation of critical incidents (eg, specific behavior exemplars) for extreme ratings should be required and must be consistent with the numerical ratings.
- Documentation requirements should be consistent among raters.

4. Legally defensible *raters*:
- Raters must have the opportunity to observe the employee firsthand.
- Use of more than one rater is desirable in order to lessen the amount of influence of any one rater and to reduce the effects of biases.

These recommendations are intended as prescriptive measures that nursing administrators can take to move toward more fair and legally defensible performance appraisals for their nursing staff. Since case law and court rulings are continually updated, these are not guaranteed "defense-proof" listings, but represent instead sound personnel practices that protect the rights of both employers and employees.

DESIGNING AN APPRAISAL SYSTEM

The process of designing an appraisal system consists of selecting from options available from each of the following:

- Measurement content
- Measurement process
- Rater definition
- Ratee definition
- Administrative characteristics

It is a challenge to make the correct choices since no single configuration of choices is optimal in all situations. The choice of each element of an appraisal system is dependent or *contingent* on the nature of the situation in which the system is to be used. The approach to appraisal system design advocated here is to systematically assess the contingencies present in a situation, called a *contingency model for appraisal system design* (Bernardin & Kane, 1991).

Measurement Content

In designing an appraisal system, there are three choices that concern the content on which performance is to be measured: (1) the focus of the appraisal; (2) criterion differentiation; or (3) performance level benchmarks.

The focus of the appraisal. Appraisal can be either person-oriented (focusing on the person who performed) or work-oriented (focusing on the *record of outcomes* that the person achieved on the job). It is not appropriate to base performance appraisal on the worth of individuals (ie, traits) but rather on the worth of their performance. Personal traits (such as dependability, integrity, perseverance, loyalty) often are not job related, invite stereotyping and other biases, and are not limited to the person's behavior during a specific period of work.

Work-oriented content, the preferred focus, involves another choice: whether to appraise (1) the period-specific projects and/or assignments carried out by the performer or on (2) the enduring duties or job functions that define the performer's job. There are two key distinctions between project-focused and job function-focused appraisals. First, results of appraisals based on job functions can be compared from one period to the next whereas project-focused appraisals are period-specific. Projects typically encompass unique combinations of activities and are not comparable from one appraisal period to the next. Job function-focused appraisals which are the norm for all staff nurses in the institution can pinpoint strengths and weaknesses of a person's performance, which is useful for developmental purposes.

Criterion differentiation. Virtually all conventional appraisal systems require raters to make a single overall judgment of performance on each project or job function although there are up to six primary criteria by which the performance in any work activity may be assessed (Kane, 1986). These six criteria are:

1. *Quality:* the degree to which the process or result of carrying out an activity approached perfection in terms of either conforming to some ideal way of performing the activity or fulfilling the activity's intended purpose.
2. *Quantity:* the amount produced, expressed in such terms as dollar value, number of units, or number of completed activity cycles.

3. *Timeliness:* the degree to which an activity is completed, or a result produced, at the earliest time desirable from the standpoints of both coordinating with the outputs of others and maximizing the time available for other activities.

4. *Cost effectiveness:* the degree to which the use of the organization's resources (eg, human, monetary, technological, material) is maximized in the sense of getting the highest gain or reduction in loss from each unit or instance of use of a resource.

5. *Need for supervision:* the degree to which a performer can carry out a job function without either having to request supervisory assistance or requiring supervisory intervention to prevent an adverse outcome.

6. *Interpersonal impact:* the degree to which a performer promotes feelings of self-esteem, good will, and cooperativeness among co-workers subordinates, clients and customers.

The appraisal design choice is whether to assess performance on each job function as a whole (ie, considering all relevant criteria simultaneously) or to assess each relevant criterion of performance on each job function separately. The overall approach is faster than making assessments on separate criteria but has the major drawback of requiring raters to simultaneously consider as many as six different criteria and to mentally compute their average. This subjective reasoning will be less accurate than those done on each relevant criterion for each job function.

When performance is rated separately on each of the criteria relevant to each job function, the result is a set of scores on various job function-criterion combinations. We refer to each of these job function-criterion combinations as *performance dimensions.* For example, Nurse A might be appraised on the "timeliness in which patient assessment is completed" and the "need for supervision in patient assessment" where "timeliness" and "need for supervision" are criteria and "patient assessment" is the job function (see Table 13–1).

Performance level benchmarks (or descriptors). Work-oriented appraisal systems require raters to compare performance on each job function or project against a set of benchmarks. These benchmarks are brief descriptions of levels of performance. These descriptions of performance levels are often referred as *performance level descriptors* (*PLDs*). PLDs may take three different forms: (1) adjectives or adjective phrases, such as "satisfactory," "effective," "below standard," or "rarely"; (2) behavioral descriptions, or "critical incidents"; or (3) outcomes or results produced by the performance.

Adjectival benchmarks are highly subjective because their interpretation can mean different things to different raters. Behavioral PLDs consist of descriptions of the actions taken by the person being appraised. It only makes sense to use behavioral benchmarks if they are causally linked to relevant outcomes. For example, Nurse A may have completed the patient assessment activities but failed to identify the priority of patient need in order to develop the most effective plan of care. Most nurse job functions have no single set of optimal behaviors. Similarly, any specific behavior may lead to different outcome levels depending on other concurrent behaviors and the effort invested. It is inappropriate to use behavioral benchmarks as PLDs, unless the appraisal is only to identify skill areas that need improvement.

TABLE 13–1. PERFORMANCE DIMENSIONS: JOB-CRITERION COMBINATIONS

1. Performance assessment on each job function as a whole

    Job Function 1: Patient assessment

    [Consider timeliness, need for supervision, criterion 3, criterion 4 . . . , criterion 6 in your rating]
      Excellent, Good, Average, Below Average, Poor

2. Performance assessment on each criteria for each job function

    Job Function 1: Patient assessment

      criterion 1: timeliness
      criterion 2: need for supervision
      criterion 3: ────

3. Performance level bench marks

    a. Adjectival bench marks
       JF1: Patient assessment
          Excellent, Good, Average, Below average, Poor
    b. Behavioral bench marks
       JF1: Patient assessment
          Identifies priority of pt need, yes/no
    c. Goal-oriented, benchmarks
       JF1: Patient assessment
          Assessment results in appropriate plan of care, yes/no

Goal-oriented PLDs (based on outcomes or results produced) are generally preferable to either adjectival or behavioral PLDs when performance outcomes are identifiable and when the person's contribution to the results can be distinguished. If neither of these are possible, behavioral PLDs should be used.

Measurement Process

The appraisal system's measurement process involves the following: rating format; accounting for situational constraints on performance; control of rating errors; and overall score computation method.

Rating format. There are three basic ways in which raters give performance assessments: comparisons among (ratee) performances, comparisons among performance level benchmarks (PLDs), and comparisons *to* benchmarks (PLDs).

1. *Comparisons among performances:* Compare the performances of all ratees to each PLD for each job function or project. Rater judgments may be made in one of the following ways:
    a. Paired comparison: Indicate which ratee in each possible *pair* of ratees performed closest to the performance level described by the PLD.
    b. Straight ranking: Indicate how the ratees ranked in terms of the closeness to the performance level described by the PLD.
    c. Forced distribution: Indicate what percentage of the ratees performed in a manner closest to the performance level described by the PLD. (Note: the percentages must total 100 percent for all the PLDs within each job.)
2. *Comparisons among benchmarks (PLDS):* Forced choice: Compare all the PLDs

for each job function and select the one or more that best describes the ratee's performance level. Rater judgments are made in the following way: Indicate which of the PLDs fit the ratee's performance best (and/or worst).

3. *Comparisons to benchmarks (PLDs):* Compare each ratee's performance to each PLD for each job function or project. Rater judgments are made in one of the following ways:
   A. Management by Objectives (MBO), graphic rating scales, behaviorally anchored rating scales (BARS), checklists: Whether or not the ratee's performance matches the PLD.
   B. Summated rating scales such as behavioral observation scales (BOS) and performance distribution assessment methods (eg, PRISM): The degree to which the ratee's performance matches the PLD.
   C. Mixed standard scales: Whether the ratee's performance was better than equal to, or worse than that described by the PLD.

The most common rating formats are the summated scale (also known as behavioral observation scales), behaviorally anchored rating scales, and management by objectives. See Bernardin and Kane (1991) for examples.

While research indicates that the rating format has little effect on rating accuracy (Landy & Farr, 1983), there is recent evidence which indicates that a format designed to prevent the rater from determining the overall rating level of the responses seems to help reduce intentional rating errors (Bernardin & Orban, in press).

In the absence of any proven advantage of one format over the others, the main basis for selecting a rating format should be congruence with the level of precision needed in the measurement and ease of use. If only rank orders of staff nurses are required, then formats using comparisons among ratee performance are adequate. However, if a higher level of precision is needed, eg, for specialty nurses, comparison to benchmarks offer the most direct approach.

Accounting for situational constraints on performance. One of the major factors that causes inaccurate and unfair performance appraisals is the practice of blaming employees for poor performance that was caused by factors completely beyond their control. Many conditions present in the job situation prevent a person from performing optimally. Personnel shortages, lack of supplies, too little time, lack of information, equipment failure, and numerous other situational factors can hinder achieving a higher performance level even though the person has the ability and exerts the effort to perform well. The current nursing shortage causes most health care institutions to have areas where nurses are short-staffed. These nurses' performances may not meet expected standards since attending to the most serious situation is the priority. Possible constraints on performance include:

1. Absenteeism or turnover of key personnel
2. Slowness of procedures for action approval
3. Inadequate clerical support
4. Shortages of supplies or materials
5. Excessive restrictions on operating expenses

6. Inadequate physical working conditions
7. Inability to hire needed staff
8. Inadequate performance of co-workers or personnel in other units upon whom an individual's work depends
9. Inadequate performance of subordinates
10. Inadequate performance of managers or supervisors
11. Inefficient or unclear organizational structure or reporting relationships
12. Excessive reporting requirements and administrative paperwork
13. Unpredictable workloads
14. Excessive workloads
15. Changes in administrative policies, procedures, and/or regulations
16. Pressures from co-workers to limit an individual's performance
17. Unpredictable changes or additions to the types of work assigned
18. Lack of proper equipment
19. Inadequate communication within the organization
20. Variability in the quality of materials
21. Economic conditions (eg, interest rates, labor availability, and costs of more basic goods and services)
22. Inadequate training

Unless there is a reason to believe that there are no situational constraints on the person's performance in the job situation, the appraisal system design should consider their effects so that ratees are not unfairly downgraded for these uncontrollable factors. The basic approach to doing this is to reduce the upper limit against which a person's performance is to be assessed from absolute perfection down to the highest level possible under the circumstances (the "best feasible" level). This is particularly difficult with systems that rank order employees since the rater has to consider each person's performance relative to what was feasible. Since judgment and information processing occurs in the rater's mind, one cannot cross-check rater judgments for error. This is an argument against the use of ranking systems. While all rating formats instruct raters to adjust ratings based on feasibility during an appraisal period, only one method, Performance Review and Information Systems method (PRISM), provides a quantitative adjustment to the ratings and asks raters to document the maximum feasible distribution of performance (Kane, 1987).

Control of rating errors. Performance appraisals are subject to a wide variety of inaccuracies and biases referred to as "rating errors." These rating errors occur in rater judgment and information processing (Bernardin & Kane, 1991; Landy & Farr, 1983) and can seriously affect performance appraisal results. There are many errors and biases, but the most common ones are:

1. *Leniency:* ratings tend toward the high end of the scale regardless of actual ratee performances
2. *Severity:* ratings tend toward the low end of the scale regardless of actual ratee performances
3. *Central tendency:* ratings tend to be toward the center of the scale

4. *Halo effect:* the rater inappropriately assesses ratee performance similarly across different job functions, or performance dimensions
5. *Rater affect* (such as favoritism, hostility): excessively high or low scores given only to certain individuals or groups based on rater attitudes toward the ratee, not based on actual behaviors or outcomes
6. *Primacy and recency effects:* when the rater is more influenced either by the first or the most recent ratee behaviors or outcomes
7. *Perceptual set:* the tendency for raters to see what they want or expect to see.

Many studies have documented the existence of these and other rating errors and biases and the interactions among them (Cardy & Dobbins, 1986; DeNisi, Cafferty, & Meglino, 1984; Murphy & Balzer, 1989). These errors can arise in two ways: as the result of unintentional errors in how people observe, store, recall, and report events or as the result of intentional efforts to fake ratings (Banks & Murphy, 1985; Kane & Lawler, 1978). The relative influence of unintentional versus deliberate rating errors is unknown since the errors are indistinguishable. The survey by Cardy and Korodi (1990) indicates that errors related to affect and intentional rating bias may be particularly troublesome in nursing.

Attempts to control unconscious or unintentional errors often focus on rater training. An assumption of rater training is that awareness of rating errors will reduce their frequency; but training has not been shown to be effective and may even reduce accuracy since one inappropriate or inaccurate rating pattern may be substituted for another (Bernardin & Buckley, 1981; Hedge & Kavanagh, 1988). However, training to improve the rater's observational and categorization skills (frame-of-reference training) can increase rater accuracy and consistency (Athey & McIntyre, 1987; Bernardin & Buckley, 1981). Frame-of-reference training forces the rater-observer to focus on job-related behaviors and outcomes and seeks to establish a common nomenclature for both observation and rating.

Research on performance appraisal indicates that there is often a significant discrepancy between a person's self-assessment and the supervisor's assessment. Bernardin and Abbott (1985) found such discrepancies predicted lower job satisfaction for nurses. Bernardin (1990) hypothesized that a large portion of this discrepancy can be accounted for by observer bias.

Training to reduce external constraints (TREC) is proposed as an intervention to reduce discrepancies in self versus supervisory evaluations by concentrating on the perceived situational constraints on the ratee's performance. The steps in TREC are as follows:

1. Supervisors and subordinates independently assess the effects of potential situational constraints on the subordinate's performance for each important performance dimension of the subordinate's job.
2. Critical incidents are written to illustrate the effects of particular constraints. Critical incidents are descriptions of specific behaviors and their outcomes.
3. Supervisors and subordinates exchange their ratings.
4. Supervisors and subordinates meet for the performance appraisal interview,

with a focus on discrepancies in ratings and acknowledged constraints on performance.

5. Specific goals are set which focus on the reduction of constraint effects with timetables for assessment. Supervisors agree to attend to acknowledged constraints or to evaluate their effects on subordinate performance.

6. Goals are evaluated pursuant to the timetable.

Research with TREC has shown it to be effective in reducing the discrepancy between self and supervisory appraisal (Bernardin, 1990) and to increase subordinate motivation and job satisfaction.

A second strategy to control rating errors is to minimize the rater's involvement in the rating process in order to also minimize the opportunity for judgmental and information processing errors to occur. Kane (1986) maintains this can be accomplished by having the rater make assessments of occurrence frequencies. By avoiding performance *judgments,* it is theorized that the biases and errors introduced by the judgment process also will be avoided. For example, such a procedure might pose a rating question such as: On what percentage of all the times that Nurse A provided orientation to the family and patient did she explain the hospital smoking policy? or On what percentage of all the times that Nurse A did patient assessments did she provide all of the necessary documentation? The responses to such questions would be mathematically converted into appraisal scores which, it is believed, will be relatively free from biases and errors. Obviously some judgment is involved with this rating approach but, compared to other rating formats, the judgment factor is minimal.

Attempts to control intentional efforts to manipulate ratings include making ratings observable and provable, cross-checks by other people, and reducing the rater's motivation to make false ratings. The organization might reduce rater motivation to intentionally manipulate ratings by rewarding raters for accurate ratings, making it more likely that they will get caught and by increasing the likelihood of punishment if caught. Making the performance appraisal process an important component of the evaluator's job results in more effective performance appraisal (Bernardin & Kane, 1991).

Overall score computation. Once performance has been assessed on all of a job's important functions, it is necessary to produce an overall score reflecting the level of performance on the job as a whole. There are two basic ways of producing an overall score:

- *Judgmental:* The rater forms a subjective judgment of overall performance, usually after completing the ratings of performance on a job's functions.
- *Arithmetic:* The rater or some other scorer mathematically computes the weighted or unweighted mean of the ratings of performance on a job's functions.

The judgmental approach to overall score computation is used by many appraisal systems. However, it can lead to overall performance judgments that bear little relation to performance on the component parts of the job. The arithmetic approach is much more likely to accurately reflect overall performance based on all job functions. The question then becomes whether to compute the average by equally weighting the ratings on the various job functions or by assigning them different weights based on their relative importance. In general, the fewer separate job components on which performance is rated, the *more* important it is to use a weighted approach. When many separate components are assessed, each is typically such a small part of the job as a whole that the error generated by weighting everything equally will be small. When there are fewer components, the influence of each on the overall score is more substantial and precise weighting becomes more essential. There are a variety of ways to derive weights for a job's components, ranging from rater consensus to empirically derived weights using statistical procedures.

Defining the Rater

Despite the fact that the immediate supervisor traditionally serves as the rater in performance appraisals, others (such as peers, subordinates, customers, clients, patients, external reviewers, higher level superiors, the ratee him/herself) usually have direct and unique knowledge of at least some aspects of the ratee's job performance. These different types of raters have been shown to provide reliable and valid performance information (Bernardin, 1986; Bernardin & Kane, 1991; Harris & Schaubroeck, 1988). The use of multiple raters could contribute to the accuracy and comprehensiveness of appraisals. Cardy and Korodi (1990) report that most nursing evaluation systems involve only one rater (presumably the nurse's supervisor).

The number of rater types to be used in rating performance depends on the number of types that can furnish *unique* perspectives on the performance of the ratees to be appraised. By "unique perspectives" we mean people in a position to furnish not only different information but also information processed through counterbalancing or less severe biases. Once the potentially useful rater types have been determined, it is necessary to decide how many different types are to be used. This decision is contingent on the following considerations:

1. *Cost/benefit:* Do the payoffs of using multiple rater types offset the costs entailed (eg, development of additional forms, rater training, allocation of additional time to administrative activity)? The assessment of this cost/benefit ratio also should consider any ancillary benefits to the use of certain rater groups. For example, would the use of staff nurses to evaluate head nurses increase the motivation or job satisfaction of the subordinate raters? Would customers (patients, family members) be more satisfied with nursing service if they were given an opportunity to evaluate performance?
2. *Logistic feasibility:* Can the completion of ratings by multiple raters be coordinated to ensure the timely completion of all ratings without disrupting regular operations?

With increasing frequency, organizations are concluding that the above considerations favor the use of multiple raters. The main reasons for this seems to be that such systems may be more accurate due to combined perspectives, are perceived to be more fair, often have ancillary benefits, particularly when subordinates and customers are involved, and are less often the targets of lawsuits and grievances (Bernardin, 1986; Harris & Schaubroeck, 1988; Wohlers, & London, 1989).

Defining the Ratee

Many people assume that appraisals are always focused on individual performance. There are alternatives to the individual as the ratee although they are not widely used. Specifically, the ratee whose performance is to be appraised may be defined at any of the following levels of aggregation:

- Individual
- Work group
- Organization subdivision (eg, section, department, or division)
- Organizationwide

It also is possible to define the ratee at multiple levels. For example, under some conditions, it may be desirable to appraise performance at the work group level for merit pay purposes and additionally at the individual level to identify developmental needs.

The conditions that make it desirable to assess performance at a higher aggregation level than the individual include the following:

1. *High work group cohesiveness:* This is the shared feeling among work group members that they form a team. Such an orientation promotes high degrees of cooperation among group members for interdependent tasks (Lanza, 1985) which are not externally coordinated by something like an assembly line. Team nursing was built on this premise. Appraisals focused on individual performance tend to undermine the cooperative orientation needed to maintain this cohesiveness and tend instead to promote individualistic or even competitive orientations.
2. *Difficulty in identifying individual contributions:* In some cases workers are so interdependent, or their individual performance is so difficult to observe, that there is no choice but to focus appraisals on the performance of the higher aggregate of which they are part.

When these conditions prevail, it is advisable to consider shifting the aggregation level of an appraisal system to a level above that of the individual.

Administrative Characteristics

Any appraisal system consists of more than raters, ratees, and appraisal devices. There are a variety of procedural or administrative features which must be put into place before an appraisal system can be considered fully formed. These features take alternative forms which should be selected on the basis of the conditions prevailing in the specific situation. The principle categories of administrative characteristics are timing of appraisals, appraisal scoring, rating medium, and method of feedback.

Timing of appraisals. Timing is the frequency of appraisals—the number of times per year and the interval between appraisals. Usually, appraisals are conducted once or twice per year, with equal intervals between them. However, other arrangements are entirely possible. For example, it may be desirable to have more frequent (eg, quarterly) appraisals if complete blocks of work regularly get completed or adequate samples of behaviors or outcomes can be obtained by the end of each quarter. Many hospitals conduct nurse appraisals as frequently as every 30 or 60 days during the first 6 months to 1 year of employment in order to monitor new employees during their probationary or orientation periods. In general, more frequent appraisals are desirable because of the increased amount of feedback about performance they furnish and because they avoid the surprises that annual appraisals often produce. It also is unlikely that a yearly appraisal can provide timely feedback to really accomplish improvements in performance (Dorfman, Stephan, & Loveland, 1986). The principal drawback of more frequent appraisals is the time and effort they require which conflicts with other work demands on raters. In deciding on frequency, appraisal system designers must strive to identify a comfortable balance between meeting the needs for feedback and conflicting with other work demands.

Intervals between appraisals may be fixed (eg, every six months, anniversary date, during last month of fiscal year) or variable. Variable intervals may be based on such factors as the occurrence of very poor or very high performance, consideration for a promotion, and project completion dates. Many organizations use both types of intervals; fixed for regularly occurring personnel decisions (eg, merit pay) and variable for appraisals triggered by unusual events.

Rating medium. The widespread use of desktop personal computers in the workplace has made the option of doing performance appraisals directly on computers a viable one. There are several advantages to using the computer as a rating medium. The results can immediately be integrated into the computerized central personnel record systems that most organizations are now using thereby eliminating the need for clerks to enter the data. The amount of paper generated, distributed, and filed is drastically reduced. Some computer programs monitor rater responses for logic and completeness which allows more sophisticated rater input that may have positive effects on rating accuracy. However, not every organization is ready for computerized appraisal systems. The choice of a rating medium for nurses, therefore, may depend on whether raters are current users of microcomputers or are receptive to the idea of computerized appraisals. The prospective gains in logic, accuracy, and ease of information manipulation need to outweigh the system acquisition costs. If these considerations stack up in favor of a computerized appraisal system, such a medium should be used.

Method of feedback. Raters may informally communicate appraisal results to ratees, or the information may be conveyed by a formal document or a postappraisal interview setting. Feedback serves an important role both for motivational and evaluative purposes and for improved rater-ratee communications (Northcraft & Earley, 1989). For example, supportive feedback can lead to greater motivation and feedback discussions about pay and advancement can lead to employee satisfaction, even controlling for performance level (Dorfman, Stephan, & Loveland, 1986). Specific feedback is more likely to increase performance than general feedback (Earley, 1988).

The biggest hazard in performance feedback may be emotional ratee reactions to the appraisal. It is inherent in human nature for people to believe that they have performed at higher levels than observers of their performance are likely to report (Fiske & Taylor, 1984). This tendency is magnified at lower performance levels where there is more room for disagreement and a greater motive to engage in ego-defensive behavior. It is no wonder, therefore, that raters are often hesitant about confronting poor performers with negative feedback and may be lenient when they do. Although role pressure on managers to give negative feedback may override this reluctance (Larson, 1986), it doesn't make the experience any more pleasant nor any less likely to evoke a leniency bias. Feedback for poor performers to systematically inform them of performance deficiencies and to encourage improvement does not always lead to improvements (Dorfman, Stephan, & Loveland, 1986). Many employees view their supervisors less favorably and may be more uncertain about their level of performance after the feedback or even build resentment leading to poorer performance (Becker & Klimoski, 1989).

Appraisal feedback can be handled in a constructive manner by providing the ratee with frequent, specific performance feedback during the appraisal period so that the appraisal results will bring no surprises at the formal appraisal interview and by incorporating a method such as TREC which involves self-assessment in the context of potential situational constraints on performance. A focus on clearly defined performance functions and criterion standards, considering possible constraints on maximal performance, should improve the performance appraisal interview.

DEVELOPING AND IMPLEMENTING AN APPRAISAL SYSTEM DESIGN

Although most institutions have appraisal systems in place, the nurse administrator needs to know how such a system is designed and may be called on to help design or redesign a system.

Developing an Appraisal System

The development of an appraisal system consists of the following five basic steps: (1) start with a job analysis; (2) specify performance dimensions and develop PLDs; (3) develop scoring of procedures; (4) develop appeal and adjudication processes; and (5) develop documentation.

Start with job analysis. The foundation of an appraisal system must consist of complete information about job content generated through a job analysis. A system developed without this information will not have the necessary ''content validity'' to resist legal challenges to its decisions and stands little chance of producing effective appraisals. (See Chapter 12, and Lang, 1988, for examples of thorough job analyses for nurses.)

Specify performance dimensions and develop PLDs. These next two steps should be carried out with maximum involvement by nurses and supervisors.

1. Specify job functions and the criteria relevant to each on which employee performance is to be appraised. These job function-by-criterion combinations will form the system's performance dimensions.
2. Compose the necessary number (depending on the specific measurement process used) of benchmarks (PLDs) for each performance dimension. Even with ranking or forced distribution it is necessary to have at least one PLD per dimension which describes the standard or ideal performance on which employees are ranked.

Develop scoring procedures. In more simplistic systems, the score on each performance dimension is simply the rating and the overall score is the average of the dimension scores. More sophisticated systems require hand or computer scoring. These may require development of scoring formulas, scoring sheets, procedures to submit raw ratings for scoring, and procedures to record the scores and to prepare score reports for the rater and ratee. Some sophisticated systems are easy to implement and provide ready-made solutions to many of these requirements.

Develop appeal and adjudication processes. Specific procedures should be developed for dealing with disputed appraisal results. Disputed appraisal results should include not only ratees disagreeing with their appraisals but also appraisals challenged by a rater's supervisor. Managerial oversight and review of the appraisal process will inevitably produce the latter challenge which is essential to keep the appraisal process honest. The oversight procedures should be specified during this step. The number of appeal stages, the composition of any arbitration panel(s), the rules of evidence, and the criteria for reaching judgments should be specified. There should also be specific provisions to protect employees against retaliation for disputing their appraisals. The development of this process should include the participation of incumbents and supervisors.

Develop documentation. At a minimum, every appraisal system needs to have the following two manuals:

1. *Rater manual* describes the process of observing performance throughout the appraisal period (ie, provide a frame of reference), how to prepare for the appraisal, the rating procedure, the scoring procedure (if any), what to do with completed ratings, how to conduct the feedback to the ratee, and any other tasks required of the rater in the appraisal process. The process of managerial review to which the appraisals will be subject also should be covered. Finally, the appeal and adjudication process should be fully described from the standpoints of defending appraisals against challenges both from ratees and from the rater's organizational superiors.
2. *Ratee manual* should describe the appraisal process, how it was developed, how ratees can get copies of the standards they will be appraised against

(unless these are automatically furnished), how to interpret the feedback report, what the scores will be used for, how to appeal their appraisal scores and the standards by which their appeal will be evaluated and finally judged, and the protection they have against retaliation for challenging their appraisals.

Implementing an Appraisal System

The process of actually putting the system into operation consists of the following steps: training, integration with the organization's human resource system, and a "shakedown cruise."

Training. This is by far the most important component of a system's implementation. Separate training sessions must be held for at least three groups:

1. *Rater training* should cover such topics as the rationale for the system, how it was developed, how the rating process works, potential problems and difficulties, interpretation of scores, managerial oversight, and the appeal and adjudication process.
2. *Ratee training* should aim to impart a full understanding of the topics covered in the ratee manual. It should also give some insight into the rationale for the system, the problems it was designed to overcome, and the benefits it is expected to produce.
3. *Decision makers and analysts* will require training in the use of the appraisal results both in individual personnel actions (eg, merit pay and bonus allocation, internal selection, adverse personnel actions, performance, and developmental counseling), as well as in the use of scores averaged over various organizational subunits, to the extent this is possible (eg, for training needs analysis, unit performance comparisons).

Additional training may be necessary for various other personnel who play specialized roles in the appraisal system, such as the staff of the scoring center, the appeals board members, and staff assigned to maintain the appraisal data base and furnish reports.

Integration with HRM records. In order to realize their potential usefulness, the results of every appraisal (whether manual or computer-based) of every employee should be entered into a computerized data base. This data base can either be part of the organization's HRM records or a separate data base, which may be desirable for security or limits to computer time.

Shakedown cruise. A final and critical step in the implementation process, and one that is all too often overlooked or deliberately skipped, is a no-fault tryout of the system, known as a "shakedown cruise." Given all the details involved in the design, development, and implementation of an appraisal system, it is unrealistic to expect that everything is going to run smoothly the first time the system is used. The system will have unforeseen problems and the only way to find and solve them without minor or major disasters is to try out the system. It should be made as realistic as possible, even down to the detail of having some employees file mock appeals. Questionnaires should be distributed to raters and ratees after the process to get their reactions and to identify trouble spots. It is vital that a new appraisal system get off on the right foot. The first time it is used "for real" should leave people with a favorable impression. If not, it may lose the level of cooperation necessary to make it work effectively.

EVALUATING APPRAISAL SYSTEM EFFECTIVENESS

Performance appraisal is the cornerstone of virtually all personnel decision making. It is the means by which the performance of the human component of an organization can be monitored. It is the guide to performance improvement efforts. It forms the basis for fair and equitable treatment of employees. With so much riding on these systems it would be highly desirable for organizations to evaluate their appraisal systems for effectiveness before adverse outcomes occur. No matter how sophisticated an appraisal system may be, if raters are disposed to subvert it, it will fail. Important aspects of rater reactions that should be assessed by questionnaire include the following:

- Ease of use
- Adequacy of training
- Sufficient time to complete appraisals
- How appraisal results correspond to rater beliefs as to the levels of ratee performance
- Effectiveness of job content coverage
- Degree of commitment to making the system work

Ratee reactions are also important. Ratees exert powerful influences on the tendency of raters to appraise accurately. If ratees feel unfairly appraised and resent the rater, it is likely that the next ratings will show a substantial leniency effect. Perhaps the ultimate challenge for appraisal systems is to produce candid appraisals that ratees perceive as fair. Ratee views of the appraisal system's fairness, informativeness, usefulness, and absence of bias therefore should be assessed by questionnaire as part of any evaluation.

SUMMARY

Three overriding themes should be recognized in this chapter's treatment of performance appraisal. First, the design, development, and implementation of a system is a highly technical endeavor in which small errors can result in major problems in the subsequent operation of a system. It is not an endeavor which can be effectively handled by following the latest fad or even by blindly copying another organization's system.

Second, introducing a new appraisal system into an organization must be considered a major organizational change. As with any change there will be vested interests in preserving the status quo which will resist the change no matter how beneficial it may be for the organization. These sources of resistance have to be overcome by reducing the reasons for their resistance.

Finally, once a well-designed system has been implemented, the work is still not done. An appraisal system has to be maintained and the only way to identify its maintenance needs is to monitor its operation through periodic evaluations. Clues and warnings about deficiencies that have developed or are developing can be gleaned from evaluations and used as the basis for modifications. Only by keeping an appraisal system fine-tuned will it continue to provide a rational basis for personnel decisions and prevent the subjective decision making that organizations can no longer afford.

REFERENCES

Athey TR, McIntyre RM. Effect of rater training on rater accuracy: Level-of-processing theory and social facilitation theory perspectives. *Journal of Applied Psychology.* 72:239, 1987

Banks CG, Murphy KR. (1985). Toward narrowing the research-practice gap in performance appraisal. *Personnel Psychology.* 38:2, 335, 1985

Barrett GV, Kernan MC. Performance appraisal and terminations.*Personal Psychology,* 40:3, 489, 1987

Becker, TE, Klimoski RJ. A field study of the relationship between the organizational feedback environment and performance. *Personnel Psychology.* 42:343, 1989

Bernardin HJ. Attributional bias in the workplace. *Human Resource Planning Journal.* 1990

Bernardin HJ. Subordinate appraisal: A valuable source of information about managers. *Human Resource Management.* 25:421, 1986

Bernardin HJ, Abbott J. Predicting and preventing discrepancies in self versus supervisory ratings. *Personnel Administrator.* 30:151, 1985

Bernardin, HJ, Buckley MR. A consideration of strategies in rater training. *Academy of Management Review.* 6:205, 1981

Bernardin HJ, Kane JS. *Performance appraisal: A contingency approach to system development,* 2nd ed. Boston, Kent Publishing Co, 1991

Bernardin HJ, Orban J. Leniency effect as a function of rating format, purpose of appraisal, and rater individual differences. *Journal of Business and Psychology.* In press

Cardy RL, Dobbins GH. Affect and appraisal accuracy: Liking as an integral dimension in evaluating performance. *Journal of Applied Psychology.* 71:672, 1986

Cardy RL, Korodi C. Nurse appraisal system effectiveness: A view from directors of nursing. *Paper presented at the annual meeting of the Academy of Management.* San Francisco, 1990

DeNisi AS, Cafferty TP, Meglino BM. A cognitive view of the performance appraisal process: A model and research propositions. *Organizational Behavior and Human Performance.* 33:360, 1984

Dorfman, PW, Stephan WG, Loveland J. Performance appraisal behaviors: Supervisor perceptions and subordinate reactions. *Personnel Psychology.* 39:579, 1986

Earley PC. Computer-generated performance feedback in the magazine-subscription industry. *Organizational Behavior and Human Decision Processes.* 41:50, 1988

Feldman JM. Performance appraisal. In: Rowland KM, Ferris GR, eds. *Research and Human Resources Management,* vol 4. Greenwich, CT, JAI Press, Inc, 1986

Fiske ST, Taylor SE. *Social cognition.* Reading, MA, Addison-Wesley Publishing Co, 1984

Ghorpade JV. *Job Analysis: A Handbook for the Human Resource Director.* Englewood Cliffs, NJ, Prentice Hall, 1988

Harris MM, Schaubroeck J. A meta-analysis of self-supervisor, self-peer, and peer-supervisor ratings. *Personnel Psychology.* 41:43, 1986

Hedge JW, Kavanagh MJ. Improving the accuracy of performance evaluations: Comparison of three methods of performance appraiser training. *Journal of Applied Psychology.* 73:68, 1988

Kane JS. Performance distribution assessment. In: Berk RA, ed. *Performance Assessment: Methods and Applications.* Baltimore, The Johns Hopkins University Press, 1986

Kane JS. Measure for measure in performance appraisal. *Computers in Personnel. 101* 31, Fall 1987

Klimoski RJ, London M. Role of the rater in performance appraisal. *Journal of Applied Psychology.* 59:445, 1974

Koys DJ, Briggs S, Grenig J. Individual states' judicial decisions on the challenges to employment-at-will. *Proceedings of the Academy of Management.* 46:255, 1986

Landy FJ, Farr J. Performance rating. *Psychological Bulletin.* 87:72, 1980

Landy FJ, Farr J. *The Measurement of Work Performance.* New York: Academic Press, 1983

Lang MJ. Nurse. In: Gael S, ed. *The Job Analysis Handbook for Business, Industry and Government,* (vol II). New York, John Wiley, 1988:1141–1162

Lanza P. Team appraisals. *Personnel Journal.* 47, March 1985

Larson JR. Supervisors' performance feedback to subordinates: The impact of subordinate performance valence and outcome dependence. *Organizational Behavior and Human Decision Processes.* 37:391, 1986

Mastie v Great Lakes Steel Corporation (1976). 14 FEP Cases 952.

Murphy KR, Balzer WK. (1989). Rater errors and rating accuracy. *Journal of Applied Psychology.* 74:619, 1989

Northcraft GB, Earley PC. Technology, credibility and feedback use. *Organizational Behavior and Human Decision Processes.* 44:83, 1989

Watson v Fort Worth Bank & Trust. S. Ct. U.S., 47 FEP 2789-2791, 1988

Wohlers AJ, London M. Ratings of managerial characteristics: Evaluation difficulty, co-worker agreement, and self-awareness. *Personnel Psychology.* 42:235, 1989

CHAPTER 14

Budgeting
and Compensation

Thomas B. Keal
Phillip J. Decker

Key Concept List

Annual operating budget
Capital expenditure budget
Personnel budgets
Budgeting concepts
Behavior of costs and revenues
Budget monitoring
Compensation systems
External competitiveness
Internal consistency
Job evaluation
Pay plans
Benefits

From a top-down perspective, a strategic plan expresses those strategies by which an organization intends to pursue its mission and goals over a relatively long planning horizon of 5 or more years. The financial part of a strategic plan is often expressed as a long-range financial plan or forecast, typically with alternative scenarios resulting from varying underlying assumptions. A common approach includes the development of assumption sets for a most likely case, a pessimistic case, and an optimistic or best case. Development of these alternatives affords the organization the opportunity to evaluate the downstream effect of varying economic conditions. In so doing, management decisions can be contemplated in advance should the economic environment vary significantly from the expected case. Management's response to the environment can be accelerated with forethought and with reasoned consideration of the effect of alternative decisions through the vehicle of the long-range financial plan.

An organization's annual operating plan articulates those objectives, tactics, and actions which support the longer-term strategic plan. The annual operating budgets and capital expenditure budgets express in financial terms the planned resources to be committed to realize the objectives of the annual operating plan through execution of tactics and actions during the year. The operating budget estimates service demand, revenues, and expenses. The sum of the operating budgets for all activities is an estimate of the organization's income statement (its results of operations) for the accounting period. The capital expenditure budget is the planned purchase of assets which will be capitalized (added to the organization's balance sheet) because the asset has a useful life greater than one year (eg, furnishings, equipment, and buildings or improvements).

The annual plan and related budgets must consider the economic environment and the limits imposed on the organization by such factors as demand, time, availability of human resources, capacity of facilities, and financial means. Sound will not move through a vacuum; neither will a budget. Accordingly, the nursing administrator should consider organizational mission, goals, and strategic direction, as well as the economic environment and the plans and objectives of other segments of the organization, during the development of annual operating plan objectives and related nursing budgets.

The budget is integral to planning. It provides an orderly and rational framework for organizing effort; it serves as a management tool for both directing and controlling effort. The budget follows a written expression of organizational objectives, expresses those objectives in financial terms, provides objective means to evaluate operations and alternatives and to control costs, and creates a greater awareness of the forces that play on an organization's activity and effort.

BUDGETING CONCEPTS

A cornerstone of budgeting is responsibility accounting, which means that each of an organization's revenues, expenses, assets, and liabilities is someone's responsibility. As a corollary, the individual with the most direct control or influence on any of these financial elements should be held accountable for them, generally congruent to the organization's management structure. The responsible manager should participate actively in the development of the budget, should have control of items charged against that budget, should receive periodic and timely reports on actual results compared to budget, and should be held accountable for the financial results of the operating unit(s).

The issue of accountability generally brings into discussion two additional and related cost concepts. Costs may be classified as controllable or uncontrollable and as direct or indirect. Controllable costs are those which are influenced by management decision, while uncontrollable costs are generally independent of management action during the accounting period (eg, taxes, interest, depreciation, and utilities). Direct costs are those which are clearly in support of a specific activity, such as salaries and supplies specifically used to provide labor and delivery care, while indirect costs are typically pools of costs not directly identified with a specific service, but arising in part because of the service. For example, payroll taxes and pension plans are indirect costs that vary with staff and salaries, and which are typically not charged directly to departmental operating budgets.

Whether departmental budgets include or exclude uncontrollable costs and indirect costs, those costs must be charged against a budget for which an individual is responsible. The focus in managing costs should be aimed principally at controllable costs although uncontrollable costs may appear on the budget report. Whether indirect costs should be allocated to departments or not is generally a question of organizational preference. Such detailed allocations are costly and time consuming and there is likely little impact of control of such costs by allocation. However, the department manager must consider all costs, including indirect and uncontrollable costs, when evaluating opportunities and alternatives, regardless of the method selected by the organization for periodic budgeting and reporting of such costs.

Proper matching of revenues and expenses is a generally accepted accounting principle that fits well with the concept of responsibility accounting. Matching relates to the timing of the recognition of revenues and expenses, as well as to the pairing of revenue earned with the costs, or expenses, incurred to realize the revenue. In a service industry such as health care, both revenue and expense are recognized as service is rendered, on an accrual basis, regardless of when the organization receives payment for service rendered, and regardless of when it will pay for the expenses incurred. Assets are capitalized in order to properly match cost with revenue. Since a bed, for example, will be used for a number of years and contributes to the ability to earn revenue over its useful life, the cost of the bed is recognized pro rata over its life, and charged against future operating budgets (income statements) as depreciation expense. Budgets must consider the timing of service demand by accounting period and the timing of revenues earned and expenses incurred as a result of meeting demand for service. Budgets are typically prepared for the organization's fiscal year, by month. Some organizations use a 52/53 week year, with 13, 4-week interim accounting periods, rather than calendar month accounting periods, so that each interim accounting or budget period is of equal length.

Equally important to the concept of responsibility accounting is the notion that a budget is an estimate or a guide, rather than a set of absolutes or limits. While a budget in a governmental setting may in fact include legal spending limits, in a business enterprise, a good budget is a best estimate of the business plan in financial terms. This concept is most important in motivating responsible managers to avoid excesses, to search for more effective means to realize business objectives, and to arrive at a budget that is reasonable and realistic at both the detail level and in the aggregate for the organization. Absent this conceptual frame of reference, the budget may cease to be an expression of the plan in financial terms. Viewed as an absolute rather than as an estimate, the budget can create adverse motivational behavior. Managers may pad budgets, burying contingency pools to avoid being penalized for exceeding the budget for unanticipated expenses arising from an imperfect plan. Worse, managers may avoid cost to remain within budget by not taking action which should be taken, because the action was unplanned and unbudgeted; the result may include lost opportunity, failure to meet goals, or risk to the organization's mission.

All plans are imperfect. The budget must be viewed as an estimate and communicated in the organization as such. Care must be taken to avoid punitive response to reasonable errors in estimates and to reasonable actions taken that result in exceeding budget estimates.

Whether enforced from the top, or encouraged conceptually, the notion of zero-based budgeting is a healthy mindset for any manager to adopt. Rather than beginning with the thought, "It should cost us 5 percent more per visit next year than this year to provide this service," zero-based budgeting requires a more critical line of thought. That is, first answer the question, "Should we provide this service?" If the service has become obsolete or no longer supports organizational mission and goals, the best budget might be zero. If the service should be continued, answer the second question, "Is there a better way to provide this service?" A better way might be one which improves quality (result or outcome) without changing cost, or which decreases cost without reducing quality. In the best of circumstances, a better way improves quality while decreasing costs. Doing the right things (effectiveness), in the right way (efficiency), yields the right result (productivity).

BEHAVIOR OF COSTS AND REVENUES

Because budgets are plans expressed in financial terms, it is imperative that the nursing executive have a reasonable understanding of the concepts underlying the behavior of costs and revenues, and the terminology commonly used to express those concepts. Costs and revenues are measured by the monetary equivalent of the resource consumed (cost) or the utility provided (revenue). *Costs* are the outlays incurred for such resources as labor, supplies, and the use of facilities, equipment, ideas, or rights. *Revenues* are the rewards realized for providing utility to the customer, in such forms as services, goods, ideas or rights.

The behavior of costs involves the concept of relevant range. Over a given relevant range of service demand volume, some costs are fixed while others are variable. For example, the daily linen usage of each patient may cost $2.00 and the disposable supplies used in a vaginal delivery, $6.00. These are true variable costs, which, like virtually all types of revenue, vary directly and on a linear basis with each unit of service regardless of the range of demand. Other costs may be fixed over some relevant range of demand, such as property insurance, an infection control department, or a nursing administration hierarchy.

Breakeven analysis is often undertaken before entering into a service or business, or to evaluate the impact of changing demand, market price, or service costs on profitability. The demand necessary to achieve breakeven on a service can be described both algebraically and graphically (Fig 14–1), based on total costs (fixed and variable) and revenue of the service. Breakeven volume equals fixed cost divided by contribu-

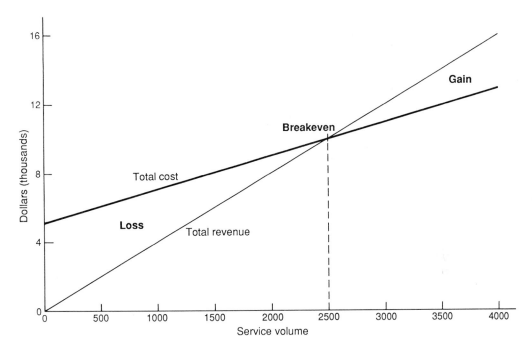

Figure 14-1 Breakeven Analysis

tion margin per unit of service, where contribution margin per unit is the difference between revenue per unit and variable costs per unit. Clearly the higher the fixed costs of a service, the higher the risk, and the higher the breakeven point, if other elements of the equation remain constant. Equally clear, the greater the contribution margin, the greater the reward for volume above breakeven, and the greater the penalty as volume falls below breakeven.

Outside the relevant range of demand, fixed costs may no longer be constant. For example, the scope of infection control service requires more than one person to function. If the level of demand is over the relevant range of the organizational budget period, the infection control function is a fixed cost; if it is within the relevant range, then infection control costs may be deemed to be step-variable, or semifixed, over the budget period.

Over a budget planning period, however, virtually all costs may be categorized as variable with demand, or fixed for the expected range of demand. A few costs may be semifixed, or step-variable, over the relevant range for the planning period. During the first quarter of a budget year, expected demand may require routine staffing of four operating suites, the second quarter five suites, the third quarter four suites, and the fourth quarter three suites. Even in such a circumstance, the ideal response to varying demand is to vary the supply of resources to exactly match demand, treating step-variable costs as true variable costs. Getting the right resources to the right place at the right time minimizes cost.

THE BUDGET PROCESS

Flexible Operating Budgets

Flexible budgets are conceptually grounded on the behavior of costs and revenues. Flexible budgeting promotes effective measurement of periodic performance against the budget plan, incorporating such concepts as variable costs, standard costs, and unit costs. Furthermore, the adoption of flexible budgeting simplifies such tasks as estimating breakeven volume, monitoring productivity, and producing what-if financial models. Under a flexible operating budget, the operating budget of a specific activity or department varies (or flexes) with the volume of service it renders. Budgeted revenues and variable expenses increase or decrease with service volume while budgeted fixed costs remain constant.

Flexible operating budgets are tied to a best measure of service output by department. For example, the patient day is likely to be the best unit of service measure for intensive, acute, subacute, and skilled nursing departments. Ideally, the unit of service selected to measure activity within a department should be relatively homogeneous. However, a more diverse population may reasonably be measured against a flexible budget if the average complexity of the unit of service is relatively stable over the course of the budget period.

The sample flexible operating budget report (Table 14–1) illustrates in summary fashion a periodic report that tabulates actual financial results versus the forecast budget and the flexible budget, for those revenues and expenses for which the operating manager is accountable. Note that the current month volume is less than forecast, while cumulative fiscal year to date volume exceeds forecast. Flexible budget revenues and variable expenses move accordingly, accounting for differences from the forecast budget that are expected because of differing volume of service. A cynic might suggest that health care expenses are variable only as volume moves up, and fixed if volume declines. However, in this example, the manager has managed actual costs to reasonably track the decline in volume in the current month, as expected in the flexible budget.

Personnel Budgets

Labor is the largest single component of health care costs. In the sample flexible operating budget report, additional data on the staffing element are reported to assist the manager in evaluating the effectiveness of effort to manage this largest component of controllable cost. The flexible salary budget is predicated on standard labor hours per unit of service (volume of labor) at a standard average cost per hour of labor (price and mix of staff). The object is to assure constant and consistent quantity of service at a predetermined level as measured by nursing care hours per patient day, for example, at the right mix of staff skill. Under optimum circumstances, the manager assures that the number and type of staff match the number and type of patients requiring care.

The staffing plan should consider variations in expected demand, by season, by day of week, and by shift. If demand is expected to vary substantially, the base or core staff of a service should be tailored to the season, the day, or the shift. Methods

TABLE 14-1. SAMPLE HOSPITAL FLEXIBLE OPERATING BUDGET REPORT

For the Cost Center: 16280 5 North Acute Care Nursing
Month of: June 1990
YTD period: Nine months
Manager: A. Sample, R.N.

	Current Month				Year to Date			
Service Demand Summary	Forecast	Flexbudget	Actual	Variance	Forecast	Flexbudget	Actual	Variance
Medicare inpatient days	484	473	473		4,800	4,703	4,703	
Other inpatient days	352	306	306		2,718	2,889	2,889	
Total patient days	836	779	779		7,518	7,592	7,592	
Over (under) forecast		−6.8%				1.0%		
Revenue/Expense Summary								
Medicare inpatient revenue	121,000	118,350	117,850	(500)	1,200,000	1,175,750	1,175,000	(750)
Other inpatient revenue	88,000	76,500	76,250	(250)	679,500	722,250	721,750	(500)
Total revenue	209,000	194,850	194,100	(750)	1,879,500	1,898,000	1,896,750	(1,250)
Per unit of service	250.00	250.00	249.04	−0.96	250.00	250.00	249.84	−0.16
Salaries	81,513	76,476	78,648	(2,173)	737,876	739,863	773,633	(33,770)
Med/surg supplies	1,933	1,802	1,856	(54)	17,390	17,561	16,523	1,038
Office/admin supplies	339	339	360	(21)	3,003	3,003	3,204	(201)
Linen and bedding	418	390	376	14	3,759	3,796	3,810	(14)
Staff training/travel	563	563	727	(164)	5,073	5,073	4,661	413
Total direct expense	84,766	79,570	81,967	(2,398)	767,100	769,296	801,830	(32,534)
Per unit of service	101.39	102.09	105.17	−3.08	102.04	101.33	105.62	−4.29
Total department margin	124,234	115,280	112,133	(3,148)	1,112,400	1,128,704	1,094,921	(33,784)
Per unit of service	148.61	147.91	143.87	−2.11	147.96	148.67	144.22	−4.12

continued

311

TABLE 14-1. Continued

For the Cost Center: 16280 5 North Acute Care Nursing

Month of: June 1990
YTD period: Nine months
Manager: A. Sample, R.N.

Service Demand Summary	Current Month				Year to Date			
	Forecast	Flexbudget	Actual	Variance	Forecast	Flexbudget	Actual	Variance
Labor Analysis								
Regular salaries	73,526	68,548	70,295	(1,746)	643,181	645,650	597,915	47,735
Overtime salaries	876	817	630	187	33,302	32,820	64,059	(31,239)
Registry labor	0	0	0	0	0	0	70,103	(70,103)
Productive salaries	74,402	69,365	70,925	(1,560)	676,482	678,470	732,077	(53,607)
Nonproductive salaries	7,111	7,111	7,724	(613)	61,394	61,394	41,556	19,838
Salary total	81,513	76,476	78,648	(2,173)	737,876	739,863	773,633	(33,770)
& total labor variance				−2.8%				−4.6%
Regular hours worked	5,803	5,410	5,535	(125)	50,763	51,263	46,122	5,141
Overtime hours worked	49	46	35	11	1,863	1,881	3,278	(1,396)
Registry hours worked	0	0	0	0	0	0	2,270	(2,270)
Productive hours	5,852	5,456	5,570	(114)	52,626	53,144	51,669	1,475
Hours worked per unit	7.00	7.00	7.15	−0.15	7.00	7.00	6.81	0.19
% efficiency variance				−2.1%				2.8%
Nonproductive hours paid	557	557	605	(48)	4,892	4,892	4,914	(23)
Total hours paid	6,409	6,013	6,175	(162)	57,518	58,036	56,583	1,453
Average hourly rate	$12.72	$12.72	$12.74	($0.02)	$12.83	$12.75	$13.67	($0.92)
% rate variance				−0.1%				−7.2%

need be considered to supplement the base staff if demand exceeds expectations or to reduce or realign staff if demand falls short of expectations.

Absent such tools as coordinated staffing, the ability to float staff among care centers, on-call staffing pools, staff regularly scheduled as part-time who extend their hours as demand requires, summer leave programs to reduce staff as demand declines, and the ability to redirect or schedule demand, the manager is unlikely to get the right staff to the right place at the right time. And it will show as actual or perceived uneven quality and as excessive costs of care per unit of service.

Budget Monitoring

Periodic personnel and operating budget reports serve as gauges to measure the effectiveness of tools in place to control staffing and costs. The information is a feedback loop, typically of monthly historical data, that may be used to detect deviations that warrant correction, or to reinforce the impression that operations are within reasonable tolerances. If the administrator is actively monitoring day-to-day operations, the information should be no surprise. Rather, it measures in objective terms the results that the administrator should have expected based on daily observation and management of the activity.

The source of actual revenue and cost reported in monthly budget performance reports is the organization's general ledger. The general ledger is typically posted monthly from totals of the detailed transactions recorded in subsidiary accounting records. The operating administrator should receive itemized reports that identify the transactions or groups of transactions that comprise the totals reflected in the monthly budget reports. These detailed reports typically include labor distribution reports for each payroll period during the month, supply utilization reports for stock issued from inventory, and purchasing/accounts payable reports itemizing purchases of services and of supplies not stocked in inventory. Departmental service volume and revenue are similarly recorded in detailed subsidiary records and are typically reported in detail to the departmental manager.

Budget Variances

Variances from budget are described as favorable, resulting in greater net income than planned, or unfavorable. Variances of actual revenue and expense from the forecast budget arise from three basic components of errors in budget estimates or assumptions. The first component, volume variances, isolates the effect of differing service volume than planned. Volume variances are reflected in the dollar differences between the forecast budget and the flexible budget. The second type, rate variances, isolates the effect of differing prices charged patients per unit of service, differing hourly rates paid employees, differing prices paid per unit of service for supplies, etc. The third type, efficiency variances, isolates differences arising from the quantity of utility provided and the quantity of resource used per unit of service.

On occasion, the term "mix variance" is used, often to describe revenue or expense differences from plan. Revenue "mix variances" generally describe differing composition of services measured under a common unit of service; for example, where patients are charged depending on acuity and the unit of service measure is patient days, a mix variance occurs if the average acuity varies from budget. Similarly, if staffing per patient day varies with acuity and the unit of service is the patient day, a staffing and expense "mix variance" occurs.

Corrective Action

Budget variances should be evaluated by the manager to identify alternative actions that might be taken to correct financial outcomes to the budget plan. Most critical are unfavorable variances in either fixed costs or in variable unit costs of service, which increase the volume of service necessary to break even. Similarly, if revenues per unit of service vary unfavorably from plan, the ability to operate profitably is impaired. In general, adverse volume variances require no action, unless determined to be a significant continuing trend. In such a case, the operating manager should consider alternatives to reduce breakeven volume either by foregoing discretionary outlays of budgeted fixed costs or by reducing variable costs per unit of service.

Favorable variances, while financially advantageous in the short run, may not be desirable in the long run. If, for example, labor costs per patient day are significantly below budget because of inadequate staffing which, in turn, may jeopardize care, corrective action is clearly required.

Whether an organization reports budget results using a flexible budget approach or not, the administrator should evaluate budget performance with an understanding of the impact of demand on revenue and expense, taking actions to support cost effective service to meet actual levels of demand.

CREATING THE BUDGET

The team who prepares the budget should include each of the line managers held accountable for service and the management of costs. Typically the budget is organized on the same basis as the management hierarchy and organization chart. It is prepared by the individual with direct responsibility with direction from the manager's supervisor, is consistent with the annual plan, and is subject to the approval process of the organization. In many organizations the budget preparation process is supported by financial management staff who may participate in varying degrees at varying stages of the process. In the final analysis, however, the line manager must participate to the degree necessary to acknowledge ownership of the departmental budget and responsibility for its execution. In today's more decentralized health care organizations, first line nurse managers often have budgetary responsibilities and the administrator's job is to oversee the process.

Preparation of the plan and budgets may involve several iterations. Early in the process the objectives and plan for the year must be agreed on and demand forecasts for the year prepared for each departmental unit. The annual plan, its objectives, the operating budget, and the capital expenditure budget are interrelated.

DEMAND FORECASTING

Demand forecasts should consider the environment, business cycles, seasonality, and interrelated organizational demand. Forecasting techniques may include such statistical methodology as time series, linear regressions, and multivariate regressions.

In any organization there are certain indicators of demand which are independent variables, while other dependent demand variables vary in some relationship to one or more independent variables. For example, hospital admissions by type may be independent demand variables, while patient days by type and by level of care may be dependent variables tied to lengths of stay. Emergency department visits, outpatient surgery cases, and clinic visits are other examples of units of service which in a given organization might be deemed independent demand variables. Inpatient demand in ancillary departments such as radiology and laboratory are clearly dependent on the amount and type of inpatients admitted.

Given a time series forecast of independent demand variables (eg, admissions by month by type), and regression analyses which produce correlating dependent variables (eg, patient days from length of stay constants, inpatient surgeries from cases per admission constants), forecast demand for each department may be developed. Demand then serves as a basis for drafting the operating budgets.

The operating budgets should consider both variable and fixed costs. Methods of operation should be evaluated to identify more effective means to provide service, historical standards and unit costs modified to accommodate planned changes in method, and the impact of assumed inflation rates incorporated into the budget. The budget product for review should facilitate comparison to recent results, incorporate and describe the effect of planned changes in approach or demand, support organizational mission and goals, and be integrated into the overall organizational plan through departmental objectives.

The annual capital expenditure budget should similarly support the overall plan and the underlying services to be provided. Under ideal circumstances capital expenditure budgeting should be framed over longer terms than annually, considering expected asset replacements and additions over a 5-year horizon or longer. Because the resources available to an organization to fund asset purchases are finite, most capital expenditure budgets require prioritization of proposed purchases based on need and economic value.

Financial feasibility analyses to evaluate the economic value of an asset purchase, or a new program or service, may take several forms. Return on investment is a term used regardless of form or method, one of which is the estimated internal rate of return on net present value of cash flow. This approach considers the time value of money, as well as the relative value of the investment decision. As with any economic evaluation this pro forma analysis measures the incremental value of the investment decision. As illustrated in Table 14-2, the anticipated cash outlays and cash receipts over the life of the asset are discounted to their value at date of purchase, and internal rate of return on the investment is calculated. Alternative purchases, or alternative financing of a purchase, may be compared using the approach as a decision-making aid.

IMPACT OF REIMBURSEMENT SCHEMES ON BUDGETING

With the creation of Medicare cost-based reimbursement in the mid-1960s, investment decisions and care decisions were cushioned from financial risk because payments

TABLE 14-2. INVESTMENT ANALYSIS: NET PRESENT VALUE OF CASH FLOW

Summary Analysis:	Year 0	Year 1	Year 2	Year 3	Year 4	Year 5	Total
Net cash (outlays) inflows	(265,000)	91,232	144,802	169,505	159,736	125,229	425,504
Present value of cashflows	(265,000)	82,938	119,671	127,352	109,102	77,757	251,820
Net present value of investment:	$251,820				Internal rate of return:		27.4%
Cash Outlays:							
Equipment purchase price	(250,000)						(250,000)
Installation costs	(15,000)						(15,000)
Annual maintenance outlays			(15,000)	(15,750)	(16,538)	(17,364)	(64,652)
Supplies, per unit		$1.00	$1.05	$1.10	$1.16	$1.22	
annual outlays		(2,400)	(3,780)	(4,410)	(4,399)	(3,890)	(18,879)
Labor, per hour		$14.00	$14.70	$15.44	$16.21	$17.02	
annual outlays		(40,768)	(42,806)	(44,947)	(47,194)	(49,554)	(225,269)
Total cash outlays	(265,000)	(43,168)	(61,586)	(65,107)	(68,131)	(70,808)	(573,799)
Cash Inflows:							
Gross revenue, per unit		$70.00	$73.50	$77.18	$81.03	$85.09	
annual revenue		168,000	264,600	308,700	307,928	272,273	1,321,502
Collection loss rate		20%	22%	24%	26%	28%	
uncollectible revenue		(33,600)	(58,212)	(74,088)	(80,061)	(76,237)	(322,198)
Total cash inflows	0	134,400	206,388	234,612	227,867	196,037	999,304
Assumptions:							
Forecast units of service		2,400	3,600	4,000	3,800	3,200	17,000

Equipment cash purchase price of $250,000, plus installation costs of $15,000; useful life 5 years;
First year maintenance under warranty; maintenance contract 6% in year 2;
Supply cost of $1.00 per unit of service in year 1;
Fixed staffing of 1 FTE daily, at year 1 hourly rate of $14.00;
Market price for unit of service $70; historical collection loss rate 20%, increasing 2% annually;
Inflation of 5% annually on both costs and prices;
Cost of capital (discount rate) is 10%.

for service rendered Medicare patients were paid at cost, as defined by regulation. With the change in the mid-1980s to prospective payment for Medicare patients on a fixed-price basis by DRG, financial risk for effective operation was returned to hospitals. Other third-party payers have followed Medicare's lead in reimbursement policies. As capital cost reimbursement is eliminated from payment schemes, asset investment decisions are similarly at greater risk.

Some hospitals have incorporated demand forecasting by DRG into their budgeting system to improve estimates of collectible patient revenue. Some of these organizations then utilize admissions by DRG as independent demand variables, forecasting inpatient departmental demand (eg, patient days, EKGs, lab tests) as dependent variables by DRG.

Some hospitals have implemented cost accounting systems to identify costs of care by DRG. Since resource consumption by DRG largely depends on physician order, efforts to control costs of care by DRG must be focused on attending and consulting physicians. Accordingly, the cost of resource consumption, rather than the amount of resource consumption by DRG, are controllable costs that departmental managers must minimize. Efforts to monitor and control the amount of resource utilization, by DRG by physician, have typically been assumed by hospital utilization review staff in concert with medical staff peer review.

In general, organizations do not allocate overhead costs, deductions from revenue, and like elements of the income statement to operating departments, since such elements of cost and such uncollectible revenue as bad debts and Medicare write-offs are uncontrollable at the operating department level. Similarly, determination of direct and indirect controllable costs by DRG has merit in evaluating relative profitability by business line. However, allocations of uncontrollable fixed overhead costs by DRG may be of lesser value since the ability to absorb such costs is largely contingent on organizationwide volume and the margins generated within each business line or department.

While DRG classifications and related reimbursement issues are interesting and of some current value, they are not congruent with most health care organization structures. Budgets should be developed along responsibility and authority lines and managers should be held accountable primarily for controllable elements of cost. Furthermore, future reimbursement is likely to be derivative of capitation contracts rather than DRG reimbursement. The greatest continuing benefit of DRG applications in budgeting appears to be demand forecasting which is likely to continue whether reimbursement schemes move toward capitation or other methodologies.

COMPENSATION

One of the largest areas in budgeting, and especially so for nursing service, is compensation of employees. Persons involved in compensation are immersed in one of the greatest challenges, that is, the efficient and equitable distribution of returns for work. There are many compensation decisions to be made in the budgeting process including how much to pay people who perform both similar and different types of work, whether to use pay to recognize individuals' experience or to reward perform-ance, and how to allocate pay between cash, benefits and services. Employees often see compensation as a measure of equity and justice in organization. They also see compensation as a return for services rendered and/or as a reward for satisfactory or meritorious work. Administrators, however, usually have two perspectives. First, they see compensation as a major expense. Labor costs often account for more than 50 percent of the total cost of a health care organization. Administrators also view compensation as a possible influence on employee work attitudes and behavior. Com-pensation obviously affects individuals' decisions to apply, to work productively, and to undertake other rational behavior on a job.

Compensation is usually defined as all forms of financial returns, tangible ser-vices and benefits employees receive as part of the employee relationship (Milkovich & Newman, 1987) and is typically categorized as direct and indirect. Direct compensa-tion is base wage and merit pay; indirect compensation is services and benefits. Base wage is the cash compensation an employer pays for work performed. It can be paid by the hour or in a salary. Salaries are paid to those workers who are exempt from regulations of the Fair Labor Standards Act and, hence, do not receive overtime pay. Workers who are covered by the overtime and reporting provisions of the Fair Labor Standards Act are called nonexempt and usually have their pay calculated on an hourly rate referred to as a wage, though some nonexempts are paid a salary and receive compensation for overtime. Merit pay rewards past work behavior and ac-complishments and is usually given as lump-sum payment as an increment to base pay. Merit pay is typically defined as a reward, but if most employees receive the same percentage merit pay, it is hard to rationalize it as a reward for performance. It is more a reward for longevity. Incentives are tied directly to performance. Short-term incentives are paying an employee for every part or service produced, such as an insurance agent paid per insurance policy written. Long-term incentives may be yearly or multiyearly and are usually paid to top administrators and professionals for long-term accomplishments.

Employee services and benefits are programs that include a wide variety of things including pay for time off, such as vacation, jury duty; services, such as cafeteria support or counseling; and protection, such as medical care, life insurance, and pen-sions. The cost of providing these services and benefits has been rising significantly. Employers pay nearly half of the nation's health care bills and health care expendi-tures have increased at rates in excess of overall inflation every year since 1970. Be-cause of this, health care costs have become an increasingly important part of com-pensation which has to be considered very carefully (Marlnaccio, 1985). Consequently, the various pay forms which make up the total compensation package paid to any given employee is a complex network. Some of the decisions as to the form of pay are made in a subsystem, such as nursing service, and some are made by the institution and controlled by the personnel office.

A Model for Compensation

A basic model of the overall compensation system explains the variables interacting in employee compensation. A pay system in any hospital is designed and managed to achieve certain objectives. The basic objectives include efficiency, equity across job, and compliance with governmental laws and regulations. These objectives are obviously broad but the efficiency objective can be stated more specifically to be: (1) improving productivity and (2) controlling labor costs. Equity is a fundamental theme in all pay systems so that employees are treated fairly, but equity is a very complex issue. Compliance to various federal and state compensation laws and regulations is a very complex issue. There are well over 30 federal laws applying to pay systems and numerous state laws that would apply for any given institution. In order to achieve these aims, there are four basic policy decisions which any employer must make: *internal consistency, external competitiveness, individual contribution,* and the *nature of the administration of the pay system.* These policies form the foundations from which a pay system is designed and administered.

Internal consistency, often called equity, refers to comparisons among jobs or skill levels inside a single institution. The focus is on paying for jobs equitably, given the contribution of that job to the organization's objectives. For example, how does the work of a unit clerk compare with the work of a computer operator or a janitor? Does one job require more skill or experience or effort than another? The major tool in internal consistency is the use of job analysis and job evaluation to determine the relative input and output of a given job so that those jobs can be compared and given an assigned wage (see Chapters 12 and 13).

External competitiveness refers to how an employer positions its pay relative to what competitors are paying. This is a particularly difficult problem today with institutions competing with each other to recruit the short supply of nurses. How much do other employers pay staff nurses? How much do we wish to pay staff nurses in comparison to all of the other employers in our geographic region? All employers make decisions regarding their external competitiveness and decide whether they will lag behind, meet, or lead other employers in their wage offers. Employers who are in attractive areas to work and live may be able to offer a lower overall compensation package than those employers in less desirable locations. It is difficult to integrate the goals for equity and the goals of competitiveness in a compensation system. Often, there are jobs in which the pay should be increased in order to attract candidates, while in the overall scheme of the institution that job may be ranked lower than positions at lower salaries.

Individual employee contribution is the relative emphasis placed on the performance or seniority of people doing the same job. The institution's policy can either be focused on performance, which would push the system toward merit pay, or it can focus on seniority which would push it toward cost-of-living increases for all employees. The issue is twofold: Should all employees receive the same pay regardless of performance and seniority? Should those who have higher performance or greater seniority receive higher pay?

Administration of the pay system includes designing a system that incorporates internal consistency, external competitiveness, and individual contribution and which will achieve the objectives set within a cost constraint. The best system that achieves equity and competitiveness will not last long if administrative costs and headaches are extremely high. The balance among the four policies is a key decision to be made in any compensation strategy. None of them can be totally ignored. Ignoring internal consistency in order to achieve competitiveness, for example, may increase the employer's vulnerability to lawsuits and may decrease employee satisfaction which affects absenteeism, turnover, and possibly unionization. An obvious issue that relates directly to staff nurses is compensation. The starting pay of nurses is now approaching what would be considered by most to be an adequate level. The pay ceiling, however, is considered too low, thus making the differentials within the system too low. This contributes to salary compression in nursing.

Internal Consistency Policies

The pay structure is made up of pay differentials between jobs and between pay levels within a particular job. Pay structures are usually designed to pay more for jobs which require more skill as well as less desirable working conditions. Sometimes jobs are priced depending on the value that is placed on the output of that job. As the work is made more democratic and as more employees are involved in decision making, salaries and benefits equalize and differentials narrow (Rosow, 1986). An important element in an internal consistency policy is the distinction between employee contribution and internal consistency. Internal consistency refers to the relationship among jobs rather than among individuals. Word processors may be paid $10 an hour whether they have graduate degrees or are vocational school graduates. Despite many different levels of entry to practice, a nurse is like all nurses under an internal consistency policy.

The obvious question is why worry about internal consistency at all? Why not pay employees what it takes to get them on a job and to stay? Why not let external market forces determine wages? One of the reasons is the motivation of many employees to be equal with others putting in equal effort, skill, and experience. It also is possible that some jobs are valued by a specific organization more or less than the rates requested for that job in the market. Regardless of why an organization chooses an internal consistency policy, the major effort is to develop a system that ensures that jobs are ranked or placed in some equitable pay structure. That system is typically job evaluation.

Job Evaluation

The typical process involved in the administration of job evaluation is depicted in Figure 14-2. The major decisions in job evaluation are to: (1) establish its purpose; (2)

Relationships among jobs
↓
job analysis
↓
job descriptions
↓
job evaluation
↓
job structures

Figure 14-2 Determining an Internally Consistent Pay Structure

decide whether to use single or multiple procedures; (3) choose among alternative approaches; (4) obtain involvement of relevant parties; and (5) evaluate the plan's usefulness. There are four basic methods of job evaluation—ranking, job classification, factor comparison, and point system—and their use depends on the circumstances and the purposes involved.

Ranking simply involves ordering the job descriptions from the highest to the lowest based on the definition of some value or contribution. This is usually a global determination. Two methods of ranking are alternate ranking and compared comparison. Alternate ranking involves ordering the job descriptions alternately at each extreme from top to bottom. Paired comparison method involves comparing all possible pairs of jobs under study. A simple way to do paired comparisons is to set up a matrix and use two numbers to identify chosen versus rejected. When all comparisons have been completed, the job with the highest number of acceptances becomes the highest ranked job and so on. Despite its ease, ranking is seldom the recommended approach. The factors in which the jobs are ranked are usually crudely or globally defined. Furthermore, the evaluators using this method must be knowledgeable about every single job in the organization. Lastly, it can only be used on a very small number of jobs. For example, 50 jobs require 1225 comparisons.

The *job classification* method involves plotting job descriptions into a series of classes that cover the range of jobs. Classes can be conceived as a series of carefully labeled shelves on a bookshelf. The labels are descriptions which serve as a standard against which the job descriptions are compared. One defines classes, identifies, and slots benchmarks for each class, then prepares a classification manual and uses that system to assign all the nonbenchmark jobs. Benchmark jobs are defined as reference points and are jobs where the content is well known, are relatively stable over time, and that known salary information is available from a comparison market. These jobs are common across a number of different employers and they represent a wide range of the job being evaluated. Most organizations use 10 to 20 classes. The federal government uses 18 classes with its personnel management schedule (GS) system.

While the classification system is not as vulnerable to legal and employee challenges as the ranking approach, classification plans do not offer much detail or work-related rationale to justify pay differentials. This lack of work-related rationale may not be very compelling to the nurse manager whose immediate problem is getting a salary increase for subordinates, but it takes on importance in an equal pay lawsuit or in an equity policy at the administrative level. There is also evidence that employers are slashing the number of classes in their plans. Rather than use diverse job titles, all workers are known as technicians or associates in some companies. A logic behind reducing classes and using universal titles is increased flexibility to overcome inefficient work rules; yet some balance between flexibility and rules is required in job evaluation.

In the *factor comparison* method, job evaluations are based on two criteria: (1) a set of compensable factors and (2) wages for a select set of benchmark jobs. This method is much more sophisticated than either the ranking or the classification system. The basic approach follows several steps. The first step is to conduct a job analysis (job analysis is discussed in Chapter 12). In most factor comparison systems, the jobs are analyzed and described in the terms of the number of compensable factors used in the plan. The second step is to select benchmark jobs. Selection of benchmark jobs is critical in that they serve as reference points and most pay levels are extrapolated out from them. The third step is to rank the benchmark jobs on each compensable factor. This differs from the ranking plan in that each job is ranked on each factor rather than as a whole job. The fourth step is to allocate benchmark wages across factors. This is done by deciding how much of the wage rate for each benchmark job is associated with mental demands, how much physical requirements, and so on across all the compensable factors. As an example, if someone makes $10 an hour, that $10 is allocated to each of the compensable factors such that mental demand may receive $2, physical requirement receives $1, and so on. After the wage for each job is allocated among the compensable factors, the dollar amounts for each factor are ranked. The job that has the highest wage allocation for mental requirements is ranked one at that factor and so on. Separate rankings are done for wage allocation to each compensable factor. At this point we have two sets of rankings. The first ranking is based on comparisons of each benchmark job to each compensable factor and it reflects the relative presence of each factor among the benchmark jobs. The second ranking is based on the proportion of each job's wages but as attributed to each factor. The next step is to see how these two rankings compare.

If there is disagreement in any point in the distributions, the rationale for the wage allocations and the factor rankings is re-examined and adjustments and rankings are all brought into line with each other. The comparison of the two rankings is simply a cross-checking of judgment. If agreement cannot be reached, then the job is no longer considered a benchmark job and is removed. Possible explanations for lack of agreement in the ranks may include union pressures for higher wages or skill shortages in the external labor markets. The sixth step is to construct the job comparison scale which involves sliding the benchmarks into a scale for each factor based on the amount of pay assigned to each factor. Such a scale will have the compensable factors across the top and the dollar amounts on the side in a matrix. The last step is to apply the scale. This scale is used as a mechanism to evaluate the remaining jobs and all the nonbenchmark jobs are now slotted into the scales under each factor at the dollar value thought to be appropriate in comparison with the benchmark jobs. Only about 10 percent of employers use the factor comparison approach (Nash & Carroll, 1975). The method is complex and very difficult to explain not only to dissatisfied employees, but also to managers who have to use it. Another problem is that the agreed on wage rates of the benchmark jobs are probably going to change because relationships among the jobs may change and the allocations of the wages among the factors must be re-adjusted, so continuous updating of the entire system is required when any one or two jobs change.

The fourth, and most popular, job evaluation system, the *point system*, is rather complex and usually requires the assistance of consultants. Once designed, the plan is relatively simple to understand and administer. Point systems have three common characteristics: (1) compensable factors; (2) factor degrees numerically scaled; and (3) rates reflected in the relative importance of each factor. The location of any given job is determined by the total points assigned to it in this system. The job's total point value is the sum of the numerical values for each degree of compensable factor that the job possesses. There are six steps to designing the point plan. The first is to conduct a job analysis. The second is to choose compensable factors. The third is to establish factor scales. The factor scale is simply a series of degrees for each factor. A major problem in determining degrees is to make each degree equal distant from the adjacent degrees (internal scaling). This is usually very difficult to do, but there are many systems for doing it. The next step is to derive the factor weights. The weights reflect differences and importance attached to each factor by an employer. There are two basic methods for establishing factor weights: committee judgment and statistical analysis. In the statistical analysis, the weights are empirically derived by statistically analyzing benchmark jobs. Once this is done, an evaluation manual can be developed showing the factors, the factor weights, and the points for each factor; and the last step is to apply that system to all the nonbenchmark jobs in the organization.

Once the job evaluation system has been developed, the organization would develop a method for administrating the job evaluation system and that may be done by committee or the personnel office. There will also be a plan for appeals and reviews and for continual evaluation of new nonbenchmark jobs. The true key to job evaluation is to build the system so new nonbenchmark jobs can be continually evaluated without having to change the entire structure of the pay system.

External Competitiveness Policies

The link between pay level decisions and operating expenses is easy to understand. Labor costs constitute a significant proportion of most health care organizations' total expenses. Other things being equal, the higher the pay level, the higher the labor costs. Furthermore, the higher the pay level relative to what the competition has to pay, the greater the relative cost to produce a similar service. So in order to be competitive in one's market, the obvious conclusion is to set the minimum pay level possible. However, other things are rarely equal. The decision to establish a relatively high pay level may make it easier for an organization to attract and retain a highly qualified nursing work force especially in a nursing shortage.

There is no single "going rate" for a job; rather, an array of rates always exists. This is because different employers adopt different policies and practices regarding external competition. One organization may not put money into higher pay levels, but put it in its recruiting efforts and pay bonuses, for example, rather than higher wages. The determination of external competitiveness by an organization is affected by labor market forces, the market forces for the product or service that it provides, its organizational system, and work force characteristics. The concept of the labor market sounds simple but is extremely complex and it is not the purpose here to explain labor economics (see Ehrenberg & Smith, 1985; Kalleberg & Sorensen, 1979). Regardless of how economists conceive of a labor market, an exchange among employers and workers is necessary and does occur. This exchange involves sharing information about job opportunities and inducements, and if the inducements and contributions offered are acceptable to both parties, some kind of a contract may be executed. The result of this labor market is the allocation of employees to job opportunities at certain pay rates. There is a very complex relationship between the demand

and the supply of labor and how it affects cost. To make the situation even more complex, the interplay between labor unions and organizations can create more job competition and change the relative importance of training and experience in the market.

Any organization must, over time, receive enough revenues to cover compensation and expenses. For health care organizations, revenues are generated primarily through the provision of service and the selling of products. An employer's ability to pay is constrained by its ability to compete, especially in the private sector. The degree of competition among service providers and the level of demand for the service are the two key market factors that affect the ability of an organization to change prices for its services. The employer's ability to finance higher pay levels through price increases depends on the product market conditions. Employers in highly competitive markets will be less able to raise prices without loss of revenues. At the other extreme, single service providers with a very strong demand will be able to raise prices if they wish. Third-party payers obviously play a major role in this interchange.

One organization may be a more desirable place to work than another institution. Also, organizations may employ different psychologies in the use of pay. Some may opt for high pay so they lead the competition where others may not. Also work force characteristics affect an employer's pay level decision and consequently its competitive position. Employees with high productivity and more experience may be able to command higher salaries than less productive or less experienced workers. Also, union affiliation affects this relationship by specifying pay levels by contract.

Setting externally competitive pay levels and designing a corresponding pay structure is very complex. It includes the need to clarify the employer's pay level policy, determine the issues to be addressed in any survey of competitors and/or labor market, design and conduct such surveys, interpret and apply survey results, and then finally design the ranges and rates of the pay system, so the process is really circular rather than linear. Surveys are used to determine what other people are paying; however, most health care institutions don't have to do that work. Most industries have associations that do salary surveys and health care is no exemption. Most hospital associations or nursing associations can provide salary data to tell you very clearly what the competition is paying on an average basis in your geographic area. This is also how benchmark jobs are chosen and pay levels for them are determined. The data from salary surveys or association reports are graphed and the benchmark jobs chosen. The data often have to be upgraded for inflation.

The *next step* is to actually design pay ranges for all the nonbenchmark jobs inside the organization. *The first step* is to develop the classes or grades that are going to be used. A grade or a class is a grouping of different jobs. Each grade is usually made up of a number of jobs which are considered substantially equal for pay purposes. They have approximately the same evaluation points. The second step is to set the midpoints, maximums, and minimums of pay for each grade. The midpoint rates for each range are usually set to correspond to the pay policy line established conceptually earlier whether the job should lead, meet, or lag the competition. The maximum and minimums are usually based on what other employers are doing and the size of the range is identified in survey data. The last step is to decide the degree of the overlap. The differences in midpoints among ranges and the range spread determine the degree of overlap between enjoining grade ranges. This can be seen in Figure 14-3. The high degree of overlap indicates small differences in the value of jobs in the adjoining grades. Such a structure results in promotions without much change in the pay rate. On the other hand, few grades result in wider midpoint differentials unless overlap between adjacent ranges permits the manager to reinforce a promotion or movement into a new range with a greater amount of dollars. At some point, the differential must be great enough to induce employees to seek or accept promotion. The problem in nursing is that all nurses typically are put into one grade and the ranges are small in number and there is lots of overlap with the minimum and the maximum being very close. Nurses do not have any incentive to move up within one organization, but rather they have an incentive to move between organizations to increase their wages.

One of the difficult issues in developing the pay system is to reconcile the differences between internal and external pressures. Often there are two different structures with two different philosophies. The pay plan must do both: be internally equitable and externally competitive for the institution to survive. Too frequently decisions are made on the basis of expediency which undermine the integrity of the entire pay system. Reclassifying a market sensitive job, such as nursing, into a higher salary grade where it will tend to remain long after the imbalance has been corrected will only create additional problems in the long run for the organization.

Compression is an example of an imbalance between external competitive pressures and internal equity. Compression is seen extensively in nursing and results

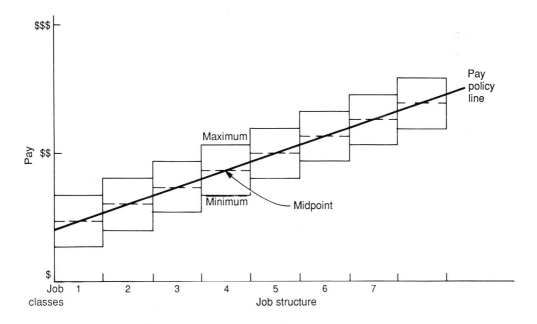

Figure 14-3 Constructing Pay Grades

when wages for jobs filled from outside the organization are increasing faster than the wages for jobs filled by promotion from within the organization. The result is that pay differentials among jobs become very small and the pay structure becomes very compressed. These internal and external conflicts need to be resolved and judgment is typically required to do so, but it is very difficult to be a competent decision maker when one is faced with a severe shortage of a critical work force. Most administrators try to balance external and internal pressures as they occur to best keep the work force within some basic cost constraint. This is obviously a much more important issue in health care today than it was before prospective reimbursement.

Benefits

During World War II, wage controls made it difficult to use salaries as a means of attracting, motivating, and retaining employees so employers competed by offering different benefits. Many benefits can be provided more cost efficiently by an organization than the individual. Group coverage for insurance and pensions, for instance, are very cost efficient. The Internal Revenue Code also has made benefits preferable to wages because many benefits are nontaxable to the employee and are deductible by the employer. Unions have also found it profitable to bargain over benefits. Once a benefit is granted, increases in service or in cost usually is absorbed by the employer with no further bargaining necessary, so the employee receives more compensation with little effort on the union's part. Finally, many benefits, such as Social Security, are mandated by the federal government.

The components of a benefits plan should complement the overall compensation program. Benefits can no longer be considered a fringe item since they constitute up to 50 percent of the total compensation package. There is little evidence that benefits are connected to any return on investment for the employer although evidence does suggest that benefits increase retention and impact on employee satisfaction. Most organizations obviously hope that the bottom line of benefits affects productivity. Consequently, an organization with turnover problems may choose to design a benefits package that improves progressively with seniority thus providing a reward for continuing service. But if benefits are considered a major part of the recruitment process used to attract good employees, the benefits program should be designed with rapid or instant eligibility provisions (eg, health insurance) and attractive vesting requirements (ie, immediate vesting in retirement plan). Because of the high increase in health care costs and the consequent increase in the health care benefit cost, many organizations have begun to redefine their criteria for cost effectiveness and have consequently reduced their health benefits or required significantly higher co-payments from employees. Three major administrative issues arise in setting up a benefits package: (1) Who should be protected or benefitted? (2) How much choice should employees have among the array of benefits? (3) How should benefits be financed? There are advantages and disadvantages to flexible benefit programs. The major advantages are that the employees can choose packages that best satisfy their unique needs, that the flexible plans help meet the changing needs of the work force, that the increased involvement in the employees improve the understanding of the benefits and there is some cost containment. The disadvantages are that employees often make bad choices and find themselves not covered for predictable emergencies. Also, employees tend to select only benefits that they will use and the subsequent high benefit utilization increases its cost.

Financing the benefits plan includes three basic alternatives: (1) noncontributory, where the employer pays everything; (2) contributory where the costs are shared between employee and employer; and (3) employee-financed where the employee pays the entire cost of the benefits. Most organizations today choose noncontributory and contributory plans although more and more are moving toward contributory.

Managing the Compensation System

Compensation is a significant part of the operating expenses of any organization. Controlling these expenses is one of the principal reasons for installing a formal pay system and including it in the budgetary process. Budgeting helps to ensure that future expenditures are coordinated and controlled, the budget becomes a plan within which managers operate, and it is a standard against which their actual expenditures are evaluated. The compensation system in organizations is no different than any other budgeting element and, in fact, is one of the most important ones. There are two basic approaches to generating compensation budgets: (1) bottom-up in which individuals' pay rates for the next fiscal year are individually forecasted in the total organizational budget; and (2) top-down in which a total pay budget for the unit is determined and allocated down to individual employees during the fiscal year. The bottom-up approach requires managers to plan the pay treatment for each of their employees. It places the responsibility for pay management on the administrator. The professional in the personnel department takes on the role of advisor. In the top-down method, unit level budgeting involves estimating the pay increase budget for an entire organizational unit and once the total budget is determined, it is allocated to each administrator who plans its distribution among subordinates.

There are many approaches to unit level budgeting. The two most common are the planned level rise and the planned compa-ratio. The planned level rise is the percentage increase in the average pay for the unit which is planned to occur. Top management sets this figure in consultation with the personnel and finance departments after considering such factors as anticipated rates of change, market data and changes in cost of living, the employers ability to pay, and the effects of turnover and promotion. The average pay at the beginning of the year is changed by the anticipated factors of change such as market adjustments, turnovers, and so on, to give the planned level rise, a percentage of increase in average pay.

Under the compa-ratio approach to budgeting, a planned compa-ratio is established as the target rather than a rise in the average pay level. The compa-ratio equals the average rate paid divided by the range midpoint. The known real difference between this approach and the planned level rise approach is that a planned compa-ratio plays a more formal role. Figures 14-4 and 14-5 show the process used in planned level-rise calculations and in compa-ratio calculations. Whichever method is used, once it is estimated it is distributed down to the subunit managers. Once again, a wide variety of methods are used to determine what percentage of salary budget each manager should receive. (There is a more complete discussion of personnel budgeting in Sullivan and Decker, 1988, Chapters 5 and 19). This discussion also includes an explanation of analyzing the cost of wage proposals.

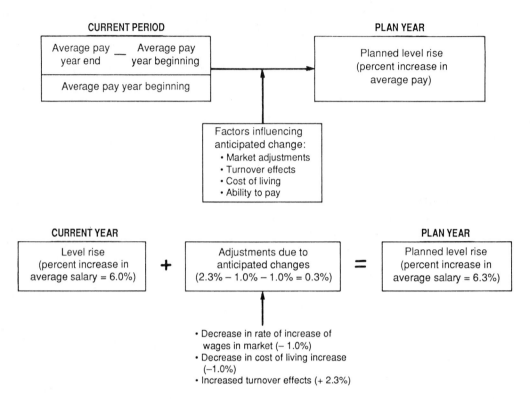

Figure 14-4 Planned Level Rise *(Adapted from Milkovich GI, Newman JM. Compensation, 2nd ed. Homewood, IL, Irwin, 1987)*

SUMMARY

The major difference between hospitals and other industries is that hospitals sell a service which is an intangible. In any service industry there is what is known as moment of truth which is that intensely personal experience the customer has when dealing with a service provider in a transaction. An airline may face 50,000 such moments of truth each day; a hospital may face hundreds of thousands. And most of those in a hospital affect a nurse. Those moments of truth add up, and hospitals that consistently score high in the patients', the patients' families, or other customers' minds will prosper. Those that consistently score low will eventually lose market share and will succumb. The major issue for a service provider is that it sells the performance of the person delivering the service. Manufacturers sell a product. As a manufacturer manages product quality, a service provider manages service performance. The individual worker, in any given task, has a margin of discretionary effort that can make the difference between a horror story and hero story. Compensation in a service industry has to be linked to that margin of discretionary effort that makes the difference between successful service provision and unsuccessful. Most health care institutions have not realized that people are not paid for time but for service performance. Therefore, compensation must be tied to a tangible, measurable issue.

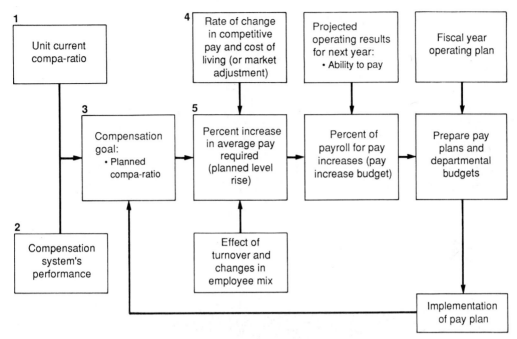

Figure 14-5 Planned Compa-Ratio *(Taken from Milkovich GI, Newman JM. Compensation, 2nd ed. Homewood, IL, Irwin, 1987)*

Furthermore, compensation of that measurable behavior must be part of a budgetary process in order to ensure cost containment and rational decision making about allocating resources. These issues relating to compensation and budgeting must also be contained in the strategic plan of the organization.

REFERENCES

Ehrenberg RG, Smith RS. *Modern Labor Economics*. Glenview, IL, Scott-Foresman, 1985

Fair Labor Standards Act. 29 C.F.R. 5, Sec A.3-A.5, 1938

Kalleberg AL, Sorensen AB. The Sociology of Labor Markets. *Annual Review of Sociology*. 12:351, 1979

Marlnaccio L. Managing the Healthcare Dollar. *Compensation and Benefits Management*. 169, Winter, 1985

Milkovich GT, Newman JM. *Compensation*. Plano, TX, Business Publications, 1987

Nash AN, Carroll SJ. *The Management of Compensation*. Belmont, CA, Wadsworth Publishing, 1975

Rosow JM. The organization in the decade ahead. Conference sponsored by Work in America Institute. Scarsdale, NY, March 3-5, 1986

Sullivan E, Decker PJ. *Effective Management in Nursing*. Redwood City, CA, Addison Wesley, 1988

Organizing People

CHAPTER 15

Staff Development and Patient Education

J. Kevin Ford
Rita Clifford

> ## Key Concept List
>
> Staff development
> Needs assessment
> Organizational, operations, and person analyses
> Training design issues
> Implementation methods and issues
> Evaluation
> Orientation
> Patient education

The educational mission of the nursing unit has several components, each essential to the productiveness of the nursing personnel. These components are intimately related to the quality of nursing care delivered in the institution. *Staff orientation* is the process by which new employees are introduced to the institution. Orientation introduces the key players, the departments, and the philosophy and missions of the institution. The new employee learns what is expected, is trained on the use of equipment, is evaluated on skills and procedures, learns the arrangement of the unit and organization, and thus acquainted, can begin patient care with professional confidence. *Inservice education* maintains and increases the nurses' skills in the provision of nursing care. This includes updating knowledge in general nursing practice as well as learning concepts and skills in specialized areas of practice. Training in management and administration also are offered for selected staff. *Patient education,* an integral part of the provision of nursing care, involves explaining to patients various procedures, possible outcomes, and proper use of medicines. It includes keeping them informed of treatment or progress, alleviating fears, and answering questions (perhaps even unasked ones). Through understanding their own situation, patients can regain a sense of control in personal well being. Current thinking holds that the better educated patients are about their health status, the more they can participate in their own care and the better the outcomes will be. Health institutions which provide consistent patient education are serving their community well.

Many hospitals are sites for the clinical practice of students in nursing. Therefore, the *coordination of nursing student clinical experience* is the province of the educational unit in nursing administration. Students make up a vast resource for nursing recruitment, a vital concern of nursing administration. A positive clinical experience which leaves the student feeling good about the unit or the hospital can be a major factor in the decision of the student to work there after graduation.

Finally, *volunteer education* rounds out the educational mission of the department. Volunteers are important players in both patient care and the smooth cost effective functioning of the institution, but they require very specific orientation, training, and supervision since their knowledge and skills are likely to be less than the employees of the agency.

Nursing administration's role in each of these educational areas is threefold. First, units or subunits with specific educational responsibility and accountability must formally exist within the organization. Second, each of these units must be funded appropriately to fulfill their responsibilities. Third, nursing administration must develop and support an atmosphere in which these training activities are accorded appropriate respect and importance. It does no good to have well-funded staff development units if staff development offerings are consistently canceled or if arrangements are not made which allow nurses to attend.

STAFF DEVELOPMENT: SHARED RESPONSIBILITY?

There are many differing approaches to the organization or delivery of staff development services. In some institutions, the nursing service unit has complete responsibility for staff development. All personnel involved, all funds required, and all arrangements made are from the nursing service staff development department. In some settings, nursing service provides development activities for other departments in the agency. In others, there is a separate department of education and training for the institution which employs nurses to provide nursing content for educational offerings. Obviously, very close coordination must exist between the nurses employed by the institution's education and training department and nursing service so that all the educational needs of the nurses will be met. Occasionally, smaller facilities, whose budgets cannot support staff dedicated solely to education, bring in outside contractors to provide educational offerings. Finally, several institutions may band together to share staff development resources. By this ''shared services'' arrangement the providers can profit from economies of scale, improvement in quality, and increased political power (McGowan & Merrill, 1983). The American Hospital Association publicly supported such efforts as early as 1975 and they have become commonplace today.

The organization of the staff development activities in each institution depends on several factors: the philosophy of the institution and administrators; available financial and personnel resources; existence of other similar institutions in the area; and the extent of cooperation or competition among them which influences whether a ''shared services'' concept is viable or desirable.

There is increasing recognition that developmental activities are key strategies for improving organizational efficiency and effectiveness. This recognition has led many health organizations to increase the resources available for development. Furthermore, the US Government and private foundations have supported development in health care through grants and contracts.

Health care providers are under increasing pressure to maintain accountability for bottom line costs relative to benefits. In this environment, the administrator must justify the cost and benefits of educational programs just like other hospital programs to gain funding, staff and administrative sanction (Blomberg, Levy, and Anderson, 1988). A professional orientation toward training and education that leads to needed, quality, beneficial programs is essential for gaining support from upper management.

The purpose of training is to maintain and upgrade current skills or provide the knowledge and skill required on the present job. Such training can occur in a formal instructional setting or can be conducted on the job. By comparison, education refers to learning basic principles that can be used to synthesize information, make judgments, and take action at some future date (London, 1989). Education is the major development tool used in society. It has traditionally been directed toward children, with a long-term orientation to meeting society's future needs. Today's educational opportunities for adults are increasing to meet the demands of a changing world.

The distinction between training, education, and development becomes blurred in the face of rapid changes occurring in health care organizations today. In addition to learning job specific skills, people in health related jobs need to be taught how to monitor their own learning as well as be prepared to learn new information as it becomes available. Consequently, many health care organizations are moving toward a continuous learning philosophy. These organizations not only offer job specific training but also stress the need to broaden knowledge and skills by completing advanced degrees. The continuous learning philosophy implies that there is always room for improvement regardless of career stage. Such a philosophy demands that employees actively participate in expanding their own skills as learning becomes an everyday part of the job (Roscow & Zager, 1988). We will use the term ''training'' here to mean all short-term educational activities performed by the healthcare institution for the purpose of staff development.

A MODEL FOR STAFF DEVELOPMENT

Training and educational activities must be planned and developed to meet the needs of individual employees as well as the health care organization. The four basic processes of training are: (1) analysis of training needs; (2) design and planning of the training program; (3) implementation of the program; and (4) evaluation of program effectiveness.

A thorough assessment of need must be conducted to determine where training is needed in the organization, what type of training is required to meet the need, and who within the organization needs training. Program design includes developing a training plan of instruction with objectives, content, and learning principles. Implementation includes a plan to stimulate learning by selecting the appropriate instructional method. Evaluation is the investigative process to determine if training is having the expected impact on learning and on the transfer of knowledge and skills from training to the job.

Figure 15-1 presents an integrated framework of these four steps or processes and the factors that can impact on training effectiveness. There should be a logical flow from the initial determination of training needs to program development, implementation, and to training evaluation. The model also indicates that training should be a continuously improving process with evaluation information used as feedback to reenergize and redesign the training system.

EDUCATION AND TRAINING NEEDS

A thorough assessment of training needs is of utmost importance to form the foundation for any training endeavor. Training needs analysis consists of three critical and interrelated components: organizational analysis, operations analysis, and person analysis (Ostroff & Ford, 1989).

Organizational Analysis

Organizational analysis involves examining the entire organization for work unit issues to determine where training is needed. This systemwide analysis includes:

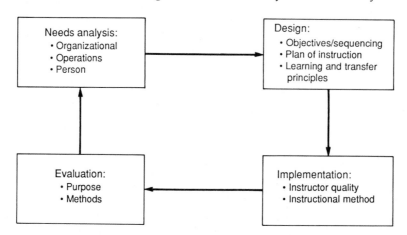

Figure 15-1. A Model of the Training Process

(1) examining whether existing goals of the organization might be better met by increasing employee knowledge or skills; and (2) determining what additional training might be needed to support the strategic or long-term goals of the organization.

Examining Existing Goals. A first step in organizational analysis is identifying the current goals of the organization and work units. This can be accomplished through interviews with administrators and managers and through various organizational publications. The second step is to determine the extent to which the current goals are being met. Efficiency indices, quality records, retention incidents, patient complaints, and supervisory performance ratings can be used. The third step is to analyze why certain goals are not being met. Organizational or work unit goals may not be met due to inadequacy of knowledge, skills, or experience. Inadequacies in these domains are amenable to training as a solution.

On the other hand, there are a variety of other situational factors which can constrain performance and thus result in goals not being met. Such items as job related information, tools and equipment, material and supplies, financial and budgetary support, services and help from other departments or work units, availability of necessary time; and physical comfort and conditions necessary for doing the job may not be affected by development (Peters, O'Connor, & Eulber, 1985).

An additional constraint can be the climate of the organization or work unit toward a particular type of training program. In particular, supervisory support for training has been cited as a key factor facilitating or inhibiting the transfer of training to the work setting (Huczynski & Lewis, 1980). If the work environment is nonsupportive of new skills, then training will not be successful.

Another possible constraint is the reward system in the organization. Kerr (1975) has described organizational policies that reward "A" while hoping for "B." For example, health care organizations may say they want employees to be safe but then set up systems to reward those who take short cuts that could lead to unsafe patient care or put the employee in danger (eg, not using gloves). Training on safety may be ineffective if the reward system in the institution is counter to the training.

Given these situational and administrative constraints, nursing administrators must determine if training is the appropriate solution for meeting goals. All too often training is offered as the solution to a problem when other situational factors are the major cause of a goal not being met.

Strategic Planning and Training. Organizational analysis must also be directed toward understanding future training needs that arise from the strategic plans of the organization. Strategic plans are the formal or informal business plans for the organization that codify what future goals (eg, for the next 5 or more years) the organization wishes to attain. For example, a proposed introduction of new technology in an emergency room (ER) has important training implications for ER nurses.

Linking strategic planning to training needs is critical if training that is timely and proactive rather than reactive to critical events is to be developed. Nursing administrators must consider scanning and acquiring information on future organizational goals as well as their own strategic plans so that training plans can be integrated with the overall strategic plan for nursing service and the organization. This integration is obviously more likely if nursing administrators participate in formulating the organization's business plan.

Operations Analysis

Once it is determined where training is needed, an operations analysis is conducted. An operations analysis concentrates on what particular nurses must do to perform the job satisfactorily. It consists of three phases: (1) determining tasks performed on the job; (2) identifying knowledges, skills, abilities, and other personal characteristics (KSAOs) needed to perform those tasks; and (3) establishing performance standards. This information is critical to determine program content and to develop educational objectives.

Task Analysis. A task analysis focuses on the work activities performed. Through individual or group interviews with nurses or other health care professionals, statements can be derived that describe the specific activities of individuals in a particular job. Information from these interviews are often summarized in terms of task statements. Task statements include a verb or performance activity, a condition and an outcome or event. Surveys then can be conducted to gather information about each task.

For example, a group of pharmacists and a group of pharmacy technicians were asked to describe the tasks of the pharmacy technician job. Through group interviews, 128 task statements were derived that defined the job of technician. Figure 15–2 presents five example task statements that define the job of pharmacy technician. Once task statements were formulated, a task survey was developed. The survey asked pharmacists and pharmacy technicians to rate each task in terms of how frequently (from not frequently at all to very frequently) the task is performed and how important (from low importance to high importance) each task is to job performance.

Example Task and Knowledge Statements

A. Task Analysis
   Operate pneumatic tube system
   Reconstitute sterile powder in a vial
   Calculate solutions with different concentrations and dilutions
   Maintain controlled substance records
   Prepare intravenous piggybacks aseptically

B. Knowledge and Skill Analysis
   Knowledge of pharmaceutical symbols
   Knowledge of drip rate calculations
   Knowledge of laws for controlled substances
   Skill in drawing drugs through a filter straw
   Skill in use of syringes and needles

Figure 15-2. The Job of Pharmacy Technician

Knowledge and Skill Analysis. A knowledge and skill analysis focuses on the underlying components of each task. It specifies the capabilities necessary to effectively perform the job (Goldstein, 1986). After a task analysis is completed, interviews can be conducted to determine the necessary capabilities needed to perform those tasks.

Figure 15–2 shows five of the 98 knowledge statements that were found through interviews to define the knowledge capabilities required to be a pharmacy technician. Similar to a task analysis, a survey was developed to acquire information about the importance of each knowledge or skill to the job.

Performance Standards. Task and KSAO analyses describe the job and its basic components. The next step is to focus on the behaviors that are expected of individuals who perform the job in question. Developing standards or expectations of performance usually begins at the task category level. Job experts can be used to develop "critical incidents," ie, behaviors that they have observed which demonstrate effective and ineffective performance on each task.

Instructions given to job experts in developing these critical incidents are to describe: (1) the circumstances that preceded each incident; (2) the setting in which it occurred; (3) precisely what the employee did that was effective or ineffective; (4) the consequences of the incident; and (5) the extent to which the consequences were in the control of the employee (Bernardin & Beatty, 1984). The incidents generated can then be rated in terms of their effectiveness and scales developed which distinguish effective from ineffective behaviors. Figure 15–3 presents example critical incidents created by nurses regarding the effectiveness of "observational behaviors" of nurses (Ostroff, 1985).

Person Analysis

The identification of tasks, underlying knowledge and skills, and performance standards provide a comprehensive analysis of a job. Person analysis assesses whether individuals are performing at expected levels (standards) and, if not, is the cause of the problem inadequate knowledge, skills, or experience with the task. The first step

---

A. Effective Behaviors

- This nurse could be expected to observe a change in a chronic nephritis patient's ability to read a newspaper
- This nurse could be expected to observe that an ambulatory patient in for study who has been out of bed most of the day demonstrates decreased activity and often can be found lying quietly in the bed

B. Ineffective Behaviors

- This nurse could not be expected to observe that a patient consistently leaves untouched a particular type of food
- Would not expect this nurse to recognize a cessation of flow of urine from an indwelling catheter

---

Figure 15–3. Example Critical Incidents

in a person analysis is to determine if a ''performance gap'' exists. A performance gap involves determining if the existing performance meets expected performance (as identified in the operations analysis). Each individual's job performance must be evaluated and compared to job standards. Performance can be evaluated through objective indices such as the amount of time for answering patient calls, the number of days absent, the percentage of time a symptom is diagnosed correctly as well as scores on a test of job knowledge. Performance is evaluated more often through ratings of performance by the individual's supervisor or through self ratings. (See Chapter 13 for more on performance evaluations.)

The next step is to determine whether any performance gaps found might be a result of inadequate knowledge, skills, or experience. For example, a recent survey of recently promoted nursing supervisors found that they felt unprepared for their new roles and needed more knowledge and skills in budgeting, communications skills, and in evaluating employee performance (Paradis, Lambert, Spohn, & Pfeifle, 1989). In other cases, a performance gap may be the result of situational factors that might constrain an individual's performance. Inadequate equipment, low staff levels, counterproductive reward systems, and work unit norms must be considered to determine if the gap can be reduced through training or other interventions.

The final step in a person analysis is for the nursing administrator or nursing educational specialist to develop (with the employee) an action plan for each individual. The action plan might include training activities, goal setting, job rotation, or other remedies to ensure that performance will meet job expectations in the future. The end result of a person analysis is the determination of who needs what types of education or other interventions to improve performance.

DESIGN ISSUES

Needs assessment provides information on where, what and who needs to be trained. Program design is the process of developing a plan of instruction (POI) for each training program to be offered. Developing a POI requires the specification of training content and the incorporation of adult learning and transfer principles.

Identifying Training Content

The content of a training program should be based on the important tasks and KSAOs identified through the needs assessment process. Prior to writing training content, one must specify training objectives and sequence those objectives.

Training Objectives. Training objectives constitute the formal description of what a trainee should be able to do once training is completed (Campbell, 1988). Identifying a complete set of training objectives provides a roadmap for training program design. There are three characteristics of a well-written training objective. First, a training objective must include the desired terminal behavior. The stating of a desired behavior begins with a verb that describes an observable action, for example, ''take the temperature of a patient.''

A second step is to specify the conditions under which the behavior will be performed. Conditions specify: (1) what the trainee will be provided when they demonstrate a behavior; (2) restrictions or limitations imposed; (3) tools, equipment, and clothing used; (4) references or other job aids to be used; and (5) the physical and environmental conditions surrounding the task (Craig, 1976). An example is, "With a digital oral thermometer, take the temperature of a patient."

The third step is to state the criterion of acceptable performance. The criterion specifies how well the trainee must be able to perform a particular task. The criterion can consist of minimum standards, time to perform, and the quality and quantity of work or service produced. For example, "With a digital oral thermometer, take the temperature of two patients to within .1 degree of accuracy."

Sequencing of Training. The next step is to sequence training objectives in such a way to enhance learning activities in the training program. The key to sequencing is to ensure that the prerequisite knowledge and skills have been acquired prior to the introduction of advanced content or skills (Craig, 1976). Consequently, the instructional sequence chosen may or may not mirror the order in which knowledge and skill is used on the job. Sequencing can be done on the basis of (1) logical order—present least difficult material first and build to the most difficult; (2) problem centered order—focus on a general problem and develop various ways to solve the problem prior to moving to another problem area; (3) job performance order—order based on the sequence in which a job or task is actually performed; or (4) psychological order—determine whether it makes more sense to move from abstract concepts to concrete examples and hands on experience or vice versa.

Once objectives are placed into a logical sequence, job experts can be used to develop lesson plans. For each training objective, experts can identify the specific facts, concepts, principles and skills needed to build competency in an area. The plans also include the method of instruction (lecture, discussion, modeling, skill practice), testing procedures to use, and how much training time is needed to accomplish each training objective. In developing a plan of instruction, adult learning principles and principles of transfer of learning should be incorporated.

Adult Learning Principles

Since adult learners are different from children, training must be designed differently to increase the adult learner's receptiveness to new learning and to increase the likelihood that learning actually will take place. Knowles (1978) suggests four basic concepts which differentiate adult from child education: (1) self-concept; (2) experience; (3) readiness to learn; and (4) time perspective. Figure 15–4 presents characteristics of adult learners.

First, adults are self-directing and enjoy planning and carrying out their own learning exercises and evaluating their own progress. Second, adults have rich and varied work and life experiences that must be incorporated into training through structured experiential or hands-on exercises rather than relying only on lecture oriented training methods. Third, adults often are motivated to learn but may lack self-confidence in a formal classroom setting. Interventions prior to training may be

Characteristics of Adult Learners	Implications for Adult Learning
Self-Concept: The adult learner sees himself as capable of self-direction and desires others to see him the same way. In fact, one definition of maturity is the capacity to be self-directing.	A climate of openness and respect is helpful in identifying what the learners want and need to learn. Adults enjoy planning and carrying out their own learning exercises. Adults need to be involved in evaluating their own progress toward self-chosen goals.
Experience: Adults bring a lifetime of experience to the learning situation. Youths tend to regard experience as something that has happened to them, while to an adult, his experience is him. The adult defines who he is in terms of his experience.	Less use is made of transmittal techniques; more of experiential techniques. Discovery of how to learn from experience is key to self-actualization. Mistakes are opportunities for learning. To reject adult experience is to reject the adult.
Readiness to learn: Adult developmental tasks increasingly move toward social and occupational role competence and away from the more physical developmental tasks of childhood.	Adults need opportunities to identify the competency requirements of their occupational and social roles. Adult readiness-to-learn and teachable moments peak at those points where a learning opportunity is coordinated with a recognition of the need-to-know. Adults can best identify their own readiness-to-learn and teachable moments.
A problem-centered time perspective: Youth thinks of education as the accumulation of knowledge for use in the future. Adults tend to think of learning as a way to be more effective in problem solving today.	Adult education needs to be problem-centered rather than theoretically oriented. Formal curriculum development is less valuable than finding out what the learners need to learn. Adults need the opportunity to apply and try out learning quickly.

Figure 15-4. Characteristics of Adult Learners and Educational Implications

needed to enhance perceptions that their efforts will lead to mastery. In addition, a recent study by Beeman (1988) found that the amount of support given by instructors and peers to nurses during education and training was an important factor in trainee perceptions of the educational experience.

Adults also have a better sense of needed improvements. It is appropriate to allow individuals to participate in determining what training they need and how new knowledge or skills can be used on the job. Finally, adults have a problem-centered time perspective which requires a problem-solving rather than theoretical orientation in training. Formal, rigid training curriculums oriented around subject areas (as for children) are less valuable than organizing program content around needs and experiences.

Principles of Learning and Transfer

A number of program design factors can affect learning and the transfer of that learning to the workplace. These factors include the readiness to learn, conditions of practice, conditions for transfer, and relapse prevention.

Readiness to Learn. Before learners can benefit from training, they must have the relevant background and experiences. It is very difficult to learn a new sequence of behaviors or add to existing skills if the component behaviors or underlying skills have not been previously learned (Decker, Clifford & Knight, 1992).

How effective a training program can be also depends on whether individuals feel they can successfully complete a training program. Research has shown that an individual's "self efficacy," or confidence, can have a large impact on task performance (Bandura, 1977). Trainees will have different expectations regarding the likelihood that effort invested in the training program (eg, participating in group exercises, answering questions, practicing skills) will result in mastery of the training content. Self-efficacy perceptions affect how likely the individual is to try new behaviors and place efforts toward accomplishing the goals of training.

Trainees might not only differ in experiences and self-efficacy perceptions but also differ in the extent to which they believe that learning and retaining knowledge and skills obtained in the training program will lead to desirable outcomes. Desirable outcomes can be internal to the person (eg, they feel that the training may increase their autonomy on the job or the number of skills that can be utilized on the job) or external to the person (eg, a raise in pay or a promotion). The more that a person sees that successful performance during training will lead to desirable outcomes, the more motivated the individual is to learn the training material.

Conditions of Practice. Conditions of practice include a number of specific design issues including massed or distributed training, overlearning, and feedback. Massed versus distributed training is the division of training into modules or segments. For example, training could be completed in one 8-hour day (massed) or over 2 hours a week for 4 weeks (distributed). Complex material learned under distributed practice is generally retained longer than material learned by massed practice.

Overlearning is the process of providing trainees with continued practice far beyond the point when the task has been performed successfully. The greater the amount of overlearning, the greater the subsequent retention of the trained material (Baldwin & Ford, 1988).

Feedback or knowledge of results is a critical element in achieving learning. Feedback given soon after the desired behavior and feedback that is quite specific in pointing out ways to improve lead to performance enhancement. As individuals gain more competency in an area, self-feedback from monitoring their own performance can become an important source of feedback. Such self-monitoring and feedback help the trainee feel more in control of their own mastery of the knowledges and skills in the training program.

Conditions for Transfer.   Transfer of training occurs when the learning has become part of long-term memory (Decker, Clifford & Knight, 1992). Consequently, training program designs should incorporate conditions that facilitate the storage of knowledges and skills into memory. Conditions for optimizing retention include the use of identical elements, stimulus variability, and general principles (Goldstein, 1986).

The notion of identical elements suggests that retention is enhanced when there is psychological and physical fidelity between the training context and the job setting. Physical fidelity involves matching the training context as closely as possible to the actual work environment conditions (surroundings, tasks, equipment). Psychological fidelity is the degree to which trainees attach similar meanings in the training and in the organizational context. To enhance psychological fidelity, training exercises could be developed that necessitate the same responses and decision making processes that the trainee should use in real nursing situations.

Stimulus variability is based on the notion that transfer is maximized when the variety of situations the trainee will face on the job are incorporated in the training program. Incorporating variability helps avoid the problem of trainees only using trained skills in a narrow range of job situations. With variability, trainees can more easily integrate novel situations on the job with those experiences that occurred in training to determine how appropriate it is to apply trained knowledge of skills to that novel situation.

A third condition is to provide trainees with the general principles underlying the particular training being completed. Retention is enhanced when the principles underlying the specific content or behavior to be learned are understood or coded along with the observable behavior. This can be done by asking the learner to apply the general principles in a variety of situations and by supplying written description of the rules that underlie the behavior across work situations.

Relapse Prevention.   Marx (1982) has adapted the transfer strategy of "relapse prevention" from the clinical literature on the treatment of addictive behaviors (Marlatt & Gordon, 1980) to organizational training. The relapse prevention model consists of both cognitive and behavioral components designed to facilitate long-term maintenance of learned behaviors. A relapse program assumes that by exposing trainees to possible future failure situations, trainees can expect and prepare for such situations in advance. This advanced mental preparation for difficult situations increases the probability that the person will apply trained skills in the face of some failures.

Trainees are asked to pinpoint situations or barriers that are likely to sabotage the use of the newly trained skills. These barriers can include "blocks" in which it appears impossible to use trained skills due to existing policies or people who are not supportive of the training. Time pressures may also limit trainee perceptions that the trained skills can be used effectively on the job. Individuals may also feel that using a new skill is risky and do not want to look foolish trying out new behaviors or skills on the job (low self-efficacy). Once these high risk situations are identified, trainees are led through exercises to develop coping strategies to deal with those high-risk situations. These exercises take the form of "what if" scenarios. For example, if there is a block, the trainees would be asked to analyze other ways to accomplish the goal of using trained skills that would not involve the apparent block. Such relapse prevention training can lead to greater commitment to try new skills on the job and maintenance of skills in the face of organizational constraints.

IMPLEMENTATION

Prior to implementing a training program, two issues must be addressed: the selection and preparation of instructors and the selection of the appropriate learning method or training technique.

Instructor Effectiveness

Critical to success of training is the instructor's effectiveness. There are five key effective teaching behaviors: (1) clarity or presentation; (2) variety; (3) task orientation; (4) engagement in the learning process; and (5) task difficulty (Borich, 1989).

Clarity includes two dimensions. Cognitive clarity means the instructor presents the material in an organized fashion. Oral clarity means the instructor presents the material without wandering, not speaking above the heads of the students, and presenting in a clear, strong voice.

Variety refers to flexibility of delivery including different training methods, such as lecture, group discussion, video, and case analyses, as appropriate for the behavioral objectives. Effective behaviors include showing enthusiasm and animation through voice, eye contact, gestures, varying mode of presentation, using a mix of rewards and reinforcers, incorporating student ideas into lesson, and using questioning techniques to stimulate discussion.

Task orientation concerns the degree to which an instructor is achievement-oriented and has high expectations for students. Effective instructors know what behavioral outcomes they want to achieve within certain time limits and push to achieve those goals.

Engagement in the learning process concerns that amount of time trainees are actually engaged in learning the material for the course. Instructor behaviors should minimize the amount of time the trainee is emotionally and mentally detached from instruction. The instructor can monitor work, move around the room, provide continuous feedback, and use material slightly above current level of functioning to engage the learner.

Task difficulty means that effective instructors know where trainees stand and develop lesson plans that challenge the trainee. These tasks are usually those in which there is a moderate to high probability of successful completion of the task. Thus, instructors with skills to present clear training include task variety, are task oriented, and actually engage students in the learning process at moderate to high rates of success lead to greater learning (Borich, 1989).

Learning Method or Training Technique

Training techniques can be divided into nonexperiential, experiential, and modeling techniques. Nonexperiential techniques are knowledge oriented and include such techniques as lecture or group discussion, audiovisual presentation, and programmed or computer-aided instruction. Experiential techniques focus more on building trainee skills and include on-the-job training and work simulations. Modeling (in person or on videotape) approaches focus on training behaviors that trainees should exhibit on the job.

Nonexperiential Techniques. The lecture method is one of the most extensively used training techniques. The objective of the lecture method is to increase knowledge. The lecture method has been criticized for focusing on one-way communication, resulting in passive learning, and for ignoring individual differences in ability to comprehend the material being communicated. Despite its shortcomings, the lecture is a very direct and low-cost way to convey knowledge-based information. When combined with other training methods, such as group discussion and case analysis, the lecture can be quite useful to enhance learning and aid retention.

With the increased complexity of health care institutions, rapid technological advances, and the number of people requiring training, attempts to make training more efficient and accelerate the learning process are more and more important. Audiovisual techniques, such as films, closed circuit television and interactive video, are often used to supplement or accompany the use of lectures. Audiovisuals allow details to be presented in a uniform manner to a large number of people in multiple locations. Audiovisuals are particularly useful in presenting training content that cannot be easily demonstrated in a live format.

Computer-assisted instruction is a recent innovation in training. Information can be conveyed and questions asked of the trainee "on line." In this way, responses by trainees can be continually analyzed by the computer to determine the appropriate pace for individualized instruction. Computer-assisted instruction also can be used to display expensive equipment through modifiable graphics and have the trainee identify parts to the equipment or identify how they would use the equipment by touching the screen or moving a "mouse" to the appropriate location on the screen. A major potential advantage of computer-assisted instruction is that the instructors can focus their energies on analyzing the data on trainee progress, determine problem areas, and help individual students who may require additional practice. As with other techniques, computer-assisted instruction should not be seen as a stand alone system as most adult learners prefer human interaction as well.

Experiential Techniques. One of the best ways to learn is through experience. On-the-job training has been the major way that new employees gain experience, skills, and knowledge under the guidance of a experienced person. On-the-job training often is effective as trainees are actually applying knowledge and skill to the actual work context. Drawbacks include the trainer's lack of coaching skills, costs involved when mistakes are made, and the lack of opportunity to perform key job tasks due to time pressures to get the job done. Under these pressures, the trainer often performs and the trainee watches which actually is modeling rather than experience.

Simulation is another way to build skills through practice. Simulations include computer simulators, games, and case study methods that attempt to mirror the physical or psychological fidelity of the job. Computer simulators allow trainees to work outside the work context but with the actual equipment used on the job. The simulator should be designed to maximize psychological (eg, noise level, time pressures) as well as the physical conditions to increase transfer of the skill to the job.

Games are simulations that attempt to represent the functioning of an organization or subunit. Trainees are provided with information and make decisions under changing conditions and with feedback from various sources. Such "games" attempt to improve the decision-making skills of administrators by helping the trainee discover the interrelationships within an organizational system and to how decisions impact on other subsystems (Camp, Blanchard, & Huszczo, 1986).

A case study approach assumes that people learn through guided discovery (Kelly, 1983). A written description of a real or imaginary situation (eg, a high level of turnover of one unit's nursing staff) is used to allow trainees to diagnose and develop alternative ways of solving the problems in the case. Trainees learn from each other, learn the value of analytical techniques and the need to consider alternative courses of action.

Behavioral Modeling. Behavioral modeling is based on the principles of social learning theory (Bandura, 1977). These principles contend that we learn most through focused observation of ourselves and others and through the reinforcements we obtain as a consequence of our behaviors or actions.

In particular, behavioral modeling includes four key activities: (1) modeling, in which trainees watch filmed or live models display the set of behaviors that are to be learned; (2) retention processes, in which trainees complete a series of formalized activities to help the trainee retain information from the model; (3) behavioral rehearsal or role play, in which the trainees actually practice the key behaviors displayed by the model under realistic contexts; and (4) feedback and social reinforcement, in which praise is given to trainees for successful behavioral rehearsal and constructive information for improvement during the next role play (Decker & Nathan, 1985). In addition, a behavioral modeling approach incorporates conditions of learning and transfer such as overlearning, stimulus variability, and identical elements to enhance learning and to facilitate transfer to the work context.

Behavioral modeling has been found to be quite effective in training manual and social skills. Latham and Saari (1979) developed a behavior modeling program for improving supervisors' interpersonal skills in dealing with subordinates. They found that the behavior modeling program was well received and more importantly led to the transfer of the behaviors to the job.

EVALUATION

Evaluation involves the development of an information gathering methodology to help decision makers make judgments. Training evaluation information is critical for determining: (1) the success of the program in meeting its stated objectives and (2) what refinements in the training are needed to improve its quality. Despite the importance of this step, training evaluation in nursing is an often talked about but seldom realized step in the training process (Milne & Whyke, 1988).

Difficulty in Conducting Training Evaluations

The lack of formal evaluation of training occurs because: (1) the focus of efforts on getting the training program "up and running"; (2) a lack of expertise in many health care organizations for developing a rigorous evaluation system for training; and (3) the difficulty and cost in developing a comprehensive evaluation system. Even when systematic evaluation is contemplated, it is often unclear to the evaluator what decision makers in the organization want to know about the training program. This ambiguity can lead to a lack of focus to the evaluation effort.

In those cases where evaluation is conducted, there are numerous obstacles that lessen the ability of the evaluator to determine if training has been successful. For example, in evaluating a nursing course on chemistry and biochemistry, Smillie, Wong, and Arklie (1984) found that the knowledge measures may not have been content valid. They also found that initial enthusiasm for a comprehensive evaluation of the program by key personnel waned as the study progressed making collecting data difficult. These difficulties in conducting a systematic and reliable evaluation often lead training staff to simply collect trainee reactions to the training experience. Although trainees can provide useful information regarding their level of satisfaction with the program and aspects of the program that could be improved, this information is inadequate to determine training success. The difficulty with evaluation can lead to the regrettable situation where many ineffective training programs continue to operate while successful ones are eliminated.

Training Purposes

The key question asked during the evaluation process is: what do we want to know about our training program? Decision makers may be interested in answering one or more of the following evaluation questions. The first three purposes focus on evaluating the quality of the training program itself while the other four focus on examining outcomes for the individual trainee and the organization.

Training Program Quality. One purpose of a training evaluation system is to determine the content validity of the training program. Content validity asks: Is the training content job relevant? It must be determined whether the content of the training program includes the most important ones to learn to perform job duties. Such an analysis includes the results from the operations analysis phase of the needs assessment process and an evaluation of the content of the training program.

A second purpose is to determine the integrity of the training program. Was the plan of instruction for the training program followed by the instructor? This analysis, often called formative evaluation, requires that a third party observe and record the training process in relation to the plan of instruction.

A third purpose is to examine training efficiency. Is the training program over-

or undertraining certain tasks? Information regarding the importance of tasks in the job and the emphasis of those tasks in the training program must be acquired. In this way, an analysis can be conducted to determine whether time is spent training for those tasks that are the most important for job performance.

Trainee and Organizational Outcomes. A fourth purpose to conducting training evaluation is to determine training validity. Did the trainees learn the material that was being presented? Information about the performance of the trainees must be collected during and/or at the end of the training program. The analysis determines the extent to which learning has taken place in comparison to a specified standard or criterion of success. Learning measures, which should be developed based on the behavioral objectives specified prior to training, include written knowledge tests, hands-on performance or skill tests, and ratings of performance.

The fifth purpose is to determine transfer validity. Are people using the knowledges and skills learned in training on the job? Information regarding performance on the job must be collected and compared to some criterion of success to determine the extent of successful transfer. A key issue is the extent to which trainee knowledge and skill has shown improvement on the job since attending the training program. Performance measures can include observation of the trainee on the job, supervisory rating of performance, and peer assessments of skill transfer.

A sixth purpose for evaluation is to determine the predictive validity of a training program. At times, training is used as a device to select, place, or promote individuals into a particular job. Does the trainee's performance level during a training program predict how well an individual will do on a job different from the one currently held? This analysis requires determining performance level at the end of training and comparing that information with how well the individual is doing in the new job.

A final purpose for conducting training evaluation is determining the costs versus the benefits of the training program. While it may be somewhat easy to calculate the costs of training (eg, trainee lost wages, cost of the facilities, instructor costs), it is usually more difficult to calculate the benefits of training. For example, what is the dollar impact of improving a nurse's care of patients. A cost-benefit analysis requires the evaluator to measure changes in behavior or organizational outcomes (eg, reduced turnover or fewer incidents) and place a dollar value on that change.

Methods of Evaluation

Research methods and experimental designs must be used to systematically examine if changes in behavior have occurred and to determine if training is the major cause of the change. One useful design for determining success of training is the pretest, posttest, experimental design. In this design, individuals are randomly assigned to an experimental or control group. The experimental group is tested prior to and after they attend a training program. The control group also completes the tests at the same times as the experimental group but does not attend the training program. With this design, it is relatively easy to determine if the experimental group has improved their skills over and above the control group. If so, it is likely that the training program is the major cause of that improvement in performance. Then one would be interested in determining the dollar cost of training in comparison to the dollar benefit of the skill improvement (see Campbell, 1988 or Goldstein, 1986).

ORIENTATION

No matter how experienced a nurse may be, starting a new job is anxiety producing. A well-planned and presented orientation can do much to ease the new employee into the workplace. Prior to World War II when our society was less mobile and nursing care simpler, nurses could adjust to the infrequent job change with relative ease. They were shown to their unit, introduced to their head nurse and started to work. Because health care organizations today have many new nurses each year and because scientific advances rapidly change nursing care, organizations must assure that new nurses are given sufficient information to allow them to function safely and effectively in the new setting. The most cost-effective way to achieve this goal is to provide a comprehensive and up-to-date orientation program.

Components of Effective Orientations

Comprehensive Plan.   Orientation is a joint responsibility of the staff development department and the unit nursing manager. The overall plan for the orientation is usually developed by the staff development department with continuing input from nursing managers, staff nurses and the orientees. Some orientation can be presented in classroom and seminar settings, but certain parts must be learned in the clinical site. Division of responsibilities among the staff development department and the nurse manager should be very clear so that no details of the orientation are overlooked. In general, staff development instructors provide information on nursing service or the institution while the nurse manager focuses upon those parts of the job related specifically to the nursing unit. In large institutions, the personnel department may provide institutionwide information. In any case, the staff development department has responsibility for monitoring the process to ensure a comprehensive orientation.

Role Models and Preceptors.   The use of role models in the orientation process can be planned, unplanned, or both. A new nurse often observes experienced nurses, admires their practices and consciously or unconsciously tries to emulate them. When the nursing care is good this can be a very effective way of orienting the new nurse to nursing or to the particular institution's procedures. In order to insure that the role model is the best example, however, formal role modeling arrangements are recommended. The most common type of arrangement is called the *preceptor model*. This model provides opportunities for orientation and socialization of the new nurse as well as being a way to acknowledge outstanding staff nurses. Preceptors should be chosen not only for their superb nursing skills but for their organizational, teaching, and interpersonal skills, and their interest in the orientation process. A highly motivated preceptor can assist the new nurse in gaining comfort and skill in the provision of nursing care in that setting and also can provide a sounding board and a "safe haven" where the novice can feel free to acknowledge inexperience or lack of knowledge. Young, Theriault, and Collins (1989) posit that this one-to-one teaching relationship is the most effective mechanism for learning. In one-to-one teaching the process can be tailored to the specific needs of the learner, immediate feedback can be given to the learner and errors can be corrected before they become habits (Young, Theriault & Collins 1989).

Preceptors are chosen by consultation with the nurse managers who have the most accurate knowledge of the skills of staff nurses. A short formal program of orientation for the preceptors should cover the purposes of the preceptor program, the role of the preceptor, principles of adult education, how to teach and provide feedback, common problems of new nurses, and methods of evaluation of the preceptee for which the preceptor will be responsible. In addition, a support person for preceptors should be identified so the preceptor will have consultation available, if needed. Formal recognition of preceptors is essential. Appointments of new preceptors published in the institution's newsletter, special name tags, and social events are only a few of the ways these nurses can be recognized for their contributions as preceptors.

Nursing faculty members may be utilized as preceptors for the newly graduated nurse. Most new graduates join the work force during the summer months when many faculty members are not employed by a school of nursing. Often these faculty members are employed in clinical settings and can perform the preceptor role with skill. One study found faculty preceptors to be highly qualified, motivated, and flexible and the program was judged to be cost effective (Greipp et al 1989). Greipp also suggests the identification of a unit based educator (UBE) as an alternative to a formal preceptor program if staff shortages exist. The UBE is a nurse already assigned to a unit, perhaps a clinical nurse specialist or a senior staff member. The UBE would be responsible for the learning needs of the new staff on the unit.

Internships. Internships differ from preceptor programs in that they are a combination of supervised experience and course work and usually are longer (up to one year) than the typical preceptorship of three to four weeks. Internships provide a protected environment for transition from student to staff nurse. Some institutions pay the intern full salary while others pay only partial salary but the intern is not considered in the staffing mix until the completion of the internship.

Peer Group Support. Formal orientation programs should build in many opportunities for informal interaction among the orientees. The development of peer group affiliations provides a source of support and encouragement, a forum for reality testing, and may be the beginning of long-term professional colleague relationships. Peer relationships may be encouraged by including times for sharing experiences, by setting a tone of mutual caring and concern, and by allowing some opportunities for social interaction at one or two points in the orientation process.

Orientation and the Nurse Shortage

Orientation programs can be helpful in addressing the nursing shortage. New graduates often believe that their first jobs will be filled with exciting new challenges and wide ranging responsibility. When they find themselves assigned fairly unde-manding entry level tasks, they may become disillusioned. Orientation programs can also hurt when new graduates are thrown directly into the fray with 7 to 10 patients. These students may burn out early and become bitter towards the grinding demands placed on them.

Excellent orientation programs also can be an inducement for new employee to choose to work in one institution over another. Especially for new graduates, it is reassuring to know that at least for a certain period of time they will still be considered ''learners.'' If the orientation is well publicized in local schools of nursing, it can be one powerful tool in the recruitment process. If appropriate relationships exist, nurs-ing faculty could have some involvement in the orientation and their high estimation of the program could be influential in student employment decisions.

Socialization as a Part of Orientation

Socialization involves transforming a person from an outsider to being one of the group. The stages of socialization are anticipatory socialization, accommodation, and role management. *Anticipatory socialization* refers to all learning that takes place prior to joining the organization. Markers are realism, (how accurate a perception of the organization is gained) and congruence, (how well matched are the needs of the per-son and the organization.). *Accommodation* occurs when the person attempts to be-come a member of the association. Markers are initiation to the task (degree of per-ceived competence to accomplish the task), initiation to the group (degree of perceived acceptance and trust by co-workers), role definition (agreement with co-workers about the specific tasks to be performed and their priority), and congruence of evaluation (how closely the employee and supervisor agree on the evaluation of the employee). *Role management* refers to struggles between home and work expecta-tions and between the employee's work group and other groups in the organization. Markers are the resolution of outside life conflicts and resolution of conflicting de-mands.

The accommodation phase of socialization is related to orientation where the in-troduction to task and group occur. Without this formal description of expectations of the job and the setting, role definition and congruence of evaluation would be unlikely. Although orientation planners do not necessarily interact with potential em-ployees, understanding the anticipatory phase can encourage recruiters to describe the real job and fitting the employee to the job. Proper socialization reduces dissatis-faction, absenteeism, and turnover, which leads to effective unit functioning. The formal orientation program is one of the major contributors to this socialization process.

PATIENT EDUCATION

Patient education has been recognized as important since the very early days of nurs-ing. However, only since the 1970s have nurses focused on their patient education role. Decker, Clifford & Knight (1992) point out several trends that have encouraged this growing attention. Today's shortened hospital stays with early ambulation, increase in long-term illnesses and disabilities, increase in malpractice suits, the need to control health care costs and increased interest in maintaining health are factors that have implications for patient education. There are also pressures from the patient for more information. The self-help movement has encouraged people to participate more and make decisions about their own health care. Patients are no longer willing to quietly accept the physician's or nurse's advice without knowing and agreeing with the rationale for that advice. Patient education plays an important part in each of these trends.

Legal Responsibilities

Not only is patient education beneficial for the patient and an accepted part of nursing practice, it is a legal responsibility of the nurse. The American Nurses Association has published numerous documents in which patient education is advocated. The ANA specifies in its Model Nurse Practice Act (ANA 1975) that patient education is an expected function of the professional nurse. In many states, nurse practice acts are modeled after the ANA Model Nurse Practice Act and therefore include the expectation of patient education. Nurses should be familiar with the Nurse Practice Act of their state to determine not only the existence of patient education expectations but other professional expectations as well.

The Joint Commission for Accreditation of Heathcare Organizations (JCAHO) discusses the need for patient education and both the American Medical Association (AMA) and the American Hospital Association (AHA) have published position statements which discuss hospitals' responsibilities for patient education. The AHAs 1982 statement says:

> A hospital has a responsibility to provide patient education services as an integral part of high quality cost effective care. Patient education services should enable patients and their families and friends when appropriate to make informed decisions about their health; to manage their illness; and to implement follow up care at home. Effective and efficient patient education services require planning and coordination, and responsibility for such planning and coordination should be assigned. The hospital should also provide the necessary staff and financial resources. (p 14)

Among the criteria for evaluating a professional in a malpractice suit is whether the care given to the patient was according to accepted standards. One of the ways attorneys find these standards is by referring to documents from the professional organizations and to the professional practice act in the appropriate state. Therefore, the staff nurse, nurse manager, and others are held accountable for patient education if it is influential in the malpractice situation. It is critically important that patient education be documented either on the patient chart or in some organized fashion so that the record of the educational process can be retrieved should it be needed.

Barriers to Teaching

Even with the recognition of the importance of patient education, there are times when it is neglected or unsuccessful. Decker, Clifford & Knight (1992) identify several barriers to patient teaching. First, is a lack of priority. When the atmosphere is not conducive for an activity to take place, then, even if there are occasions in which it could be practiced, it is unlikely to occur.

> Specific ingredients essential in establishing patient education as a priority are: (a) development of a philosophy for patient education by the organization and by nurses; (b) commitment from hospital administration for support of patient education in terms of allocation of time, budget, and staffing; (c) inclusion of accountability for patient teaching as a component of performance evaluation; (d) rewards for doing it and sanctions for not doing it; and (e) provision of reinforcement and recognition for teaching efforts and accomplishments. (p 352)

The most often cited barrier to patient teaching is lack of time. In many situations, nurses have very heavy patient loads due to inadequate staffing. It is very difficult to imagine scheduling time to teach one patient about safe foot care when the nurse is concerned about basic physical care for an overwhelming number of other patients. The nurse manager should encourage the staff nurse to discard the view that patient teaching must be done only in a time set aside just for the teaching. Teaching may be done at the same time the nurse is providing other kinds of care for the patient.

Another barrier identified is lack of communication. Each staff member should know what the patient needs to learn. This will allow reinforcement of content from many sources and should increase retention of knowledge. The patient's educational needs should be a part of the plan of care and documented in the written care plan. Any teaching done must be documented in the patient's record. Lack of knowledge and lack of confidence about ability to teach are also barriers to patient education. Efforts should be made to increase the staff nurses knowledge about health/illness topics and to equip them with teaching learning techniques. Nurses can attend inservice programs, workshops, or other kinds of educational programs. Positive reinforcement for successful teaching promotes the patient education program, since recognition for a job well done helps to ensure continued efforts.

Many nurses exhibit a lack of training skill. They may not know exactly how to teach the patient and this lack of skill is a barrier to patient education. Teaching involves communication skills, being sensitive to patient needs, and knowing how people learn, in addition to having the specific content knowledge. These training skills may be learned by observing an excellent teacher, self-study or by attending specific courses and/or workshops on teaching.

Other barriers identified are lack of family involvement in teaching activities, lack of continuity, poor patient motivation, the patient's physical condition, and psychosocial adaption to illness. The nurse manager should monitor the patient education occurring (or not occurring) on the unit and assist the staff nurses in identifying and addressing any barriers that become evident.

Rankin and Stallings (1990) identify three types of learning which lead to behavior change: cognitive (knowledge and information), affective (attitudes and values) and psychomotor (skills and performance). In determining learning methods, one must consider these types of learning as well as whether the teaching will take place with an individual, in a group, or in an established teaching protocol in a hospitalwide program. Learning strategies include lecture, group discussion, demonstration, role play/return demonstration, testing, program instruction, and media. Media comes in many forms such as reading materials, videotapes, audiotapes, computer-assisted instruction, graphics, overhead projection, chalkboards, displays, flipcharts, bulletin boards, photographs, drawings, models, and games/simulations. See Rankin and Stallings (1990) for an indepth discussion of teaching strategies.

How to Set Up a Patient Education Program

Decker, Clifford & Knight (1992) suggest that one way to overcome some of the barriers to patient education is to set up a multidisciplinary patient education planning group. Including physicians should help overcome physician resistance and the committee can develop a philosophy of patient education, specify staff expectations about patient teaching and develop staff nurses' knowledge and skills in patient teaching. Such a committee could provide peer motivation and support for patient teaching. Teaching can be carried out by all professionals in contact with a patient, but, a single professional should have the responsibility for assessing the learning needs, planning the learning content and assuring that the teaching is done. Careful communication and documentation is essential. If barriers to teaching exist in regard to allocation of hospital resources, this committee could be influential in identifying this problem and lobbying for reallocation.

Materials do not have to be developed in each institution. Hundreds of voluntary agencies disseminate information about diseases or conditions. Their materials are usually well developed and up-to-date and be obtained usually without cost. Incorporating these materials in the patient education efforts can be very cost-effective.

Staff development departments are excellent resources for patient education programs. They regularly update staff nurses on health/illness content and new technologies and procedures. The focus could broaden to include educational programs on teaching/learning principles, patient teaching strategies and evaluation methods. The department can assist in the development and implementation of hospitalwide patient education programs and offer input and support to clinical experts developing patient education materials. The expertise of these educational specialists could be used for individual consultation either by the nurse manager in regard to unitwide patient education concerns or by staff nurses in regard to individual patient education needs. These positions are most often found in the staff development department and serve several purposes. They allow a more cost-effective approach by averting duplication of materials and programs and by centralizing the implementation and evaluation of patient education programs. The patient education coordinator also could be a resource for the nurse manager and the staff nurse.

SUMMARY

In summary, patient education is an integral part of patient care. It is the nurse manager's responsibility to see that educational needs of all patients are identified and attempts are made to satisfy these requirements. A supportive atmosphere created by the nurse manager adds greatly to the odds of overcoming the barriers which can stymie the best intentions of professionals. Lindeman (1988 and 1989) summarized all known nursing research on patient education from 1965 to 1986 (149 studies). She concludes, ''The effectiveness of patient education as a nursing intervention is clearly established'' (Lindeman, 1989, p 53). With this kind of analysis, it is clear that good patient care must include patient education.

REFERENCES

American Hospital Association. *Hospital Responsibility for Patient Education.* AHA, 1982, p. 14

American Nurses Association *American Nurses Association: Model Nurse Practice Act.* Kansas City, ANA Publication Code: NP–52M 5/76, 1979

Baldwin TT, Ford JK. Transfer of training: A review and directions for future research. *Personnel Psychology.* 41:63, 1988

Bandura A. *Social Learning Theory.* Englewood Cliffs, NJ, Prentice-Hall, 1977

Bass BM, Vaughn JA. *Training in Industry: The Management of Learning.* Belmont, CA, Wadsworth, 1966

Beeman P. RNs' perception of their baccalaureate programs: Meeting their adult learning needs. *Journal of Nursing Education.* 27:364, 1988

Bernardin HJ, Beatty RW. *Performance Appraisal: Assessing human behavior at work.* Boston, Kent, 1984

Blomberg R, Levy E, Anderson A. Assessing the value of employee training. *Health Care Management Review.* 13:63, 1988

Borich GD. *Air Force Instructor Evaluation Enhancement: Effective Teaching Behaviors and Assessment Procedures.* AFHRL Technical Paper (88–15). Brooks AFB, TX, 1989

Bray S, Cummings C, Peduzzi T. A comprehensive system to enhance the staff role in patient education. *J Nurs Staff Development.* 5:6, 261, 1989

Camp RR, Blanchard PN, Huszczo GE. *Toward a More Orgainzationally Effective Training Strategy and Practice.* Englewood Cliffs, NJ, Prentice-Hall, 1986

Campbell JP. Training design for performance improvement. In: Campbell JP, Campbell RJ, Associates eds. *Productivity in Organizations.* San Francisco, Jossey-Bass, 1988

Craig RL., ed. *Training and Development Handbook.* New York: McGraw-Hill, 1976

Decker PJ, Clifford R, & Knight L. Staff development and patient education. In: Sullivan E, Decker PJ, eds. *Effective Management in Nursing,* 3rd ed. Menlo Park, CA, Addison-Wesley Publishing Company, 1992

Decker PJ, Nathan B. *Behavior Modeling Training: Principles and Applications.* New York, Praeger Scientific Publishing, 1985

Goldstein IL. *Training in Organizations: Needs Assessment, Development and Evaluation.* Monterey, CA, Brooks/Cole, 1986

Greipp M, Whitson S, Gehring L, McGinley M. An innovative approach to orientation: Faculty preceptors. *J Nurs Staff Development.* 5:6, 269, 1989

Huczynski AA, Lewis JW. An empirical study into the learning transfer process in management training. *Journal of Management Studies.* 17:227, 1980

Kelly H. Case method training: What it is, how it works. *Training.* 46, February, 1983

Kerr S. On the folly of rewarding A, while hoping for B. *Academy of Management Journal.* 18:769, 1975

Knowles MS. *The Adult Learner: A Neglected Species,* 2nd ed. Houston, TX, Gulf, 1978

Latham GP, Saari LM. The application of social learning theory to training supervisors through behavioral modeling. *Journal of Applied Psychology.* 64:239, 1979

Lindeman C. Patient education. In: Fitzpatrick J, Taunton, R, Benoliel J, eds. *Annual Review of Nursing Research,* vol 6. New York: Springer Publishing Company, 1988

Lindeman C. Patient education: Part II. In: Fitzpatrick J, Taunton, R, Benoliel J, eds. *Annual Review of Nursing Research,* vol 7. New York: Springer Publishing Company, 1989

London M. *Managing the Training Enterprise.* San Francisco, Jossey-Bass, 1989

Mager RF. *Preparing objectives for instruction,* 2nd ed. Belmont, CA, Fearon,1969

Marlatt GA, Gordon JR. Determinants of relapse: Implications for the maintenance of behavior change. In: Davidson PO, Davidson SM, eds. *Behavioral Medicine: Changing Health Lifestyles.* New York: Bruneer/Mazel, 1980, 410–452

Marx RD. Relapse preventions for managerial training: A model for maintenance of behavior change. *Academy of Management Review.* 7:433, 1982

McGowan R, Merrill R. *Shared Training and Development Services for Hospitals.* Chicago, American Hospital Association, 1982

Milne D, Whyke T. New measures for the formative and summative evaluation of a post-basic psychiatric nursing education course. *Journal of Advanced Nursing.* 13:79, 1988

Ostroff CL. *Cognitive categories of raters in performance appraisal and their relationship to rating accuracy.* Unpublished Master's Thesis, Michigan State University, 1985

Ostroff CL, Ford JK. Assessing training needs: Critical levels of analysis. In: Goldstein L, ed. *Training and Development in Organizations.* San Francisco: Jossey-Bass, 1989

Paradis LF, Lambert JL, Spohn BB, Pfeifle WG. An assessment of health care supervisory training needs. *Health Care Management Review.* 14:13, 1989

Peters LH, O'Connor EJ, Eulber JR. Situational constraints: Sources, consequences, and future considerations. In: Rowland KM, Ferris GR, eds. *Research in Personnel and Human Resources Mangement,* vol 3. Greenwich, CT, JAI Press, 79–114, 1985

Rankin S, Stallings K. *Patient Education,* 2nd ed. Philadelphia, JB Lippincott Company, 1990

Roscow JM, Zager R. *Training: The Competitive Edge.* San Francisco: Jossey-Bass, 1988

Smillie C, Wong J, Arklie M. A proposed framework for evaluation of support courses in nursing curriculum. *Journal of Advanced Nursing.* 9:487, 1984

Sullivan EJ, Decker PJ. *Effective Management in Nursing,* 2nd ed. Menlo Park, CA, Addison-Wesley, 1988

Young S, Theriault J, Collins D. The nurse preceptor: Preparation and needs. *Journal of Nursing Staff Development.* 5:3,127, 1989

CHAPTER 16

Managing Problem Employees

Tonda Hughes
Jim Breaugh

Key Concept List

Staff performance dimensions
Diagnosing performance problems
Coaching
Discipline
Dehiring
Handling employee complaints
Chemical dependency of nurses
Intervention with and re-entry of impaired nurses
Stress and burnout

In health care, as in other organizations, employees do not always perform at the level desired. While most employees cause little difficulty for the institution, employees who do perform poorly create significant problems. For example, the failure of a staff nurse to follow established hospital procedures for disposing of needles following injections may put the nurse, as well as other hospital personnel, at risk. If an institution has employees who fail to meet performance expectations, or standards of performance, it can have adverse consequences on patients, other staff, the nurse, administrator, and the institution.

Given the potential for harm created by "problem employees," the importance of managing these problems should be evident. However, before an effective strategy for addressing substandard employee performance can be developed, the cause of the problem behavior must be determined so that appropriate action can be taken. Without an accurate understanding of the antecedents of the problem, inappropriate corrective strategies may be used. For example, attempting to motivate an employee with the threat of discharge when the problem is lack of ability is not only inappropriate but ineffective.

Once one has determined the cause of the problem behavior, a strategy such as coaching or formal disciplinary action must be used swiftly to effectively address the problem. The nurse administrator, responsible for management of nursing staff, must examine institutional policies for the effect on performance problems. For example, a poorly designed sick-leave policy can lead to excessive absenteeism and thus create significant staffing problems. To initiate changes in institutional-level policies, the nurse executive must collaborate with other institutional departments and the chief executive officer of the institution.

The first section of this chapter will provide information to assist a better understanding of deficient staff performance. A model for determining the cause of performance problems is discussed and specific suggestions for alleviating problem behaviors resulting from different causes included. The problem of chemical dependency in nursing is presented along with suggestions to help the administrator deal with impaired employees. Finally, stress and burnout in nursing is discussed and suggestions to reduce stress are given for both the institution and employees.

DEFICIENT STAFF PERFORMANCE

The job performance model presented in Fig. 16–1 provides a simplified framework for understanding some of the common causes of performance deficiencies. This job-performance model suggests that an individual's performance on the job is largely a function of the person's motivation and ability.

Figure 16–1 delineates six performance dimensions likely to be viewed as important by the nurse administrator. Although there is conceptual overlap in these performance categories, separate designation helps to emphasize the importance of each.

The nurse administrator should keep several factors in mind when using this

EMPLOYEE PERFORMANCE	=	f (MOTIVATION	and	ABILITY)
Daily job performance		Compensation		Recruitment
Absenteeism		Benefits		Selection
Lateness		Job design		Training
Rule violations		Supervisory style		Special programs
Accidents		Recruitment and selection		
Theft				

Figure 16–1. A Simplified Model of Job Performance *(The items listed under the headings of performance, motivation, and ability are not intended to be all inclusive)*

model. First, a health care institution should establish and communicate clear descriptions of "problem behavior." Second, behavior considered problematic in one department may be acceptable in another department. Finally, some behaviors are viewed as serious only when repeated, whereas others are deemed serious following one incident.

Understanding Performance Problems

Motivation. Not surprisingly, many problem behaviors result from a lack of employee motivation. Motivation is influenced primarily by the organization's compensation system, benefits program, job design, style of supervision, and methods of recruitment and selection (see Fig. 16-1).

Having a performance-based compensation-reward system has been demonstrated to have a direct impact on employee motivation. For example, when across-the-board salary increases are given and staff nurses see their salaries as relatively unaffected by their behavior, compensation will not be a strong motivator of performance.

Benefits can also influence employee performance and behavior. Most institutions offer their employees paid sick leave. Typically, institutions offer programs that have the following elements: (1) for every X days worked, employees accrue a specific number of paid sick days; (2) there is a maximum number of sick days that an employee can accumulate; (3) notification of the supervisor or employer is required to be paid for a sick day; and (4) employees who leave the organization without using accumulated sick leave, "lose" these sick days. There is no payment or reward for not using the sick days accumulated.

Not surprisingly, most institutions with sick leave policies such as the one just described, experience relatively high rates of employee absenteeism. Employees tend to use sick leave once they have accumulated the maximum allowed just prior to leaving the organization. The reasons for such "problem absenteeism" should be obvious.

The number of institutions offering "wellness" programs for employees has increased significantly in the past two decades. Although there is not yet sufficient data on the effectiveness of such programs, some evidence indicates that such programs do, in fact, improve employee attendance (Rhodes & Steers, 1990).

Another type of benefit program is employee assistance programs. Such programs recognize that performance problems such as excessive absenteeism, or lowered productivity may result from an employee's personal problems such as family situations, depression, or alcohol or other drug dependence rather than a lack of motivation.

In addition to compensation and benefit policies, several other factors, over which the employer has some control, may also affect employee motivation (see Fig. 16-1). Challenging and interesting jobs motivate employees (Lawler, 1986). Efforts to ensure that nurses are rewarded for their performance can significantly increase motivation. For example, nurses who are encouraged to share their expertise with less experienced nurses and physicians are more likely to take greater pride in their abilities and work hard to teach others what they know.

Given the central role the administrator plays in determining the overall character of nurses' jobs, one's supervisory style can have a major influence on staff motivation. Nurse administrators can do a great deal to create a performance-oriented motivational climate. Encouraging employees to participate in decisions that affect their practice (eg, shared governance) has been found to increase motivation (Lawler, 1986).

Wanous (1980) has shown that providing realistic job information can increase employee satisfaction and reduce employee turnover. When given accurate information about a position, job candidates can "self-select" out of jobs that are not seen as offering opportunities they value. In addition, methods of screening such as interview work sample questions (see Chapter 12) can be used to screen out prospective employees who are not likely to be motivated by what a position offers.

EMPLOYEE ABILITY

Although employee performance problems often result from lack of motivation, frequently, poor performance is caused by lack of ability. Some employees, although motivated, are unable to meet organizational expectations. As is true with employee motivation, there are a number of methods to improve the overall level of ability of employees. Three of the most obvious and effective ways are *recruitment, selection,* and *training.*

Recruitment efforts that focus on programs and schools with a proven record of providing well-prepared graduates helps to ensure an overall higher level of performance ability in the staff. Realistic information must be given during the recruitment process to allow potential employees to assess the fit between their abilities and the responsibilities of the job. Further, institutions that use more structured methods of selection (eg, structured interviews) and training (eg, behavioral modeling), are more likely to employ nurses who have the ability to meet the job requirements.

Understanding the factors that lead to substandard employee performance is important in making an accurate diagnosis of the cause of employee performance problems. It is not an easy task, however.

DIAGNOSING PERFORMANCE PROBLEMS

Figure 16–2 presents questions for diagnosing the cause of an employee performance problem. By answering these various questions, different strategies, such as coaching, are suggested for addressing specific performance problems. To diagnose a problem effectively, both realistic "standards of performance" and an accurate picture of the current performance of the staff member are needed. An administrator whose expectations are too high will have difficulty motivating staff. In addition, it is equally

KEY BEHAVIORS: *Diagnosing and remedying performance problems (ask all of these questions in order to decide the cause of the problem)*

1. Is the performance deficiency a problem? Will it go away if ignored? (Generally ignore problems which are temporary).
2. Is it due to lack of skill or motivation? How do I know? (Observed in past, used reward/sanction to get performance, tested).

IF SKILL:

3. Is it a complex skill (formal training) or simple skill (coaching)?
4. Is there a cost/time constraint such that selecting a new person is the answer? Can I simplify the job? Can I transfer/demote employee?

IF MOTIVATION:

3. Is desired performance punished? (If so—remove punishment)
4. Is desired performance rewarded? (If no—point it out)
5. Does the employee value the rewards/see them as equitable? (If not—change them)

Figure 16-2. How to Diagnose and Solve a Performance Problem *(From Decker PJ*, Healthcare Management Microtraining. *St. Louis, Decker & Associates, 1982. Copyright 1982 by Phillip J Decker. Used with permission)*

important to understand the importance of accurate and timely documentation, (eg, regular performance appraisals and records of noteworthy performance).

Once one has concluded that a performance problem exists, whether the problem demands immediate attention must be determined. If immediate attention is required, the administrator must then determine whether the problem is caused by lack of ability or lack of motivation. Figure 16–2 provides a framework to help the administrator decide whether a particular deficiency in skill can be remedied through formal or informal training. If a skill-based performance problem cannot be eliminated through training (see Chapter 15), the administrator must consider other alternatives. For example, the job specifications may be changed or the nurse transferred, demoted, or terminated.

If the performance problem is attributed to motivation rather than ability, a different set of questions must be addressed (see the bottom of Fig. 16–2). Specifically, whether the employee believes the behavior leads to punishment, reward, or no action must be determined. Furthermore, although one may dismiss the possibility that employees view "good performance" as resulting in punishment, this is sometimes the case. For example, if the "reward" for conscientiously coming to work when scheduled to work on holidays rather than calling in sick is to be scheduled for future holidays, than good performance is linked with punishment.

The administrator should attempt to rearrange the reward system so that staff see a strong link between valued outcomes (eg, desirable work schedules) and meeting performance expectations. Unfortunately, creating a performance-reward climate will not eliminate all problem behaviors. When the use of rewards is not effective, it will be necessary to use formal coaching, or, in some cases, discipline. The use of coaching and discipline are discussed in more detail later.

In attempting to differentiate between lack of ability and lack of motivation, an assessment of past performance is useful. If the nurse has previously performed at an acceptable level, it is likely that the problem results from lack of motivation. (This assumes the standard of performance has not been raised or that the nurse's abilities have not decreased.) In contrast, if the nurse has never performed at an acceptable level, the problem may stem from lack of ability. Different intervention strategies should be used depending on whether the problem results from a lack of motivation or a lack of skill.

The objective in determining an appropriate intervention should be improvement in problem behavior rather than punishment. Problem behaviors frequently cause administrators to feel anger or resentment toward the employee but retribution is inappropriate when attempting to correct performance deficiencies.

Many administrators are reluctant to confront problem employees because of fears regarding potential liability. Although employees' civil rights must always be respected (see Chapter 11 on employment law) this should not preclude appropriate responses to performance problems. Discipline is the immediate superviser's responsibility who should work closely with the nurse executive and the human resources department. All staff should be treated fairly and equitably. Different responses to staff can lead to claims of discriminatory treatment. As noted earlier, it is important to accurately document problem behavior.

A final topic of great importance in staff performance is administrator credibility. Having credibility with one's staff is critical to effective administration. An administrator should not make promises or threats without being willing to follow through. An administrator who is viewed as lacking credibility will have little influence on staff motivation. In determining whether an administrator is credible, staff rely heavily on past experience.

One of the ways an administration can protect credibility is to check with the organizations's administration or other departments (eg, human resources) before making commitments. It is far better to determine beforehand whether an action will be supported than to back down after making a promise or committing to a disciplinary action.

STRATEGIES FOR RESPONDING TO PROBLEM BEHAVIOR

In order to encourage maximum performance, rewards for above average performance are necessary. However, regardless of reward systems or the level of skill a manager possesses, there will be times when a staff member's behavior does not meet expectations. At such times, coaching is required.

Coaching

Experience has shown that by following a sequence of prescribed behaviors managers can improve the likelihood that a coaching session will improve an employee's future performance. Figure 16–3 lists these key behaviors for coaching.

Before entering into a coaching session, the specific reason for the meeting should

1. State the problem in behavioral terms; immediately focus on the person.
2. Tie problem to organizational and/or personal consequences.
3. Ask employee why the behavior occurred. Try to bring the reasons for the problem into the open.
4. Ask for suggestions on how to solve the problem. Listen openly.
5. Discuss the employee's ideas or, if none are offered, lead the employee to your own preferred solution by asking if it has been tried.
6. Agree on steps each of you will take to solve the problem. Write them down. If appropriate: Ask for employee's commitment to the above steps.
7. Agree on and record a specific follow-up date.

Figure 16-3. Key Behaviors for Coaching *(Taken from Decker PJ,* Healthcare Management Micro-training. *St. Louis, Decker & Associates, 1982. Copyright 1982 by Phillip J Decker. Used with permission)*

be thought out carefully to avoid having multiple goals for the session. A well-planned coaching session is written down. It is important to anticipate how the nurse will react, so that an appropriate response can be formulated. Remember also that coaching works best when problem behaviors are responded to in a timely manner.

At the onset of the meeting, the problem should be clearly stated so that the nurse knows specifically which behaviors were inappropriate and why it is important to correct them. For example, rather than saying "you are rude to patients," specific examples will likely be more effective, eg, "you walked out of the room while Mr. Thomas was talking to you." The second coaching strategy is designed to motivate the nurse to correct the problem behavior. The nurse needs to understand why following a rule, a procedure, or a way of behaving is important. Too often, managers assume that staff know why the expected behavior is important when they do not. The third coaching strategy gives the staff member a chance to explain why the unacceptable behavior occurred. Although the reason may seem apparent, the nurse should always have an opportunity to explain her or his position. The information gained should help the manager decide how to proceed with the session. For example, if the problem behavior occurred because a newly hired nurse was unfamiliar with hospital rules and regulations, the manager may decide to review with the nurse what is correct in this situation, as well as other rules and regulations.

For most problem behaviors, the nurse should be asked for suggestions about how to prevent the behavior from recurring (coaching behavior #4). If the suggestions offered are useful, the manager may proceed to coaching behavior #6. However, if the nurse's suggestions are unsound, the manager should express specific concerns with the suggestions and ask for alternatives. Employees are likely to be much more committed to solutions to which they had input. Thus, if at all possible, the nurse should be given an opportunity to try her/his solution.

The last two steps of the coaching process are straightforward. Having agreed to steps that the nurse (and in some cases the supervisor) will take to solve the problem, these actions are written down. In addition, a follow-up date is set for assessing and discussing progress toward improving the performance problem. These two steps parallel the motivational technique of goal setting.

It is important that a manager not blindly follow the coaching behaviors as outlined in Fig 16–3. The manager should select a response appropriate for each particular situation. For example, if the problem is minor or a first-time occurrence, outlining specific steps to be followed and scheduling a follow-up meeting may be unnecessary.

During coaching sessions nurses may well discuss personal problems believed to contribute to their difficulty at work. In this case caution must be used so that the coaching session does not become a counseling session. The manager should convey both concern and willingness to help the nurse with the problem. The manager, however, is not the staff's therapist and should refer the employee to more appropriate sources of help (eg, the employee assistance program). Managers should remember that personal difficulties may contribute to problems at work but do not excuse them. Patients have a right to expect appropriate care regardless of the personal problems of staff. Thus, the nurse manager must balance concern for the nurse with responsibility for ensuring safe patient care.

Employee Discipline

Few managers or executives enjoy confronting and disciplining employees. Nevertheless, confrontation and discipline are sometimes unavoidable, particularly when repeated coaching fails to solve the problem, or when a critical rule or regulation has been violated. It is important to remember that the primary function of discipline is not to punish, but to motivate appropriate behavior in the future.

Different sets of key behaviors are necessary for disciplining an employee (see Fig 16–4) and for responding with a rule violation (see Fig 16–5). These two sets of key behaviors closely parallel the key behaviors for coaching.

When employee discipline is necessary, it is important that the nurse manager work closely with the nurse executive and the human resources department. This close coordination increases the likelihood that disciplinary actions will be administered in a legally sound and fair manner.

The following precautions can help increase the likelihood that discipline is perceived as fair:

---

1. Define the problem in terms of lack of improvement since the previous discussion.
2. Ask for and openly listen to reasons for the continued behavior.
3. Explain why the behavior cannot continue.
4. If disciplinary action is called for, indicate what action you must take and why.
5. Agree on specific steps to be taken to solve problem (write them down).
6. Set a follow-up date and outline further steps to be taken if the problem is not corrected.
7. Assure the employee of your interest in helping him/her to succeed.

Figure 16–4. Key Behaviors for Disciplining Employees *(Taken from Decker PJ*, Healthcare Management Microtraining. *St. Louis, Decker & Associates, 1982. Copyright 1982 by Phillip J Decker. Used with permission)*

1. Prepare before the meeting (eg, is the employee aware of the rule, how employee will react, has the rule been consistently enforced).
2. Without hostility, describe the behavior which violated the rule.
3. State the rule which has been violated.
4. Ask for and listen openly to the employee's reasons for the behavior.
5. Explain why the behavior cannot continue (and offer your help in solving the problem, if you think it would be useful).
6. Set and record a specific follow-up date.

Figure 16-5. Key Behaviors for Dealing with a Rule Violation *(Taken from Decker PJ*, Healthcare Management Microtraining. *St. Louis, Decker & Associates, 1982. Copyright 1982 by Phillip J Decker. Used with permission)*

1. Establish a clear set of rules and regulations.
2. Communicate these rules and regulations (preferably in writing) to each employee. Some employers have every employee sign a statement documenting that they have read the rules and regulations.
3. Develop a set of progressive penalties for violating a rule or a regulation. For example, for minor violations (eg, smoking in a nonsmoking area), penalties may progress from an oral warning, a written warning, a one-day suspension, a three-day suspension, to dismissal. For a major rule violation (eg, physical abuse of a patient), the initial penalty would be more severe (eg, a three-day suspension or termination).
4. Develop an appeals process for a person who believes the discipline process was unfair. In some institutions, penalties are appealed to a higher-level manager. In other institutions, there are "appeals boards" made up of a cross-section of employees. In institutions where nurses are unionized, arbitration may be available.

The preceding four disciplinary precautions are largely the responsibility of the institution. The following guidelines are more directly applicable to nurse managers.

1. *Get the facts before acting.* Do not make assumptions. It is important that the employee have a chance to present her or his side of the story.
2. *Do not act while angry.* It is very difficult to be improvement oriented when angry.
3. *Discipline in private.* Public reprimand is humiliating and reflects lack of respect for the employee.
4. *Make the offense clear and specify what is appropriate behavior.* In responding to a performance problem, the manager should make clear the problem behavior as well as the appropriate behavior. In this meeting, the supervisor should also inform the employee of the consequences of repeated problem behavior.
5. *Do not suddenly tighten your enforcement policy.* If a rule has not been previously enforced, sufficient warning should be provided before enforcement is begun. All staff should be informed of the date on which enforcement of the rule will begin. An explanation of the rule should also be given.

6. *Enforce rules consistently.* Nothing destroys staff morale more quickly than an inconsistent enforcement of rules. If rules are enforced sometimes and not others, staff are understandably confused. More importantly, if the manager holds some employees accountable for adhering to the rules and regulations but not others, a charge of discrimination may result.

Dehiring

When a nurse's behavior is sufficiently disruptive, termination must be an alternative. However, termination is serious and may be followed by a number of undesirable responses (eg, threat of lawsuit or grievance, an increase in an institution's unemployment compensation rate, stressful and time-consuming hearings, and replacement costs). Given the potentially undesirable correlates of the termination process, institutions often prefer that a disruptive employee voluntarily withdraw from employment. By closely documenting an employee's poor performance and consistently enforcing rules for all staff, a health care institution may "encourage" a nurse to find employment elsewhere. Such "dehiring" allows the nurse to leave without a record of termination. At the same time, it allows the institution to avoid the negative consequences sometimes associated with discharging an employee. However, although this procedure may be acceptable for some performance problems, it should not be used when evidence exists that the nurse's practice is impaired due to alcohol or drug dependency. Allowing chemically dependent nurses to seek employment elsewhere without confronting the problem simply transfers the problem to another institution. In states with mandatory reporting laws, it is illegal not to report impaired practice.

Documentation

The importance of adequate documentation of employee performance problems should now be apparent. In coaching, an accurate record of past performance helps the supervisor establish a track record and a baseline for future performance appraisal; when discipline is the selected response, accurate documentation is essential. Without a clear record of performance the manager may not have the needed support to act. In addition, lack of clear documentation may hinder an organization's defense should a grievance or lawsuit result from the action.

Managers should be alert for out-of-the-ordinary behavior. If performance is noteworthy in a positive sense, managers take note of the behavior and the employee is praised. Similarly, when an employee's behavior is unacceptable, the manager documents the behavior and then follows up with coaching or discipline. The procedures required for documenting noteworthy employee behavior should not be a time-consuming procedure; otherwise, managers will not do it.

Handling Employee Complaints

Although the major thrust of this chapter has been on the manager's responsibility in initiating responses to performance problems, employees may themselves have complaints they wish to discuss. Figure 16–6 presents a sequence of key behaviors that have been found to be effective in handling complaints from employees.

1. Listen openly.
2. Do not speak until the person has had his or her say.
3. Avoid reacting emotionally (don't get defensive).
4. Ask for his or her expectations about a solution to the problem.
5. Explain what you can and cannot do to solve the problem (if appropriate).
6. Agree on specific steps to be taken and specific deadlines.

Figure 16-6. Key Behaviors for Handling Complaints *(Taken from Decker PJ*, Healthcare Management Microtraining. *St. Louis, Decker & Associates, 1982. Copyright 1982 by Phillip J Decker. Used with permission)*

CHEMICAL DEPENDENCY

Substance abuse and dependency have reached epidemic proportions in the United States. In business and industry, problems related to excessive drug and alcohol use have reached such proportions that most major corporations offer insurance benefits that include provision for drug and alcohol treatment and many have developed employee assistance programs.

Ironically, health professionals have been reluctant to acknowledge and deal with chemical dependency within their own professions. Only recently has the problem of what is popularly referred to as "impairment" among health professionals been addressed. The American Nurses Association Task Force on Addictions and Psychological Dysfunctions defines "impaired practice" as a professional's inability to meet the requirements of the professional code of ethics and standards of practice because of excessive alcohol or drug use, addiction, or psychiatric illness (ANA, 1984).

A profession has a responsibility to monitor the practice of its members to protect the safety of the public. In keeping with this imperative, the profession of nursing must ensure safe, high quality nursing care while caring about the nurses who are members of this profession (ANA, 1984). Despite this imperative, scant research has been conducted on the topic of chemically impaired nursing practice and few institutions have developed policies and procedures to guide response to chemically dependent nurse employees.

IMPACT OF IMPAIRED PRACTICE

Because of the dearth of research focusing on the problem of impaired nursing practice, estimates of the prevalence of alcohol and drug dependency among nurses are difficult to make. Using general population data, the American Nurses Association estimates that about 6 to 8 percent (about 120,000 to 160,000) of the registered nurse population has a problem related to the excessive use of alcohol or drugs (ANA, 1987).

Regardless of the prevalence of impairment in nurses, the impact is significant. The potential for harm to the public, to the profession, and to individual practitioners when nurses become impaired is great.

Substance abuse and addiction have been linked to illness, accidental death and suicide in nurses. The association between suicide or suicide attempts, and chemical dependency among nurses is well documented (Bissell & Haberman 1984; McMahon, 1986; Haack, 1989).

In addition to individual suffering and the social impact of impaired practice, the economic cost to employers is great. For example, estimates indicate that alcohol dependent employees cost employers about 25 percent of their annual salaries. Compared with other employees, they are estimated to have 2.5 times as many absences of 8 days or more at a time, receive three times as many benefits for accidents and sick leave, and file five times as many compensation claims (Wrich, 1980).

Estimates of the cost of replacing a nurse range from $1500 (Hoffman, 1985) and $3000 (Sullivan, 1986), to more than $9000 (LaGodna & Hendrix, 1989). Following a comprehensive analysis to examine the cost of impaired practice, LaGodna and Hendrix (1989) estimate the total costs to an institution to be $17,867. This figure includes the cost of initial counseling and documentation, institutional investigation, termination, board of nursing reporting and procedures, counseling remaining unit staff, and replacing the nurse. Given the current and projected shortage of registered nurses, the loss of these nurses from the profession is particularly disturbing.

POLICIES AND PROCEDURES

Professional Response

The responsibility for dealing with impaired practice caused by the excessive use of chemical substances was first formally acknowledged in nursing in 1982 when the American Nurses Association House of Delegates adopted a resolution "to address health problems that compromise nurses' ability to function within the standards and code of conduct for professional practice" (ANA, 1984). The resolution called for the development of guidelines for state assistance programs, the encouragement of nurses' employers to offer appropriate services prior to disciplinary action, and the establishment of mechanisms to collect and disseminate information related to the problem of impairment among nurses (ANA, 1982).

Currently, approximately 28 state nurses' associations have peer assistance programs in place, and an additional 20 states have formed committees or are in the process of developing some form of assistance program (Naegle, 1989). State programs vary considerably in focus and level of activity. Some provide only education and referral, while others have developed relatively comprehensive programs of assistance.

Several states (eg, California, Florida, Kansas, New Mexico, and Texas) have already implemented programs whereby nurses who voluntarily enter treatment can avoid the usual disciplinary procedures. These programs, often referred to as "diversion programs," are voluntary, nonpunitive alternatives to disciplinary action that provide help for the alcohol or drug dependent nurse while ensuring that patient care is not adversely affected. Diversion programs are designed to remove the nurse from practice during the active phase of dependency and to monitor practice for a designated recovery period. In other states (eg, Louisiana), the state nurses association has established a similar, though less formal, alternative to disciplinary action via a memorandum of understanding with the board of nursing. The philosophy underlying these alternative programs asserts that chemical dependence is an illness and that a rehabilitative rather than a punitive approach is more effective in trying to solve the problem.

Approximately one half of the states in the United States have mandatory reporting laws. These laws require that any nurse whose practice is impaired by the use of alcohol or other drugs be reported to the state licensing board. In states that do not have alternative programs, mandatory reporting laws are viewed primarily as punitive and have not proved effective in regulating practice.

Institutional Response

Just as the profession is responsible for setting standards of practice, individual institutions set performance expectations through the development of policies and procedures, quality assurance guidelines, and performance evaluation criteria. Standards are effective only when explicitly stated and communicated to all levels of nursing staff. Clear standards of performance facilitate early identification of problems and documentation of substandard performance and are recognized as key in identifying nurses who are abusing alcohol or drugs or who are chemically dependent (Abbott, 1987).

Although it is now recognized that chemical dependency affects a large number of nurses, few hospitals and other health care agencies have policies for dealing with the problem (Hughes, 1989; Department of Management and Budget, 1988). A recent survey of top-level nurse administrators from acute care hospitals in one midwestern state found that only 41 percent of the hospitals surveyed had written policies related to impairment caused by the excessive use of alcohol or other drugs (Hughes, 1989).

While there have been definite improvements made over the past several years, responses to chemically dependent nurses are still often punitive or inadequate (Hughes, 1989; Lachman, 1988). Although professional ethics dictate that nurses intervene whenever patient safety is at risk and many states require nursing administrators to report chemically dependent nurses to the state licensing board, chemically dependent nurses are frequently not confronted, or they are confronted only after the situation can no longer be ignored (Bissell & Haberman, 1984; Lachman, 1988). At that point the impaired nurse may be asked to resign or be dismissed, often without the alcohol or drug problem being acknowledged. When this occurs, the nurse is free to seek employment elsewhere and the problem is simply transferred to another institution.

Thus, the absence of institutional policies or guidelines acts as a fundamental barrier to intervention and, as such, allows chemically dependent nurses to become progressively worse, places clients at increased risk of harm, and exposes employers to greater risk of liability. In contrast, policies based on a rehabilitation model adopted in some hospitals (Durburg & Werner, 1989) benefit all involved. Such policies reflect the view of chemical dependency as a treatable health problem and thus assists rehabilitation of the chemically dependent nurses and ensures patient safety by closely monitoring the nurse's practice during recovery or by temporarily reassigning the nurse to a nonclinical position.

IDENTIFYING THE CHEMICALLY DEPENDENT NURSE

Signs and Symptoms

While the manifestation of signs and symptoms differ depending on the individual nurse and the drug used, a number of similarities exist including changes in job performance, and physical, personality and mental status changes.

Job Performance. Changes in job performance include excessive use of sick time, especially a pattern of sick leave requests following days off; absence without notification or "last minute" requests for time off; long lunch and coffee breaks; and unexplained absences from the unit. This pattern is not the same for the drug dependent nurse who is illegally obtaining drugs from the hospital. Rather, this nurse will *rarely* be absent and will in fact volunteer for extra shifts, and may linger on the unit even when not on duty. Also common is sloppy record keeping, including illegible or illogical chart entries.

Physical Changes. Physical changes observed may include a general deterioration in appearance as well as evidence of frequent injuries such as bruises or cigarette burns.

Personality and Mental Health Status Changes. The chemically dependent nurse may exhibit emotional lability (irritability or frequent mood swings), frequent inappropriate verbal or emotional responses, decreased mental alertness, confusion, forgetfulness, or lapses in memory. A formerly gregarious nurse may become increasingly withdrawn, declining invitations to join colleagues for lunch or activities outside work.

Figure 16–7 list signs and symptoms that may be observed in nurses who are dependent on alcohol or other drugs.

INTERVENTION

Many of the signs and symptoms listed in Fig 16–7 may be manifested by nurses who are experiencing severe emotional distress unrelated to chemical dependency. Whatever the cause of impaired performance, documentation of specific job performance problems provides the most effective tools for intervention.

For problems related to substance abuse, the intervention must be carefully planned and carried out. Naegle (1985) offers the following suggestions for interventions involving chemical dependency.

1. The intervention is planned on behalf of the nurse with the goal of restoration of health, protection of the consumer, and maintenance of nursing standards.

Background Indicators

Background indicators include:

Family history of alcoholism or drug abuse
History of frequent change of worksite, in the same or other institutions
Prior medical history requiring pain control
Prior reputation as conscientious and responsible employee

Behavioral Signs

Behavioral signs include:

Increasing isolation from colleagues, friends, and family
Frequent complaints of marital and family problems
Frequent reports of illness, minor accidents, and emergencies
Complaints from others about the person's alcohol or drug use and/or poor work performance
Evidence of blackouts
Mood swings, irritability, depression, or suicide threats and/or attempts (which may be caused by accidental overdose)
Strong interest in patients' pain control, the narcotics cabinet, and use of pain control medications
Frequent trips to the bathroom or other unexplained, brief absences
Request for night shifts
Social avoidance of staff; eating alone; isolation
Elaborate or inadequate excuses for tardiness or absence, including long lunch hours or use of sick leave immediately after days off
Difficulty meeting schedules and deadlines
Illogical or sloppy charting

Physical Symptoms

Physical symptoms include:

Shakiness, tremors of hands
Slurred speech
Watery eyes, dilated or constricted pupils
Diaphoresis
Unsteady gait
Runny nose
Nausea, vomiting, diarrhea
Weight loss or gain
Increasing carelessness about personal appearance   *(continued)*

Figure 16–7. Indications of Addictions *(From Sullivan E, Bissell L, Williams E.* Chemical Dependency in Nursing: The Deadly Diversion. *Menlo Park, CA, Addison-Wesley, 1988)*

2. The intervention is based on objective observations and documentation.
3. The intervention is planned with the assistance and consultation of an individual knowledgeable about impaired practice.
4. The intervention is carefully planned. Decisions concerning who is to participate and when the intervention is to occur are made in advance. Two individuals working together are usually best able to confront a nurse's denial and maintain objectivity.

Narcotics Discrepancies

Nurse managers and staff should suspect the probability of drug diversion if any of the following occur:

Frequently incorrect narcotics counts
Apparent alteration of narcotics vials
Increased number of patient reports of pain medication ineffectiveness
Discrepancy between patient reports and hospital records of pain medication (eg, patient reports he takes pain medication only during the day, records indicate nighttime administration as well)
Discrepancies in physician's orders, progress notes, and narcotics records
Large amounts of narcotics wasted
Numerous corrections on narcotics records
Erratic patterns of narcotics discrepancies (these may be timed with the addicted nurse's work schedule)
Significant variation in quantity of drugs required on a unit

Additional Signs and Symptoms

Additional signs and symptoms specific to a nurse who may be abusing narcotic drugs include:

Rapid mood change from irritation to depression to euphoria
Use of long-sleeved clothing continuously, even in warm weather
Change in work schedule
Appearance on the unit on days off
Request of assignment that facilitates access to drugs
Disappearance into the restroom immediately after accessing narcotics cabinet

---

Figure 16–7. (continued)

5. Resources and options for treatment are determined in advance and offered to the nurse at the time of the intervention.
6. The intervention should always be planned with consideration of the nurse's rights including confidentiality and legal council.

Although nurses at all levels are responsible for responding to chemical impairment among colleagues, nurse administrators have the authority to advise a nurse that failure to seek treatment will result in notification of the state licensing board.

RE-ENTRY

Despite understandable hesitation on the part of employers to hire recovering chemically dependent nurses, reports indicate that successful re-entry to nursing practice can be accomplished with effective intervention, treatment, and support (Lachman, 1988; Sullivan, Bissell, & Williams, 1988). Most institutions that knowingly employ recovering nurses usually do not allow them to return to work or begin work until they have successfully completed a course of treatment. While the amount of time required for treatment varies based on the severity of the impairment, financial resources of the nurse, and philosophy of the treatment providers, nurses are rarely allowed to return to work in less than 6 to 8 weeks following entry into treatment.

After return to work, recovering nurses, particularly recovering drug dependent nurses, are often temporarily restricted from handling narcotics and are usually monitored for periods ranging from 6 months to 2 years. The most common monitoring methods include close supervision of performance, restrictions related to handling narcotics, and random urine screens for the presence of drugs. In addition, attendance at nurse support groups or 12-step groups such as Alcoholics Anonymous (AA) or Narcotics Anonymous (NA) also are frequently required.

Contracts that specify guidelines for re-entry following treatment are increasingly being used in hospitals that employ recovering nurses. Figure 16–8 is an example

---

_____ Hospital Employee Assistance Program
Agreement Between Employee and _____ Hospital

I, _____, agree to the following conditions upon my continuing employment at _____ Hospital. These conditions will apply for a period of two years, beginning on _____ and ending on _____.

1. If it should be determined that I am using any mood-altering chemicals (except with the agreement of my therapist and under the direction of a physician who will keep the Employee Assistance Program informed as to reason and specific period of time), I will be immediately terminated and reported to the State Board of Nursing.

2. I agree to cooperate in any random urine check requested by _____ Hospital. The results will be sent to the Employee Assistance Program. If at any time mood-altering substances are found, my employment will be terminated immediately and I will be reported to the State Board of Nursing.

3. I agree to follow the prescribed program of aftercare, including attendance in A.A. I will be responsible for providing documentation of attendance to the Employee Assistance Program and if I do not comply, either in attendance and/or documentation, my employment will be terminated immediately and I will be reported to the State Board of Nursing.

4. If I should voluntarily terminate from _____ Hostital, I agree to keep the Employee Assistance Program informed as to my compliance with prescribed program of aftercare, my address and place of employment. I further agree to inform my new employer of my condition and request my new employer to keep the Employee Assistance Program at _____ Hospital informed of my progress. Unless other arrangements are made which are mutually agreeable to the new employer and the Employee Assistance Program at _____ Hospital, and if the above conditions are not met, I will be reported to the State Board of Nursing.

These four conditions have been read and agreed upon by:

_____   _____
(Employee signature)   (Date)

_____   _____
(Director of Nursing-_____ Hospital)   (Date)

_____   _____
(EAP Coordinator-_____ Hospital)   (Date)

Figure 16–8. Sample "return-to-work" contract (_Return-to-work contract. Used with permission from Sullivan EJ, Bissell L & Williams E._ Chemical Dependency in Nursing, _Menlo Park, CA: Addison-Wesley, 1988_)

of a "return to work" contract. Most contracts or agreements for recovering nurses returning to work require total abstinence from all chemical substances (alcohol and other drugs). Acceptable use generally includes only medications prescribed by a physician with the knowledge of the person(s) responsible for monitoring the recovering nurse's performance.

Most contracts do not include provisions for relapse and in those that do, termination is often mandated (Hughes, 1988). Chemical dependence is a chronic, progressing, and sometimes recurring health problem; therefore, relapse must be recognized as a potential hazard. Contracts that do not address relapse or require termination following relapse deny that it may take more than one attempt to maintain abstinence. A more supportive, and perhaps more effective, approach details the consequences of relapse as well as steps to be taken to assist the nurse should relapse occur. This approach encourages early intervention and provides the nurse with needed help while at the same time safeguarding patient care.

If the nurse repeatedly relapses or fails to adhere to other stipulations of the contract termination of employment must be the consequence. The nurse must also be reported to the state licensing board to ensure that the problem is not simply transferred to another institution. In addition, every effort should be made to get the nurse admitted or readmitted into treatment.

Return-to-work contracts are usually applicable only at the institution where they are initiated. That is, recovering nurses are generally required to remain at the same institution throughout the period of the contract. If the nurse must change jobs prior to the end of the contract, a report must be made to the state licensing board.

Most nurse administrators grapple with the problem of chemically impaired practice. Numerous personal, institutional, and professional consequences ensue from chemically impaired practice. The most powerful means of minimizing these consequences is the quick, supportive response of colleagues and administrators. Such a response depends on the ability to recognize chemical dependency, the existence of policies to guide response, and adequate resources to implement the response.

STRESS

Nature of Stress

Stress can be defined as a disruption of homeostasis resulting from internal or external events that disturb the normal flow of life (Selye, 1956). For example, heat, cold, anger, fright, conflict, frustration, and physical exertion create specific demands on the body and each call for highly individualized responses. However, all these sources of stress share a common element—they require readjustment through adaptive functions that re-establish normalcy or equilibrium. Stress is not inherently negative or undesirable; however, perception of ability to control stressful events is crucial to healthy coping or adaptation.

Since Selye's pioneering work on stress, a number of other researchers and theorists have contributed to our understanding of stress and its effects on health. For example, work by Lazarus provided considerable support for the belief that stress involves both the person and the environment (Lazarus & Cohen, 1977).

Stress in Nursing

Job-related stress is not unique to the nursing profession. One need only review the literature to discover that stress and burnout are eminent concerns of most professions, particularly those that are "helping professions." Nursing, however, is thought to have a unique combination of stressors. Nurses, perhaps more than any other professional group, confront pain, grief, dying, and death on a daily or even hourly basis. These factors, combined with the role conflict and role ambiguity inherent in the work of nurses, greatly increase the likelihood of excessive stress. Furthermore, the high work pace demanded of nurses because of medical and technological advances and frequent inadequate staffing can quickly turn stress into burnout.

Figure 16–9 gives a stress model developed by Decker (see Sullivan & Decker, 1988). This model outlines the antecedents of stress that are particularly relevant to nurses and includes consequences of stress and the intervening constructs of role ambiguity and role conflict.

Antecedents	Intervening Constructs	Consequences
Organizational Factors		*Negative*
Job tasks		Stress
Physical environment		Health problems
Supervisor behavior		Marital problems/divorce
Institutional factors		Alcoholism/drug abuse
Changing environment		Lower performance
Societal/nursing traditions		Lower job satisfaction
Self-worth		Lower self-esteem
Intraprofessional divisiveness		Absenteeism/turnover
	Role Ambiguity	Career dissatisfaction/change
Interpersonal Factors		*Positive/Coping*
Role messages		Role redefinition
Trust/respect for senders		Share roles
Multiple roles		Integrate roles
(nurse, manager, parent, spouse)	Role Conflict	Confront role senders
		Redefine role
Individual Factors		
Rate of "life change"		Personal reorientation
Ability to perform roles		Reactive coping
Self-esteem/self-perception		Increased performance
Tolerance for ambiguity		Increased efficiency
Other personality traits		Prioritize tasks/goals

Figure 16–9. Stress Model Source: *Phillip J Decker and Eleanor J Sullivan. Effective Management in Nursing, 3d, Menlo Park, CA, Addison-Wesley, 1992. Used by permission)*

ANTECEDENTS OF STRESS

Organizational Factors

Although stress in the nurse's workplace stems from a number of sources, staffing and workload are among the most common sources of organizational stress identified by nurses (Mann & Jefferson, 1988). For example, a survey of more than 1200 staff nurses at a large university hospital found that workload was significantly related to stress and job dissatisfaction and was cited by significant number of respondents as a reason for nurses leaving the profession (Weisman, Alexander & Chase, 1981). Similar findings were reported in a study of MICU nurses (Mann & Jefferson, 1988).

Overload was the most frequently cited source of job stress for top level nurse executives (Scalzi, 1988). Overload in this study was conceptualized as (1) conflicting expectations from hospital administrators and the nursing department; (2) too large a span of control, (3) too many expectations for the job in general; and (4) difficulties related to managing personnel.

Continuing demands for cost-containment, coupled with greater patient acuity, have created increasingly heavy work demands on nurses. The nursing shortage has further complicated this situation by making it difficult or impossible to provide adequate staff to all units in some hospitals. The pressure for nurses to perform more efficiently, with fewer staff, undeniably creates significant stress for staff nurses and managers.

Institutional factors that can lead to stress include lack of supplies and properly functioning equipment, excessive paper work, and working with auxiliary departments and personnel such as laboratory, pharmacy, and dietary (Humphrey, 1988). In addition, although nurses have major responsibility for patient's well-being, they have little authority relative to other professionals employed in health care institutions.

Furthermore, dramatic changes in hospitals and other health care delivery systems have created additional stress for nurses. Rapid changes in technology including computerization and the use of highly sophisticated monitoring equipment require a high level of technical skills. Malpractice suits, previously almost exclusively the concern of physicians or hospital administration, now involve more nurses, more directly. In addition, increased pressure from external agencies such as third-party payers, accrediting bodies, and licensing agencies have made nurses' jobs more difficult, conflicting, and stressful.

Friction or tension, within limits, reflects a healthy work environment and provides the challenge necessary to keep a job interesting. However, excessive tension, or tension that continues for extended periods without the buffer of external support will eventually have detrimental effects on staff morale and productivity (Pines, 1982). For example, supervisor behavior has been identified as an important factor in either exacerbating or mitigating the stress experienced by nurses (Constable & Russell, 1986). Similarly, peer support is believed to be an important factor in buffering the effects of work stress. Because of their perception of themselves as providers rather than receivers of care, health professionals may have difficulty reaching out to others for emotional support (Patrick, 1979).

Individual Factors

Life events are among the individual factors that cause stress. Holmes and Rahe (1967) consider the following ten events to be among the most serious causes of stress: (1) death of a spouse; (2) divorce; (3) marital separation; (4) jail term; (5) death of a close family member; (6) personal injury or illness; (7) marriage; (8) being fired; (9) marital reconciliation; and (10) retirement. Although widely used, life events scales such as the one developed by Holmes and Rahe have been criticized for lack of relevance to certain groups (Rabkin & Struening, 1976), including women (Norbeck, 1984). In addition, some critics have argued that a measure of day-to-day problems more accurately reflects levels of stress (Lazarus, 1981).

The individual's perception of stressful events is key in determining the effect of these events. It is widely recognized that many people experience stressful events with no obvious deleterious effects. Kobasa, Maddi, and Kahn (1982) identified a set of personality characteristics they believe buffer the effects of stress. According to these researchers, stress-resistant people tend to be ''hardy,'' that is, they have a specific set of attitudes toward life—an openness to change, a feeling of involvement in whatever they do, and a sense of control over events. Rich and Rich (1987) studied 200 female staff nurses and found the personality traits constituting hardiness to be important stress-resistant resources in preventing or reducing burnout.

The personality traits labeled Type A and Type B behavior and their relationship to health problems have also received considerable attention among stress researchers. The Type A personality, commonly associated with heart disease, is aggressive, ambitious, competitive, and compelled to achievement, while Type B personalities are more relaxed and easygoing. Type A personalities are less able than Type B personalities to manage frustration and are more likely to become stressed or angry when they perceive their efforts to be unsuccessful or unfairly compromised by others. Because Type A behavior is thought to be common in nurses (Cronin-Stubbs & Velor-Friedrich, 1981), nurse managers should recognize the influence of different personality characteristics on individual nurses' experience and tolerance of frustration and stress.

Role Conflict and Role Ambiguity

Role stress is a general concept that encompasses conditions in which role demands are vague, difficult, or impossible to meet (Burke & Scalzi, 1988). Role conflict and role ambiguity, types of role stress, are endemic in the work of nurses and are widely recognized causes of stress. Nurses' success in dealing with these role related problems may well determine the overall effects of work related stress. Nurses are required to assume a number of widely divergent roles—caretaker, counselor, teacher, supervisor, mediator, and coordinator of patient care—often without the authority or recognition that should go with these roles.

Role conflict occurs when inconsistent, incompatible, or inappropriate demands are made. The nurse who experiences role conflict feels pulled in several different directions. For example, a nurse supervising a unit that is short-staffed often feels conflict about whether to complete administrative responsibilities or to assume clinical responsibilities. Role conflict may also occur when a nurse's values or ethical beliefs conflict with those of supervisors or supervisees.

Role ambiguity is similar to role conflict in that the nurse experiences stress because of conflict; however, this conflict results from unclear job performance expectations and responsibilities, authority, or accountability. Inadequate information or conflicting expectations about one's role or responsibilities can create significant stress.

Multiple roles are a source of stress for most women, including nurses. Societal views and expectations of women may make nurses disproportionately at risk for high levels of stress and burnout. That is, most nurses are women who not only have full-time jobs but frequently have a great deal, if not total, responsibility for the maintenance of their homes and families. Thus, both halves of their lives are spent caring in some way for the needs of others. Added to this are the demands created by shift and weekend work required in the majority of nursing jobs.

CONSEQUENCES OF STRESS

Excessive stress, whether the source is organizational, interpersonal, or individual, left unchecked, can create a host of physical and mental problems. In fact, Humphrey (1988) notes that most standard medical textbooks attribute anywhere from 50 to 80 percent of all diseases to stress-related origins.

Among the physical health problems commonly associated with stress are hypertension and heart disease, gastrointestinal problems including peptic ulcer and colitis, migraine headaches, backache, weight loss or weight gain, and injuries caused by accidents. Common mental health problems associated with stress include anxiety, depression, and burnout. In addition to the individual costs of stress, organizations suffer inestimatable costs including those related to lowered productivity, patient errors, and increased absenteeism, accidents, and injuries.

Coping Strategies

Lazarus (1974) outlines the following four methods of coping with stress: (1) direct-active—changing the source of stress, confronting the source of stress, finding positive aspects in the situation; (2) direct-inactive—ignoring the source of stress, avoiding the source of stress, or leaving the stressful situation; (3) indirect-active—talking about the stress, changing oneself to adapt to the stress, getting involved in other activities; and (4) indirect-inactive—drinking or using drugs, becoming ill, and collapsing.

The direct-active and indirect-active methods are generally the most positive and productive strategies for handling stress. Examples of coping strategies used with these methods include using assertive behavior, talking about the situation with supervisors, physicians, or coworkers, leaving the unit, or taking time off from work.

When these options are not available or when these strategies are unsuccessful, other less healthy coping strategies are employed. These strategies, if overused, can lead to depression, burnout, and chemical dependency (Haack, 1985).

BURNOUT

While few people agree on the exact definition of burnout, almost all agree that it is a process, not an event. Although the process of burnout is subtle and may be manifested in a number of ways it is believed to have at least three basic and consistent elements: emotional exhaustion, shift toward negative attitudes, and a sense of personal devaluation that occurs in response to work-related stress (Patrick, 1979). Nurses who work in high stress units such as oncology, burn, or intensive care units may be more vulnerable to burnout.

Emotional Exhaustion

Stress is inherent in nurses' day-to-day work environment. Responsibility for sick patients and the need to make important decisions quickly on a regular basis requires considerable emotional resources. A nurse in the early stages of burnout typically suffers from emotional fatigue. In an effort to conserve needed resources this nurse will frequently withdraw emotionally from patients and families. If stressful interpersonal contact cannot be limited, the emotionally fatigued nurse may experience emotional exhaustion (Maslach, 1982).

Shift Toward Negative Attitudes

Distancing themselves from patients and others is one way nurses who are experiencing emotional fatigue or exhaustion may attempt to cope with their work situation. Although effective for short-term coping, continued distancing leads to detachment. Detached nurses treat patients, families, and co-workers in a mechanical, unfeeling manner.

Personal Devaluation

Self-worth and self-esteem are damaged by negative attitudes. Feeling negatively about clients and others leads to guilt about the care being delivered, which further erodes self-esteem and results in feelings of professional and personal inadequacy.

Burned out nurses become noticeably less idealistic and enthusiastic and more rigid. Work performance deteriorates markedly, and they are frequently absent or late for work and may even resign their positions or leave the nursing profession altogether. The cost of hiring and training a new nurse is estimated to be more than $9000.00 (LaGodna & Hendrix, 1989). As with most health problems, prevention is a less costly and preferable approach to burnout among employees.

STRATEGIES FOR REDUCING STRESS AND BURNOUT

Following are some of the features of hospitals having healthy work climates that can improve job satisfaction and help to prevent burnout among nurses (Working conditions, 1981).

- A head nurse with a baccalaureate or master's degree has full responsibility (including hiring) for personnel on units.
- Assigned staff plan their own work schedules including days off, shifts worked, and so on.
- Nurses on day and night shifts have equal input into the total nursing care program.
- Inservice training is planned so nurses can meet their education needs.
- Pay differential is provided for day and night shifts so enough nurses would choose nights, and day nurses would not have to rotate to other shifts.
- Collaboration among other units and hospitals enables nurses to have a choice of opportunities to update skills.
- Salary increases should be tied to performance and recognition of good work.
- Nurses have input into all policies affecting them, including nursing practice, patient care, and personnel benefits.
- Nurses share planning for patient care with physicians and other health care administrators, and take part in decisions about patient discharge or movement to another care unit.

Nurse administrators can use this list to assess the work environment in their institutions. Other factors to consider when assessing stress among staff include whether the organization has:

1. Clear lines of authority. Organizations that have a clear and single flow of authority are believed to be more satisfying for employees and to result in more effective performance than organizations without such clear lines of authority (Burke & Scalzi, 1988).
2. Clear roles and responsibilities. Classical organizational theory prescribes that all positions within an organization have specified tasks and responsibilities. When nurses do not know what is expected of them, how their performance will be evaluated, or what they have the authority to decide, they will experience stress, will hesitate to make decisions, and will generally perform less effectively.
3. Staff involvement in decision making. Involving nurses in the decision-making process, particularly in decisions that directly involve them, can not only assist in arriving at more effective solutions to problems, but can also help to increase staff satisfaction and productivity.
4. Clearly written and communicated goals, philosophy, and purpose of the institution.
5. Clear standards of performance (see Chapter 13).
6. Mechanisms for recognition and rewards. In addition to providing adequate salaries and benefits, recognizing quality work or an outstanding service record through written or verbal acknowledgement can do much to boost the morale of staff.
7. Available resources for referral of staff who are having difficulty managing stress. It is important to assure that resources are available either through an

employee assistance program, the human resources department, or collaboration with an outside agency for staff who need help dealing with stress.

8. Facilitation of support among staff. Good working relationships among colleagues has been identified as one of the most important elements in staff morale (Pines & Kafry, 1978). Emotionally supportive environments enhance positive communication and cohesion among staff.

The above factors are important to consider in developing strategies for dealing with institutional or organizational problems that may cause stress. However, apart from these institutional factors, nursing is fraught with stressors. Therefore, to stay healthy and to avoid burnout, nurses at all levels must develop individual strategies to manage stress. Lachman (1983), in a book on stress management for nurses, identifies the following key strategies for nurses to use in minimizing work-related stress: (1) Insure adequate relaxation time for healing and rejuvenation. One of the most useful methods for dealing with stress identified by nurses is spending time and energy on activities and interests unrelated to work. Such activities include hobbies, sports, and recreational activities. (2) Train the body to withstand stress through exercise. The method of exercise is not as important as engaging in some form of exercise on a regular basis. Regular exercise has been shown to be a potent stress reducer. (3) Increase self-awareness. Scully (1980) identifies unrealistic expectations for self as one of the four main sources of stress for staff nurses. She maintains that expecting too much of oneself can lead to burnout faster than any other single stressor. Yet, this is likely the stressor over which the nurse has the most control. Nurses must recognize and accept their limitations and learn how to care for themselves.

Nurse managers and administrators can do much to facilitate these individual strategies by providing regular time off from work, instituting mechanisms that promote and foster supportive relationships within and between units, and offering workshops and exercise programs for nurses who are interested in those methods of stress reduction. It must be remembered, however, that no one prescription can be used to alleviate the stress of all nurses. Stress is, to a great extent, a personal experience.

Without "sweating the small stuff" nurse managers and administrators can do much to protect nurses from undue stress. Creating an environment that enhances nurses' health is a strategy that will benefit not only nurses and the institutions that employ them, but will ultimately benefit patients as well.

SUMMARY

- Chemically impaired practice is a problem encountered by most nurse managers and nurse administrators.
- The costs of impaired practice are considerable and include costs to the nurse, the institution, and the profession.
- Policies and standards are important to guide response to chemically dependent nurse employees.

- Successful re-entry of recovering nurses into practice can be accomplished with effective intervention, treatment, and support.
- Stress results from internal or external events that disturb the normal flow of life.
- Nurses are thought to experience a unique pattern or combination of stressors.
- Excessive stress, left unchecked, can result in a host of physical and mental health problems, including burnout.
- Costs of burnout to the individual, institution, and the profession are great.
- Individual and institutional strategies can be initiated to reduce the effects of stress and help prevent burnout.

REFERENCES

Abbott CA. The impaired nurse. Part II: Management strategies. *AORN* 46:6, 1104, 1987

American Hospital Association. (January). US hospitals facing severe shortage of nurses. *American Hospital Association News Release.* Chicago, Author, January 1987

American Nurses Association House of Delegates. *Action on alcohol and drug misuse and psychological dysfunctions among nurses,* Resolution #5, adapted June 29, 1982

American Nurses Association. Impaired nursing practice (media backgrounder). *ANA News.* Kansas City, ANA, March 1987

American Nurses Association. *Addictions and Psychological Dysfunctions in Nursing: The Profession's Response to the Problem.* Kansas City, ANA, 1984

Bissell L, Haberman PW. *Alcoholism in the Professions.* New York, Oxford University Press, 1984

Breaugh J. Understanding & Effectively Managing Absenteeism and Turnover. In: Sullivan EJ, Decker PJ, eds. *Effective Management in Nursing,* 2nd ed. Redwood City, CA, Addison-Wesley, 387–410, 1988

Burke GC, Scalzi CC. Role stress in hospital executives and nursing executives. *Health Care Management Review.* 13:3, 67, 1988

Constable JF, Russell DW. The effect of social support and the work environment upon burnout in nurses. *Journal of Human Stress.* 12:20, 1986

Cronin-Stubbs D, Velsor-Freidrich B. Professional and personal stress. *Nurse Leadership.* 4:19, 1981

Department of Management and Budget. *Hospital-based drug diversion by nurses in Michigan.* Report prepared for the Michigan Department of Licensing and Regulation, Bureau of Health Services. Michigan, Division of Management and Budget, 1988

Durburg SK, Werner J. Reentering the professional practice environment. In: Haack MR, Hughes TL, eds. *Addiction in the Nursing Profession: Approaches to Intervention and Recovery.* New York, Springer Publishing Co, 1989: 148–172

Haack M. *Antecedents of the impaired nurse: Burnout, depression, and substance use among student nurses.* Unpublished doctoral dissertation, University of Illinois at Chicago, 1985

Haack MR. *Future directions in research and prevention.* In: Haack MR, Hughes TL eds. *Addiction in the Nursing Profession: Approaches to Intervention and Recovery.* New York, Springer Publishing Co, 1989: 218–237

Hoffman FM. Cost per RN hired. *Journal of Nursing Administration.* 15:27, 1985

Holmes TH, Rahe RH. The social readjustment scale. *Journal of Psychosomatic Research,* 11:213, 1967

Hughes TL. *Chief nurse executives' responses to chemically dependent nurses.* Unpublished doctoral dissertation, University of Illinois at Chicago, 1989

Humphrey JH. *Stress in the Nursing Profession.* Springfield, IL, Charles Thomas, 1988

Kobasa S, Maddi S, Kahn S. Hardiness and health: A prospective study. *Journal of Personality and Social Psychology.* 1:168, 1982

Lachman VD. *Stress Management: A Manual for Nurses.* NY, Grune & Stratton, Inc, 1983

Lachman VD. The chemically dependent nurse. *Holistic Nursing Practice.* 2:4, 34, 1988

LaGodna G, Hendrix J. Impaired nurses: A cost analysis. *Journal of Nursing Administration.* 19:13, 1989

Lawler EE. *High involvement management.* San Francisco, Jossey-Bass, 1986

Lazarus RS. Psychological stress and coping in adaptation to illness. *International Journal of Psychiatric Medicine.* 5:321, 1974

Lazarus RS. Little hassles can be hazardous to health. *Psychology Today.* 15:58, 1981

Lazarus RS, Cohen JB. Environmental stress. In: Altman I, Wohlwill JF, eds. *Human Behavior and the Environment: Current Theory and Research.* New York, Plenum Press, 1977

Mann EE, Jefferson KJ. Retaining staff: Using turnover indices and surveys. *Journal of Nursing Administration.* 18:17, 1988

Maslach C. *Burnout: The Cost of Caring.* Englewood Cliffs, NJ, Prentice Hall, 1982

McMahon JM. Characteristics of chemically dependent nurses in a large metropolitan area in the state of Texas. (Doctoral dissertation, University of Houston, 1986). *Dissertation Abstracts International.* 47:11A, 3987, 1987

Naegle MA. Creative management of impaired nursing practice. *Nursing Administration Quarterly.* 9:3, 16, 1985

Naegle MA. Professional issues, ethical constraints, and legal considerations. In: Haack MR, Hughes TL, eds. *Addiction in the Nursing Professional: Approaches to Intervention and Recovery* New York, Springer Publishing Co, 1989: 1–19

Norbeck JS. Modification of life events questionnaire for use with female respondents. *Research in Nursing and Health.* 1:61, 1984

Patrick PKS. Burnout: Job hazard for health workers. *Hospitals.* 53:87, 1979

Pinder CC. *Work Motivation.* Glenview, IL, Scott, Foresman and Company, 1984

Pines A. *On burnout and the buffering effects of social support.* In Farber BA, ed. Stress and Burnout in the Human Service Professions. New York, Pergamon Press, 1982

Pines A, Kafry D. Occupational tedium in the social sciences. *Social Work.* 23:299–307, 1978

Rabkin JG, Struening EL. Life events, stress, and illness. *Science,* 194:1013–1020

Rhodes SR, Steers RM. *Managing Employee Absenteeism.* Reading, MA, Addison-Wesley, 1990

Rich VL, Rich AR. Personality hardiness and burnout in female staff nurses. *Image.* 19:63, 1987

Scalzi CC. Role stress and coping strategies of nurse executives. *Journal of Nursing Administration.* 18:34, 1988

Scully R. Stress in the nurse. *American Journal of Nursing.* 80:911, 1980

Selye H. *The Stress of Life.* New York: McGraw Hill. 1956

Sullivan EJ. Cost savings of retaining chemically dependent nurses. *Nursing Economics.* 4:4, 179, 1986

Sullivan EJ, Bissell L, Williams E. *Chemical Dependency in Nursing: The Deadly Diversion.* Menlo Park, CA, Addison-Wesley, 1988

Sullivan EJ, Decker PJ. *Effective Management in Nursing,* 2nd ed. Redwood, CA, Addison Wesley, 1988

Wanous JP. *Organizational Entry.* Reading, MA, Addison-Wesley, 1980

Weisman CS, Alexander CS, Chase GA. Determinants of hospital staff nurse turnover. *Medical Care.* 19:431, 1981

Working conditions cause nurses to leave. *American Nurse* 12:10, 5, 1981

Wrich JT. *The Employee Assistance Program.* Hazeldon: MN, Hazeldon Press, 1980

Management of Groups

David P. Gustafson

Groups are a fact of life in all organizations; they are the basic building blocks for organizations. Nursing administrators spend much of their time in group settings meeting with staff, with other administrators or in committees and task forces. Many administrators consider groups as major wasters of time but groups can be sources of effective decision making, a means of sharing information, and a method of social coordination and integration among units. The purpose of this chapter is to help nursing administrators more effectively to understand the nature of groups and group processes, how to influence organizational success, and what nurse administrators can do to influence groups and improve their effectiveness in working with groups.

This chapter focuses on formal groups such as command groups, task groups (or teams), task forces and committees, and informal organizational groups. Informal groups such as family, social, special interest groups, and therapy groups will not be included.

GROUPS DEFINED

A group is two or more individuals who interact with each other on a relatively continuous basis, are psychologically aware of each other and perceive themselves as a group (Schein, 1970) The top administration team of a health care organization which includes a nursing administrator is an example of such a group. Others include nursing education committees, nursing policy and procedures committees, hospital disaster committees, hospital procedures committees, and patient care evaluation committees.

Command groups are organized to do certain organizational tasks. The supervisor of the group has line authority over the members. A task group is several persons who work together to do certain tasks. Sometimes a task group is also a command group but often there are several task groups in a department, or there are task groups which include members from several departments (eg, patient care team which includes a nurse, a physician, a dietitian, and a social worker).

Special groups, such as committees or task forces, are formed to deal with specific issues involving several departments. A committee which is responsible for safety or a task force assigned to develop better procedures are two examples.

Formal groups are classified as vertical versus horizontal groups and permanent versus temporary groups. Vertical groups include members from different levels in the organization while horizontal groups include individuals at similar levels in the organization either within a specific department across several departments in the organization. Committees, task groups, and task forces can be either vertical or horizontal while command groups are vertical groups. Likert (1961) suggests that an important role of command group members is to serve as links with other groups in an organization. The group leader links that group to groups higher in the organization, while other group members link it with lower level groups in which they serve as leaders. These links facilitate problem solving and lead to higher productivity and job satisfaction.

Permanent groups are those with unlimited life while temporary groups are those established for a specific purpose and then disbanded after completing the designated task. Command groups, teams, and committees usually are permanent groups while task forces are usually temporary. Each of these different types of groups presents opportunities and difficulties to the leader and the organization.

Informal groups arise from the interaction of people within the organization. They are informal in the sense that they are not formally recognized by the organization and they are not part of the formal organizational structure. Because informal groups are important in satisfying the needs of group members, it is necessary for nurse administrators to understand how they emerge, how they influence member performance and satisfaction, and how they can be influenced by the nurse administrator.

Group Leadership

Leadership roles in a group are very important. These leadership roles can be either formal or informal. For example, the nurse administrator may lead a command group but also serve as a leader in an informal grouping of nurse administrators or may be appointed to head a task force or chair a committee. The leader's influence on group processes and the ability of the group to work together often determines whether the group will be effective in accomplishing organizational and personal goals. This chapter will discuss how nursing administrators can effectively manage groups by presenting a model of group processes and then discussing group decision making, teams and team based organizational development, and the management of committees and task forces.

GROUP PROCESSES

A modified version of Homans' (1950; 1960) model of groups is shown in Figure 17–1. This model identifies the factors "external" to the group: tasks, technology, and work design, the formal administrative and reward system and the background

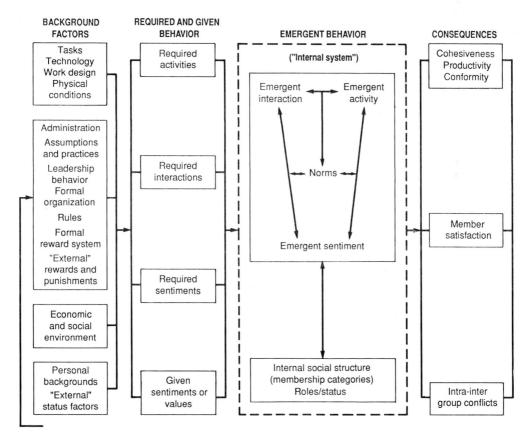

Figure 17–1. A Model of Group Behavior *(Source: Homans G. The Human Group. Social Behavior: Its Elementary Forms. New York, Harcourt Brace Jovanovich, 1950. New York, Harcourt Brace, 1961)*

characteristics of the group members. These external factors affect the "internal" system of the group: the emergent behavior of the group members and the group's social structure. These in turn influence the cohesiveness and productivity of the group as well as the satisfaction and growth of the group members. Homans also distinguishes between those things that are "required," which come from the external system, and those things that "emerge" and are part of the internal system.

The three essential elements of Homans' framework are activities, interactions, and sentiments. Activities are the observable things people do such as talk, move, and write. Interactions are the activities of one person which correspond to the activities of another person. Oral communication is an example of interaction (assuming listening is taking place) where the behavior of one person, the sender, corresponds to the behavior of the other, the receiver. Interaction can also be nonverbal. For example, a highly skilled surgical team can perform complex operations with only a minimum of verbal communication. The third important element is sentiments. These are the values, attitudes, and beliefs held by an individual. They can be both positive and negative. Also see Goodman (1986) for the development of groups.

Phases of Group Development

A second model that helps to understand groups is the group development model. According to Tuckman (1965) groups, whether formal or informal, go through certain stages of development. In the initial stage, *forming*, group members are cautious in approaching others, become familiar with each other, and begin to develop an understanding of the requirements of group members. At this stage the members are often quite dependent on the group leader. As the group begins to develop the second stage, *storming*, occurs where conflict arises among the members of the group on issues which are important to the members and they vie for power and status. In the third stage, *norming*, the group begins to define what is or is not acceptable behavior, and the group becomes organized into an effective unit. In the *performing* stage, the energy of the group members is channeled into the work, good communication occurs among the members, and they have a relaxed atmosphere of sharing. The fifth stage is either *adjourning* (the group has achieved its purpose) *or reforming* when some major change takes place in the membership of the group or in the environment of the group causing the group to be recycled through the previous four stages.

Some of the "external" factors can affect this development process. People who are physically close to each other because of the work design or who are emotionally close because of similar backgrounds are apt to interact more frequently and develop shared interests. People who interact frequently with others are likely to develop positive feelings toward each other. People with the same sentiments or with positive feelings toward each other are likely to interact more frequently. Smaller groups facilitate this interaction process.

Norms

Norms, developed in the third stage of Tuckman's group development process, are considered by Homans to be the most important element in the internal system. Norms are the informal rules of behavior shared and enforced by the group members.

Norms are sentiments group members have about what are acceptable versus unacceptable activities, interactions, and sentiments. Whenever humans interact together in organizations they are likely to form cohesive groups and develop strong norms as how their members ought to behave. Nurses and other health care employees are no exception. Norms for nursing staff might be to take care of no more than nine patients on a medical unit or two in intensive care on a given day or to check for coverage with another staff member before leaving the unit.

Schein (1970) defines two different types of norms in groups: pivotal norms where adherence to the norm is a requirement for continued membership in the group and peripheral norms where it is desirable for members to conform to them but not essential. One pivotal norm groups establish is how hard a group member should work. Norms, especially productivity norms, may conflict with the formal rules of the organization and are an important source of intragroup and intergroup conflict.

Norms (Feldman, 1984) are likely to be enforced by a group if they facilitate group survival, make predictable what behavior is expected of members, help the group avoid embarrassing interpersonal problems, or if they express central values of the group and clarify what is distinctive about the group's identity. There are progressive stages in enforcing group norms (Leavitt & Bahrami, 1988). Group members can use rational argument by presenting reasons for the norms to the deviant. If this does not work, members can use seductive techniques reminding the deviant how important the group is to the person. The next stage is attack. This can be verbal or physical and can include sabotaging the deviant's work. The final stage is ignoring the deviant. Leavitt and Bahrami suggest it is more difficult for a deviant to acquiesce to the group as these stages progress. Agreeing to rational argument is easy but agreeing after attack is very difficult. When ignored, acquiescence may be impossible because nobody listens to the deviant's surrender.

Group Roles

Norms apply to all group members while roles are specific to positions in the group. A role is a set of expected behaviors that fit together into a unified whole and relate to an individual's position with a group. Specific roles in groups include: the task leader, the maintenance or social or emotional leader, the friendly helper, and the newcomer. Roles in the group can also be divided into regular group members, deviants, and isolates as to whether they comply with the group's norms or not.

The most important role in a group is the leadership role. Leaders are appointed by the organization for most formal groups. Command groups, by definition, are led by a formal leader. Usually someone is appointed by the formal organization to head a team, committee, or task force. Leaders in informal groups emerge. Some factors contributing to emergence of leadership in small groups include the ability to accomplish group goals, group sociability, good communication skills, self-confidence, and a desire for recognition.

Roles and role behavior can lead to role ambiguity and role conflict. Several definitions are useful to understand this process. A role set is the people who share expectations of appropriate behavior for a given role. The sent role is the set of expectations which members of the role set send to the individual; the received role is the individual's perception of that sent role; and the enacted role is the way the individual actually behaves.

Role ambiguity occurs when the individual lacks clear information as to the expectations of the role set. This often leads to stress, dissatisfaction, and poor performance. Intrapersonal conflict occurs when the sent role is inconsistent with the individual's personal values, beliefs, or preferences. This can also lead to stress.

Intersender role conflict occurs when different role senders have conflicting expectations. This can occur in groups when the group's norms are in disagreement with the organization's policies, procedures and rules. For example, the organization could have a rule against not taking lunch hours but group members might expect nurses to give up lunch time when during busy periods. This situation would lead to role conflict as different role senders—the organization and the group—have different expectations about what is correct behavior. Usually the individual is more likely to be influenced by the norms of a cohesive group than the edicts of an organization.

Interrole conflict occurs when there are incompatible demands from different roles, when role behavior acceptable in one role setting, such as in an informal group, is not compatible with role behavior acceptable, for example, to the formal organization.

Status

Status is the social ranking of individuals relative to others in a group because of the position they occupy in the group. Status often comes from factors the group values the most such as achievement, personal characteristics, the ability to control rewards, or the ability to control information. But level of education, age, or social class do not necessarily lead to high status within a group; rather status is usually enjoyed by members who most conform to group norms. Higher status members often have more influence than lower status members in group decisions. Status incongruence occurs when the factors contributing to group status are not congruent, for example, when a younger less experienced person is appointed as the group leader. New nursing graduates have experienced this incongruence when they have been assigned to supervise experienced nursing assistants. Status incongruence can have a disruptive impact on a group.

Communication in Groups

Groups serve as important channels of communication in organizations. The group serves to disseminate information in the organization. Other group members are often the source of information about what is going on in the organization. Groups that have gone through the stages of development will achieve mutual acceptance and its group members will communicate openly with one another. This will lead to increased confidence and even more interaction within the group. Competition in a group, however, can lead to less communication. Important leadership roles are gate keeping, attempting to keep communication channels open, facilitating the participation of all group members, and suggesting procedures for discussing group problems.

GROUP CONSEQUENCES

Behavior in groups is purposeful and rational to the group members even though it might not seem so to outsiders. There are several consequences to group behavior: cohesiveness, conformity, productivity; member satisfaction; and conflict. These factors are highly interrelated but will be discussed separately.

Cohesiveness, Conformity, and Productivity

Cohesiveness is the degree to which the members are attracted to the group. It is the "glue" holding the group members together. It includes how much the group members enjoy participating in the group and how much they are willing to contribute to the group. Cohesiveness is related to homogeneity of interests, values, sentiments and background factors. Several propositions on group interaction and cohesiveness are shown in Table 17–1.

Cohesive groups are more likely to develop where there are shared values and beliefs, where individuals have similar goals and tasks, where individuals have to interact together to achieve these tasks, where there is proximity in both time and distance (ie, group members work in the same unit and on the same shift), and where group members have specific needs that can be satisfied by the group. Groups in these situations are likely to develop strong norms that influence the behavior of group members through enforcement by the group.

One of the background or external factors influencing a group's internal system and its level of cohesiveness is the formal reward system. If group members have equal treatment, similar pay, and similar jobs, especially where their jobs require interaction among the members, the group will tend to be more cohesive just as unequal treatment, unequal pay, different jobs and little job interaction will lead to lower group cohesion. Characteristics of the group members will also influence whether a group becomes cohesive. Similarities in educational experiences, social class, sex, age, and ethnicity that lead to similar sentiments will strengthen group cohesiveness.

Cohesiveness is related to social pressure and conformity. Highly cohesive groups can demand and enforce conformity to its norms regardless of their practicality or effectiveness. This makes it more difficult for the administrator to influence the staff. An example in nursing is the value placed on technical skill and "doing" and less value on using interpersonal skills to teach patient self-care (eg, home care for a colostomy).

Groups establish norms of how hard members should work. In highly cohesive groups where powerful norms are established on how hard members should work there will be uniformity among group members' productivity. When cohesiveness is low, wide differences can exist in employees' productivity. Groups can restrict productivity especially when they oppose the organization's leaders.

Groups can affect absenteeism and turnover. Groups with high levels of cohesiveness exhibit lower turnover and absenteeism than groups with low levels of cohesiveness. Cohesiveness influences member satisfaction and intragroup and intergroup conflict. Cohesiveness can also lead to a phenomenon called "group think," which is discussed later.

TABLE 17-1. PROPOSITIONS ON GROUP INTERACTION AND COHESIVENESS

The greater the opportunity/requirement for interaction, the greater the likelihood of interaction occurring (Homans, 1950, 1961).

The more frequent the interaction among people, the greater the likelihood of their developing positive feelings for one another (Homans, 1950, 1961).

The greater the positive feelings among people, the more frequently they will interact (Homans, 1950, 1961).

The more frequent the interactions required by the job, the more likely that social relationships and behavior will develop along with task relationships and behavior (Homans, 1950, 1961).

The more attractive the group, the more cohesive it will be (Festinger, Schacter, & Black, 1950).

The more cohesive the group, the more influence it has on its members. The less certain and clear a group's norms and standards are, the less control it will have over its members (Festinger, Schacter, & Black, 1950; Homans, 1961).

The greater the similarity in member attitudes and values brought to the group, the greater the likelihood of cohesion in a group (Homans, 1961).

Group cohesion will be increased by the existence of a superordinate goal(s) (an overarching goal to which group members subscribe) subscribed to by the members (Sherif, 1967).

Group cohesion will be increased by the perceived existence of a common enemy (Blake & Mouton, 1961).

Group cohesion will be increased by success in achieving the group's goals (Sherif & Sherif, 1953).

Group cohesion is increased in proportion to the status of the group relative to other groups in the system (Cartwright & Zander, 1968).

Group cohesion will be increased when there is low frequency of required external interactions (Homans, 1950).

The more easily and frequently member differences are settled in a way satisfactory to all members, the greater will be group cohesion (Deutsch, 1968).

Group cohesion will increase under conditions of abundant resources.

The more cohesive the group, the more similar will be the output of individual members (Homans, 1950).

The more cohesive the group, the more it will try to enforce compliance with its norms about productivity.

The greater the cohesion of the group, the higher productivity will be if the group supports the organization's goals, and the lower productivity will be if the group resists the organization's goals (Zaleznik, Christensen, & Roethlisberger, 1958).

A cohesive group will by definition have a high overall level of satisfaction.

Source: Cohen AR, Fink SL, Gadon H, Willits RD. Effective Behavior in Organizations. Homewood, IL, Irwin, 1988: 100–112

Member Need Satisfaction

The reasons for joining groups vary from individual to individual but, basically, individuals join groups to satisfy their needs. Generally groups are able to satisfy the five general needs of affiliation, security, esteem, reality testing, and task accomplishment.

Groups provide an opportunity to:

1. Share experiences
2. Develop a sense of belonging or identity
3. Relate to others

4. Avoid being lonely
5. Reduce boredom
6. Lesson tensions by venting emotions
7. State our opinions
8. Test our assumptions about reality

Groups can also help us perform tasks, especially organizational tasks which we cannot perform alone or provide information necessary for task accomplishment. Groups provide us with security and social support. The group can be used to protect members from outside forces through the "safety of numbers." Unfortunately, groups can also be tyrannical toward members and ruthless toward nonmembers and contribute to conflict in the organization.

Intragroup Conflict

Intragroup conflict can occur when group norms or standards are violated or changed. For example, in an organization undergoing decentraliztion, head nurses might be expected to change in various ways, such as not taking patient care assignments or wearing a lab coat over street clothes. This change might conflict with group norms, which require that all staff give patient care, and could stimulate internal conflict for head nurses who have perceived themselves as caregivers. Another potential source of intragroup conflict with which a nurse manager must deal is the introduction of new members into a cohesive group by making sure that the new member is accepted and made part of the group.

Intergroup Conflict

Intergroup conflict arises between groups having differing goals, where one group's goals can only be achieved at the expense of another group's goals (win–lose competition) or where one of the parties has the ability to interfere with the attainment of goals by the other group (Klein & Ritti, 1984; Organ & Bateman, 1986). These types of conflicts can range from small day-to-day ones to broader issues. For example, a smaller day-to-day issue might be when the radiology department wants patients sent to x-ray in gowns without metal snaps on the sleeve because the snaps show on the film. Nursing staff prefer these snaps because they make it easier to change gowns on patients receiving intravenous fluids. Neither side wants the bother of changing gowns prior to x-rays and believes the other should do this task. A broader issue might be that the administration's goal is to control salary expenses while nursing's goal is to upgrade staffing with a resultant increase in salary costs. The conflict between unions and management is another example.

Intergroup conflict can occur when there is competition between groups for limited resources, group members have different values and norms, they are dependent on each other (especially where there is asymmetric dependency by a high status group on members from low status groups such as physicians and nurses), and when there are overlapping task assignments so it is difficult to determine responsibility for a task (credit or blame). Intergroup conflict affects group cohesiveness. Groups which experience winning increase in cohesiveness. The "we" feeling increases when groups achieve their goals (Sherif, 1967). Winning can lead to complacency, however, if a group wins frequently. Losing in intergroup conflict decreases cohesiveness, especially if a group loses frequently, and leads to a challenge or change in leadership— a "fire the losing manager syndrome."

Intraorganizational Conflict

Groups or departments which are differentiated from each other due to differences in structure, time orientation, interpersonal orientation, or subenvironment orientation can be in conflict (Lawrence & Lorsch, 1967). For example, some units in hospitals such as dietetics and housekeeping tend to have mechanistic structures, financial services and accounting have bureaucratic structures while nursing has a professional structure. Psychiatric units have long-time orientations while the emergency room has a very short-time orientation. Some hospital units, such as personnel or public relations, have strong interpersonal orientations while laboratories have strong task orientations. Administrative units such as finance, have an orientation toward the economic environment while units such as radiology have a more technical or scientific subenvironment orientation. The more differentiated these groups or departments are the greater the potential for conflict, especially if they must work together to perform their tasks and if one unit is highly dependent on the other unit. Similarly, there may be conflicts between those units providing support services and those units providing patient care.

GROUP DECISION MAKING

There are both advantages and disadvantages in using groups for decision making. Characteristics of the problem and the characteristics of the people influence group effectiveness (Maier, 1967). The greater the complexity of the problem the more likely that a group, rather than one individual, has the resources to deal with the problem. Groups possess greater knowledge and information than any of their members. Groups offer more approaches to solve a problem. Rather than suffering from tunnel vision as some individuals do, groups have a greater variety of training and experiences and approach problems from more points of view. Where an individual might continue using a particular approach, a group of individuals is more likely to try several approaches. Groups are more effective when there is task interdependency. For example, problems crossing group boundaries or presenting procedural change need input from the various departments involved. Participation in problem solving also increases acceptance and understanding of a group's decisions.

Group decision making also has disadvantages including goal displacement, extra time and resources, and possible conflict among members. Social loafing and free riding can occur in groups (Harkins, Latane, & Williams, 1980). Social loafing refers to the tendency for individuals to produce below their maximum capabilities in a group. Free riding occurs when a loafer receives the full benefits of group membership. Groups can also be influenced by group think and risky shift, concepts to be discussed later.

When to Use Groups for Decision Making

Vroom and Yetton have developed a model for deciding whether to use a group for decision making (see Vroom & Jago, 1988). This model is shown in Figure 17–2 along with the important questions that need to be answered in determining which leadership styles are feasible. These feasible leadership strategies are shown in Table 17–2.

DECISION TREE

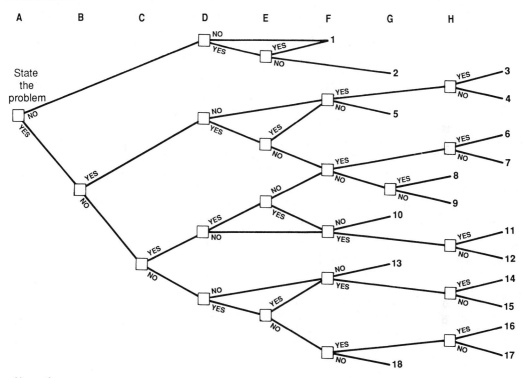

Alternatives

The feasible set is shown for each problem type for group (G) and individual (I) problems:

1. G: AI, AII, CI, CII, GII
   I: AI, DI, AII, CI, GI
2. G: GII
   I: DI, GI
3. G: AI, AII, CI, CII, GII
   I: AI, DI, AII, CI, GI
4. G: AI, AII, CI, CII, GII
   I: AI, AII, CI, GII
5. G: AI, AII, CI, CII
   I: AI, AII, CI
6. G: GII
   I: DI, GI
7. G: GII
   I: GI
8. G: CII
   I: CI, GI
9. G: CI, CII
   I: CI, GI
10. G: AII, CI, CII
    I: AII, CI
11. G: AII, CI, CII, GII
    I: DI, AII, CI, GI
12. G: AII, CI, CII, GII
    I: AII, CI, GI
13. G: CII
    I: CI
14. G: CII, GII, DII
    I: DI, CI, GI
15. G: CII, GII
    I: CI, GI
16. G: GII, DII
    I: DI, GI
17. G: GII
    I: GI
18. G: CII
    I: CI, GI

Figure 17–2. Model for Determining What Decisions to Delegate and to Whom *(Source: From Vroom VH, Jago AG. Decision making as a social process: Normative and descriptive models of leader behavior.* Decision Sciences. *5: 743, 1974)*

TABLE 17-2. DEFINITIONS OF COURSES OF ACTION IN DECIDING WHEN TO DELEGATE AND TO WHOM

For Individual Problems

AI   You solve the problem or make the decision yourself using information available to you at that time.

AII You obtain any necessary information from the subordinate, then decide on the solution yourself. You may or may not tell the subordinate what the problem is in getting the information from him or her. The role played by your subordinate in making the decision is one of providing specific information you request, rather than generating or evaluating alternative solutions.

CI   You share the problem with the relevant subordinate, getting his or her ideas and suggestions. Then you make the decision. This decision may or may not reflect your subordinate's influence.

GI   You share the problem with one of your subordinates and together you analyze the problem and arrive at a satisfactory solution in an atmosphere of free and open exchange of information and ideas. You both contribute to the resolution of the problem, with the relative contribution of each depending on knowledge rather than formal authority.

DI   You delegate the problem to one of your subordinates, providing him or her with any relevant information you possess, but giving him or her responsibility for solving the problem alone. Any solution the subordinate reaches will receive your support.

For Group Problems

AI   You solve the problem or make the decision yourself using information available to you at that time.

AII You obtain any necessary information from subordinates, then decide on the solution to the problem yourself. You may or may not tell subordinates what the problem is in getting the information from them. The role played by your subordinates in making the decision is one of providing specific information you request, rather than generating or evaluating solutions.

CI   You share the problem with the relevant subordinates individually, getting their ideas and suggestions without bringing them together as a group. Then you make the decision. This decision may or may not reflect your subordinates' influence.

CII You share the problem with your subordinates in a group meeting. In this meeting you obtain their ideas and suggestions. Then you make the decision, which may or may not reflect your subordinates' influence.

GII You share the problem with your subordinates as a group. Together you generate and evaluate alternatives and attempt to reach agreement on a solution. Your role is much like that of a chairperson, coordinating the discussion, keeping it focused on the problem, and making sure the critical issues are discussed. You do not try to influence the group to adopt "your" solution and are willing to accept and implement any solution that has the support of the entire group.

DII You delegate the problem to a group of subordinates in which you do not participate. You provide them with any relevant information you possess, and give them authority to solve the problem as a group. Any solution they reach will receive your support.

Source: Vroom VH, Jago AG. Decision making as a social process: Normative and descriptive models of leader behavior, Decision Sciences, 5, *743, 1974*

The decision of which leadership style to use from this feasible set would depend on the answers to these questions: is there sufficient time for the group to make the decision, will the costs of group resources used to make the decision be more or less than the benefits from a possible improvement in the quality of the decision or the benefits from the acceptance of the decision, and can it be used as an investment in developing the group's decision making skills for the future?

Generally groups should be used for decision making when there is time for a group decision but with a deadline, the problem is complex or unstructured, the group shares the organization's goals, there is need for acceptance of the decision (or at least understanding of the decision) to implement it properly and the process will not lead to unacceptable conflict among group members.

Types of Decision-Making Groups

There are several different types of decision making in groups. These include: ordinary interacting groups, nominal group technique, brainstorming groups, statistical aggregation, and the Delphi technique (Murninghan, 1981; Levine & Moreland, 1990). The latter four techniques have been developed to overcome the disadvantages of ordinary group decision making.

Ordinary interacting groups usually begin with the group leader stating the problem followed by an open, unstructured discussion. Normally the final decision is made by consensus, but the decision could also be by vote of the majority, by vote of a significant minority, by an expert, by the leader, or by some authority figure after the group makes a recommendation. Interacting groups enhance the cohesiveness and esprit de corps among group members. Participants are able to build strong social ties and there will be commitment to the solution decided by the group. These groups often are affected by domination of one or a few members and are very dependent on the skills of the group leader. Often excessive time is spent dealing with social or emotional relationships reducing the time spent on the problem and making it difficult to come to a consensus.

Ordinary groups are most effective when they have five or seven members. If a group becomes too large, participation rates drop, while a group smaller than five might not have adequate resources to make decisions. The composition of the group also determines a group's effectiveness. Heterogeneous groups will have more resources but be harder to lead while homogeneous groups will have fewer resources to draw on and be more likely to be influenced by group think.

Two techniques that allow the input from various individuals while avoiding some of the disadvantages of ordinary groups are the nominal group technique (NGT) and the Delphi technique. The nominal group technique, developed by Van de Ven and Delbecq (1974), is a structured group decision-making process. The format consists of individuals first generating their ideas independently and silently on a task or problem in writing. Then individuals present their ideas in a round-robin procedure with the ideas recorded in summary fashion on a blackboard or flip chart. After all the ideas have been presented they are discussed for clarification purposes and then members are asked to vote for the alternatives they prefer using the group's decision rule.

In the Delphi technique the participants are physically separated and do not meet face to face. Judgments on a particular topic are systematically gathered and collated through a set of carefully designed sequential questionnaires interspersed with a summary of information and opinions derived from previous questionnaires. The process can include many iterations but normally does not exceed three. This technique relies on the input of experts who are widely dispersed geographically. It often is used to make predictions about the future based on current scientific knowledge. This technique is useful when expert opinions are needed and the experts are geographically separated but it is costly and time consuming.

On fact finding problems with no known solution, the NGT and the Delphi technique are superior to the ordinary group technique; group member satisfaction is highest in the NGT (Van de Ven & Delbecq, 1974). Both the NGT and the Delphi technique keep particular members from dominating the discussion and allow participants ample opportunity to think through ideas independently.

Like the Delphi technique, statistical aggregation does not require a group meeting. Individuals are polled regarding a specific problem and their responses are tallied. It is a very efficient technique but is limited to a narrow range of problems, those for which a quantifiable answer can be readily obtained. One disadvantage is that there is no opportunity for group members to strengthen their interpersonal ties.

In brainstorming, people are encouraged to generate as many diverse ideas as possible without consideration of their practicality or feasibility. A premium is placed on generating lots of ideas as fast as possible and on coming up with unusual ideas. In addition, and most important, members do not critique the ideas as they are proposed. Evaluation takes place after all the ideas have been generated. Members are encouraged to "piggyback" on each other's ideas. These sessions are very enjoyable, but are often less successful because the members violate the three rules, and as a result, the meetings shift to the ordinary interacting group format. The NGT can be used to overcome some of the problems of the brainstorming technique but is not as exciting to the participants.

Skunk Works
Another type of group found to be effective to develop innovative ideas is called "skunk works" (Peters & Waterman, 1982). A small group of individuals, often 8–10 "zealots," go off in a corner, out of sight of management, and develop some new product or process. They are headed by a champion, often a technical genius who wants to prove that the rest of the organization is wrong. They are usually a small group of highly committed members who communicate well with each other. These groups are often more effective than many larger groups.

Risky Shift and Group Think
Group decision making can be affected by the phenomena of risky shift and group think. Risky shift is when groups make more risky decisions than an individual acting alone (Napier & Gershenfeld, 1985). Several factors play a role in this process. Individuals who lack information about alternatives may choose to select a less risky decision but after group discussion of the various alternatives may feel more comfortable

about a less secure alternative and agree to that decision. This could be due to persuasive argumentation from others and social comparison (Levine & Moreland, 1990). The group setting also allows for diffusion of responsibility. If something does go wrong with the decision, others can also be assessed the blame or risk. In addition, leaders may be greater risk takers than individuals and there may be a social value attached to risk taking. A nursing administrator should be aware of this phenomenon but risky shift may be less of a problem in health care institutions because society values risk taking less where health is concerned.

The second phenomenon affecting group decision making and related to risky shift is group think. Group think occurs when group members are highly attracted to a group and want to remain so much a part of the group that they tend to think alike, want to achieve consensus and harmony, and fail to engage in critical thinking. The symptoms of group think include:

1. Illusion of invulnerability
2. Shared stereotypes
3. Rationalization
4. Illusion of morality
5. Self censorship
6. Illusion of unanimity
7. Direct pressure on deviants
8. Mind guarding

These symptoms of group think interfere with critical thinking and can make group decision making ineffective. Janis has suggested several approaches to prevent group think. These are also shown in Table 17–3.

Dialectical Inquiry

Another technique resulting in less group think includes the use of dialectical inquiry. Dialectical inquiry uses a formal debate between advocates of a plan and others who propose a counterplan. This technique formalizes conflict by allowing disagreement while reducing some of the emotional aspects of conflict, and encourages the exploration of alternative solutions (Cosier & Schwenk, 1990). Because it is emotionally neutral, this approach can be used regardless of participants' feelings. The benefits from this method come from the presentation and debate of the basic assumptions underlying proposed courses of action. False or misleading assumptions become apparent during the debate. The process promotes better understanding of problems and leads to higher levels of confidence in decisions. The method also has some drawbacks. It can lead to an emphasis on who won the debate rather than what the best decision is. It can also lead to compromise. It tends to work best when making decisions with high uncertainty and low information availability.

These various techniques can help reduce group think in cohesive groups. It is important for administrators to understand that conflict is not always dysfunctional and dissent must be allowed if good decisions are to be made.

TABLE 17-3. GROUP THINK

Group think occurs in *cohesive groups,* those in which members have strong, positive feelings toward their group and are highly motivated to remain part of that group. In such groups, there is a strong sense of *solidarity,* which makes the group strive for agreement and often prevents it from seriously considering problems or possible consequences. Members of cohesive groups often simply fail to use *critical thinking.*

Major Symptoms of Group Think	
Illusion of invulnerability	This allows the group to feel complacent and secure in any decision it might make.
Shared stereotypes	The strong "we" versus "they" feeling of a cohesive group toward an adversary group tends to foster this symptom of group think.
Rationalization	A tightly knit group begins to pool its resources to devise certain rationalizations that help group members maintain their self-respect.
Illusion of morality	A belief in its own morality that allows a group to disregard any ethical or moral objections to its behavior.
Self-censorship	The tendency of individual members to restrict any doubts they might have.
Illusion of unanimity	Members do not express their doubts, even if they have them, because they assume that everyone else's silence implies agreement, and they are reluctant to disrupt the unity of the group.
Direct pressure	When a deviant member does speak out in a group—and this happens rarely—direct pressure is applied to the dissenting member; he(she) is reminded that the group's aim is agreement, not argument.
Mind-guarding	This is the action of protecting the group from disturbing ideas or opinions.

continued

TEAMS AND TEAM BUILDING

Teams are groups established to perform certain organizational tasks requiring the diverse skills, and the interaction and cooperation of the team members to achieve these tasks. Not all work groups are teams. For example, co-acting groups or competing groups are not teams. In co-acting groups the members perform their tasks independently of each other. The members might perform similar individual tasks which do not require the individuals performing these tasks to interact or cooperate with each other. In competing groups the members are in competition with each other to perform their tasks. In competing groups members compete for recognition or compete with other group members to obtain the resources to accomplish their individual tasks.

Many of the same processes occur in groups whether they are teams, informal groups, command groups, task forces, or committees. There are a few critical differences in these groups. Task forces and committees tend to make recommendations while teams have command or line authority to perform organizational tasks and to make specific decisions. There are also important differences between task forces and standing committees. Task forces are temporary and usually are disbanded once they

TABLE 17-3. Continued

Preventing Group Think

1. The leader of a policy-forming group should assign the role of critical evaluator to each member, encouraging the group to give high priority to airing objections and doubts. This practice needs to be reinforced by the leader's acceptance of criticism of his or her own judgments in order to discourage the members from soft-pedaling their disagreements.

2. The leaders in an organization's hierarchy, when assigning a policy-planning mission to a group, should be impartial instead of stating preferences and expectations at the outset.

3. The organization should routinely follow the administrative practice of setting up several independent policy-planning and evaluation groups to work on the same policy question, each carrying out its deliberations under a different leader.

4. The group should from time to time divide into two or more subgroups to meet separately, under different chairpersons and then come together to hammer out their differences.

5. Each member of the policy-making group should discuss periodically the group's deliberations with trusted associates in his or her own unit of the organization and report back their reactions.

6. One or more outside experts or qualified colleagues within the organization who are not core members of the policy-making group should be invited to each meeting on a staggered basis and should be encouraged to challenge the views of the core members.

7. At every meeting devoted to evaluating policy alternatives, at least one member should be assigned the role of devil's advocate.

8. Whenever a policy issue involves relations with a rival group time should be spent surveying all warning signals from the rivals and constructing alternative scenarios of the rivals' intentions.

9. After reaching a preliminary consensus about what seems to be the best policy alternative, the policy-making group should hold a 'second chance' meeting at which every member is expected to express as vividly as they can all their residual doubts and to rethink the entire issue before making a definitive choice.

Source: Janis, IL. Groupthink: Psychological Studies of Policy Decisions and Fiascos, *2nd ed. Boston, Houghton Mifflin, 1982: 262–271*

achieve their goals. Task forces are usually formed to analyze special nonrecurring problems and membership is usually based on knowledge and expertise while committees are more permanent in nature and deal with re-occurring problems. Membership on committees is usually based on organizational position and role while membership of a team depends on the specific skills the individual can offer to accomplish the team's task. The management of task forces and committees is discussed in more depth later in this chapter.

Teams can be lateral, vertical, or diagonal in member composition. That is, they can be composed of members from the same work group (eg, surgical intensive care), from different levels in the organization (eg, all RNs) or from different departments in the organization (eg, therapy team). They can have both a short life or exist over long periods of time. Some of the specific difficulties teams experience (as do other types of groups such as task forces and committees) include goal confusion, hidden agendas, territoriality, disagreement over procedures, competition among team members, intragroup conflict, intergroup conflict, and a nonsupportive climate. Four conditions are necessary for the development of effective teams: (1) the group must have mutually agreed objectives; (2) group members must depend on each other's experiences, abilities, and commitment; (3) group members must be committed to team effort; and (4) the group must be accountable as a unit within the organization (Patten, 1979).

Team Building

Team building is a popular organizational change and development (OD) technique which can be used to overcome some of these specific problems of teams. Wilson (1985) suggests some specific exercises to resolve conflicts in groups, to release tensions, to promote trust and self-disclosure, and to promote cohesion among group members (See Table 17–4).

These team building techniques can be used to improve performance of the team and also to overcome one of the most important difficulties in managing teams (and task forces) in organizations which is that teams are expected to perform at a high level immediately and usually do not have time to go through the normal stages of group development. Teams, to be effective like any other group, must go through the development (form, storm, norm, and perform) very quickly; these activities can help. These techniques can also be used to intervene in traditional work groups which are experiencing problems.

The first stage in team building is diagnosis. In this stage questions are asked about the group's climate including its mission and goals, procedures and decision-making style, group members' roles, interpersonal relationships including the members' feelings about each other, and the group's relations with other groups.

Diagnosis requires answering certain questions about the group's goals, roles, procedures, intragroup and intergroup relations. Do the members understand and accept the group goals? Is there any goal confusion? Goal confusion occurs when the team is unsure of their goals or there is disagreement over these goals. Do the members have any hidden agenda which interfere with the group's goal attainment? Hidden agenda are the individual goals of the group members which are not shared with the group as a whole and keep the members from being committed and enthusiastic team members.

Is the leadership role being handled adequately? Does each member understand and accept his or her role in the group? How does the group make decisions? How does it handle conflict? Are conflicts dealt with through avoidance, forcing, accommodating, compromising, competing, or collaborating methods? What feelings do the members have about each other? Do they trust and respect each other? What is the relationship between the team and other teams in the organization?

Only after diagnosing team problems can efforts be taken to improve functioning. There are specific actions a team leader can take to build and maintain an effective team such as engaging in team building exercises from the sources discussed above. Survival exercises are useful for bringing the group together in an unusual setting to learn about itself, its processes, and its decision-making procedures. Survey feedback can be useful. Members respond to an anonymous survey asking questions similar to those discussed above. The results are discussed by the group and action steps are agreed on to overcome these problems. After a period of time another survey is taken to see if change has occurred and whether the process needs to be repeated. An

TABLE 17–4. A SAMPLING OF EXPERIENTIAL EXERCISES

Type of Exercise	Expected Outcome
Warm-ups	
Batting balloons	Become acquainted; move into Child Ego State
Saying "Hello" nonverbally	Prepare for self-disclosure
Saying "Hello" with crayons and paper	Become acquainted
Sharing nicknames	Become acquainted
Verbal introductions in dyads with roleplay	Become acquainted
Kinetic techniques	
Freeze tag	Awareness of the process of asking for help
Family sculpture	Awareness of one's position in the family system
Breaking into the circle	Awareness of being isolated
Movement Techniques	
Fantasies	Awareness of one's immediate feelings
Exploring space	Letting "go" to explore unknown space
Dyad sculpturing	Experiencing the feeling of controlling others or being controlled
Passing on a movement	Experiencing directing or controlling others
Lifting and rocking a member	Experiencing giving up control to others
Improvisation	Awareness of one's immediate feelings
Protective techniques	
Bataca swords	Safe expression of anger
Body bag/punching bag; pillows	Safe expression of anger
Lifting and rocking a member	Reduction of tension
Parachute toss	Reduction of tension
Behavioral rehearsal	
Roleplaying	Increasing repertoire of possible responses to situations
Sociodrama	Expand repertoire of role performance
Psychodrama	Explore individual intrapsychic phenomena within one's role
Group building	
Verbal exchanges in dyads	Increase group cohesion
New games	Increase group cohesion
"Spider web" and yarn	Increase group cohesion
Group mural, collage, poem	Increase group cohesion
Blind walk	Promote trust and self-disclosure
Passing a member around	Promote trust

Wilson M. *Group theory/process for nursing practice,* Bowie, MD: Brady Communications Company, Inc. (Prentice-Hall), 1985

outside intervention specialist can be brought in to conduct team building sessions which can include holding a confrontation meeting to identify problems.

MANAGING TASK FORCES

Task forces are groups established to work on problems or projects that cannot be easily handled by the organization through its normal activities. Often task forces must deal with problems crossing departmental boundaries. There are a few critical differences between task forces and other groups. For example, the members of a task force have less time to build relationships among each other, and, since they are temporary in nature, the need for long-term positive relationships might be lacking. The fact a task force has been formed can represent a criticism of the regular organization leading to tensions among task force members and between a task force and other units in the organization. The various members of a task force usually come from different parts of the organization and, therefore, have different values, goals, and viewpoints.

There are specific actions a leader can take to increase task force effectiveness. Many of these actions are also useful for conducting normal committee meetings. According to Ware (1983), these can be grouped into four categories:

1. Preparation prior to the first meeting
2. Conducting the first meeting
3. Managing subsequent meetings and subgroups
4. Completion of the task force's report

In addition to these categories general guidelines for conducting meetings and the leadership of meetings will also be presented.

Preparation Prior to the First Meeting
Prior to the task force's first meeting the leader must determine the objectives of the task force, its membership, the task completion date, how often and to whom the task force would report while working on the project, and the group's authority including the task force's budget, availability of information, and ability to make decisions. The task force leader should be in contact with the administrators who commissioned it so its mission can be clarified. One administrator may attend the first meeting to give the task force its "charge" including anticipated outcomes and deadlines for completion.

Task force members should be selected on the basis of their knowledge, skills and personal interest in the task, their time available to work on the task, and their organizational credibility. They should also be selected on the basis of their interpersonal skills. Those who enjoy group activities and will not dominate the group's efforts are especially good members.

Conducting the First Meeting
The goal of the first meeting is to come to a common understanding of the group's task and to define the group's working procedures and relationships. Task forces must rely on the general norms of the organization to function. The task force leader should legitimize the representative nature of participation on a task force and encourage members to discuss the task force's process with other members of the organization.

During the first meeting everyone should be encouraged to participate. The leader should be careful to be neutral and should prevent a premature consensus. Working procedures and relationships among the various members, subgroups, and the rest of the organization need to be established. The frequency and nature of full task force meetings and the number of subgroups must be determined. Ground rules for communicating must be established along with norms for decision making and conflict resolution.

General Guidelines for Conducting Meetings

In order to conduct a successful meeting, the leader should spend time thinking about the purpose of the meeting, preparing an agenda, determining who should attend, making assignments prior to group meetings including determining who should take minutes, and selecting an appropriate time and place for the meeting. An agenda should be prepared ahead of time and sent to the participants. The ideal committee size is between five to seven persons. Having too few members or too many can limit the effectiveness of a committee or task force. It is helpful if members have similar status, as large status differences among committee members can impede communication among group members.

Meetings should be held where interruptions can be controlled and at a time when there is some natural time limit to the meeting such as late in the morning or afternoon where lunch or dinner make natural time barriers. In addition, meetings should start and finish on time. Starting late positively reinforces latecomers while punishing those arriving on time or early. Locking the door at the appointed time or ''fining'' latecomers can discourage such behavior.

Leadership of Meetings

A leader can play an effective role in conducting meetings by insuring that the twelve leadership roles shown in Table 17–5 are present. Even though a leader's personality and value systems might make it difficult to perform all of these leadership roles, the leader is still responsible to make sure that these various tasks and group relations functions do occur, even if they are performed by some other members.

A leader can also increase effectiveness by not letting one person dominate the discussion, by separating idea generation from its evaluation, by encouraging members to refine and develop the ideas of others (a key to the success of brainstorming), by recording problems, ideas, solutions on a blackboard or flip chart, by frequently summarizing information and the group's progress to date and encouraging further discussions, and by bringing disagreements out into the open where they may be reconciled. The leader is also responsible for drawing out the members' hidden agenda (personal needs individuals bring to a group which are not disclosed to the group but influence the members' contributions to the group) so these do not interfere with group decision making.

Moore (1988) provides some summary guidelines for leading group discussions:

- Set a warm, accepting, and nonthreatening climate.
- Define all terms and concepts.
- Foster cooperation in the group.
- Establish group goals and identify major objectives.
- Allocate time for all decision-making steps.

TABLE 17-5. THE TWO MAJOR TYPES OF FUNCTIONS

Every group leader has two major functions. They are: (1) TASK functions and (2) GROUP RELA-TIONS functions.*

The purpose of the TASK functions is to keep the group working on the task or project at hand, ie, getting the group work done.

The purpose of the GROUP RELATIONS functions is to maintain constructive group relations among the members and to keep diverse individuals working together as a team. This means dealing with individual and group feelings and attitudes which may prevent the progress of the group toward its goals.

TASK FUNCTIONS

INITIATING: Proposing tasks or goals; defining a group problem; suggesting a procedure or ideas for solving a problem.

INFORMATION OR OPINION SEEKING: Requesting facts; seeking relevant information about group concerns; asking for suggestions or ideas.

INFORMATION OR OPINION GIVING: Stating a belief; providing relevant information about group concerns; giving suggestions or ideas.

CLARIFYING: Elaborating, interpreting, or reflecting ideas and suggestions; clearing up confusions; indicating alternatives and issues before the group; giving examples.

SUMMARIZING: Pulling together related ideas; restating suggestions after group has discussed them; offering a decision or conclusion for the group to accept or reject.

CONSENSUS TESTING: Sending up "trial balloons" to see if group is nearing a conclusion; checking with group to see how much agreement has been reached.

GROUP RELATIONS FUNCTIONS

ENCOURAGING: Being friendly, warm, and responsive to others; accepting others and their contributions; regarding others by giving them an opportunity for recognition.

EXPRESSING GROUP FEELINGS: Sensing feeling, mood, relationships within the group; sharing one's own feelings with other members.

HARMONIZING: Attempting to reconcile disagreements; reducing tension; getting people to explore their differences.

MODIFYING: When his own idea or status is involved in a conflict, offering to modify his own position; admitting error; disciplining oneself to maintain group cohesion.

GATE-KEEPING: Attempting to keep communication channels open; facilitating the participation of others; suggesting procedures for sharing opportunity to discuss group problems.

EVALUATING: Evaluating group functioning and production; expressing standards for group to achieve; measuring results; evaluating degree of group commitment.

Source: Benne K, Sheats P. Functional role of group members, Journal of Social Issues. 4:2, 41–49, 1948

- Lead the discussion so that all members have an opportunity to contribute.
- Help integrate the material and ideas that have been generated.
- Help group members identify the implications of the ideas.
- Help the group evaluate the quality of the discussion.

Managing Subsequent Meetings and Subgroups

In running a task force, especially when several subgroups are formed, the leader should hold full task force meetings often enough to keep all members informed of the group's progress. Unless a task force is small (five to seven persons), subgroups are mandatory. The leader must not be aligned too closely with one position or subgroup too early in the deliberations. Interim project deadlines should be established and the task force and subgroups held to these deadlines. The leader must be sensitive to the conflicting loyalties created by belonging to a task force. One of the leader's most important roles is to communicate information to task force members and to the rest of the organization.

Completion of the Task Force's Report

In bringing a project to completion, a written report summarizing the findings and recommendations to the commissioning administrators must be prepared. Drafts of this report should be shared with the full task force prior to presentation to administrators. A two-meeting approach should be used to present the task force's report to administrators. The first meeting is to present the report without making any decisions on the report. This gives a chance for administrators to read and respond to the report before having to make a decision on it. It is especially important for the task force leader to personally brief key administrators prior to presentation of the report to reduce defensive reactions to the report.

SUMMARY

Groups influence organizational success so it is important for nursing administrators to understand the nature of groups and group processes, and what they can do to influence group effectiveness.

The types of groups important in nursing administration include formal groups such as command groups, task groups (or teams), task forces and committees, and informal organizational groups. A group is two or more individuals who interact with each other, are psychologically aware of each other and perceive themselves as a group.

Groups' internal structures, including its norms and roles, are influenced by external factors such as tasks, technology, work design, formal administrative and reward systems, and backgrounds of the group members. Groups develop through the five stages: form, storm, norm, perform and adjourn or reform. Cohesive groups establish strong norms which influence the behavior of group members, especially in productivity. Groups help satisfy member needs of affiliation, security, esteem, reality testing, and task accomplishment.

Groups can contribute to conflict in an organization especially intergroup conflict because of different group goals or values. Groups can be effective in making decisions especially if they are small, there is time to use a group technique and member acceptance or understanding of the decision is needed.

There are several different types of decision making in groups: ordinary interacting groups, nominal group technique, brainstorming groups, statistical aggregation and the Delphi technique. The nominal group technique tends to be superior to the others because it is effective and cheap and member satisfaction is high.

Group decisions can be affected by risky shift, the tendency for groups to accept more risk than the average member, and group think, the tendency for cohesive groups to fail to engage in critical thinking. OD based team building can be effective in developing teams. Task forces can be effectively managed by a nurse administrator who understands group processes and the critical stages of task force development.

REFERENCES

Benne K, Sheats P. Functional roles of group members. *Journal of Social Issues.* 4:2, 41, 1948

Blake RR, Mouton JS. Reactions to intergroup competition under win-lose competition. *Mngmt Sci.* 420, July 1961

Cartwright D, Zander A. *Group Dynamics: Research and Theory.* New York, Harper & Row, 1968

Cohen AR, Fink SL, Gadon H, Willits RD. *Effective Behavior in Organizations.* Homewood, IL, Irwin, 1988

Cosier RA, Schwenk CR. Agreement and thinking alike: Ingredients for poor decisions. *Acad Mngmt Ex.* 4:1, 69, 1990

Deutsch M. The effects of cooperation and competition upon group process. In: Cartwright D, Zander A, eds. *Group Dynamics: Research and Theory.* New York: Harper & Row, 1968

Feldman DC. The development and enforcement of group norms. *Acad Mngmt R.* 9:47, 1984

Festinger L, Schacter S, Back K. *Social Pressures in Informal Groups: A Study of a Housing Project.* New York: Harper & Row, 1950

Goodman PS, et al. *Designing Effective Work Groups.* San Francisco, Jossey-Bass, 1986

Harkins S, Latane B, Williams L. Social loafing: allocating effort or "taking it easy," *Journal of Experimental Social Psychology.* 16:457, 1980

Homans G. *The Human Group.* New York, Harcourt, Brace, Jovanovich, 1950

Janis IL. *Groupthink: Psychological Studies of Policy Decisions and Fiascos,* 2nd ed. Boston, Houghton Mifflin, 1982

Klein SM, Ritti RR. *Understanding Organizational Behavior,* 2nd ed. Boston, Kent, 1984

Lawrence PR, Lorsch JW. Differentiation and integration in complex organizations. *Admin Sc Q.* 12:1, 1, June 1967

Leavitt HJ, Bahrami H. *Managerial Psychology,* 5th ed. Chicago, University of Chicago Press, 1988

Levine JM, Moreland RL. Progress in small group research. *Annual Review of Psychology.* 41: 585, 1990

Likert R. *New Patterns of Management.* New York, McGraw-Hill Book Book Co, 1961

Maier NRF. Assets and liabilities in group problem solving: The need for an integrative function. *Psychological Review.* 74:4, 239, 1967

Murninghan, K. Group decision: What strategies to use? *Management Review.* 70:55, 1981

Napier RW, Gershenfeld MK. *Groups: Theory and Experience,* 3rd ed. Boston, Houghton Mifflin, 1985: 247–255

Organ DW, Batemen T. *Organizational Behavior,* 3rd ed. Plano, TX, Business Publications, 1986

Patten TH. Team building part 1: Designing the intervention. *Personnel,* 56:1, 11, January/February, 1979

Peters TJ, Waterman RH. *In Search of Excellence,* NY: Harper & Row, 1982

Schein EH. *Organizational Psychology,* 2nd ed. Englewood Cliffs, NJ, Prentice-Hall, 1970

Sherif M. *Group Conflict and Cooperation: Their Social Psychology.* Boston, Routledge & Kegan Paul, 1967

Sherif M, Sherif CW. *Groups in Harmony and Tension.* New York, Harper & Row, 1953

Tuckman BW. Developmental sequences in small groups. *Psychological Bulletin.* June: 384, 1965

Van de Ven AH, Delbecq AL. The effectiveness of nominal, delphi, and interacting group decision making processes. *Acad Mngmt J.* 17:4, 605, 1974

Vroom VH, Jago AG. Decision making as a social process: Normative and descriptive models of leader behavior. *Decision Sciences.* 5: 743, 1974

Vroom VH, Jago AG. *The New Leadership.* Englewood Cliffs, NJ, Prentice Hall, 1988

Ware J. Managing a task force. In: Schlesinger LA, Eccles RG, Gabarro JJ, eds. *Managing Behavior in Organizations.* New York, McGraw-Hill, 1983: 116–126

Wilson M. Group Theory/Process for Nursing Practice. Bowie, MD, Brady Communications Company, Inc. (Prentice-Hall), 1985

Zaleznik A, Christensen CR, Roethlisberger FJ. *The Motivation, Productivity and Satisfaction of Workers.* Boston, Harvard Business School, 1958

CHAPTER 18

Collective Bargaining and Labor Relations

Charles L. Joiner
Glenda S. McGaha

Key Concept List

Labor movement history
Wagner Act, as amended
Union certification process
Contract bargaining
Grievance procedures
Impasse resolution

Labor is the expenditure of physical or mental effort to make services and goods available. Employees who produce the goods and services that constitute the output of any industry are known as the labor force. Managers are those employees who have responsibility for organizing and directing the labor force to produce the industry's output. The issues impacting the relationship between the labor force and management are many, varied, and sometimes difficult to resolve to mutual satisfaction. In the United States, organizations of employees, called labor unions, originated primarily for the purposes of communicating with management about wages, hours of work, and conditions of employment. Philosophically, the labor force believed that through a process of collective bargaining, the union could facilitate communication between employees and managers to produce improvement in the labor force–manager relationship. From this relatively simple idea, labor relations began and evolved into the complex human relations challenge it is today.

   In recent years, unionization of the health care industry has accelerated. Along with this acceleration has come an increase in the impact of this movement on nursing and nursing management. This chapter will discuss collective bargaining in nursing by examining the history of unions, reviewing the history and trends in labor law, reviewing trends specific to nursing and finally, examining the role of the nursing executive in labor relations. Chief nurse executives will benefit from an understanding of these concepts regardless of the union or nonunion status of their particular facility. The issues which ultimately may result in formal organization or union representation of an employee group exist in every labor–management relationship. Effective management of this relationship from both parties will accomplish the goals of any organization with or without a union present.

HISTORY OF LABOR MOVEMENTS IN THE UNITED STATES

Although union activity can be traced back to the late eighteenth century, not until the late 1800s did activity increase to noticeable amounts in the United States. In 1886, the American Federation of Labor (AFL) was formed and later in the early 1900s, merged with the Knights of Labor from Philadelphia (Sloane and Witney, 1981). In 1905, the International Workers of the World (IWW) was formed and in 1913 the US Department of Labor was established. In spite of these events, however, union activity prior to 1930 was confined predominantly to skilled crafts and was met by strong antiunion attitudes from employers and government.

In the 1930s, spurred by federal legislation following the depression, membership in unions increased substantially from 11 million members to an estimated 14.5 million members by 1945. These members consisted mostly of blue-collar, manufacturing workers, with membership in this group peaking in 1945, at 35 percent of the work force. Since that peak, the proportion of blue-collar workers has declined steadily to today's average of less than 20 percent. Coupled with the decline of blue-collar worker participation, union organizations have attempted to organize service organizations such as those in the health care system. Although scattered evidence of unionization of health service can be found in health care industries in the early 1920s, this trend was not significantly present until the mid 1960s.

The acceleration of the labor movement in the health care industry can be attributed to several influences. First, federal legislation which established labor laws was amended in 1974 to include health care organizations. Second, health care organizations have increased dramatically in size and complexity, remaining very labor intensive with a host of employee relations problems. Third, health care institutions have become more profit oriented, forcing more management control. Finally, societal focus on civil rights issues in the 1960s and influences such as changes in family structure and the role of women have supported unionization among health care workers.

HISTORY OF LABOR MOVEMENTS IN NURSING

Hospital unionization already was on the increase before the 1974 labor law amendments. The majority of agreements existed in either government owned or investor owned hospitals already regulated by state labor laws, the National Labor Relations Act or Executive Order (1962). The percentage of health care organizations having at least one collective bargaining unit by 1973 had risen to 14.4 from 7.7 in 1967 (Gifford, 1974).

The labor movement in nursing parallels the development of unions in the total health care industry. Roots of the movement can be traced philosophically to 1893 when the American Society of Superintendents of Training Schools for Nurses was established to promote the general welfare of nursing. In 1887 the Nurses' Associated Alumnae of the United States and Canada was formed for nurses in education and service. In 1911, this association became the American Nurses Association (ANA).

In 1946, the ANA initiated the Economic Security Program to enable state associations to bargain collectively. However, the association's ability to bargain from a position of strength was hampered by the "no strike" pledge adopted at the program's beginning. In 1968, the ANA membership rescinded the "no strike" policy which cleared the way for associations representing nurses to utilize work stoppage as a tool in the bargaining process. Enactment of the 1974 labor law amendments and the change in the ANA work stoppage philosophy stimulated unionization efforts in nursing. The Service Employees International Union, the National Union of Hospital and Health Care Employees, and the Federation of Nurses and Allied Health Professionals began organizing units of registered nurses. Along with the American Nurses Association (ANA), these unions currently represent approximately 140,000 registered nurses across the nation (Rakisch, 1985). The ANA, with its state associations (SNAs) currently represents the largest number of registered nurses with some 700 outstanding contracts.

LABOR LAW HISTORY AND TRENDS
FOR HEALTH CARE INSTITUTIONS

The philosophical and procedural basis for the collective bargaining process is defined and established by several pieces of legislation known collectively as "the labor laws." The National Labor Relations Act (NLRA) is the foundation for the labor laws of the United States. The NLRA, often called the Wagner Act, was adopted in 1935 and has been amended by the Taft-Hartley Act of 1947, the Landrum-Griffin Act of 1959, and Public Law 93-360 (the Health Care Amendments) in 1974.

The Wagner Act authorized formation of the National Labor Relations Board (NLRB) to administer the provisions of the act. The NLRB monitors procedures in the negotiation process between labor and management. The monitoring functions of the NLRB foster adherence to this philosophy through the decisions rendered when labor or management conduct is protested. Instances of alleged misconduct are investigated. Case examples exist which suggest the NLRB and the courts expect both parties to be accountable for good faith bargaining, to facilitate open communication in the process, and compromise until agreement is mutually satisfying (LLR, 3115, 3135.70, 3105, 3130.6, 3143.38). The Wagner Act encompassed all institutions with impact on interstate commerce. The status of nonprofit health care institutions was left to the interpretation of the courts. Proprietary institutions and nursing homes were considered within the jurisdiction of the act. Since by definition governments are not employers, federal, state, and municipal hospitals were specifically exempted from the jurisdiction of the Act (Rakisch, 1973).

Under the protection of the Wagner Act, unions flourished in industries of virtually all types, creating a host of problems regarding the regulation of union and management relations. Industries had to contend with many jurisdictional strikes caused by disputes between competing unions. Some labor leaders, because of their new and unbridled power, refused to bargain in good faith (Rakisch, 1973). The Wagner Act proved to be inadequate to curb these and other abuses of the bargaining process. Therefore, in 1947 Congress passed the Labor Management Relations (Taft-Hartley) Act. It is this legislation that has become the backbone of the nation's labor laws (Rakisch, 1973).

The Taft-Hartley Act amended the Wagner Act by listing specific unfair labor practices. In addition, it specifically exempted nonprofit health care institutions from coverage under the act. The status of other types of health care institutions did not change.

With the passage of the Taft-Hartley Act in 1947, the move toward equalizing power between unions and employers continued, with a move to regulate union unfair practice toward members and employers. Further explaining specific procedures, Taft-Hartley promoted a balance of power and fair conduct between both parties. In 1974, the legal framework governing health care organizations was clarified with the deletion of the "nonprofit hospital exclusion clause." This legislation opened the door for organization of the large, service-oriented, labor intensive, health care system. Thus, the labor movement had grown to include major manufacturing, goods oriented industries and service oriented, health organizations as well.

In 1959 Taft-Hartley was amended by the Labor-Management Reporting and Disclosure (Landrum-Griffin) Act. Among its many provisions, this act requires employers, including voluntary nonprofit health care facilities, to submit a report to the US Secretary of Labor detailing the nature of any financial transactions and/or arrangements that are intended to improve or retard the unionization process (Rakisch et al, 1985). It also provides a bill of rights for union members.

Until 1967 the courts determined which proprietary health care institutions and nursing homes had an impact on interstate commerce and thus came under the NLRA on a case-by-case basis. As a result of several court cases, the NLRB in 1967 determined that proprietary health care institutions with an annual gross revenue of at least $250,000 and nursing homes, regardless of ownership, with an annual gross revenue of at least $100,000 were covered by the Act (Rakisch et al, 1985).

With voluntary hospitals comprising the largest sector of the health care industry, it was only a matter of time until they too fell under federal legislation. Their shift in status occurred in 1974, when Congress passed PL 93-360 to amend the labor relations act. These amendments, which extended the coverage of the labor laws to include all health care institutions under nonpublic ownership and control, defined a health care institution as any "hospital, convalescent hospital, health maintenance organization, health clinic, nursing home, extended care facility, or other institution devoted to the care of sick, infirm, or aged persons'' (Rakisch et al, 1985).

The 1974 amendments include unique provisions for health care organizations in contract notices, notification preceding a strike, conciliation of labor disputes, and individuals with religious convictions (Pointer & Metzger, 1975). Specifically, these unique provisions extend the notification period when a work stoppage is threatened, extend the time frame following a decision to strike to allow for patient care considerations, allow for appointment of an impartial board to help resolve disputes, exempt from membership those employees with conflicting religious beliefs and forbid organizing in areas of patient access. (Pointer & Metzger, 1975).

Most authors agree that the 1974 amendments spread unionization in health care but the impact was not as explosive as predicted (Rakisch et al, 1985). In fact, between 1960 and 1970, unionization of hospitals grew more rapidly (+ 17.7 percent) than during the 1970–1980 period (+ 5.6 percent). Federal hospitals have the highest percentage of unionization; 86 percent have at least one contract. Religious, nonprofit, nongovernmental have the lowest at 16 percent. Overall, approximately 27 percent of all hospitals were unionized by 1980 (Kaynard, 1981). In general, the larger the size, the greater the probability for unionization. Geographically, the south has remained the least likely part of the country for unionization with less than 20 percent of all hospitals having a contract in place.

MANDATORY AND VOLUNTARY SUBJECTS

The labor legislation defines subjects to be included in the bargaining process and agreement. The NLRA (sections 8,9, 1935) defines mandatory subjects to include issues of pay rate, wages, hours, conditions of employment, existing agreements, overtime, discharge, suspension, layoff, recall, seniority, discipline, promotion, demotion, assignments, and protection of health in employment. Voluntary subjects are those that may be proposed but not insisted on as a condition to an agreement. While not as easily recognizable as mandatory subjects, these include issues omitted in the mandatory definition. Examples of voluntary subjects may be clauses limiting union size or membership, secret ballot vote requirement, and exclusivity of union representation.

INSTITUTIONAL VULNERABILITY

Successful union campaigns are the result of management failure. Most often, the failure is not defined in terms of behavior of the chief executive officer, or board member but rather as failure on the part of the most immediate supervisor. Although the chief nurse executive is ultimately responsible for management failure, the most direct link to the staff nurse is the head nurse. Unions originated because of a need for the labor force to communicate more effectively with management. Institutions then, that ignore employee-supervisor relations, are vulnerable to organization by a union. Institutions with unions in place are also vulnerable to further deterioration of relations if they fail to develop sound employee relations.

Conversely, institutions that consider the benefits and conditions inherent in a typical union contract in thier policies often avoid the need for a union. If seniority, wages, promotional opportunities, and grievance processes typical of union contracts are addressed routinely by institutional policy and supported by sensitive management, institutional vulnerability is dramatically reduced or nearly absent. Specific discussion of these policies follows later in the chapter (see also Bade and Stone, 1985).

CERTIFICATION PROCESS

Before a union can represent any group of health care workers, including nurses, it must be recognized as the certified, exclusive bargaining agent for that group. The bargaining unit determination and election processes are set with the NLRB. The actual petition can be filed by a group of employees, one single employee, or an individual representing a labor organization on behalf of the employees. At least 30 percent of the employees must indicate their support of the petition. The NLRB then conducts an investigation to determine that the facts of the petition are true, the jurisdiction is present, the union is qualified, if named, and finally whether any barriers exist to an election (Pointer, 1974). Once eligibility is established, an election is conducted according to NLRB guidelines. In an approved bargaining unit, a majority of the employees will determine the outcome. If the union loses, it must wait one year before another petition can be filed.

ORGANIZING PROCESS

The process of organizing a unit is usually begun through the work of a leader from the interested union. This individual often specializes in human relations, is well acquainted with the culture in the institution, and interacts easily with the employees. He or she is sensitive and aware of the policies affecting the worker, from the worker's viewpoint. In most instances, the organizer is experienced at organizing workers and is usually trained by the union to accomplish the task successfully. Success for the union means increased revenue from dues and membership, so the goal is a financial one.

Through a process of assessment of the community and the institution, establishing employee leaders inside the institution and finally, through distribution of materials to employees, the organizer will attempt to get the required recognition and certification. Recognition may occur voluntarily, but if not, a petition for election must be filed or the union must obtain signed, authorization cards from a majority of employees to act as the bargaining agent. The union will attempt to initiate meetings away from the facility, visit employees at home, distribute publicity via handbills and advertising, and predict for employees that management will respond negatively.

BARGAINING PROCEDURES

The bargaining process, according to Metzger (1978), suggests that successful bargaining is built around:

1. Advance planning of strategies
2. Choosing one, experienced spokesperson to present management's full position
3. Authorizing the spokesperson to "make a deal" for management

These factors, along with the personalities of the negotiators, influence the outcome of the bargaining situations.

Most sources agree that the key factor in determining the eventual settlement is the makeup of the negotiating team. Much depends on the individual skills and judgments brought into the bargaining arena by the negotiators. Logically the major responsibility for negotiating a contract should be with the management executive who has day-to-day responsibility for employee relations. The chief executive responsible for nursing will most likely be involved in this process. In many instances, an immediate supervisor or department head with appropriate rapport and experience will be a member of the team. However, regardless of who negotiates, selection will follow analysis of the issues and strategic planning from top management in the organization. The chief executive officer of the institution will not usually serve on the team.

Most union negotiators are well versed in negotiating techniques. The union negotiating team may include the president of the local, vice-presidents, and employees of the institution who have been elected by their fellow workers to represent them in the negotiations. This committee is often comprised of the delegates who have been elected to handle the day-to-day problems and, therefore, are knowledgeable about grievances and arbitrations of preceding years. More often than not they are the institution's most outspoken proponents of the union. In most instances, the principal spokesperson for the union is the local president. In addition, both sides are usually represented by a specialized attorney.

Strategies for Bargaining

An institution approaching a bargaining situation must prepare for the experience seriously. Management should gather detailed information about each issue in question, employee benefits and salary levels, seniority, previous arbitrations and details of any other contracts negotiated by the union in question. Specific detailed information regarding negotiation, NLRB regulations and procedures should be reviewed in advance.

Following data gathering, decisions should be made to identify compromise issues, nonnegotiable issues and the exact limits of the proposed contract. The management team should consider the implications of work stoppage on the institution, the employees, and the union. The climate of the negotiation process will be determined by many factors. Among the most important are the personalities of the negotiators, the history of the contract, and the preparation of management (Bade & Stone, 1951).

Key Contract Clauses

Once an agreement is written it becomes a guideline for operation. Four areas or clauses are usually specifically negotiated and included as standard for any agreement. These include union security, management rights, seniority, and no-strike/ no-lockout. Union security statements protect the union's existence in the facility. Management rights statements assign specific areas of authority for management. Statements about seniority focus rewards based on length of service and are often resisted by health care organizations who want to reward employees for productivity. Finally, no-strike clauses outline conditions defining a strike situation.

CAUSES OF LABOR–MANAGEMENT PROBLEMS

The fundamental differences between the goals of management and labor create conflict that cannot be totally explained as simply as a desire for higher wages, shorter working hours or better working conditions. The issues of management rights and efficiency in patient care versus human value create an inherent tension. Management always will assert its rights to prescribe modes of action and levels of productivity. Yet, labor unions question whether management should have complete power over the work force. Organized labor attempts to gain more control from management by obtaining a voice for employees about working conditions and terms of employment. The question of management's right to govern is paralleled by the question of human value versus efficiency in patient care. To achieve management's goals and objectives, it must maintain efficiency through increased productivity and cost containment. Conversely, the union seeks to improve members' standards of living. Neither side is totally right or wrong in its demands; unfortunate circumstances often trigger conflict. For example, a management wishing to improve the existing benefit package may be prevented from doing so by union pressures to increase wages.

Evidence of this type of conflict is mounting almost daily in health care. Added pressures as a result of the shortage and reimbursement concern over the quality of care issues are encouraging labor and management friction. Although little published empirical data are available, the ANA asserts nurses are beginning to see increased value in collective bargaining as a means to solve wage disputes and improve quality practice (Champlin, 1989).

WHY EMPLOYEES JOIN UNIONS

Employees often unionize because of three issues: wages, dissatisfaction with work benefits, and their perceptions about the organization as a place to work. Brett (1980) found that employees join unions because they are dissatisfied with working conditions and perceive a lack of influence to change those conditions and that the potential for dissatisfied employees to organize a union depends on whether they accept the concept of collective action and believe that unionization will yield positive, rather than negative, outcomes.

In health care, other factors have contributed to unionization. For example, civil rights legislation has stimulated changes in attitudes about being represented by a union. Union membership is often not considered as unprofessional as it once was (Phillips, 1974; Stanton, 1971). The level of satisfaction with wages, job security, fringe benefits, treatment by supervisors, and chances for promotion was significantly correlated with a vote for union representation.

There are some interesting commonalities in the attitudes of health care workers who seek union representation. Although not all-inclusive, the studies show that money and fringe benefits are not always the only issues important to employees. Other, less tangible factors such as poor communication, poor supervision, bad working conditions, and inconsistently enforced personnel policies carry considerable weight.

One reason workers frequently mention for joining unions is failure by management to treat them fairly, decently, or honestly. Employees view management as fair, decent, and honest if it recognizes the needs of individuals and treats people with dignity. Issues such as wage disputes, respect, and recognition for loyalty and service to the institution are related to the individual's need to be recognized and to be treated fairly.

Why Nurses Join Unions

Studies indicating why nurses join unions are limited. Those available indicate that nurses generally join unions for the same kinds of reasons as any other worker. Nurses often organize to make management listen to their grievances. This aspect was more important to the majority of nurses than improved wages and benefits in Godfrey's (1978) assessment. What is interesting about her findings is the identification of the issues nurses wanted management to recognize and "listen to." Fifty-nine percent of the nurses in the study wanted management to listen to and address "quality of patient care" issues as well as stating that the failure of the manager was the reason for joining the union. Champlin (1989) reported that the recent trend in contracts negotiated for nurse bargaining units is toward including clauses about temporary staffing ratios, staff mix, involvement in practice committees, nursing standards for practice and safety for patients and patient care workloads. These trends add further support for the impact of patient care issues on nurses' desire to organize.

STRATEGIC LABOR-MANAGEMENT RELATIONS

Strategic labor-management relations are concerned with maintaining a positive labor relations climate regardless of whether the organization is unionized or not. The fundamental principles are applicable, even if simply focused on maintaining good relations between management and organized labor.

With well over 3 million workers, the health care industry represents one of the largest work force population groups in the United States. Nursing is the largest single occupational group within the population and as a rule, the largest single group of employees in any health care institution. The health care industry also represents one of the largest pools of nonunion employees, and, therefore, is a prime target for union organizers. Logically, nurses are likewise an attractive target because of size alone. Coupled with other factors, such as wage and salary compression and the growing shortage of nurses, increases the likelihood of unionization. The nurse administrator, along with directors and managers, is responsible for influencing the environments he or she supervises in a positive way.

Management strategy regarding its desired relationship to labor organizations should be formulated as a part of overall policy development. The decision to seek representation from an organized union is employee motivated and initiated as a response to existing conditions in the organization. The chief nurse executive is responsible for the creation of the working environment and should understand how that environment is assessed by union organizers from the outside looking in.

What the Union Organizer Wants

In most instances, employees in any organization will attempt to resolve difficulties through internal mechanisms until those prove unsatisfactory. The union organizer usually first appears via employee invitation after much prolabor work has already been completed from inside.

The chief nurse executive must understand that the union will choose to evaluate a given organization based on several factors. Previous union activity in the facility, management's response, and personalities of members of the organizing team will determine the exact nature of the assessment. However, certain areas of any institution are vulnerable to the organizer. These include staff working on shifts where there are few supervisors, situations where conflict is present and observable, wage inconsistencies between personnel, and situations where salary compression is evident. Incentive pay, overtime, and benefit discrepancies are also examined. The organizer typically attempts to identify any issue where organizational conflict may exist. In addition, organizers of nursing groups are sensitive to quality patient care concerns.

Trends in contracts for organized nurses include clauses regulating the quality of clinical care through a variety of mechanisms. Patient practice committees, concern with staffing expertise and mix, and concern over standards are a few of the subjects nurses bargain to influence. Logically then, an organizer would be sensitive to situations where nurses were not allowed input into practice regulation, patient care quality improvement or decision making. The administrator should ensure that staff nurses have regular mechanisms for influencing patient care policy and quality. In addition to understanding the assessment tactics of the union organizer, the nurse executive should also consider the elements of strategic labor-management relations. Policies and practices designed through the use of these concepts will enhance existing relationships in the workplace, regardless of union status in the facility.

Employee Attitude Assessment

When conducted correctly, surveys of employee's attitudes are a practical method for development of management's understanding of the work environment. A simple survey, scheduled regularly, which clearly differentiates both positive and negative attitudes should reassure employees of management's continual concern for their needs. In addition, when combined with consistent formal and informal upward communication at all levels of the institution, the result should be a positive change in the attitudes of employees and the development of a management system for dealing with personnel problems before they become critical. Corrective action from management, as well as ongoing communication regarding employee concerns, is essential if the assessment process is to be judged meaningful. Employees must clearly identify the relationship between their concerns, the communication of the concerns and management's response or the assessment process will fail. The symbolism represented in the failure of management to respond promptly and adequately can severely damage labor-management relations.

Employee Development

Administration is ultimately responsible for training the staff. An investment in an active employee training program is a strong indication of the value management places on staff satisfaction and growth. In recent years, the nursing profession has seen the revival of career ladder programs within hospitals in an attempt to provide a boost for employee satisfaction and development. Management should recognize the value of providing training opportunities as incentives, as well as the link between these training opportunities and performance appraisal and reward. (See Chapter 15 on staff development.)

Employee Value Systems

Research has identified as many as seven different employee value systems, varying from tribalistic to existentialist (Hughes, 1976). Each system is unique in some way, to the person, and will vary considerably among professional and nonprofessional classifications. The value system of a particular staff member will influence his or her response to a specific type of reward or policy in the institution. Management must provide a variety of alternatives to specific problems or issues confronting the staff. Analysis of the organizational culture and the predominant values of the staff should be included in the management data base when policies are developed. In general, both professional and nonprofessional staff respond positively to consistency, honesty, and open communication. Participatory decision making, especially with professional staff, can facilitate the development of incentives and policies. Flexible work scheduling, earned time programs, job sharing, job enrichment, and cafeteria benefits packages are examples of programs aimed at addressing the myriad of value systems inherent in an employee community.

First-Line Managers

The nurse administrator must recognize the importance of first-line managers (head nurses) and other supervisors in preventing serious labor problems. Although the chief nurse executive is ultimately responsible for the manager-staff nurse relationship, the first-line manager represents management in a most immediate way on a daily basis. If these managers do not have good management skills, the institution is inviting unionization. The chief nurse executive should be sensitive to early identification of manager-staff difficulty. Confidential, planned evaluation of the manager by staff is essential. The administrator should assess the skill level of the supervisor or head nurse, not as a clinician, but as a manager and provide training for management functions accordingly.

Performance Appraisal

Positive, development oriented evaluation of employees is likewise essential. Evaluation of the individual staff member should be planned, scheduled, consistent, and confidential. Simplicity and honesty will support an environment where high morale will flourish.

A nurse manager's avoidance of an honest appraisal of the nonproductive employee simply demonstrates to all workers that the reward system is inequitable or that productivity is not rewarded. This can be interpreted logically as evidence that the nonproductive actually are rewarded more than productive in relation to their effort. In many instances, the administrator will delegate performance appraisal to the most immediate supervisor. The appraisal system must be administered by that supervisor consistently. The best appraisal system is as weak as the people who operate it. In addition, failure to assess the competence of the persons providing care will result in loss of staff morale, and increased liability for the institution. (See Chapter 13 for more on performance appraisal.)

Disciplinary Policies and Procedures

Management must take great care in applying disciplinary policies and procedures consistently. Consistent and fair application normally can prevent unnecessary employee relations problems and grievances. Basically, management must have "just cause" for imposing discipline. The following parameters can be used for determining just cause:

1. Was the disciplinary rule reasonably related to efficient and safe operations?
2. Were the employees properly warned of potential consequences of violating the rule?
3. Did management conduct a fair investigation before applying the discipline?
4. Did the investigation produce substantial evidence of guilt?
5. Were the policies and procedures implemented consistently and without discrimination?
6. If a penalty resulted, was it related to the seriousness of the event as well as the past record of the employee? (Did the punishment fit the crime?)

Grievance Procedure

Employees should be able to complain formally about perceived problems without fear of subjective reprisal. Although any grievance procedure is open to problems of interpretation and application, some basic factors can be applied equally in evaluating the system from the employees' perspective whether unionized or not.

1. Employees should understand the mechanics of filing a grievance and where they can go to ask questions about any step of the system. The procedure should be written.
2. When a grievance is filed, it should receive prompt action.

3. The grievance process should include a way to access the process when the immediate supervisor is the problem.

If employees realize that a fair grievance procedure is available and management is attempting to prevent unnecessary problems, the result should be a decreased number of complaints, fair and objective processing of those that are filed, and employees feeling that management is concerned about employee needs.

Administering the Contract

Once a collective bargaining agreement has been completed and negotiations concluded, implementation of the agreement is a key responsibility of the parties. Several frequently used procedures may appear complex to both the manager and employee. An explanation of the procedures governing discipline, grievance, and arbitration follows.

Discipline

Generally the collective bargaining agreement will impose limitations on the disciplinary powers the nurse manager may exercise. Ironically, most of the limitations usually imposed are consistent and even desirable for an effective human relations' policy. For example, although management still has the right to impose discipline, the administration of it must involve due process for the employee. The nurse manager must utilize a sound procedure based on due process to correct the employee's negative behavior. The disciplinary actions must be progressive, documented, and consistent. Management must keep records of each reprimand, warning, layoff, and discharge. An action to discharge must be for just cause.

Grievance Procedure

The grievance procedure is usually extremely important in the collective bargaining agreement. Consistent and fair adjudication of grievances is the hallmark of sound employee–employer relations.

Most procedures contain several steps designed to support objectivity and fairness as well as due process for the employee. The typical steps are:

1. Presentation of grievance to the immediate supervisor.
2. When the grievance involves the immediate supervisor, presentation to a department head or manager outside the unit.
3. Presentation of the grievance with a union official, and a labor relations representative from the organization.

Metzger (1979) provides the following checklist for managers involved in administering the grievance procedure:

1. Listen. Permit the presentation of the full story by the employee and/or the delegate.
2. Try to understand. Uncover the how, who, what, when, where, and why of the grievance.
3. Separate fact from emotion. This requires painstaking investigation.

4. Refer to policy and contract provisions. These are the rules of the road. Do not attempt to rewrite policy and the bargaining agreement at this stage of the game. The role of the supervisor is to interpret such policy and contract provisions as they pertain to the grievance at hand.

5. Remember that your decision may set a precedent. A decision in one case has a direct bearing on subsequent cases.

6. Consult with others. It is not a sign of weakness to check with other supervisors who may have had similar grievances, and to check with the personnel department.

7. Explain your decision fully. It is essential to get employee commitment and understanding. Therefore, be explicit and honest in communicating your decision. (p 265)

Arbitration

Provisions for the use of arbitration to resolve contract interpretation disputes during the life of the contract appear in more than 90 percent of all collective bargaining agreements. Arbitration is the final step in the grievance procedure.

Voluntary arbitration is quasi-judicial in nature. When two parties are unable to resolve a dispute by mutual agreement, they submit the particular issue to an impartial person for solution.

There are several types of voluntary arbitration clauses dealing with contract administration disputes. The most common provides for both parties to select an arbitrator each time a dispute arises. The selection of a separate arbitrator for each issue has the marked advantage of securing a qualified individual to rule on a particular type of dispute (Metzger, 1970).

A less widely used voluntary arbitration clause provides for a permanent arbitrator system. That is, the parties agree on the identity of an impartial arbitrator who will handle all arbitrations during the life of a specific agreement. This has the distinct advantage of providing both parties with a carefully selected individual who has earned the respect of both labor and management. The arbitrator's decision is final and is binding on both parties.

The first principle of effective arbitration in contract administration is joint agreement between management and the union on the type of arbitration desired. Even more critical is the question of the limits or non-limits on what matters shall be submitted to the arbitrator. In deciding which matters should be submitted to the arbitrator and the arbitrator's authority, contractual definitions must be considered. The arbitrator's authority is limited by the agreement. Typically the arbitrator is responsible for interpreting or applying a specific clause in the contract. The arbitrator is precluded from adding to or deleting from any clause contained in that agreement. Some contracts limit the arbitration process to specific issues and not to all clauses contained in the collective bargaining agreement.

In submitting contract interpretation disputes to an arbitrator, both parties risk losing the decision on matters they deem to be important but this is a small price to pay for uninterrupted service. The advantages of continuing operations while deciding disputed claims arising from interpretation of the contract are obvious. Arbitration neither diminishes nor detracts from the collective bargaining process. Rather, it is an extension of the bargain arrived at during the negotiations. It is an administrative tool for living with the contract. Having adopted the arbitration process voluntarily, both parties are more likely to accept the decision which emanates from the arbitrator.

SUMMARY

Collective bargaining agreements are on the increase in nursing. Working conditions, changes in health care delivery payment, the shortage of nurses and the increasing sophistication of nursing associations suggest the trend will continue. In order to function effectively in this new environment, the nurse manager must integrate a knowledge of labor law, labor movement history, union operation, and sound management practice to respond to the challenges.

REFERENCES

American Arbitration Association. *Labor Arbitration, Procedures and Techniques.* New York, American Arbitration Association, 1981

Bade, WJ, Stone M. *Management Strategy in Collective Bargaining Negotiations.* New London, CT, National Foremen's Institute, 1951

Brett M. Why employees want unions. *Organizational Dynamics* (American Management Association). 48, Spring 1980

Buerhaus PI. Not just another nursing shortage. *Nursing Economics.* 5:6, 267, Nov/Dec 1987

Champlin L. More RNs see value in collective bargaining. *American Nurse.* 21:10, 9, Nov/Dec 1989

Clelland R. Grievance procedures: Outlet of employee, insight for management. *Hospitals.* 41:18, 60, Aug 1967

Cook SA. The neglected art of negotiation. *The Daily Record,* Baltimore, January 19, 1972, 1

Dunlop JT, Hely JJ. *Collective Bargaining,* rev. ed. Homewood IL, Irwin, 1955: 53

Gifford CD, ed. *Directory of US Labor Organizations,* 1978–1979 Edition. Washington, DC Bureau of National Affairs, 1974

Gillies, DA. *Nursing Management: A systems approach,* 2nd edition. Philadelphia: WB Saunders, 1989

Godfrey MA. Job satisfaction—or should that be dissatisfaction? *Nursing.* Apr–May–June, 1978

Goodfellow M. If you aren't listening to your employees, you may be asking for a union. *Modern Hospital.* 113:4, 88, October 1969

Goodfellow M. Checklist: How the union organizer rates your institution. *Risk Management.* 1, December 1972

Guidebook to Labor Relations. Chicago, Commerce Clearing House, 1985: 315

Hospital Financial Management. Keeping your employees' morale up takes more than money. 28:11, 24, November 1974

Hospital Progress. Goals and trends in the unionization of health care professionals. 53:2, 40, February 1972

Hughes L. *Making Unions Unnecessary.* New York, Executive Enterprises Publications, 1976: 43

Imberman AA. Communications: An effective weapon against unionization. *Hospital Progess*. 54:12, 54, December 1973

Joiner CL, Blayney KD. Career mobility and allied health manpower utilization. *Journal of Allied Health*. 157, Fall 1974

Justin JJ. *How to Manage with a Union*. New York, Industrial Relations Workshop Seminars, Inc, 1969: 294–295

Kaynard SM. Health care industry under the National Labor Relations Act. In: Metzger N, ed. *Handbook of Health Care Human Resources Management*. Rockville, MD, 1981: 537–569

Lewis HL. Wave of union organizing will follow break in the Taft-Hartley dam. *Modern Healthcare*. 1:2, 25, May 1974

Lorenz FJ. Nursing administration and undivided loyalty. *Nursing Administration Quarterly*. 6:2, 67, 1982

Matlack DR. Goals and trends in the unionization of health professionals. *Hospital Progress*. 53:2, 40, February 1972

McClelland J. Professionalism and collective bargaining: A new reality for nurses and management. *Journal of Nursing Administration*. 13:11, 36, 1983

Metzger N. Labor relations. *Hospitals*. 44:6, 80, March 16, 1970

Metzger N. Voluntary arbitration in contract administration disputes. *Hospital Progress*. 51:9, 1970

Metzger N. *The Health Care Supervisor's Handbook*. Rockville, MD, Aspen Systems, 1978

Metzger N. *Personnel Administration in the Health Services Industry*, 2nd ed. New York, Spectrum, 1979

Metzger J, Ferentino J, and Kruger K. *When Health Care Employees Strike*. Rockville, MD, Aspen Systems, 1984

Metzger, N, Pointer DD. *Labor-Management Relations in Health Services Industry: Theory and Practice*. Washington, DC, Science and Health Publications Inc, 1972: 360.

Milliken RA, Milliken G. Unionization -Vulnerable and outbid. *Hospitals*. 47:20, 56, Oct 16, 1973

National Labor Relations Act, 298 U.S. 238, 1935

Phillips DE. Taft-Hartley: What to expect. *Hospitals*. 48:13, 18a, July 1, 1974

Pointer DD. How the 1974 Taft-Hartley amendments will affect health care facilities. *Hospital Progress*. 55:10, 68, October 1974

Pointer DD, Cannedy LL. Organizing of professionals. *Hospitals*. 48:6, 70, March 16, 1974

Pointer DD, Luttman P. Collective bargaining and professionalism: Incompatible ideologies? *Nursing Administration Quarterly*. 6:21, Winter 1982

Pointer DD, Metzger N. *The National Labor Relations Act—A Guidebook for Health Care Facility Administrators*. New York, Spectrum, 1975: 272

Rakisch JS. Hospital Unionization: Causes and effects. *Hospital Administration*. 10, Winter 1973 Vol 18

Rakisch, J, Longest B, Dar K. *Managing Health Services Organizations*, 2nd ed. Philadelphia, WB Saunders, 1985

Reed KA. Preparing for union organization. *Hospital Topics*. 48:4, 30, April 1970

Rutkowski D, Rutkowski BL. *Labor Relations in Hospitals*. Rockville, MD, Aspen Systems, 1984, 3

Sargis N. Collective bargaining: Serving the common good in hospitals. *Nursing Management*. 16:2, 23, 1985

Sibson RE. Why unions in the hospital? *Hospital Topics*. 43:8, 46, August 1965

Sloane A, Witney F. *Labor Relations*. Englewood Cliffs, NJ, Prentice-Hall, Inc, 1981

Stanton ES. The Charleston hospital strikes. *Southern Hospitals*. Vol. 10, 39, March 1971

Stanton ES. Unions and the professional employee. *Hospital Progress*, 55:1, 58, January 1974

US Congress. S. Rep. #93-766, 93d Cong., 2d Sess. 5 (1974); H.R. Rep. #93-1051, 93d Cong., 2d Sess. 7 (1974)

Organizing for Production

CHAPTER 19

Technology and Physical Facilities

Roger O. Lambson
Scott D. Ramsey

Key Concept List

Facilities management
Evaluation of space and facilities
Facilities planning
Technology
Computer networks
Integrated hospital information systems
Construction management

The hospital, clinic, laboratory or office is a place to work and, yet, it is much more. In addition to housing people, these spaces accommodate a broad spectrum of furniture and equipment—the tools required to carry out specific jobs. While we do not often stop to analyze the facilities in which we work, each space has its unique character and personality; some are comfortable and efficient, others are formal and foreboding. In this chapter we will introduce and explore physical facilities and space as a tool to support patient care functions and as a valuable resource. A discussion of some of the issues involved with facilities evaluation and management will enhance understanding of the operation, planning, construction, and renovation of health care facilities. The chapter also provides a basic overview of organizational technology. The term itself is defined, and Perrow's model is offered as a framework for recognizing and understanding different types of technology. In the health care environment, technology is often complex, expensive, and rapidly changing. It offers profound opportunities and challenges for the nursing administrator. In today's world, it is critical for administrators to be able to understand and manage technological innovation and to recognize its potential impacts in the work place. Current and emerging technologies both in the office and patient care environments are presented and discussed and their interplay between productivity, work flow, and the physical layout of facilities is examined.

FACILITIES MANAGEMENT

The range of topics which could be discussed under the heading of facilities management is very large. Here, we will focus on the evaluation of space and facilities, not only to understand the issues involved in the management of this valuable resource, but also as the basis for planning renovations or the construction of an entirely new facility.

The politics of space, if studied and practiced, provides a powerful management tool which can be used in many different settings. Everyone has heard the phrases ''key to the executive washroom,'' ''the corner office,'' ''matched wood furniture,'' ''the reserved parking space,'' ''the master key,'' or ''the private telephone line.'' Each of these items is a real or perceived icon of status or power in most office settings. The size of one's desk, its placement at the entrance of a room, as one in a group of desks in the middle of a room, or next to a window with a pleasant view again connotes some real or perceived level of status within the organization. Similarly, the size of one's office or research laboratory and its location within the building may reflect seniority or power. Just as the size and security of the territory marked by the household cat is guarded and defended, so it is for people within many organizational settings. Appreciation of the fact that the amount and location of space is viewed by many as being as important as budget or staff size is a first step toward understanding the management of facilities.

The level of an office's finish and furnishings is, along with its size and location, another perceived statement of territory. Wallpapers are a step above painted drywall but the addition of chair rail and hardwood wainscotting would add an even higher level of finish. Ceiling types range from no ceiling finish to a vaulted, concealed-spline tile system with indirect lighting. Sealed concrete and vinyl tile may be at one end of the spectrum of floor coverings while custom inlaid carpeting would be at the other. The types of lighting fixtures, door hardware, and electrical cover plates which are chosen to finish an entire facility or different spaces within the building will significantly influence the project budget and its perceived status. Such amenities as built-in bookcases, exotic wood desks, leather, high-backed chairs, side tables with lamps, sofas, and original art further extend the range of options for level of finish and establish a hierarchy of territories with the organization. While these example best characterize corporate or academic office settings, similar parallels can be easily constructed for ambulatory care facilities, hospitals, or nursing homes.

Just as the level of architectural finish and furnishings of an individual office or entire facility helps formulate impressions and establish levels of expectation about the interactions conducted therein, the location of a particular office or activity may intentionally or inadvertently transmit equally strong messages. For example, the location of the affirmative action office in a remote part of the basement suggests that the organization may not be totally committed to the practice of equal opportunity in hiring or promotion. The relative locations of nursing services, medicine, and hospital administration within the hospital may also say a lot about the status of and working relationships among these personnel groups. A hospital with a history of personnel problems would do well to question whether the quality and location of office spaces for particular groups might be a contributing factor in these personnel problems.

It is important for the nurse manager and executive to appreciate the very powerful impact almost every aspect of a facility has on its occupants and visitors. For the visitor, impressions begin with the neighborhood setting, the building's architecture, its landscaping, signage and ease of access. The level of housekeeping and maintenance of parking areas, walks, and entrances also establish a level of expectation. Such impressions continue in the front lobby, corridors, elevators, and stairwells en route to an office, clinic, or patient room. As with people, a facility has no second opportunity to create a first impression. These impressions and expectations can have a profound influence on human behavior, personal interactions, professional productivity, and patient outcomes.

EVALUATION OF SPACE AND FACILITIES

Given the very subjective and often emotional reactions to discussions about space, the administrator would be well advised to enter into such discourses well prepared. For most medium to large organizations, a computerized space inventory may prove beneficial to the institution's facility planner, the director of facilities operation, line managers, as well as the administrator. Such inventory can be entered and maintained on a personal computer. A record is created for each room in the facility which contains such common information as the building name in which the room is located, the room number, its size, its type or description, one or more major functions which are carried out in the room, and perhaps the names of the departments and individual users to whom the room is assigned. Other fields of the record might include the identifier of the air handling unit serving the space, the last date the room was painted, carpeted, or rehabbed, or the identity of the housekeeping section responsible for cleaning the room.

Such a space inventory system, particularly when electronically linked to other institutional databases, can be a powerful tool in the hands of the nurse manager, facility manager, and administrator. For example, the director of facilities operation could use the space inventory to develop a schedule for painting the facility or to compare housekeeping costs for different buildings within the complex. If a record of the number of patients seen in each clinic was maintained, the space inventory could provide an opportunity to objectively compare the "productivity" of different clinical services. In a research setting, the space inventory would enable the manager to measure the productivity of any particular investigator or unit by calculating such values as the number of generated extramural research dollars per square foot of research laboratory space or the number of research publications per unit of space assigned to that individual or department. Such objective measures facilitate comparisons between organizational units and remove much of the subjective and emotional nature of space evaluations. They provide an objective basis for decisions about space assignments, reassignments or determinations of the amounts of space needed to support a specific level of productivity for the organization.

On the other hand, some managers would argue that detailed inventories and calculated productivity measures are not needed if the organization has developed or adopted a detailed set of *space standards*. Using this approach, tables may have been developed listing a specific office size for nursing managers, a slightly larger office for nursing directors, and another standard for the chief nurse executive. Similar listings or standards can be prepared for research laboratory space, work areas for secretaries, accountants, directors, department heads, and so on. One major deficiency of such approach to space management is that most buildings do not have either the number or range of room sizes to match the prescribed standard. Another problem is that such formulas become very complicated if they attempt to allocate space based on the amount of work area required to perform a specific task or set of tasks. Unless the organization is very large and the work tasks very circumscribed, space allocations based on job title will be frustrating and have little management utility. On the other hand, evaluations of *space utilization* based on quantifiable output measures provide the manager with powerful tools for the allocation or reallocation of space based upon productivity.

Periodically, executives should also give some attention to evaluating the *functionality* of their facilities. A building or space within a building may be aesthetically pleasing but, for many reasons, the functions which are carried out in the facility are compromised. Poor traffic patterns for people and materials, inadequate lighting, too much noise, and poor ventilation are but a few of the factors that influence the efficiency and effectiveness of the facility. While the original architectural and engineering designs have a major influence on the long-term functionality of a facility, specific space assignments and locations of individual activities and people within the facility and their spatial relationships with functionally related units are also very important determinants of how well a facility works.

Whether planning a new facility or evaluating an existing one, it is useful to draw functional maps to track the movements of different groups of people, paperwork, supplies, or trash. Such maps will facilitate decisions about where to locate different activities. For example, it may make good sense to locate classrooms on the basement, ground or first floors of a building to avoid having large numbers of students rely on elevators for vertical transport at the time of every class change. Similarly, offices which deal with the public might best be located near the front entrance for the convenience of customers and to avoid needless corridor congestion.

Another aspect of a facility's functionality is an evaluation of how different offices, units or activities spatially relate to one another within the facility. Are the nursing stations, as well as clean and soiled utility rooms, located central to the patient rooms to enable the most direct and efficient interaction between the patient and staff? Is the copier, laser printer, and coffee machine equally accessible to all support staff? In yet another setting where both formal and informal interaction of nursing staff is encouraged, do office locations encourage interactions? Are there designated areas with comfortable seating near the coffee machine or copier where staff are likely to congregate? The allocation and furnishing of space specifically for such purposes can significantly facilitate staff interaction and markedly improve the functionality of most health care, teaching, and research facilities.

The facility requirements of new technologies are often overlooked. Installing personal computers or similar video display terminals without considering the possible glare of overhead fluorescent lights on these screens is one example. Failure to consider such environmental factors such as lighting, noise, ventilation or temperature, will compromise employee effectiveness. On the other hand, whenever such functional deficiencies are identified, serious consideration should be given to undertaking a renovation project to alleviate these problems.

Lighting of the facilities is often accorded little attention by either the designer or the facility manager. While light fixture selection and operating costs may be considered during the design of the facility, rarely is the potential impact of light, as an architectural element, or light, as a contributing factor to worker stress or productivity, studied or discussed. Too often, when such issues are reviewed, it is late in the design process and many opportunities have been lost for introducing and incorporating natural light or for combining structural elements with light fixtures to create comfortable and effective illumination patterns. Light shafts, light wells, light shelves, skylights, and glazed atrium spaces are but a few examples of the methods by which the architect can introduce natural light deep into a building's core, to spaces internal to rooms with an outside window.

Increased use of video display terminals has focused attention on the need for lighting which reduces or eliminates the glare on the computer screens. A fortunate byproduct of these considerations is the increased use of *indirect lighting* to establish an overall ambient illumination level and *task lights* to provide a higher level of light for the specific work being performed. Such lighting practices not only lower lighting power consumption but also reduce glare and visual stress. An added benefit of thoughtful lighting is the enhancement of architectural forms which, like background music, helps establish an ambience or mood which can enhance productive personal interactions, which are so important to most teaching, patient care and professional transactions.

Security

An unfortunate consequence of our increasing population and the often congested, urban setting of many corporate, teaching, and patient care facilities is the need for security systems. In many facilities such systems begin with remote-controlled video surveillance cameras which monitor parking lots, parking garages, major entrances and corridors. A second level of security is sometimes established with magnetic access cards issued to the staff. The computers which control such access systems can be programmed to enable a particular identification card to open one or a series of doors only during particular times of day and specific days of week. Each event is recorded by the computer which can also use such information to replace a timeclock for payroll management purposes. The same card can also be used to control access to parking facilities, to check out a book from the library, or to record charges at the cafeteria. An added benefit of such systems is that the computer can be programmed to deny access to terminated employees or for a card which has been reported stolen or lost.

Combination locks or video camera monitoring with remote electronic access controls are other alternatives to standard locks and keys for limiting building access or denying access to specific rooms within a facility. The installation of vision panels in all room and corridor doors as well as maintaining adequate lighting levels in all exterior and occupied interior spaces will further enhance facility security and the safety of staff and visitors.

Temperature and Ventilation

Of the broad range of problems with which the facility manager must deal, there are few which demand more time and energy to resolve than matters of temperature and ventilation control. The building's heating, ventilation, and air conditioning system (HVAC) must maintain temperature and humidity levels within a relatively narrow range through extremes of summer and winter weather conditions for a diverse set of spaces within a building, each with a particular solar load, prevailing wind condition and heat generated by a variety of electrical equipment or a varying number of occupants. It should not be surprising that such systems are often complex and may comprise 40 percent or more of the project budget to construct and consume a large portion of the building's utility budget. Recognition of these facts should encourage thoughtful and regular evaluation of the effectiveness and efficiency of HVAC systems. It should also serve to remind the executive of the importance to delineate, during the earliest stages of planning, all activities and equipment that will be accommodated within each space of the new or renovated facility. Carefully developed descriptions will better ensure that sufficient capacities are designed and constructed.

HVAC systems can "make or break" a facility. For this reason, special attention should be given to hiring the most qualified professional engineers and mechanical contractors available when planning a remodeling project or a new facility. It is beyond the scope and purpose of this discussion to review in any detail such matters as room versus zone temperature controls, computerized energy management systems, set-back or programmable thermostats, motion detectors which activate fan systems, turn-on lights, flush toilets, or operate faucet controls, the R-values of different insulating systems, or the merits of installing energy recovery systems. Nonetheless, these terms are introduced with the suggestion that the administrator recognize them.

When planning new or renovated construction, the facility designer and construction team should openly discuss the system's operating costs and review whether such systems are cost-effective over the expected life expectancy of the facility. *Life-cycle cost evaluations* performed during the planning process can be powerful determinants of the best systems to purchase and install. For a facility which is expected to support the organization's mission for 20 to 30 years, the costs to operate and repair the building's mechanical systems cannot be ignored. Their importance is further magnified when one considers the potentially negative impact of poor HVAC and lighting systems on worker comfort and productivity. Over the expected life of most health care facilities, such costs could certainly exceed the original cost to design, purchase, and install the highest quality HVAC and lighting systems.

Similar attention should be given during the planning and design phases of a project to the selection of construction and finish materials. There are marked differences in initial cost, durability, and maintenance costs of different building products. Each material also has its own aesthetic quality and will contribute to the final "image" of the facility. Unfortunately, the project budget has a major influence on the selection of construction materials used and since decisions about interior finishes often come late in the planning process, aesthetic and durable products are often compromised by inadequate funding. The issue is extremely important to nursing staff and reinforces the need for nursing executives to be involved at the earliest stages of planning to help ensure that aesthetic and easy-to-maintain finishes are budgeted for the project. As with mechanical systems, the tangible and intangible costs of the building's exterior skin and interior finishes cannot be ignored and must be essential planning considerations.

Flexibility and Adaptability of Space

Recognizing the likelihood that neither specific people nor technology will be long-standing tenants of a new facility, it is probably a mistake to customize spaces for either. Generic designs that will serve the broadest range of activities and constructed such that they can be easily modified are basic steps toward a flexible and adaptable facility. Providing adequate space for and easy access to all of the building's mechanical, electrical, and telecommunications systems will greatly facilitate making expected modifications and significantly reduce future costs to accommodate almost certain changes. Said in other terms, *anticipating change,* whether it be change in mission, of goals and objectives, or change in technology is a critical lesson for the nurse executive. Reality is that 2 to 5 years will elapse from the time a project is conceived until construction is complete and the space occupied. In such a time interval, some key project personnel involved will have moved on, a new diagnostic technology will have emerged and must be accommodated, or a new administrative entity will have been created to meet accreditation requirements. When a time frame of 25 to 30 years is superimposed on the planning board, it is clear that activities and equipment not yet imagined will have to be accommodated in the "new" facility. If advances in telecommunications, information processing, medical imaging, and treatment continue their pace of the recent past, it is clear that practice activities and facilities requirements of all the health care professions will soon be very different. New building spaces will be needed and new building systems will be required long before the facilities being occupied today or being planned for tomorrow are no longer functional. Because of this reality, it is important to anticipate change and to build into any new or renovated facility as much *flexibility* and *adaptability* as the budget will allow without compromising the known specific functions and activities for which the space is being constructed.

On the other hand, it is costly to design and construct facilities where it is possible to quickly and cheaply convert space designed to support one activity to support a different function. One approach seen in the business world is to construct large, open, box-type structures. In such structures, modular, demountable wall units, open landscaping office furniture systems, or inexpensive drywall partitions can be erected and removed, as needed. In hospital and ambulatory care facilities with extensive plumbing and other mechanical system requirements, flexibility is sometimes achieved by constructing an interstitial space between each occupied floor. Such spaces allow for the distribution and extensive modification of ventilation and other mechanical systems without major disruption of adjacent spaces. A combination of these two approaches can be seen in intensive care units where there are few fixed dividing partitions and the considerable electrical and computer cabling, medical gases, and suction requirements are delivered to the bedside through ceiling-hung support columns.

TECHNOLOGY

In the health care environment, technology is complex, expensive, and rapidly changing. It also offers some rather profound opportunities for the nursing administrator. In today's world, it is critical for administrators to be able to understand and manage technological innovation, and to recognize its potential impacts in the work place.

This section of the chapter provides a basic overview of organizational technology. The term itself is defined, and Perrow's model is offered as a framework for recognizing and understanding different types of technology. In addition, current and emerging technologies both in the office and patient care environments, are presented and discussed. Finally, the interplay between these technologies and productivity, work flow, and actual physical layout of facilities, is examined.

Technology Defined

For many, technology is represented simply by the office personal computer hardware or the electronic gadgetry we see in patient rooms. It is, however, important to think of technology as something more than equipment. Broadly defined, technology is "the process by which an organization converts inputs into outputs" (Robey, 1986, p 137). As it pertains to health care and nursing, technology is the process by which inputs (sick people) are converted to outputs (well people). Under this definition, a hospital's technology is literally everything that takes place during a patient's stay. While this definition is perhaps too broad for this discussion, the conversion process principle emphasizes the strong relationships between technology and all of the various elements in the workplace.

One can, however, distinguish between overall technology (the basic task of the organization), subunit technologies, and the tools and techniques associated with individual job technologies (see Fig 19–1). It is at the department or individual job level that technology as a concept is most readily identified (and its implications understood) by administrators.

Technology can also be thought of as work-flow, or the tools, equipment, and work-related tasks within an organization used to transform inputs into outputs (Daft & Steers, 1986). Using the work-flow concept, the importance of technology is emphasized in the following ways:

1. The organization's work-flow has specific implications for the organization structure and management systems used to facilitate and control that work-flow.
2. Much of the increase in productivity and efficiency can be attributable through technological innovation.
3. Technology impacts the design of individual jobs.
4. Technology affects tasks associated with individual jobs, which in turn influence human needs and satisfaction (Daft & Steers, 1986, pp 149–250).

Sociologist Charles Perrow viewed technology as functions of variety and analyzability. Variety refers to the range and diversity of work activities; analyzability to the well-defined versus ill-defined nature of activities (Daft & Steers, 1986). As Fig 19–2 shows, these variables can be displayed in a two-by-two matrix, describing four major technology groups: routine, engineering, craft, and nonroutine. As variety be-

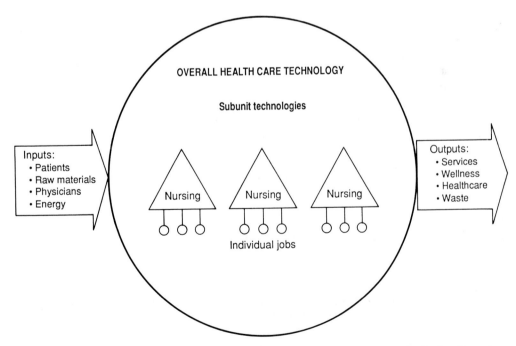

Figure 19-1. Levels of Technology within the Organization *(Source: Robey D.* Designing Organizations. *Homewood, IL, Irwin, 1986)*

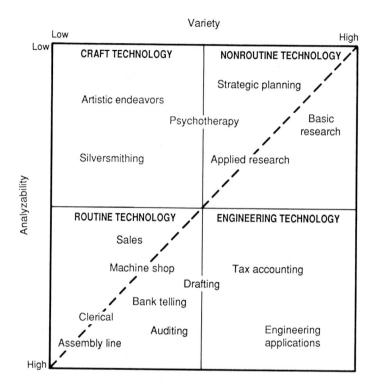

Figure 19–2. Perrow's Technology Framework *(Adapted from Perrow C. A framework for the comparative analysis of organizations.* American Sociological Review. *32: 194–208, 1967, and Daft RL, Macintosh N. A New approach to design and use of management information.* California Management Review. *21: 82–92, 1978)*

comes greater and the ability to be analyzed becomes lower, technology becomes increasingly uncertain. In nursing, work activity can generally be considered high in variety with moderate to low analyzability, yielding a nonroutine technological framework.

Using Perrow's model in the nursing environment, the relationships between technology and departmental structure, design, and management become clear. The nonroutine technology associated with nursing translates into decentralized decision-making, a fair amount of job discretion, frequent verbal and written communication, a high degree of continuing education and on-the-job training, and performance evaluation by output quality (Daft & Steers, 1986).

MICROCOMPUTERS, PRINTERS, AND APPLICATIONS SOFTWARE

The introduction of microcomputers into the office and patient environments has placed a considerable amount of low cost computing power on the desk-top, to a lesser extent at the nursing station and, occasionally, at the bedside. Computers monitor changes in patient conditions, record nursing and medical interventions and can interface with other information systems. Even the most basic micro-computer provides word processing, spreadsheet, data management and file storage capabilities. The most recent generation of microcomputers, with expanded memory, storage, and processing power, allows individuals to do desk-top publishing, graphics, and complex project management. Affordable laser printers provide high-quality output.

Videodisc technology, high-power microcomputers, and applications software have made possible the dynamic and flexible combination of text, graphics, animation, audio, and video into organized presentation formats with interactive capability. These work stations are beginning to have a tremendous impact on the use of computers as teaching and learning tools. Schools of nursing have already begun to use this technology to teach students detailed procedures, to more effectively stimulate health-care situations, and to generally complement the standard lecture/classroom/ laboratory learning experience. Nursing administrators are recognizing the role that this multimedia computer technology can have in the continuing education and development needs of the staff.

Local Area Networks

Small and medium-sized work groups of microcomputer users can be linked together in a local area network (LAN) configuration (Fig 19–3). The central mode of the LAN, called a file server, is usually a high power microcomputer. Applications software can be installed on the file server and accessed by the individual modes on the network. On a LAN users can elect to operate in stand-alone mode or be part of the network, where work-group information (documents, data, electronic mail, or schedules) can be shared. Users can also share the use of peripherals such as modems, printers, and plotters. The principal benefit of LAN technology is this sharing of information and equipment across the network that in stand-alone mode would be inefficient and not cost effective.

Minicomputers/Mainframes

Similar in concept to LANs, minicomputer systems typically serve as departmental processors for specific functions. An example would be a clinical laboratory system

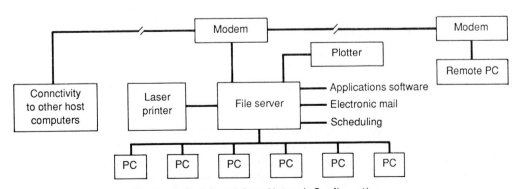

Figure 19–3. A Local Area Network Configuration

that runs on a minicomputer attached to a number of "dumb" terminals (unlike microcomputers, these terminals have no computing intelligence) and printers. This system serves many of the basic functions of the clinical laboratory (eg, billing, inventory, ordering, and so on).

Applications that require a large number of terminals sharing one or more institutional databases usually run on a mainframe system. Because mainframes are so large and complex, a core staff consisting of managers, programmers, and technicians is needed to operate and maintain these systems.

Connectivity/Layered Processing

In the 1960s and 1970s, mainframes and minicomputers, with their parallel processing environments, were predominant in most large hospital computer settings. With the introduction of microcomputers and LANs in the 1980s, a mix of these four types of computing now appears to be the norm. Using the concept of layered processing, managers are responding to the challenges of creating and maintaining a comprehensive health care network out of this "hodgepodge." Microcomputers, for example, are not only capable of solving computing problems of limited scope but can also become nodes on a hospitalwide network. Vendors are providing the hardware, software, and connectivity necessary to allow micro, mini, and mainframe computers to communicate with one another. The layered processing approach allows organizations to work with existing equipment and infrastructure to seek solutions for more comprehensive computing systems instead of relying on vendor-specific solutions. Further discussion of these concepts occurs in the Hospital Information System section later in this chapter (see also Romano, 1990).

TELECOMMUNICATIONS

Much of the connectivity that allows layered processing to occur systemwide has been made possible through advances in telecommunications. The same set of twisted pair wiring that carries voice also transmits data and limited video images. Larger band widths and fiber optics allow the transmission of live video and high-resolution images (such as x-rays) between remote sites. The potential benefits of teleconferencing and performing "remote" patient consultations are enormous.

Other telecommunications devices that help piece together the varied pieces of the computing puzzle include high-speed modems, modem pools, and information systems network (ISN) switches. In the near future health care professionals must be able to use these telecommunications and computing tools to access remote systems and acquire information in a timely manner.

Bedside Technology

In nursing, collecting and recording patient health data is both important and time consuming; in fact this information is often documented at the bedside and later transcribed at the nursing station (Hughes, 1988). Hospitals have begun to install patient information recording devices at the bedside. Examples include portable hand-held terminals, portable interactive terminals, data collection storage devices, PCs, and stationary terminals. Some of these devices simply store patient data (it is later downloaded to the central computing system); others have a direct connection to the central system through an information jack or wall outlet in the patient room.

Optical Disk Storage Systems

Hospitals routinely grapple, albeit clumsily, with the issues of storing patient records and other paper documents. In many organizations valuable space is used both on-site *and* off-site (at considerable expense) for this function. In addition, every administrator has his or her favorite story about how critical records or documents simply disappeared, only to reappear several months later at a most unlikely location (or, worse, never to reappear again).

Optical disk storage systems is an emerging technology capable of compressing up to 50,000 page images, or 2.5 gigabytes, on a 12″ compact laser disk. The system uses a scanner, computers, a laser disk drive, software, and laser printing to store, index, retrieve, and print documents. Document retrieval can take as little as 30 seconds. While still expensive, optical disk storage system costs are expected to decrease over the next several years as administrators look for ways to cope with paper storage problems.

TOWARD AN INTEGRATED HOSPITAL INFORMATION SYSTEM

All of the technologies described previously are being blended together in most large health care environments toward the development of an integrated hospital information system (HIS). Figure 19–4 illustrates the individual pieces and modules, accessible through communications technologies, that make up a fairly typical HIS.

The HIS serves two major functions: to improve access to information and to facilitate needed communications between units within the organization. Modules of an HIS include patient record information, admissions/discharge/transfer data, order entry/results reporting, drug profiles, care planning, personnel/staff planning, and financial data (Peterson & Jelger, 1988). Figure 19–5 displays an infocentric review of the health care environment affected by a functioning HIS (O'Desky, 1988).

On a more practical level, the HIS can have a tremendous impact on work flow and productivity in the patient care setting. A patient record can be accessed from several places at the same time via computer instead of spending valuable time locating that record when it is needed. Orders for tests and procedures can be more efficiently scheduled and coordinated and results more accurately reported in an HIS environment than with manual, paper systems. The emerging technology of artificial intelligence in creating expert systems allows the computer to ''review'' patient procedures that have been scheduled, ''ordering'' other necessary procedures, then ''informing'' the nursing station of what it has done (O'Desky, 1988). Procedure manuals and drug reference guides can be installed in the system and accessed when needed. Using information generated about patient numbers, loads, and acuity, supervisors can more efficiently schedule staffing to meet these needs. Theft and diversion of

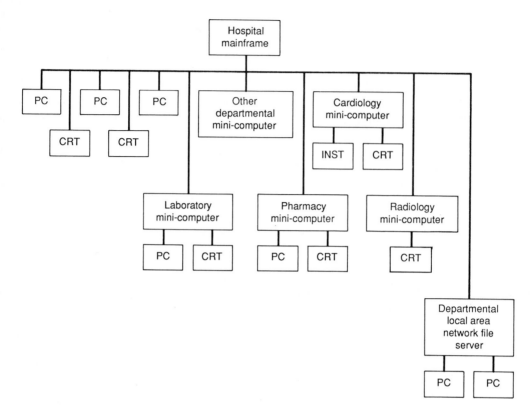

Figure 19-4. Component of the Hospital Institution System

equipment and supplies can be reduced through HIS inventory control. Patients can be presented with one itemized bill instead of separate bills from four or five service departments. Chapter 21 includes an indepth discussion of computer use for reporting and documentation.

NURSING ADMINISTRATION AND THE IMPACTS OF TECHNOLOGY

Now that several technologies (and the opportunities they afford the nursing profession) have been presented, we turn to the equally important issue of the impacts these technologies have in the work place.

When planning for change that involves technological innovation or modification, nursing administrators need to be aware of the issues raised by the following questions:

Is the Technology Appropriate for the Application Being Considered?

Administrators are occasionally afflicted with "tunnel vision"; that is, specific problems are addressed in piecemeal fashion where a more thorough analysis might show

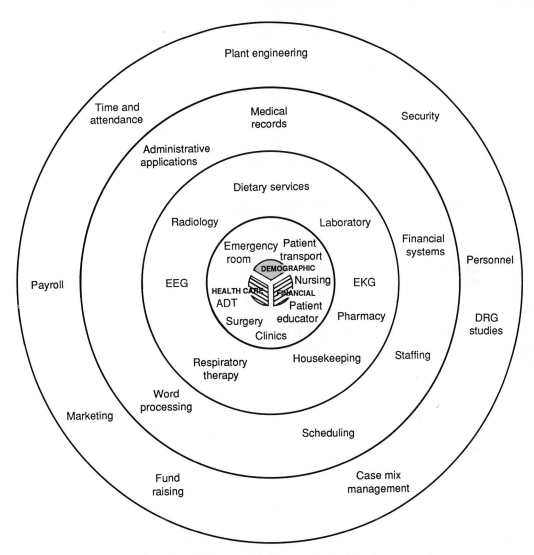

Figure 19-5. An Infrocentric View of the Health Care Environment

that the problem exists elsewhere within the organization or affects other people within the same administrative unit. This problem most frequently manifests itself in the form of using stand-alone microcomputers to work with precisely the same kinds of data that others elsewhere are using. This data redundancy might be better addressed with a LAN or some other connectivity approach.

What Are the Impacts of the Proposed Technology on Overall Work Flow?

The introduction of technology affects the way people perform their job functions. Aside from anticipated increases in efficiency and productivity, administrators need to carefully analyze whether or not new technology will create unrealistic demands or expectations in work flow.

What Are the Impacts of Technology on Individual Jobs?

Technology can significantly alter the range of tasks performed by individual workers. Microcomputers can, for example, allow a clerical worker who previously only entered data the opportunity to manage and manipulate sophisticated spreadsheets and data bases. By the same token, installing a computer terminal at a nursing station or bedside may make unwelcome demands on nurses not previously required to perform data entry.

What Kinds of Resistance Might Develop to Changes in Technology?

Workers are resistant to technology for at least two reasons. First, technology represents change. People are reluctant to change the ways they perform their jobs unless it can be clearly demonstrated that the new technology is not life threatening and offers improved capabilities. Second, technology may change the pattern of social interaction among workers. As insignificant as this detail may first appear, employees consider it extremely important.

Will the Technology Be Fully Utilized?

Given that technology can be a costly and fleeting investment (the "productive" lives of most technologies do not exceed 5 years) administrators must be creative in assessing the many and varied ways that it can be applied. For example, how many people within the unit will use it? How often will it be used? Can the technology be made available to others outside the department? How many different functions or tasks can the technology be used for?

How Is Technology Chosen?

Choices involving technology are not always made under optimal conditions. As possible recipients of technology, nursing administrators need to push hard to become active participants in the selection process. As innovators of technological change, nurse administrators would be wise to involve experts within the organization (eg, data processing, telecommunications), as well as representatives from departments who stand to be impacted by the proposed technology. Organizations that do this preplanning occasionally find out that similar technologies have been applied or are being planned elsewhere in the organization. Obvious benefits result when these inquires are made.

Who Installs, Supports, and Maintains Technology?

Installation, support, and maintenance can have as large an impact on the organization as the use of the technology itself. There are three basic scenarios:

1. *Vendor support:* Technology purchases from a private vendor may also be supported and maintained by that vendor. These services are, of course, provided at a cost; any contractual agreement between the vendor and organization should clearly specify the scope of services provided. For example, does

support include training or technical assistance? Does the maintenance agreement include providing upgrades? Is the support service agreement one charge for all services or is it based on time and materials provided by the vendor? To what extent will "core" technology departments (eg, computing services, telecommunications) be involved?

2. *Core department support:* Most mainframe (HIS) related technology, telecommunications services, and some microcomputer support are provided by core departments within health care settings. As with private vendors, it is important to identify, prior to implementing a technology, the types of service and support forthcoming from these units, as well as any financial charges involved.

3. *Departmental support:* The decentralized nature of some types of technological applications offers individual departments within an organization a great deal of flexibility in their choices. For example, the rather dramatic increase over the past several years in microcomputers and LANs reflects the increased power, sophistication, and affordability of the hardware and the applications that run on them. The recent emphasis on microcomputing has frequently left central core departments like computing services without the financial and staff resources necessary to support the technology. Department heads find themselves in the position of paying more for technology than previously, often in the form of hiring one or more technology-related personnel to support equipment and applications. The notion that the underlying costs of supporting technology may be more expensive then the technology itself must be recognized and planned for by nursing administrators.

How Long Will the Technology Last?

As was mentioned previously, most health care technologies have a life of 3 to 5 years. This fact underscores the point that technology is no longer a one-time capital investment. It has become a growing part of the department's and organization's annual budget.

What Are the Relationships between Technology and Facilities?

The impact of technology on facilities can be direct or indirect. These impacts are indirect when technology affects work flow, which in turn affects the physical layout of facilities. Examples of the interplay between technology and facilities include the following:

- Technology occasionally "creates" the need for an entirely new type of space, as evidenced by videoconferencing facilities, microcomputer classrooms, or shared microcomputer workstations.
- Technology can have an impact on the amount of space used for storage. Our previous discussion of optical disk storage systems technology noted its potential positive impact on storage now allocated to paper records.
- Office automation can make the flaws associated with poorly designed office systems more noticeable: lack of acoustic privacy, poor lighting, low air quality, inadequate ventilation, noise, and cable proliferation (Turnage, 1990).

- The emergence of integrated electronic computer and telecommunications networks places less emphasis on the need for private, contiguous office space and more emphasis on the need for shared use spaces, including conference, training, and other meeting rooms (Turnage, 1990). Space becomes a much more flexible, dynamic resource in a well-designed, networked, office systems setting where co-worker proximity is not an issue. In fact, communications technology now allows some employees to spend portions of their time working at locations remote from the traditional office (such as home).
- For projects involving the construction of a new building or major renovation of an existing structure, strong consideration should be given to wiring or rewiring so that voice, data, and video signals can be transmitted between most locations affected by the project. This should be done even if there are no short-term plans to apply technology that would make optimal use of these wiring systems. From a time and cost standpoint, major construction/renovation projects offer an efficient way to wire for the future.

Our purpose in emphasizing the scope of relationships between technology and the health care workplace is to demonstrate how important it is to be a knowledgeable, active participant in technology-related matters. In the final analysis, to recognize the full range of impacts means that as health care professionals we guide, control, and productively manage technology. In failing to do so, we instead allow technology a measure of control over our working lives.

FACILITIES PLANNING

The administrator may be involved in planning renovation or construction of physical facilities. This section presents major concepts in facilities design and construction to help administrators understand the process when and if they need it. The first step in any renovation or construction project is to develop a *program statement* which becomes the definition of the project, to serve as the initial instructions for the architect and engineers, and is often used to obtain approval funding for the project. Careful development of this document will help avoid misunderstandings and misdirection in later phases of the project.

A program statement outlines the need for the project and its mission. The tasks to be performed and who will perform them in the new facility should be described in detail. Hours of operation, work flow, and movement of patients and materials through the facility should be described. This will help determine the numbers and types of spaces anticipated in the new facility. The proposed building site, utilities and other available services should be discussed. Structural and functional relationships between the proposed facility and adjacent facilities and operations should be outlined in considerable detail. Quality descriptions of functions to be carried out in the facility are critical. Clarity in articulation of the ambience to be achieved as well as detailed descriptions of building systems, construction materials, and expected levels of finish will both expedite the planning process and help assure an outstanding facility. While facility programming services can be purchased and may be advisable for certain projects, the fact remains that the health care professionals are the most qualified to articulate the functions and operating parameters of the proposed facility.

The Process

As a manager, there are fewer decisions beyond the hiring of staff that will have more lasting impact on the organization than the selection of the team needed to plan a major renovation or a new facility. The life of a facility, from conception to replacement, in the vast majority of cases, will be significantly longer than most of the professional careers of the planners, and in many cases, beyond their biological lives of many of its occupants. The accumulated costs of inefficient work flow and pedestrian traffic patterns, of compromised productivity because of poor lighting or of increased stress for lack of proper acoustical control can indeed become very large. Thoughtful directions provided by the owner to the best designers available will result in a well-designed facility and will pay handsome dividends in worker satisfaction and productivity for many, many years.

Each organization's administrative/management framework is different which makes it impossible to prescribe a common set, either by postion or title, of participants to be involved in the planning process. Nonetheless, there are some likely candidates who can be identified. Obviously, a leader of the planning team is critical. This individual should be senior enough in the organization to have the respect and support of the chief executive officer, to clearly understand the history and mission of the organization, and be an excellent communicator. The ability to solicit, synthesize, and articulate input from many organizational levels as well as speak the language of design consultants is an important asset for the team leader to possess. Equally as important on the team is the staff member who will devote a significant level of effort collecting specific information needed for the planning effort, recording and organizing institutional input, and otherwise tracking the project.

Each and every major group who will use the new facility will expect to have a seat on the planning committee. For large or complex organizations, such representation is neither possible nor practical. Instead, three to five individuals should be identified for their objective thinking skills, institutional perspective and commitments and, importantly, listening and communications skills. Most five-to-seven person planning committee should be charged by the chief administrator of the institution to develop a comprehensive program statement for the project drawing input from all levels of the organization. It should be clearly stated in the charge that an early draft of the program will be broadly disseminated throughout the organization for review and comment and that the final program statement will be published following final approval by the administrator and appropriate board of directors. Board discussion and input throughout the planning process should not only help establish a base of institutional support for the project, but also facilitate development of the catalog of details which will be needed by the architect and engineers to prepare the plans and specifications.

Integrated Design Team

The processes and procedures which are followed to translate an architectural program statement into a set of detailed drawings and specifications are as varied as the projects involved. However, the thoughtful organization and management of an *integrated design team* by the CEO provides a high level of assurance that the contributions of each member of the team to the project are maximized. In general terms, the integrated design team consists of one or more representatives of the owner or organization, the project architect, the structural engineer, the mechanical/electrical engineer, the general contractor or construction manager, and any special consultants hired to assist with the design. Examples of these special consultants include interior designers, laboratory or hospital planners, landscape architects, and acoustical or lighting specialists.

While the architect is often assigned the leadership role of such a planning group, coordination of the integrated design team can be assigned to any member of the group. The success of an integrated design process is communication among the members of the team and the active involvement of *all* members of the team in *all* major project meetings, from the first discussion to interpret the program statements through the design development phase of the project. It is important for all members of the team to clearly understand the program and to hear the chief administrator's representative discuss each component of the program statement. Particularly early in the design process, almost every idea and decision made by one member of the team will affect another member's area of responsibility. Because of the "everything affects everything else principle," open and honest communication between all team members is essential to ensure that the consensual design of the group represents the best compromises possible. Such professional negotiations will result not only in a facility of the highest quality afforded by the budget but also provide a significant amount of education for all team members in the process. A significant byproduct of the integrated design process is a more sophisticated design team for the next project.

DESIGN AND CONSTRUCTION PROCESSES

Design-Build

One approach for building a new facility is to negotiate the project directly with a builder. The program statement is discussed with one or more reputable builders who are invited to submit project proposals. The builder then prepares *concept drawings* and a proposed *project budget*. Through interviews, evaluation of concept drawings, budget proposals, and references, a builder is selected and asked to prepare a detailed *scope of work*. The work scope details the facility to be constructed and the not-to-exceed cost of the specified facility. The proposal from the builder is an extremely important document in that it becomes the catalog of components which the builder has agreed to provide.

The builder, with a negotiated contract in hand, prepares architectural and engineering drawings for the project with the help of inhouse staff or other hired professionals. Unless specified by the administrator, these drawings may not be as detailed as those required for other construction processes. In the design-build process, the administrator/CEO must have a high level of trust in the builder that the quality of materials, systems and workmanship provided will be satisfactory because the administrator may not have a detailed project specification in advance of signing an agreement with the builder. For this reason, close inspection of other facilities constructed by the builder and careful evaluation of the builder's references is essential.

The major advantage of the design-build process is time saved by working directly with the builder and allowing him or her to proceed with the project in advance of having every detail drawn or material specified. The direct interface between the administrator and builder also facilitates decision making and the resolution of problems during construction and thus often advances the date of occupancy. The major disadvantage of the design-build approach is the absence of detailed plans and specification which the owner can review in advance of initiation of construction. All details of the final product may not be known at the time construction begins. Such uncertainty can be disastrous for complex projects; for projects with an inadequate program statement, or where there is any question about the quality or reputation of the builder. The design-build approach is not for the inexperienced or faint-of-heart administrator.

CONSTRUCTION MANAGEMENT

In the traditional design, bid and construction process, the administrator contracts with an architect for the design of a facility and the preparation of plans and specifications which are then used by general contractors to prepare bids to construct the project defined in those plans and specifications. Just as the architect contracts with a structural engineer, a mechanical engineer, an interior designer, and other specialists needed to design specific components of the building, the general contractor solicits prices from subcontractors to build a specific component of the building or install a particular building system. The sum of the prices provided by the subcontractors for each of the building's components plus the general contractor's overhead and profit becomes that contractor's bid to erect the new building. Included in the price is the responsibility to provide overall coordination of all subcontractors and the supervision of all work. The architect and engineers who have legal responsibility for their designs also monitor the construction to ensure that the designs are being followed and that the materials specified are properly installed.

Construction management services can be purchased and used as an adjunct to the traditional design process, as a method of contracting for construction, or both. If construction management (CM) services are purchased for the design phases of the project, construction specialists (often members of large construction firms) review and monitor the plans and specifications for the owner as they are being developed. The responsibilities of construction managers at these early stages of the project are to provide independent cost estimates of the facility being designed and, by virtue of their building experience, provide judgments about the constructability of the design, the likely time required to build the project, as well as provide value engineering.

Value engineering is a process where the construction manager evaluates the cost of each structural and building system being proposed against the cost of an alternative system, materials or construction method which may achieve the same or similar purpose. Such comparisons provide the owner an opportunity to make objective cost-benefit decisions about each component of the facility.

If the construction management approach is selected for the construction phase of the project, the CM and owner agree to a not-to-exceed guaranteed maximum price (GMP) at the time the designers complete plans and specifications. The CM then assumes the role of general contractor, soliciting subcontracts for building components, and providing overall project management for the owner. Such total management, in addition to the standard monitoring provided by the project architect and engineer, is increasing in popularity as a method to ensure the success of projects, particularly complex ones.

Bid and Construction

In the classical design-bid-construction process, *invitations for bids* are advertised in the newspaper or in special trade publications. Complete sets of project plans and specifications are studied by both general and subcontractors. The general contractor negotiates prices for each component of the project and then assembles a composite project *bid price* which is sealed in an envelope and submitted at a specific time and place for the *bid opening.* In its most simple form, each bid is publicly opened, read aloud, and recorded. The contract is then awarded to the low bidder assuming that the contractor meets specified bonding and insurance requirements.

For certain complex projects where costs are difficult to estimate or in situations where the bid market is volatile, the owner and designers might define certain components of the project as *add alternates* and request that contractors provide a base bid for the basic building and separate costs for each of several specified alternates. Such strategy may provide the administrator an opportunity to obtain some extra features or install higher levels of finish if the base bids turn out to be lower than estimated. In an unfavorable bidding market, this same strategy may enable the administrator with a fixed budget to construct the basic building and add frills later when additional funds become available.

In almost every project budget a certain amount of money is set aside as a *contingency* to cover unknown expenses or to make changes to the plans and specifications during the construction process. One example of an unknown expense would be the discovery under the new building of hidden layers of rock or an abandoned underground storage tank. Since neither of these conditions were known and thus not addressed by the plans and specifications the administrator must bear the cost of their removal. Contingency funds are used for such unanticipated discoveries during construction.

A second reason for budgeting contingency funds is to have funds to pay for *change orders.* Change orders arise during construction when it becomes necessary to change the plans or specifications. For example, if during a tour of the construction site, the administrator notes that the windows in all of the patient rooms are being installed at 42″ above the floor thereby making it impossible for most patients lying in bed to easily see the ground, the administrator may decide to lower all of the windows to a more acceptable level. For each requested modification, the architect is asked to prepare new drawings and specifications which are then submitted to the contractor who is asked to provide a price to make the requested change. For the example given, the cost reported by the contractor will be major. Not only will the administrator be asked to pay for removal of the work already installed and to reinstall the windows at the new lower level, but the contractor will also ask for compensation for the time lost, as well as a long list of other project items which must now be redesigned, purchased and installed. In general, the cost of change orders far exceeds their cost had the item been included in the original plans and specifications. The administrator has little leverage to negotiate the price of changes with the contractor, choices are to pay the asking price or to abandon the idea of making the change and construct the project according to the plans and specifications bid by the contractor. In some circles, the change order-process is called a license to steal. The significant lesson from this discussion is that there is no better investment than thorough planning, competent designers, and careful review of all plans and specifications prior to bidding the project. Any shortcuts will, at best, result in a less than outstanding facility; at worst, poor planning will cost significantly more.

Construction Phase

It is common practice throughout the construction process for the owner, architect, engineer, general contractor and each subcontractor to meet on a regular basis, usually weekly, to review the process of construction and to resolve coordination problems. Such *progress meetings* are important to the smooth completion of the project. When the general contractor and all of the subcontractors have finished their work and the general contractor declares that the project is complete, the administrator, architect and engineers systematically inspect the new facility and prepare a *punch list* of all items which need to be completed or corrected before the building is accepted. At the time the items on the punch list are corrected, the project is declared *substantially complete* and the administrator assumes *beneficial occupancy* and may move into the facility. At this time the *warranty* period begins. During the warranty period, usually one year, the builder is responsible for correcting building or system failures.

As noted above, the project architect and all consulting engineers have a contractual responsibility to monitor the construction to ensure that the building is being built according to the plans and specifications. However, such monitoring is often minimal and the administrator may find it beneficial to hire someone with construction experience to spend full time on the job site inspecting the work and ensuring that the materials specified are properly installed.

SUMMARY

Space and facilities are far more than a place where people work and patients are cared for. Spaces, depending on their location, unique design and level of finish become powerful statements of personal and organizational status. Thoughtful design and construction of facilities and spaces within facilities can help create a specified image as well a level of expectation that can influence the outcome of personal interactions.

All facilities, whether new or renovated, are created through a variety of planning and construction processes. However, the cornerstone of all planning efforts is the program statement, a detailed articulation of the activities to be conducted in the new facility and how those activities relate to one another, both functionally and spatially. Because of the importance of this document to any project, careful attention needs to be given to the team charged with its preparation as well as to the processes by which relevant information needed for the plan collected from throughout the organization. Shortcuts in this phase of the planning can be as disastrous and costly as a willingness to hire less than the most qualified design professionals available. Almost as important is organizing an integrated design team and ensuring that all members of the group work together lockstep until all of the design decisions have been finalized. The individual who has an institutional perspective, an experienced understanding of the politics of space and an appreciation of basic building systems, and factors which influence functionality, such as the importance of anticipating change, will be an invaluable member of the project's planning and design teams. Awareness of the many elements which can enrich the image and functionality of a space or entire building can be enhanced through practiced observation and evaluation of such matters as human interactions, pedestrian and work flows, lighting patterns and use of building materials. Such awareness can be an important and powerful tool in the hands of an administrator interested in maximizing the utilization of valuable space and facilities as well as enhancing the quality and functionality of space to maximize the long-term productivity of those who use the facility.

REFERENCES

Daft R, Steers R. *Organizations: A Micro/Macro Approach*. New York, Scott, Foresman, & Co, 1986

Hughes S. Bedside information systems: State of the art. In: Ball MJ, Hannah KJ, Jelger UG, Peterson H, eds. *Nursing Informatics: Where Caring and Technology Meet*. New York, Springer-Verlag, 1988

O'Desky RI. A neural view of computing for nurses. In: Ball MJ, Hannah KJ, Jelger UG, Peterson H, eds. *Nursing Informatics: Where Caring and Technology Meet*. New York: Springer-Verlag, 1988

Peterson H, Jelger UG. Hospital information systems. In Ball MJ, Hannah KJ, Jelger UG, Peterson H, eds. *Nursing Informatics: Where Caring and Technology Meet*. New York: Springer-Verlag, 1988

Robey D. *Designing Organizations*. Homewood, IL, Irwin, 1986

Romano, CA. Innovation: The promise and the perils for nursing and information technology. *Computers in Nursing*. 99, May/June, 1990

Turnage JJ. The challenge of the new workplace technology for psychology. *American Psychologist*. 45:172, 1990

CHAPTER 20

Purchasing and Materials Control

John J. Short
Pam Duchene

Key Concept List

Material management
Product standardization
Competitive bidding
Par stock replenishment
Stockless or just-in-time programs
Unit dose systems

The work of health care professionals mandates that their equipment and supplies be available 100 percent of the time. This requires systems to manage and control the acquisition and distribution of these materials. This is *material management* which Housley (1978) describes as the management and control of goods, services, and equipment from acquisition through disposition. Material management can encompass purchasing, receiving, central stores, mail services, central sterile processing, laundry services, pharmacy stores, print shop, and forms control.

Presented in this chapter are the basic elements of hospital material management with concentration on purchasing and material control in the patient care setting. Basic operational principles and current developments in material management will be explained. Finally, a section on drug control is presented.

The advent of prospective payment and managed care contracting have greatly increased the importance of material management in health care organizations. With cost-based reimbursement, the emphasis of the material manager was to ensure adequate inventories with little regard for the associated costs (eg, inventory stockpiling, obsolescence). This focus has changed dramatically.

Most nurses are aware of the logistical impact of material management; the availability of equipment and supplies plays an integral role in their efficiency and effectiveness. Few, however, are aware of the *financial* impact of material management. Housley (1978) estimates that the material manager may influence as much as 46 percent of the entire hospital budget. Furthermore, a typical 300 to 400 bed hospital's annual supply budget averages over $11.2 million (American Society for Hospital Materials Management, 1987).

PURCHASING

The purchasing function in any organization is responsible for the procurement of all goods and services for that organization. The various activities performed in purchasing goods and services include (a) evaluating new products and services; (b) evaluating suppliers; (c) placing orders for goods and services; (d) processing supplier invoices; and (e) troubleshooting problems.

Purchasing is an interactive process dependent on consistent communication between the user department, the supplier, and the purchasing department. Organizational policies and procedures guide the purchasing process and define responsibility for new product evaluation, supplier selection, purchasing decisions within defined dollar limits, purchase order issuance, and invoice payment. Effective policies and procedures optimize the purchasing function by recognizing that different sources of expertise are required. For example, the responsibility for issuing purchase orders is best left to the purchasing department due to the legal and organizational issues involved. Product evaluation, however, is best performed by nurses and other key users.

The Purchasing System
A typical hospital purchasing system revolves around the effective use of purchase requisitions and orders to ensure that the right product is delivered to the right place at the right time and at the right price.

Purchase Requisition. The purchase requisition is the principal communication between nursing service and purchasing. It is for internal use only and contains the basic instructions and requirements for the purchasing department to follow to place a particular order (eg, product, supplier, price, delivery date, ordering department name and charge information, and approval signature).

Purchase Order. The purchase order is a legal agreement between the hospital and the supplier, and should be designed as such. It is the principal communication between the organization and the supplier concerning an order, and should answer all questions concerning the order (eg, name and address of the organization placing the order, purchase order number, order date, expected delivery date, ordering department, quantity/unit of issue, price, and delivery/invoicing location). Additionally, standard terms and conditions of the purchase order should be included to afford protection to the hospital in the event of a dispute. Areas typically addressed by terms and conditions include: order acceptance, warranty, indemnification and insurance, provisions for changes or cancellation, and loss or theft. Refer to Housley (1978) for a more thorough description. Once finalized, the purchase order is transmitted to the supplier, with additional copies distributed to the receiving, accounts payable, user, purchasing, and accounting departments. Authority to issue purchase orders must be tightly controlled and typically is limited to the director of purchasing or material management.

Purchasing Practices in the Hospital Setting

Items which are purchased in almost any setting fall into one of three broad categories; consumable supplies, capital equipment, and contracted services.

Consumable Supplies. Consumable supplies (eg, medical, surgical, and office supplies) are low cost items (less than $300 to $500) with a useful life of one year or less. They are listed on the hospital financial statements as expenses, and do not contribute to the hospital's asset base or depreciation pool.

Evaluating Consumable Supplies. Individuals who evaluate supplies for purchase often tend to focus specifically on price. Value and utility, however, are more significant issues, and incorporate such nonprice factors as quality specifications, labor requirements, regulatory requirements, supply availability and acceptable substitutes. Such factors are often overlooked in purchasing decisions until a problem develops.

The knowledge and expertise needed to adequately evaluate products used in the patient care setting is unlikely to reside in any one individual. For this reason, a product standardization committee is often formed. This committee typically evaluates new products and identifies standard products for use throughout the hospital. It is comprised of a cross-section of hospital departments to ensure that the expertise needed for product evaluation is available. Committee responsibilities typically include the identification, evaluation, and implementation of new products, reduction of duplicate items via product standardization, and elimination of obsolete products.

Therefore, the committee charge should be from the administrator, as appropriate support by upper management is paramount in ensuring the success of this committee. Failure to provide such support reduces the committee's effectiveness. Institutional policy should require that any new patient care product be evaluated by the product standardization committee. Individuals introducing a new product must provide a brief summary of its expected benefits and costs to the committee. Most institutions have a standard form for this purpose. Once the committee has received and screened the new product request, one of three actions is taken: acceptance, rejection, or evaluation.

Immediate acceptance is rare and only granted for requests submitted with extensive product research and evaluation. Likewise, outright rejection is unusual unless it is evident that there is no apparent benefit to accepting the product. Product evaluation is the most common committee action. Several steps are necessary to ensure that an evaluation is fair and effective. First, key user groups should be identified. Second, similar products from other suppliers should be investigated to ensure that the best product is selected. Third, an evaluation methodology must be developed which includes the identification of test sites, data collection methods, and inservice training plans. Finally, decision criteria based on cost and quality factors must be established (see Fig 20–1). Cost/quality tradeoffs must be analyzed in depth in order to make an effective decision. While consideration of cost is often straightforward, quality assessment may be subjective, increasing the complexity of decision making. The ability to provide savings which can offset price increases should be assessed and quantified. For example, a more expensive product may require less nursing time, or a less costly item may require the purchase of costly adjunct supplies.

In addition to evaluating product requests from user departments, the product standards committee must be proactive in seeking cost saving opportunities by periodically evaluating items in use in the institution. Frequent assessments of the storeroom inventory must be performed in order to identify products which are not being used or have become obsolete and can be removed from the inventory.

Competitive Bidding

Items of a more generic commodity (eg, tape, gauze, gloves, disposable gowns, eggcrate mattresses) do not require extensive professional evaluation prior to purchase, and may not need the involvement of the product standardization committee. Purchasing decisions involving these items are usually managed via a straightforward *competitive bidding* process. The competitive bidding process involves several steps. First, the institution must forecast its annual usage of the product. Next, minimum acceptable product specifications must be determined. Products which do not meet these specifications will be excluded. Third, supplier terms and conditions must be identified in order to specify supplier performance criteria. Finally, a list of acceptable bidders must be developed. Many organizations set requirements that any purchase in excess of a predetermined dollar amount be competitively bid. Others leave that decision to the purchasing department's or the user's discretion. In either respect, health care professionals must be aware of the merits of competitive bidding in hold-

	Cost		
Quality	Increase	Same	Decrease
Increase	?	Accept	Accept
Same	Reject	?	Accept
Decrease	Reject	Reject	?

Figure 20–1. Product Standardization Decision Matrix

ing down supply costs. The competitive forces introduced by bidding provide one of the most effective means for an institution to hold down its supply costs.

Evaluating Capital Equipment

Health care institutions compete in an industry in which the availability of high tech equipment can have a major impact on its ability to attract patients, physicians and nurses and to deliver current, comprehensive patient care services. Nurse executives find themselves in the position of constantly evaluating and recommending purchase of new state-of-the-art equipment. As the availability of capital funds decreases with changes in reimbursement levels from government and private payors, nurse executives must ensure that major equipment purchase decisions are prudent.

Capital equipment is defined as any piece of equipment which costs in excess of a defined dollar amount (usually $300 to $500) and has a useful life of greater than one year. It is carried on the balance sheet as a depreciable asset and contributes to the depreciation pool. Equipment other than buildings and land is usually depreciated over a 10-year period in most not-for-profit hospitals. Most of the principles of purchasing capital equipment are the same as those for purchasing consumable supplies. Some differences do exist and these are discussed in this section.

In a capital equipment purchasing decision, the most costly mistake is not in paying too much for the equipment, but rather in buying a piece of equipment that never meets expectations. Every nurse executive can undoubtedly recall an example of an expensive piece of equipment that was purchased and ended up gathering dust in a storage closet. For this reason, a great deal of time and effort must be spent evaluating the piece of equipment, a responsibility best left to the users.

An on-site evaluation is one of the most effective aids to evaluate equipment. A supplier's refusal to allow an on-site trial should arouse suspicion of poor equipment performance, poor market penetration, general unavailability of the equipment, or obsolescence. Also included in the purchase agreement should be a clause providing for payment on acceptance or the withholding of a sizable portion of the final invoice payment until the equipment is performing successfully. A large outstanding balance is very effective at convincing the supplier to resolve any difficulties after the equipment is delivered. References from other hospitals that use the equipment in a similar application or environment should be verified. Finally, performance guarantees, where the purchase order language specifies performance criteria to be met over a defined period of time (eg, 30 days to 1 year) can be useful in preventing the purchase of an inadequate piece of equipment. Failure of the equipment to meet performance criteria will result in a refund or other remedy.

Often, institutions are in a position of evaluating similar equipment from multiple suppliers. The effects of competition provide further incentives for the supplier to ensure that the equipment will perform as expected. The institution must, once again, look beyond the price tag in order to gather an accurate picture of the true cost of the equipment. Other factors that can significantly impact on the equipment's total cost include: service costs, warranty period, freight charges, required supplies and peripheral equipment, and facility or environmental requirements. Additionally, in these days of leveraged buyouts, hostile corporate takeovers, and company reorganizations, some background knowledge of both the manufacturer and the distributor of a product (they are often different companies) is essential. Companies in poor financial condition or companies which have recently been bought or sold are more likely to make major changes in product lines, which may leave the institution with an obsolete piece of equipment.

Once the "non-price" factors have been addressed, the institution can begin negotiating the purchase price. The most important resource in this phase is *information*. The hospital is usually at a disadvantage during price negotiations because pricing information for specialized medical equipment is generally not available. All equipment manufacturers establish list prices and discounting policies for their product lines, but this information is rarely available to the institution. Some suppliers have been known to quote prices at levels well above the recommended list price. Erratic discounting practices create a "buyer beware" mentality and arouse suspicions of attempts to "dump" a product. The negotiation base of an institution may be improved through joining a purchasing group or service which negotiates directly with manufacturers or gathers data on purchase prices across a large cross section of institutions.

Contracted Services

Many institutions choose to hire outside companies to provide services within the institution. These services may include professional services, such as nursing, medical, laboratory, or data processing, or they may include facility services, such as housekeeping, laundry, or maintenance. Contracted service agreements vary widely and can apply to virtually every service performed in the institution. Some of the variables in contracted services include scope of service, ownership of employees, payment mechanisms, and liability and insurance requirements. These variables will be discussed as they apply to nursing agencies.

Scope of Service. Agreements may be limited to management or consulting services, or may include full provision of services. Given the nursing shortage, nurse executives may depend on service agreements with agencies to keep patient beds open. The Johnston R. Bowman Center for the Elderly, a specialized geriatric care hospital and part of Rush-Presbyterian-St. Luke's Medical Center, recently opened a new 10-bed geriatric medical unit through the use of contract nursing services. The agreement called for the unit to be managed by the hospital's gerontological nursing leadership, while the unit was staffed by agency nurses. In opening the unit, the department chairperson obtained competitive bids from various staffing agencies, and selected one agency to staff the unit contingent on the agency's ability to provide adequate numbers of nurses. Within one month, the agency failed to provide sufficient staff. The unit continues to function, but multiple agencies are required to supply enough nurses for safe patient care.

Ownership of Employees. Most management contracts keep staff level employees on the hospital payroll while all supervisory and management employees are on the contractor's payroll. This practice is in contrast with nurse staffing agencies where the nurses remain employees of the agency, not the hospital. The intense competition for nurses has resulted in the adoption of policies to prohibit or restrict employment of agency nurses by hospitals using agency services.

Payment Mechanism. A wide variety of payment mechanisms exists in the contracted services arena and ranges from a flat rate for services rendered to full-time and materials billing. Nursing agency rates vary according to shift, day of the week, and specialty, and payment is typically expected on a weekly or biweekly basis. Agency rates may be as much as three times the hourly salary of hospital employed nurses, which may lead to resentment of the agency nurses, who tend to receive lighter patient loads, without expectations to complete care plans and other responsibilities. Many contracted services agreements contain performance incentives such as guaranteed labor hours or fee caps. Care must be taken to ensure that these incentives do not encourage the contractor to behave in a manner which is in conflict with hospital goals and objectives.

Liability and Insurance. Provisions must be made in the event that a negligent act by a contractor employee results in a risk of liability for the hospital (or vice-versa). Most contracts specify limits of liability and requirements for liability insurance by the contractor. Staffing agencies carry liability and malpractice insurance, but nurse executives must verify licensure, insurance coverage, and performance ability of all agency nurses with patient care responsibilities.

Contracted services have become very common in some areas as hospitals have rethought the question: What business are we in? However the contract is structured, care must be taken to ensure that the contractor is acting in the best interest of the hospital at all times.

Trends in Purchasing Practices

Cost control pressures in the health care industry have resulted in a great deal of change in purchasing practices. Two of the most significant developments have been the increase in membership in purchasing groups and in the negotiation of corporate purchasing agreements with major suppliers.

Group Purchasing Organizations. Many institutions have joined one or more group purchasing organizations (GPOs) in an effort to consolidate their purchasing power with several other institutions. Most GPO's are formed by a hospital alliance or association and include anywhere from a few local member hospitals to hundreds of members nationwide. The GPO negotiates favorable contracts with selected suppliers by using the leverage of high volume purchases from its members. Pressure may be placed on member institutions by the GPO to adopt products of the suppliers with whom the GPO has negotiated contracts, thereby limiting freedom of the nurse executive to select products.

Corporate Purchasing Agreements. In an effort to increase market share, many suppliers are offering corporate purchasing agreements. These agreements vary widely, but the essential elements include a commitment by the institution to increase purchases from a supplier in return for lower prices, rebates, or some other form of financial benefit.

Both group purchasing organizations and corporate purchasing agreements enable institutions to consolidate purchases under a smaller range of vendors. Hospital mergers and multi-institutional corporations now make the larger entity able to purchase in bulk with resulting lower prices. Such consolidation may increase negotiating leverage, but may cause a reduction in competitive forces. Institutions can optimize their purchasing effectiveness by competitively bidding through multiple corporate agreements and group purchasing organizations.

MATERIAL CONTROL

The first section focused on the purchasing process of bringing goods and services *into* the hospital. This next section will focus on material control, or the set of systems and procedures used to manage the use of supplies once they are *inside* the hospital. These systems and procedures must address: requisitioning, delivery and distribution, storage, replenishment, control, patient charges, and cost allocation.

Institutions maintain both "official" and "unofficial" inventories. Official inventory is counted as assets on the financial statements and is defined as the inventory of supplies that is held in the central storeroom, pharmacy, dietary, and central sterile processing areas. Once items are dispensed to user departments or consumed, they are considered expenses. Unofficial inventory, on the other hand, is the inventory of supplies ordered and controlled by user departments, and is expensed immediately. As third-party insurers move away from cost-based reimbursement, the advantages of maintaining unofficial inventory diminish. Modern inventory control methods call for a drastic reduction in unofficial inventory levels in order to help increase cash flow.

Another factor in inventory control is that some items are charged directly to patients, while others are charged to hospital departments. Patient charge items add a charge to a specific patient's bill and also expense the item to the appropriate department. Usually the department which receives the revenue will also receive the expense for the item in an effort to match revenues and expenses. Increasing the number of patient charge items increases the complexity of the hospital billing process and the risk of lost patient charges, but it also increases the hospital's revenue and allows better tracking of supply use. The revenue generating advantages of patient charge items, however, are decreasing as more third-party payors are changing to per-diem, per-case, or capitation reimbursement methods. Also, insurance audits reveal that many items charged are not used by the patient to whom they are billed and are being challenged on an increasingly frequent basis.

The overall objectives of any material control process are to maintain inventory supply, minimize inventory cost, and provide information for decision making.

Inventory Supply

Most institutions use one of two standard official inventory supply methods in patient care areas: par stock replenishment or exchange cart.

Par Stock Replenishment. This method requires establishing maximum supply or par levels, for each official inventory item used in the department. Storeroom personnel routinely check the supply levels and replenish each item up to its par level.

Par stock replenishment systems provide a framework for gradually increasing the number of items which are brought into the official inventory. They also provide data on item usage and decrease the amount of required storage space. However, the systems may be labor intensive and require a centralized storage space for organization.

Exchange Cart. This method involves the use of wheeled storage carts to hold the department's supply inventory. Supplies are stocked at predetermined levels on these carts and are replenished via total cart replacement. The old exchange cart is returned to the storeroom and restocked for the next delivery.

The principal advantage to an exchange cart system is the improved distribution efficiency of storeroom personnel. A single visit to the user department is required for stock replenishment and the amount of time required for exchange is minimal. However, the system requires an investment in carts, usually two per area served, and the carts require storage space.

Inventory Control

The need for adequate supplies at all times in the hospital setting must be balanced with the need to minimize stockpiling of inventory. Stockpiling ties up precious financial resources in nonproducing assets, and may lead to increased usage and waste of supplies. Additionally, it risks carrying supplies that will become obsolete or outdated and uses large amounts of storage space.

Performance Measures

Various methods of measuring inventory control performance are used by hospital administrators and material managers. These include *inventory turnover ratio* and *inventory dollars per bed*. Inventory turnover ratio is the total dollar amount of all official inventory issues divided by the average inventory value for the year. The inventory turnover ratio provides a measure of how well inventory is being turned over from the central storeroom, with a high inventory turnover ratio (nine to twelve) indicative of good inventory management.

The inventory dollars per bed calculation is often used for comparing hospitals within a given bed-size category. It is derived by dividing the average inventory value for the year by the total number of equivalent occupied beds in the hospital. Operating beds are used instead of licensed beds, and units with low supply use (eg, psychiatry, nursery, rehabilitation, and skilled care) are excluded.

Inventory Control Methods

The material manager's performance in maintaining the appropriate balance between the opposing needs for adequate supplies and minimal inventory levels will have a significant impact on the hospital's daily operations as well as on the hospital's financial performance. For these reasons, inventory control must be approached in a systematic fashion.

Most institutions carry anywhere from 500 to 1200 items in the central storeroom. One method of simplifying the approach to the large number of storeroom items is to perform an *ABC analysis*. An ABC analysis ranks storeroom items on the basis of their total dollar impact (See Fig 20-2). The material manager then focuses control efforts on those items that have the greatest financial impact on the hospital. Items comprising 70 percent of total storeroom costs are ''A'' items; items comprising the next 20 percent of total storeroom costs are ''B'' items; and the remaining items are ''C'' items. Separate policies and procedures may be set for each of the three classifications of inventory. These policies and procedures may differ in how they address areas such as budgeting, forecasting, inventory levels, method of supply reordering and replenishment, competitive bidding practices, and use of alternate products.

Inventory Supply and Replenishment.   Any ordering system must address two basic questions: When to reorder? How much to order?

When to Reorder.   Determination of a reorder point requires knowledge of the anticipated lead time for the arrival of new supplies and of the amount of the item that will be used while the new order is in transit (see Fig 20-3). A decision must be made regarding the need to carry ''safety stock'' or a substitute in the event of a delayed shipment or an unexpected surge in demand.

How Much to Order.   Determining the appropriate quantity of an item to order must balance two opposing forces: purchasing a large enough quantity to secure the best

Item Number	Description	Unit Cost	Issues	Total Cost	Cumulative Percent	Class
14059	Infusion cassette	4.00	30455	121820	3.3	A
15296	Latex exam gloves	7.25	16422	119060	6.5	A
25896	Copier paper	21.75	3761	81802	8.8	A
12356	Underpads	2.02	35991	72702	10.7	A
50024	.02% Dextrose	41.40	146	6044	70.1	B
25874	Sterile bedpan	.75	8057	6043	70.3	B
47852	Posey jackets	15.41	116	1788	90.0	C
18899	Vacutainer, red	4.38	402	1761	90.1	C
25863	Eraser	.16	20	3	99.9	C
Total dollar volume, all issues				$3,688,546		

Figure 20-2. Example of an ABC Analysis

Item	4 × 4 gauze sponge
Issue unit	package
Annual usage	6,935 packages (19/day)
Unit price	$1.39/package
Average lead time between deliveries	7 days
Safety stock	76 packages (4 days supply)
Ordering cost	$4.50 per line item
Holding cost	33% of inventory value

Reorder Point

Reorder point = (19 pkgs/day) 7 days + 76 pkgs = 209 pkgs

Economic Order Quantity (EOQ)

EOQ = square root of [2(6935pkgs/yr) × 4.50/line item] divided by ($1.39/pkg) 33%
  = square root of 136,069.32
  = 368 pkgs or 31 cases of 12 pkgs

Figure 20-3. Reorder Point/Economic Order Quantity Calculation

price and purchasing a small enough quantity to ensure maximum inventory turn-over. One of the most widely used techniques is the economic order quantity (EOQ). EOQ provides a method of balancing order quantities with inventory holding costs to yield the lowest total cost for a particular item.

Information Management

Material managers have at their disposal a wealth of information for facilitating decision making. Trends in third-party reimbursement are causing hospitals to pay closer attention to the cost of delivering care. Many hospitals are implementing systems which will monitor and report cost performance by diagnostic category, by DRG, or by patient in an effort to improve financial accountability. The "new wave" of purchasing and inventory control systems call for integration with other hospital systems for budgetary control, resource consumption, asset depreciation, and other related areas. Systems integration will be the theme for material managers in the future.

Trends in Inventory Management. As stated earlier, hospitals are faced with increasing pressures to improve financial performance by reducing inventory levels. The benefits of stockpiling inventory due to cost based reimbursement are diminishing and, as a result, hospital material managers are turning to their counterparts in manufacturing industries for ideas. Some principles of inventory control which have come from the manufacturing setting include "stockless" or "just in time" purchasing, and consignment purchasing.

The basic concept of stockless, or just-in-time programs (the terms are often used interchangeably) involves a supplier maintaining a full inventory of the hospital's supplies and delivering small shipments of supplies, presorted by functional area, in 24-to-48-hour intervals. This type of program is best suited for items which are used in large amounts and are considered commodity items (eg, tape, gauze, sutures, trays). Stockless programs can reduce inventory holding costs and receiving time. Additionally, just-in-time purchasing may provide better tracking of daily supply use and can streamline ordering procedures. However, stockless/just-in-time programs have a few disadvantages. They require a great deal of up-front work to establish item usage histories, identify substitute items (in case of stockouts) and to develop ordering procedures. Such programs often result in higher unit prices since they require more handling and assumption of risk by the supplier, and they make verification of receipts difficult since items are packed by user area and are often in irregular quantities.

Consignment Purchasing. Consignment purchasing programs are often used for infrequently used products, carry a high cost, and are required on short notice (eg, cardiac pacemakers, bone prostheses). Under a consignment program, the supplier places a full inventory of products in the hospital, but retains title to the goods. The hospital only pays for the products when (and if) they are used. Such a program allows the hospital to carry a full inventory of specialized products without investing large amounts of financial resources in this inventory. The products are stored on hospital premises and are available on demand.

Potential disadvantages to consignment purchasing exist. The additional handling and assumption of risk by the supplier will probably result in higher product costs. Secure, insured storage areas with limited accessibility are required since product damage or theft may result in financial liability for the hospital. Finally, care must be taken to ensure that competitive products are not excluded from choice simply because they are not available on consignment.

DRUG CONTROL

Distribution and Control

Hospitalized individuals receive an average of 9.1 medications during an inpatient stay in the United States making the hospital pharmacy a pivotal therapeutic service (Vestal, 1984). According to the American Society for Hospital Pharmacists (ASHP), pharmaceutical service should include the control, distribution, and procurement of all pharmaceutical supplies and medications used within the hospital (Hassan, 1986). ASHP also notes that the provision of current, accurate drug information is a critical service of the pharmacy, and that it is the responsibility of hospital staff pharmacists, nurses, and physicians to facilitate quality assurance of drug therapy through the development of policies and procedures. JCAHO standards hold that hospitals shall maintain pharmaceutical services led by qualified pharmacists and shall supervise the storage, preparation, dispensation and administration of medications.

Hospital Formulary System. The past few decades have seen radical changes in health care. One area of the hospital in which this is evident, clearly, is that of the hospital pharmacy. The role of the hospital-based pharmacist has changed from drug chemist to clinician. Contemporary concerns of hospital-based pharmacists revolve around clinical activities, in addition to the safe, efficient, and economical purchase, storage, and distribution of medications.

The quantity of pharmaceuticals available for clinical treatment is beyond the scope of any pharmacy. It is impractical and costly for pharmacists to attempt to carry every drug the medical staff may order for patient treatment. To promote effective and efficient drug utilization, hospital pharmacy and therapeutics committees are charged with establishing a hospital formulary system to identify which drugs to stock in the pharmacy. In completing this selection, committee members attempt to select medications that will be used frequently or are needed on an emergency basis and to reduce redundancy in drug ordering. Based on decisions of the pharmacy and therapeutics committee, a hospital formulary is developed and published within the hospital to ensure availability to medical and nursing staff. For each drug listed, the hospital formulary typically includes generic and trade names, the American Hospital Formulary System number, active ingredients, and types of drugs available in stock.

Because implementing a hospital formulary imposes limitations on the availability of pharmaceutical supplies that are stored in the hospital, a frequent issue is the ordering of medications not carried in stock. Implementation of a hospital formulary system also may result in liability risks. Within limits of their professional judgments, pharmacists are legally responsible for complying with physicians' medications orders and nurses are expected to administer them. Problems do not result if therapeutically equivalent brand name drugs are substituted for physician ordered generic or chemical name agents. However, when brand name drugs not available in the formulary are ordered, the pharmacist must verify with the physician that substitution is acceptable prior to dispensing an equivalent drug. The common practice of obtaining blanket approval for the formulary from the medical staff leaves the pharmacist open to liability risks. A better solution is to have prescription blanks printed with the clause ''may substitute with generic equivalent''. If physicians do not desire a substitution, they need only delete the clause, indicating that substitution is not acceptable.

Once a hospital formulary is determined and approved, it needs to be under continuous evaluation and monitoring by the pharmacy and therapeutics committee. Members of the committee review all drugs included in the formulary, and determine which preparations need to be deleted or added to the system, and which require monitoring, or are to be available for a restricted time period. Additionally, the committee recommends which members of the medical staff may use and prescribe the drugs.

A primary advantage of using a hospital formulary system is cost efficiency through purchasing control. Rather than stocking multiple chemically and therapeutically equivalent drugs, the pharmaceutical purchasing agent purchases one of a group of therapeutically equivalent medications at a higher volume, enabling price reductions. Such pharmacy cost savings should be conveyed to patients through lower pharmaceutical charges. A second benefit of a hospital formulary system is that medication instruction for physicians, nurses, and patients can be geared to those drugs listed in the hospital formulary and may result in more focused instruction.

The hospital formulary system may cause concern among physicians, as the physician is no longer able to have orders filled immediately for drugs not listed in the formulary. Physicians are asked to comply with the formulary system as much as possible in order to preserve its benefits. Physicians who are not members of the pharmacy and therapeutics committee may feel inadequately represented and may resent the decisions of the committee members. Unfortunately, nurses often bear the brunt of the physician's frustrations with the formulary system. A final limitation to hospital formulary systems occurs when pharmacy administration fails to pass the cost savings resulting from volume purchasing on to the patient. This limitation, however, is not a failure of the concept, but rather a result of the manner in which the system is implemented.

Unit Dose System. As pharmacy stocking practices have changed dramatically with the implementation of hospital formulary systems, medication dispensing procedures have been modified through the evolution to unit dose systems. The trend is to move from floor stock systems associated with high medication error rates (Calder, 1982) to unit dose programs.

Currently, 85 percent of US hospitals use some form of unit dose system (Koska, 1989). In unit dose systems, drugs are ordered, stocked, dispensed, administered, and charged in single units of use (Hassan, 1986). Given the current shortage of nurses, a primary benefit of unit dose systems is the reduction in nursing time required for medication preparation. This is true, particularly, if the unit dose system includes intravenous fluids in addition to other medications. The economic benefits of the unit dose system transcend beyond reduction of nursing hours to include decrease in pilfering and waste of floor stock, accurate charging for doses used, and elimination of credits for unused medications, because patients are charged for only those doses used. As unit dose systems eliminate the need for floor stock, waste and theft of stock drugs is reduced, and floor space required for drug storage is gained. Original medication orders are triple checked first by pharmacists prior to dispensing the unit dose medications, then by the pharmacy technician filling the prescription, and finally by the nurse administering the drug. The result is a direct patient benefit of drug error reduction and elimination (Calder, 1982).

The unit dose system can be effective with either a centralized or decentralized pharmacy department. In a centralized system, single use units sufficient for 24 hours of medication administration are dispensed daily to each nursing unit directly from the hospital pharmacy through a medication cart exchange and through use of a pneumatic tube. Decentralized systems, usually found in large hospitals with multiple buildings, involve satellite pharmacies located throughout the hospital with pharmacy technicians responsible for delivery of single use units daily to the nursing units.

A principle rationale for implementing a unit dose system is for accurate accounting of medications used. The system is associated with increased expenses, however, in pharmacist time required to check all medication orders and all unit dose deliveries made to the nursing units. Unit dose systems impose time lags between the ordering of medications and drug administration that did not exist with floor stock. In nursing units, such as critical care settings, where medication adjustments are made frequently, or drugs are needed on an emergency basis, such time lags may compromise safe patient care. In such situations, the best solution may be a blend of unit dose and floor stock systems with emergency drugs available as floor stock.

Computerized Systems. Perhaps the newest trend to revise pharmacy distribution and control systems is computerization (Cornell, 1983). Rather than reviewing a lengthy list of drugs available in the hospital formulary, physicians and nurses indicate a needed drug through the computer, and ascertain immediately whether or not the drug is carried in stock and how it is approved for use. Although computerization of the hospital formulary does not eliminate the frustration a physician may express because the drug desired is not included, the message can be relayed faster, and the pharmacist called more quickly to order the necessary medication. Hospital formulary systems may be computerized to provide a tickler system for pharmacy and therapeutics committees with regard to continuous review of the drugs listed in the systems. Computerized records of medication errors may be linked to the formulary system to cue the pharmacy and therapeutics committee into problematic drug situations.

Comprehensive computerization systems are available for medication ordering, administration, and documentation. In such systems, the unit clerk enters a drug order, the nurse reviews and signs the order, the pharmacy technician fills the order, and the pharmacist checks the order with the medication dispensed, and the nurse administers the drug. Computerized systems may identify drugs that require frequent laboratory monitoring, reminding physicians, nurses, and pharmacists to check laboratory values for possible adverse drug reactions. Such systems may prompt clinicians to check for potential interactions, including drug-drug, and drug-food interactions. Additionally, drug interactions may be computerized with regard to clinical significance and all allergies the patient may have are recorded and cross-checked with medication orders.

An additional pharmaceutical computer application, MEDSTATION, an automated narcotic and PRN system is in use at Barnes Hospital (St. Louis, Missouri). The Pyxis Corporation developed the system which is accessed by nurses through a security code. To obtain a patient medication, the nurse keys in an identification number, patient number, and medication choice, thereby opening the appropriate medication compartment. The system eliminates the need for narcotic keys and manual narcotic checking systems. At Barnes, the system has resulted in better patient care through reducing delays and errors in narcotic administration. Additionally, it is linked into automatic billing and has led to an improvement in the charge capture percentage.

Interdisciplinary Pharmaceutical Management

Pharmacy and Therapeutics Committee. The charge of this committee is to promote safe pharmaceutical therapy with resulting optimal patient care. The pharmacy and therapeutics committee membership is comprised of a least three physicians representing different specialties, and one or more nurses, administrators, and pharmacists, the director of whom commonly serves as acting or recording secretary. The nurse administrator may find the pharmacy and therapeutics committee of assistance when questions regarding the nursing role in drug administration occur. The committee recommends policy implementation, modification, and deletion regarding drug therapy to hospital, medical and nursing administration. The pharmacy and therapeutics committee is responsible for review of threats to safe medication administration, including: adverse or untoward drug reactions, medication errors, new brand and generic drugs, floor stock drugs, and emergency drug lists. The committee identifies emergency drugs and narcotics that are to be kept on the nursing units.

New and Investigational Drugs. With drugs that are newly released by the Food and Drug Administration, the pharmacy and therapeutics committee need to identify if chemically and therapeutically equivalent drugs are currently available in the pharmacy stock. If, however, the new drug meets a clinical need not addressed by other stock medications, the committee may advise that it be added to the hospital formulary. The pharmacy and therapeutics committee should consider any unique aspects of the new medication, and should recommend an educational program for safe administration of the drug.

The issues with investigational drugs are less clear. Requests to use investigational drugs should be reviewed by the pharmacy and therapeutics committee following approval by the facility's human investigations committee. If the study is scientifically sound and meets clinical, ethical, and legal standards, including the standard for informed consent and ability to withdraw from the study, both committees may approve the use of the investigational drug.

Medication Errors

Classification System. There are conflicting reports regarding the national medication error rate, with estimates ranging between 0.008 percent (Sherman & Clinefelter, 1989) and 20 percent (Koska, 1989). A primary obstacle to the determination of medication error rates is the lack of standard error definition. For example, in a study of 11 teaching hospitals, the criteria for correct administration time ranged from doses given immediately before or after the scheduled time to doses given within 1 hour before or after the time (Sherman & Clinefelter, 1989). Medication errors can be placed into nine categories of error (see Table 20–1): omission, unauthorized (or wrong) drug, incorrect administration technique, and wrong dose, dosage form, route, rate, time, or preparation.

Appraisal and Policy. Nurse administrators, with the pharmacy and therapeutics committee, must establish clear, specific, and objective criteria defining medication error. Determining clear criteria will enable the nurse executive to identify error rates and trends in errors. Corresponding with such operational definitions, the nurse administrator develops policies for reporting incidents, and guidelines for consideration of disciplinary action and identification of learning needs. In order to track medications accurately, error or incident reports contain information regarding the time, date, and individual responsible for the error. Information on the specific drug error

TABLE 20-1. CATEGORIES OF MEDICATION ERROR

Error Type	Description
Omission error	Failure to administer an ordered dose of medication
Example:	Digoxin 0.125 p.o. daily is ordered and one dose is omitted
Wrong dose	Failure to administer the dose of medication ordered
Example:	Tylenol #3 (2) p.o. q 4 hours PRN for severe headache is ordered and Tylenol #3 (1) p.o. is given
Wrong dosage	Failure to administer the medication ordered in the correct dosage form
Example:	Neosporin opthalmic ointment q 4 hours is ordered and Neosporin opthalmic solution is administered
Wrong route	Failure to administer the medication by the route ordered
Example:	Valium 5 mg IM q 4 hours PRN agitation is ordered and Valium 5 mg p.o. is given
Wrong rate	Failure to administer the medication at the rate ordered
Example:	D5.45NS IV @ 100cc/hour is ordered and D5.45NS IV is infused at 50cc/hour
Wrong time	Failure to administer the medication at the time prescribed
Example:	Mefoxin 100mg IV q 8 hours is ordered and is given at 6am and 10pm during a 24 hour period
Wrong preparation	Failure to reconstitute or dilute the drug correctly
Example:	Amoxil suspension 250mg/5cc p.o. TID is ordered. The powdered Amoxil (7.5g) is diluted with 10cc bacteriostatic water.
Unauthorized (wrong) drug	Administration of a medication that has not been ordered
Example:	The patient has developed a fever of 101.5F and the physician is not answering by phone or pager. ASA 5 gr is given p.o.
Incorrect administration technique	Administration of a medication at the correct site and by the appropriate route, but with an improper technique
Example:	Imferon 10mg IM Z track is ordered and Imferon 10 mg IM is given

needs to include the specific drug order and the drug, dosage, form, route, and strength administered or omitted. Individuals (physician and nursing supervisor) to whom the error was reported are noted. Reports include untoward reactions experienced by the patient, and corrective actions taken to prevent a reoccurrence of the error type. Reports are completed in a factual, objective format, without fault or blame finding (Tobias, 1988). Completion of the report in a judgmental fashion will result in a review of one individual's perception and opinion of the incident, rather than the error itself.

Incident reports of medication errors, once prepared and reviewed with the physician and nursing supervisor, are forwarded to the risk management department. Error reports, with names deleted, are reviewed by the pharmacy and therapeutics committee for needed preventive or corrective actions. During the pharmacy and therapeutics committee's review of the incident reports, the committee members should keep in perspective that the rationale for incident reports is twofold: to prevent a re-occurrence and to identify educational needs (Tobias, 1988).

Risk Management

The rate of medication errors has been found to be altered through changes in distribution and control of drugs and with systems such as unit dose systems. Computerized medication administration records resulted in a decrease in medication error rates by 18 percent (Adams, 1989). Unit dose systems were found to keep medication error rates between 2 and 5 percent (Koska, 1989). An all RN staff and primary nursing are associated with lower error rates (Sherman & Clinefelter, 1989).

The single, most powerful method of reducing medication error rates is through careful reporting, tracking, and follow-up of medication errors. Through such tracking, a variety of risk factors for medication errors have been identified. The absence of a hospital pharmacist is a risk factor. At least 50 percent of US hospitals do not have a staff pharmacist (Hassan, 1986). Such hospitals may be able to use a consultant pharmacist, share pharmacy services, or purchase pharmacy services from a pharmacy or larger health care facility. Insufficient lighting in drug administration areas and inadequate labeling of medication packages are two other contributors to medication errors. Medication carts are conveniences that result in time savings for nurses but may result in drug error if used at night in hallways where lights are dim. Package labeling (even in unit dose systems) needs to include the drug name, brand (if applicable) and generic, strength, route ordered, and precautions (Cohen, 1989).

A primary risk factor affecting potential medication errors is the lack of sufficient policies for medication incident reporting (Tobias, 1988). Some nurses will fill out a medication incident report when replacement of a pill is necessitated due to dropping a tablet. Others may not complete a report unless the patient's status has been compromised, such as through infusion of a 12-hour intravenous infusing in 3 hours. One method of increasing the efficiency of incident review mechanisms is through categorizing the errors. In one facility, medication errors are sorted into three categories, with category I indicating minimal or no intervention required, category II reflective of the need for localized response to correct the error, and category III associated with a potentially life-threatening error and requiring immediate contact of the facility's insurance carrier or legal authorities (Brandt, Demi, Gerke, & Lee, 1988). Such a system does not reduce the number of error reports, but can increase the speed with which serious errors are identified for corrective action.

Disciplinary Action. Nurse executives may view medication error reports as educational opportunities (Rasic, Boedicker, & Lyon, 1989). However, excessive or potentially life-threatening errors may indicate unsafe performance and the need for disciplinary action or termination. Unfortunately, many hospitals do not have systematic processes for discipline following medication errors, resulting in inconsistent follow-up for errors. In Canada, a firm stance is taken toward medication errors, with disciplinary action considered any and every time a medication error is committed (Harnden, 1988). Such a position is inhibitive to honest error reporting. Assuring nurses that no disciplinary action will be taken for medication errors fosters inadequate concern regarding errors. A medication error analysis system is needed to facilitate consistent and prudent disciplinary follow up to error patterns.

Nurse administrators of one facility advocate the use of a point value system (Rasic, Boedicker, & Lyon, 1989). In the system, points are derived from the type of error, outcome, and length of time between errors. Disciplinary action corresponds with the number of error points the individual nurse has received. The system enables tracking of nurses with high error rates yet avoids penalization of nurses for honest reporting of inconsequential errors, such as a 15 minute delay in administration of a daily medication.

Although it is essential for promotion of safe and high-quality patient care that medication errors be linked to disciplinary action, it is prudent for nurse administrators to recognize creative methods of error prevention. To illustrate, on a 44-bed geriatric rehabilitation unit, two individuals named J. Brandt were hospitalized. Both were female and over the age of 65. To prevent potential errors, primary nurse of one J. Brandt posted a large notice in the nursing conference area that stated, "Did you realize that there are *two* Mrs. J. Brandt's? Joyce Brandt is in 644 B and June Brandt is in 650 A." The notice appeared to be unit trivia, but was written for the purpose of preventing errors. It was attention getting to alert nurses, therapists, transporters, and physicians of the similarity in patient names. The notice served its purpose and no medication errors occurred. The nurse responsible for taking the preventive action received recognition in his evaluation and at department meetings for displaying the type of professional concern and creativity that create a high-quality care environment.

Dispensing During Evening and Night Shifts

One frequent problem that nurse administrators face is the lack of constant pharmacist-supervised pharmaceutical service. The availability of a 24-hour, 7-day a week pharmacy with pharmacist services is rare in any but the largest medical center. Since all hospitals provide nursing service even during hours when the pharmacy is closed, the responsibility for dispensing medications during pharmacy off-hours sometimes falls to the nursing supervisor. Since it is not within the scope of nursing practice to dispense medications, this substitution of pharmacists with nurses is at best dangerous and, in some areas, is illegal. Night cabinets, often constructed in the wall of the pharmacy for efficient servicing, minimize the risks associated with the absence of a pharmacist and provide for drug inventory control, but are costly to install. A less costly method of providing a night cabinet involves a portable floor to ceiling cart that is lockable but can be kept in an area more accessible to nursing supervisors or charge nurses for after-hours needs.

Another means of accessing the pharmacy to obtain nonfloor stock drugs is through physician services. While there are no legal restrictions prohibiting physicians from dispensing medications, physicians may object to spending time searching the pharmacy for products. Since the salary of most physicians exceeds that of staff pharmacists, this practice may not result in cost savings. Other alternatives include extending pharmacy hours, purchasing pharmacist services from a community pharmacy, or larger medical center, or placing pharmacists on-call for during off-shift hours.

Employee Selection

Employees who will be working with pharmacy and central supply stock are entrusted through the facility and public to prevent drug and supply confiscation and misuse (Daniels, 1986). The risks of employing dishonest individuals in the pharmacy and central supply areas may be minimized through careful screening and reference checks. Security screening of prospective employees can be completed by the local and state police (Daniels, 1986). Since arrest records have been found to be discriminatory to minority group members, it is best to use conviction record. To avoid charges of invasion of privacy, the candidates for positions need to sign a release for the security search. (Information on selection can be found in Chapter 12.)

SUMMARY

Effective nursing care delivery depends on the availability of necessary supplies and drugs. Given the financial impact of material management and purchasing, it is imperative that nurse executives have a solid comprehension of the areas. Dramatic reductions in patient care costs may be made through efficient purchasing and hospital formulary use.

REFERENCES

Adams C. Computer-generated medication administration records. *Nursing Management.* 20:7, 22, 1989

American Society for Hospital Materials Management. *1986–1987 National Survey Results and Performance Indicators,* Chicago, American Hospital Association and Coopers and Lybrand, 1987

Brandt M, Demi M, Gerke M, Lee E. A severity index for medication errors. *Nursing Management.* 19:8, 80I, 1988

Calder G. Purchasing, distribution and control of hospital medicines. In: Lawson D, Richards R, eds. *Clinical Pharmacy and Hospital Drug Management.* London, Chapman and Hall, 1982: 355–378

Cohen M. Medication errors: Extra label may prevent mixing mix-up. *Nursing Management.* 19:2, 12, 1989

Cornell J. *Computers in Hospital Pharmacy Management.* Rockville, MD, Aspen Systems Corporation, 1983

Daniels C. Recruitment and selection. In: Noel M, Bootman J, eds. *Human Resources Management.* Rockville, MD, Aspen Publication Systems, 1986: 1–11

Harnden L. Disciplinary responses to nurses medication errors. *Dimensions in Health Service.* 65:4, 26, 1988

Hassan W. *Hospital Pharmacy,* 5th ed. Philadelphia, Lea and Febiger, 1986

Housley C. *Hospital Material Management.* Germantown, MD, Aspen Systems Corporation, 1978

Koska M. Drug errors: Dangerous, costly, and avoidable. *Hospitals.* 63:11, 24, 1989

Lamnin M. *Quality Assurance in Hospital Pharmacy: Strategies and Techniques,* Rockville, MD, Aspen Systems Corporation, 1983

Rasic E, Boedicker M, Lyon M. A new system for managing medication errors. *Nursing Management.* 20:5, 102, 1989

Noel M. Effective discipline. In: Noel M, Bootman J, eds. *Human Resources Management.* Rockville, MD, Aspen Systems Corporation, 1986: 111–126

Sherman J, Clinefelter K. Medication variances: A multihospital comparison. *Nursing Management.* 20:5, 56, 1989

Tobias R. The incident report. In: Hamman J, Ziengenfuss J, Williamson J, eds. *Risk Management Trends and Applications.* Sarasota, FL, American Board of Quality Assurance and Utilization Review Physicians, 1988: 41–63

Vestal R. *Drug Treatment in the Elderly.* Australia, ADIS Health Science Press, 1984

CHAPTER 21

Reporting, Documentation, and Computers

Linda Fournier
Ann Minnick
Sandra Robertson

Key Concept List

Information management
Automated systems
Reporting formats
Forms appraisal
Report writing

OVERVIEW: MANAGEMENT OF INFORMATION

The introduction of computers has made it possible to compile information on a scale that was only imagined 50 years ago. Although technology has made it possible to store ever-increasing amounts of data, the ability of the human to consider a number of facts simultaneously has not improved significantly. The successful administrator of the late twentieth century must decide how to address this overwhelming data load. For the nurse executive, the decision is one of professional survival. The failure to have important pieces of information, the inability to retrieve extant data in a timely fashion, and the reliance on faulty data can all lead to decisions that are disastrous to an organization's viability. In addition, expenditure of valuable resources on the collection of superfluous or duplicative information can result in the waste of increasingly scarce professional nursing time.

The Whys of Data Collection

The purposes of any health care information system are: (1) to provide a basis for rational decision making; (2) to substantiate claims regarding the type, quantity, and quality of service to legal, payor, and accreditation representatives; and, in a related context; (3) to document the resources utilized in the provision of these services. In a variation of the theme of "keep your eye on the ball," the nurse executive should spend the bulk of time allotted for the consideration of an institutional information system on the uses of the data. Decisions regarding what information to collect and when to collect it logically follow the results of this consideration (Fig 21-1). How to collect the data should probably be the last item of consideration.

Unfortunately, the process in many institutions is the exact opposite of this approach. The executive may be tempted to accept that the needed information merely should be available faster, or less expensively, or in a new format. Hiring consultants to provide information on "how" to collect data (eg, design or sell software or computers) reinforces this mistake. The result can be a new information system that produces garbage at five times the previous rate. There is no attempt to identify what information would be helpful if only it were gathered. Unfortunately there is no exploration of other (noncomputerized) ways to exchange data. In some situations, there may be cheaper or more effective methods.

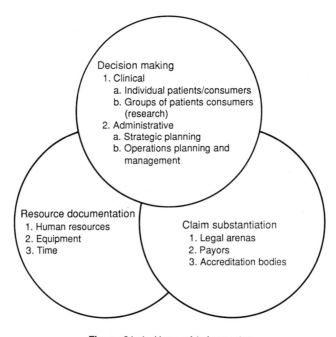

Figure 21-1. Uses of Information

One way executives can avoid the temptation to begin to immediately worry about bites, bytes, or multitask work stations is to force themselves to develop lists of how the data lodged in an information system will be used. The change to the plural of executive in this paragraph is not by chance or poor editing. The management group needs to have an active role at this critical juncture. By its very nature, information needs to exchanged. The purposes for which each manager needs information may differ. One example is the age of the employees. A human resource manager may need to know the birthdate of each employee for the determination of pension accruals, whereas the nursing information center may wish to know the age distributions of the staff in order to develop more effective recruitment campaigns. Information systems are too expensive to meet the needs of only one member of the institution.

If an information system is too important to be left to one manager, it is also too important to be left to only managers. All users of information need to begin to identify the purposes to which data are to be put. In reality, this means that every level of the organization needs to have a way in which to communicate to the information system designers the purposes for which they use information. Although the way in which users have this type of input will vary with an organization's culture, brainstorming sessions, nominal group process, or study sections may be useful.

The description of the purposes need not be done in a vacuum. The decision making of health care revolves around two interrelated concepts: clinical judgments and administrative determinations. The clinical judgments are based on data that result from testing and observation of the client and information that comes from testing and observation of persons with similar problems, ie, through research. Administrative determinations include those related to the use of human and physical resources. The two areas overlap at the point at which administrative determinations affect clinical outcomes and vice-versa. The ability of an information system to improve the executive's accuracy in predicting how an action in one area (eg, change in nurses' staffing patterns) will influence another (eg, the incidence of patient falls) is the ultimate test of an information system. Well-designed automated systems facilitate the integration of this type of information.

Philosophies of Documentation

Documentation, which is the commitment of information to a retrievable form, is influenced greatly by institutional philosophies. For example, an individual hospital may decide to adopt a policy of "charting by exception" for its clinical record keeping. Another may modify problem-oriented charting for use by health care professionals. In some agencies, all professionals may contribute to the same set of notes; in others, discrete forms may be developed for each provider type. Beliefs about how to organize nursing knowledge further influences an institution's approach. For example, in one agency, client data may be recorded around a framework of nursing diagnoses. In another, the use of "client problems" may result in markedly different documentation procedures and retrievable information.

Sharing data generated by such divergent means is a challenge to providers who are referring clients from one agency to another and to researchers and policy makers.

An important advancement in this vital area is the concept of a uniform minimum health data set (UMHDS). The Health Information Policy Council (1983) of the US Department of Health and Human Services has defined a UMHDS as:

> A minimum set of items of information with uniform definitions and categories, concerning a specific aspect or dimension of the health care system, which meets the essential needs of multiple data users. In concept, if a common minimum data set could be identified, defined, uniformly recorded and made available to multiple users through a variety of collection mechanisms, then problems of data uniformity, availability, validity, reliability, and costs of collection and use could be significantly reduced. (p 3)

Many nursing professional leaders have recognized the need for nurses to be proactive in developing a nursing minimum data set (NMDS) that can be a part of the UMHDS. One of the benefits of this advocacy is that it recognizes that an information system must contain data pertinent to the practice of nursing just as there are data about the practice of medicine. Other advantages of a NMDS are those attendant to uniform definition of terms. A NMDS would also do much to improve examinations of the validity and reliability of the information nurses use.

Werley and Lang (1988) have organized the major issues that surround attainment of a NMDS. Space does not permit a complete description of their work; however, the major issues that they have identified include: (1) conceptual considerations in NMDS development; (2) role of existing information systems; (3) data requirements; (4) addressing the needs of the multiple settings in which nursing is practiced; (5) governmental, payor, and accrediting bodies' responses; and (6) relationship of NMDS with control of practice, standards, quality, and health policy. Every nurse executive should be familiar with the directions for future actions suggested by Abdellah (Werley & Lange, 1988). Only through the active support of nurse executives will a NMDS become a reality.

Another consideration for the nurse executive is the development of a data base management system focusing on administrative information. The advantages of an effective data base management system (DBMS) for the nurse executive are clear. A carefully selected system will save administrative and/or secretarial time and energy in gathering information concerning unit, staff, and patient/client characteristics, reduce the amount of physical information storage space required, reduce redundancy often found in administrative data sets, enhance integrity of the data, and ease the work of maintaining and updating files of information. The most important contribution of a computerized DBMS for nursing practice is its capacity to provide the nurse executive with an effective tool for assessing the unit's or institution's historical and concurrent strengths and limitations. It can provide a summary of previous budgetary and staffing patterns and facilitate the projection of future needs. The combination of management information and patient outcomes within clinical data bases facilitates generation of research questions, which, when answered, will contribute to improved professional practice and administration.

Management's increasing need for large amounts of data and the use of information technology in nursing has opened up a new field of specialization called nursing informatics. Nursing informatics combines nursing with the disciplines of information management and computer science. The emergence of nursing informatics as a new specialization is due in part to advances in computing and computer technology, increasing awareness that the constantly expanding knowledge base of health care and nursing is difficult to manage using traditional methods, and to a growing conviction that the process of expert decision making will be as important to modern nursing as is the foundation on which clinical decisions or research plans are made (National Library of Medicine, 1986).

The increased use of computer technology in the past few years supports the notion of "nursing experts" in the field of computer technology. In the past decade many hospitals installed computers, with the most common uses centered on financial operations such as billing and payroll. Computer applications for nursing evolved more slowly over this period. Many hospitals developed stand-alone applications for scheduling, documentation, and care planning. Today, however, automation of nursing functions has gained increased attention as the shortage of professional nursing staff has escalated. There is also growing emphasis on productivity. The role of the nurse is being examined and ways to enhance utilization of nurses' time are being explored.

One of the first patient care computer applications was seen in patient monitoring in intensive care areas. One currently finds modifications of the intensive care type technology on many general care units. It is not uncommon to find "at risk" patients being mechanically monitored. There is also an explosion of patient care systems that focus on documentation of patient information. There are numerous care planning modules that will meet any requirements that the nurse executive demands.

Software companies are anxious to assist institutions in the development of applications that will benefit the company as well as the hospital. Technological improvement has given impetus to the development of interactive systems that allow the use of multiple data bases. An automated information system can coordinate the activity of a patient without the need to develop a paper trail, for example: (a) the physician orders a medication; (b) the order is received by the pharmacy; (c) the pharmacist prepares the medication; (d) there is an automatic charge to the patient's bill; (e) there is an automatic change in the pharmacy inventory file; (f) the medication is sent to the unit labeled with the appropriate "warning" information; and (g) the nurse administers the medication and records it on the patient's computer file—the time is automatically recorded as well as the name of the nurse making the recording.

One of the buzz words of automation today is integration. No single department can afford an independent system; it must be part of a total package. It should also be recognized that health care users are professionals; they are not professional users. They know their job and how to do it, but they may not know about computers. The literature discusses "computer resistance." If computer systems are designed to adapt to the way a professional works rather than making a professional adapt to the way a computer system works the "resistance" would be overcome.

The primary responsibility for the development of a new system or improvement of an existing system rests with management. The *users* must know what they want of a system—*users* should be in control of the system.

EVALUATING AND IMPROVING CURRENT INFORMATION SYSTEMS

The successful nurse executive needs to plan for regular formative and summative evaluations of information systems. Four concepts form the basis of this evaluation. The first is the adequacy of the data provided. Are any data not collected or reported in an unusable form? An example of the latter case is the provision of staffing data in 30-day segments but the reporting of bed occupancy information is in calendar months. The executive who is attempting to reconcile staffing and usage late in the budget year will find the task difficult if not impossible in such a situation.

A second area is accuracy. Are there human or technical factors that might be influencing the data's veracity? An example of the former is the purposeful adjustment of patient acuity ratings to attain better staffing resources. Although the use of independent observers on a random basis might stem this practice, the nurse executive needs to re-examine the institutional culture that causes employees to resort to this practice. An example of the latter case is the misprogramming of multipliers in budgeting formulae. If the fraction used to estimate the percentage of additional staffing coverage that needs to be allotted for vacation, absenteeism, holidays, and maternity leave is entered incorrectly by one department, the projection for labor for the entire year will be inaccurate. The nurse executive will thus be in the unenviable position of either defending budget overruns for a year or accounting for why he or she asked for so much money.

The timeliness of receipt of data for decision making should also be evaluated periodically. Although it is easy to decide that the staffing data need to be received by a certain time each morning and to determine that they have been delivered late two out of three times, it is more difficult to step back from the immediate situation and evaluate timeliness in terms of transaction maintenance, operational planning and control, and strategic planning.

Transaction maintenance requires data that assist in carrying out both health care and business functions. Treatment scheduling, billing, and staff schedules are examples of these types of data. The data must flow in a relatively short time frame if they are to provide a basis for activities throughout the institution. Operational planning and control functions are no less vital despite the relatively longer time periods between data receipt. Typical reports such as expense summaries and budget variation analyses are usually received on a monthly or quarterly basis. Decision making may be improved if the same types of data are received more often. Strategic planning requires not only the compilation of the transactional and operational planning and control data but also data from outside the institution. Strategic planning demands information on scientific, demographic, and economic trends and policy and operating alternatives. Often these data are not collected until the executive announces that there will be a strategic planning initiative; a scramble for data then commences.

A final area for evaluation is cost, a concept which includes both human and technological elements. Among the human resource costs are those associated with staff training and for collection, entering, and analysis of data. Managers of these staff and consultants are additional expenses. Equipment and facilities costs are only two of the technological elements that contribute to cost. Software, maintenance, utilities, and supplies are other significant items that should be included in a cost evaluation.

Armed with data from this evaluation, the nurse executive may sally forth to improve the existing systems. Principles that will ensure success are:

1. Consider whether modular implementation of improvement is best. Attempting to do all things at once often results in nothing being accomplished.
2. Secure the broadest representation possible on the implementation team. If there is no provision for input from all levels of the nursing division and departments external to nursing, isolated systems and their attendant problems of double costs at half the benefit will result.
3. Although broad representation is essential, ask yourself as you appoint the committee what role each member will fill. Enormous teams spend enormous amounts of time getting and staying organized.
4. In picking a chair for the committee, give preference to the candidate who can manage rather than one who only has expertise in computers and information technology.
5. Continue to show support for the team as the process unfolds. A strategy that has dual rewards is to have the team share plans with other members of the executive staff. The team is rewarded with recognition and feedback; the executive staff gets repeated messages that they are responsible ultimately for the use of the systems and are involved in its planning and implementation.
6. As you receive reports from the implementation team, continue to ask yourself, why do we need this and what does it cost?
7. Require the chair of the committee to account for progress according to a mutually negotiated project time frame. Change takes time; however, open-ended projects lead to a dangerous cynicism on the part of future users.

NEW INFORMATION SYSTEM DEVELOPMENT AND MANAGEMENT

Today's nurse executive has a major role in the development and management of new information systems. In a large nursing department, areas subordinate to the chief nurse executive may be charged with assisting in this assignment. The informed nurse executive cannot, however, be content with mere delegation. Rowland and Rowland (1985) present an extensive analysis of factors the nurse executive should consider in making decisions regarding information systems.

An important addition to this list of factors, however, is the need to consider what informational needs are shared across departments. An integrated system, usually referred to as a hospital information system, is generally more effective than individual (eg, nursing, medicine, financial, maintenance, laboratory) systems. Due to technological improvements, the integrated system can be built around broad clinical and institutional needs and, in fact, is usually constructed around the various combinations and permutations of patients' care experiences.

This type of system is rapidly supplanting the older system of individual documentation that typically included forms such as the Kardex, progress sheet, treatment record, medication form, and scheduling records. Although the information found in these forms is still collected, those data can be more easily related to the actions of other health professionals, institutional services, and costs. For example, a computer screen may be developed that looks markedly like the formerly separate treatment record; however, in an integrated system, the cost of the supplies used in the treatment (previously found on a supplies charge slip) and the outcome of such treatments (previously found on the progress sheet) can be related. In addition, the storeroom clerk can be simultaneously alerted that certain supplies have been consumed; thus appraised, this individual can send replacement supplies thereby saving nursing time.

ORGANIZING INFORMATION: REVIEW OF FORMATS

Reporting formats serve as the structural communication link within a health care organization. There are various types of reporting formats used to accommodate the key information needs of the setting. Table 21–1 provides an overview of the types of forms and reporting formats likely to be incorporated in various hospital settings. The table illustrates the domain(s) (legal, financial, accreditation/regulatory, and/or administrative) which necessitate the use of a respective form and/or reporting format.

Accountability

The accountability of health care institutions, physicians, and nurses has changed dramatically in the last decade. This is largely due to the increased number of successfully litigated claims, along with the increased dollar amounts awarded in settlements; and to the judicial and legislative decisions that have placed the responsibility for patient safety on health care providers, both at the individual and institutional level.

Quality assurance (QA) is one method to address accountability requirements. (See Chapter 23 for a discussion of QA.) It is a process to monitor and evaluate the quality of care and services provided within a health care organization.

The Nursing Audit

The nursing audit is one method to monitor and evaluate nursing care delivery. Typically, the nursing audit consists of evaluating nursing care based on documentation found in the patient record. Three audit approaches can be used: the organizational audit, where facilities, staffing, and procedures are examined; the process audit, where the quality of care provided to patients in the organization is reviewed; and,

TABLE 21-1. EXAMPLES OF TYPES OF FORMS AND PURPOSE FOR THEIR USE

Form Type	Purpose for Their Use			
	Legal	Financial	Accreditation/ Regulatory	Administrative
Patient Record Forms				
Patient ID forms	X	X	X	X
History & physical forms	X	X	X	X
Medical orders	X	X	X	X
Clinical observations	X	X	X	X
Procedural reports	X	X	X	X
Consent forms	X	X	X	X
Referral forms	X	X	X	X
Discharge summary	X	X	X	X
Personnel Forms				
Employment application	X	X		X
Hire/processing forms				X
Physical exam record				X
Compensation forms	X	X	X	X
Fringe benefit forms	X	X	X	X
Regulatory review (Licensure, Certification, etc)	X		X	X
Employee attendance	X			X
Performance appraisal	X		X	X
Problem-Oriented Forms				
Occupational health	X	X	X	X
Risk management	X	X	X	X
Utilization review	X	X	X	X
Quality assurance	X		X	X
Nursing Audit Forms	X		X	X
Process of care audits	X		X	X
Outcome audit	X		X	X
Budget Forms				
Capital budget		X		X
Operating budget		X		X
Actual to budget comparisons		X		X
Annual Reports	X	X	X	X
Minutes of Meetings				
Departmental/unit			X	X
Standing committees			X	X
Staff meetings			X	X
Ad hoc committees			X	X
Other				
Staffing schedules		X	X	X
Patient acuity		X	X	X
Productivity assessments		X		X

the outcome audit, where the health status of the patient becomes a significant criterion for evaluation.

From a quality assurance perspective, the division or unit reviews nursing care to determine how well nursing is meeting the standards of practice it purports. From an organizational perspective, the review assesses the degree to which nursing has minimized adverse risk to patients for injury or untoward outcome.

JCAHO recommends the outcome audit for nursing audits. The Commission assumes that professional standards have been employed by the nursing division during a patient's hospital stay if the end result is adherence to professional standards.

The nursing outcome audit can also serve as a means to examine key indicators of care in order to evaluate the impact on patient care and clinical performance, to initiate periodic adjustments in structure, operations, and monitors, and to determine whether aspects of the QA program (involvement of staff, channels of communication and the degree of documentation) are appropriate. Table 21–2 provides an abbreviated example of a nursing audit for a mastectomy patient. Care standards are listed according to the phases of the patient's hospital stay. By reviewing the medical record, the individual performing the audit can identify if deficiencies exist in the provision of nursing care for this type of patient. The results of the audit are shared with unit staff, so that an action plan can be formulated to correct the deficiencies identified by the audit.

Risk Management

Risk management is a planned program of loss prevention and liability control. The purpose of a risk management program is to identify, analyze, and evaluate risks that pose safety threats to patients or financial threats to the organization, followed by a plan for reducing the frequency and severity of injuries, accidents, and potential liabilities for the institution (see Chapter 23).

Components of a risk management program include: identifying, reviewing, analyzing, monitoring codes, eliminating and reducing risks, reviewing, identifying needs, evaluation and providing periodic reports.

In implementing an effective internal reporting system for risk management, the risk manager, together with the respective professional staff groups should review the current system for its effectiveness. Their review should focus on the following concerns:

1. Is the present format adequate? Do the present forms capture all the essential data? Are safeguards in place to ensure the confidentiality in the system?
2. Is there an administrative policy delineating the steps to be followed in internal reporting from discovery of the incident to the appropriate follow-up and resolution of incident, including purpose, responsibility, routing, and any special considerations?
3. Is there a focal office for timely internal review and follow up? Does a mechanism exist for reporting special situations on a 24-hour, as needed, basis? If not, can a more informal system be developed to provide the necessary documentation of patient incidents?

TABLE 21-2. ABBREVIATED NURSING AUDIT: MASTECTOMY

Criteria	Standard 100%	0%	Care Elements/Exceptions	Instructions
Admission				
1. Assessment to include patient understanding of reason for surgery; past health history: current health problems & medications currently taken; patient resources/social support systems available at home.	X			Progress/nurses notes; admission assessment; documented prior to surgery
2. Patient verbalizes understanding of surgical procedure and results	X		Patient unable to understand; family member verbalizes understanding	Admission assessment; progress/nursing notes; understanding documented prior to surgery
3. Patient verbalizes understanding of postoperative care	X			Progress/nursing notes; understanding of postoperative care documented prior to surgery
a. importance of post-op exercises (turning, coughing, incentive spirometry, early ambulation)				
b. explanation of tubes, IV, and wound suction				
c. resumption of diet				
d. availability of pain medication				
e. importance of arm exercises				

continued

TABLE 21-2. Continued

Criteria	Standard 100%	Standard 0%	Care Elements/Exceptions	Instructions
Interim				

Relief from pain	X		Management
			1. Instruct patient to report episodes of post-op pain
			2. When patient reports pain
			  a. administer analgesia within 15 minutes of report of pain,
			  b. document relief of pain,
			  c. wean to oral analgesics within 48–72 hours post-op
				Progress/nursing notes
				Medication record

Atelectasis/Pneumonia Prevention & routine observation (# 1-4)	X	X	1. Turn, cough, deep breath Q 2 hrs for 48 hrs, then Q 4 hrs till up ad lib 2. Use incentive spirometry Q 1 hr for first 48 hours while awake 3. Ambulate within 12–24 hours and at least QID until up ad lib Detection 4. Check breath sounds every 4 hrs for first 24 hrs, then every shift or until afebrile and chest clear	Progress/nursing notes Graphic record, x-ray report

488

		Documentation
Atelectasis/pneumonia		
Management		Progress/nursing notes
5. Report to MD within 8 hours: a. temperature > 101 b. rales not clearing with cough c. persistent dry cough or productive cough with purulent sputum		
6. Set patient at bedside to cough & deep breathe q 2 hours (Check with MD about IPPB treatment if patient unable to maintain clear chest)		
Lymphedema Prevention & routine observation (#1-3)		
1. Post-op, elevate affected arm	X	
2. Initiate exercise program on day of surgery with passive range of motion exercises to affected arm		
Detection:		
3. Check extremity for edema every 8 hrs; notify surgeon if edema occurs		
Discharge		
Afebrile	X	Graphic sheet: temperature below 100.0 degrees F. 24 hours prior to discharge.
Able to abduct & raise arm above shoulder level	X	Nurses notes: notation of ability to move arm; or instructions in progressive exercises

4. Has the importance of a thorough reporting system and the rationale behind the design of the present system been conveyed to the organization's professional staff through orientation and in-service programs?
5. Is there a systematic process whereby incidents are reviewed (a) at the time of submission to ensure the adequacy of documentation and to effect appropriate follow-up and (b) to analyze cumulative data to determine patterns or trends indicative of a need for corrective action?
6. Has a risk management committee been established to provide multidisciplinary input into the analysis? Is there an active physician involvement on this committee?

The risk management committee is responsible for the overall planning and decision making involved in risk management. Figure 21–2 presents an organizational model of a risk management program.

The nursing department is involved in patient care 24 hours a day and is critical to the success of a risk management program. The predominant high risk areas for adverse outcome or injury in health care settings fall into five categories: (a) medication errors, (b) falls, (c) complications from diagnostic or treatment procedures, (d) patient or family dissatisfaction with care, and (e) refusal of treatment or to sign consent for treatment. Medical records and incident reports serve as the source to document hospital, physician, and nurse accountability. Incident reports are used to analyze the frequency, severity, and causes of incidents within these risk categories.

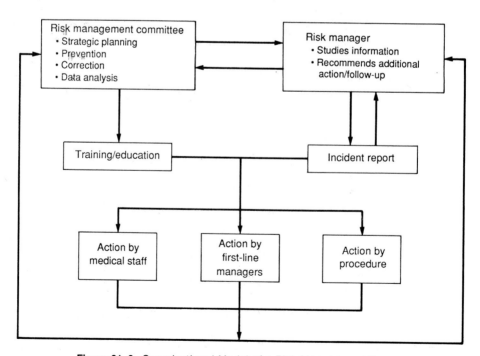

Figure 21–2. Organizational Model of a Risk Management Program

Analysis of these reports form the basis for intervention. Figure 21-3 is an example of an incident report form.

Incident Reports

Comprehensive and accurate reporting in the patient's medical record and in the incident report are critical to protect the institution and its caregivers from litigation. A reportable incident includes any unexpected or unplanned occurrence that affects or could potentially affect a patient or family member.

The process of reporting incidents involves the following:

1. *Discovery*. Physicians, nurses, patients, families, or other hospital employee may report actual or potential risk or untoward events.
2. *Notification*. Risk management receives the completed incident report within 24 *hours* of the incident. Telephone contact may be made earlier, to hasten follow up in the event of a major incident.
3. *Investigation*. The risk manager or representative immediately investigates the incident.
4. *Consultation*. The risk manager consults with the physician, risk management committee member, or both.
5. *Action*. The risk manager/representative clarifies any misinformation to the patient or family, explaining exactly what happened. The patient is referred to the appropriate source for help and for compensation for any needed service; the latter is offered, if indicated.
6. *Record*. The risk manager ensures that all records, including incident reports, follow up, and action taken, as indicated, are filed in a central depository.

The following are examples of events in the various risk categories.

Medication Errors, Including Administration of Intravenous Fluids. An incident report is warranted when a medication or intravenous fluid is omitted, given to the wrong patient, given at the wrong dosage or wrong time, or given via the wrong route. Administration of the wrong fluid or medication must be also be reported.

Example. Augmentin IVR was to be given at 1200. Error was discovered at 1400; the IV rider was immediately hung and infused. The physician was notified. The IV rider infusion time schedule was changed to reflect the altered time of administration.

Diagnostic Procedure. Any incident occurring before, during, or after such procedures as an x-ray, lumbar puncture, biopsy, blood sampling, or other invasive procedure is grouped as a diagnostic procedure incident.

Example. Upon return from x-ray, an elderly patient was noted to have a large black and blue mark over the left buttock. The area was painful to touch, however, the patient was too confused to comment about what happened in x-ray. The physician was notified.

RUSH PRESBYTERIAN-ST.LUKE'S MEDICAL CENTER
NOTICE OF UNUSUAL INCIDENT
CONFIDENTIAL

DO NOT PLACE IN PATIENT CARE RECORD
PRINT CLEARLY

1. ADDRESSOGRAPH PLATE OR I.D. HERE   PATIENT ☐   VISITOR ☐   OTHER ☐

2. DATE OF INCIDENT   3. TIME OF INCIDENT   AM ☐   4. LOCATION OF INCIDENT
                                                     PM ☐

5. ADMITTING DIAGNOSIS   6. ATTENDING PHYSICIAN   7. ADMITTING PHYSICIAN NOTIFIED
                                                              YES ☐ NO ☐   TIME _____   AM ☐
                                                                                                 PM ☐

8. PERSON REPORTING INCIDENT   DEPARTMENT   POSITION

9. WITNESS TO INCIDENT

   NAME: _____ ADDRESS: _____ PHONE: _____

   NAME: _____ ADDRESS: _____ PHONE: _____

10. ACTIVITY ORDERS BEFORE INCIDENT
       BEDREST ☐   SIDERAILS: FULL ☐
       UP AD LIB ☐   HALF ☐
       UP WITH ASSISTANCE ☐   UP ☐
       RESTRAINTS ☐   DOWN ☐
    SEDATED OR TRANQUILIZED WITHIN FOUR (4) HOURS TO INCIDENT?   YES ☐   NO ☐

11. INCIDENT FACTS/DATA:
    _____
    _____
    _____
    _____

12. INCIDENT REPORTED TO: TIME NOTIFIED: AM ☐   TIME RESPONDED: AM ☐
    SUPERVISOR: PM ☐   PM ☐

                                             TIME NOTIFIED: AM ☐   TIME RESPONDED: AM ☐
    PHYSICIAN: PM ☐   PM ☐

                                             TIME NOTIFIED: AM ☐   TIME RESPONDED: AM ☐
    OTHER: PM ☐   PM ☐

13. EXAMINED BY PHYSICIAN:
                                                                                          AM ☐
    _____   _____ DATE: _____ TIME: _____ PM ☐
        PRINT NAME   SIGNATURE

14. PHYSICIAN STATEMENT:
    _____
    _____
    _____
    _____

    FOLLOW-UP

       X-RAY (TYPE) _____ CONSULT ☐   LAB ☐   NO INJURY ☐   OTHER ☐

15.
                                                                                          AM ☐
    PREPARER'S SIGNATURE _____ DATE: _____ TIME: _____ PM ☐
                                                                                          AM ☐
    SUPERVISOR'S SIGNATURE _____ DATE: _____ TIME: _____ PM ☐

16. OBJECTIVE/BRIEF PROGRESS NOTE DOCUMENTATION?   YES ☐ NO ☐

ROUTING INSTRUCTIONS: 1. SUBMIT ORIGINAL TO CARE DIRECTOR IMMEDIATELY.
                       2. FORM MUST BE RECEIVED BY THE OFFICE OF RISK MANAGEMENT WITHIN 24 HOURS OF OCCURRENCE.
                       3. SECOND COPY MAY BE RETAINED BY DEPARTMENT ORIGINATING REPORT.

SERIOUS INCIDENTS CALL DIRECTLY TO OFFICE OF RISK MANAGEMENT: X7823 OR 8034 OR PAGE 83-6023 OR 82-5043
OFFICE USE ONLY   WP

FORM 032S REV. 4/81   THIS FORM MAY NOT BE DUPLICATED

Figure 21-3. Confidential Notice of Unusual Incident *(Used with permission, courtesy of Rush-Pres-byterian St. Luke's Medical Center, Chicago, Illinois)*

Medical-legal Incident. When a patient refuses treatment ordered and prescribed, or refuses to sign a consent, the situation is categorized as a medical-legal incident.

> Example. Patient indicated that he was no longer in need of medical care and asked to be discharged. Physician notified and came to explain potential ramifications if treatment was discontinued. Patient continued to prompt for discharge. The AMA (against medical advice) form was explained to the patient. The patient signed the form and left at 15:30 PM.

Patient or Family Attitude Toward Care. When a patient or family member indicates overall dissatisfaction or interference with care and the situation cannot be resolved, an incident report is filed.

> Example. Mr. Gray arrived on the postpartum unit at 10 PM (two hours after visiting hours were over) demanding to see his girlfriend stating that it was imperative he give her something. He became verbally abusive, threatening staff members when they refused to let him see her. Mr. Gray remained unwilling to leave and became more belligerent in his interaction with the staff. Hospital security was notified to escort Mr. Gray from the area.

Documentation on the incident report should describe the incident as factually as possible. It should also include all pertinent factors relating to the incident and the action taken immediately following the incident, such as physician notification, and the need for additional diagnostic workup. Nursing management may include additional information related to follow-up regarding the incident.

The facts of the incident should be briefly documented in the patient record. The medical report should never be used for making derogatory comments or indicating expressions of anger. These types of comments are inappropriate and serve no useful purpose.

INFORMATION SYSTEM REQUIREMENTS: HUMAN RESOURCE DATA

For a health care organization, the human resource pool represents its greatest asset. Without an adequate manpower supply, one consisting of a resource pool of highly qualified, competent professionals and technical staff, and adequately trained support staff, the organization would be unable to provide high quality patient care services.

An effective personnel management information system can assist the nurse executive to (1) maintain the structural standards set forth by the organization; (2) document the resources utilized in the provision of nursing services; and (3) facilitate decision making regarding strategic planning of manpower needs at the staff and managerial levels of the organization. Table 21–3 lists the major types and purposes for various personnel forms comprising a personnel management information system.

At the individual level, these forms or recording formats trace an individual's

TABLE 21–3. PERSONNEL FORMS

Form Type	Purpose
Job description	Set forth duties and responsibilities of the position
	Statement of characteristics needed to perform job successfully
Interview guide	Tool used to determine applicant's ability to carry functions of the position
	Glean "persona" of applicant for
	—organizational ability
	—ability to explain
	—action thinking
	Tool to predict applicant's effectiveness on the job
Employment application	Detail of work and educational experiences over career
	Tool to predict applicant's future effectiveness as an employee
Health records/pre-employment examination forms	Screen applicants with major impairments that may impede successful job performance
	Identify applicants with unfavorable attendance records or potential excessive claims against insurance companies
Payroll/compensation forms	Record employee compensation, tax liability, benefit deductions and accruals
Orientation program forms	Introduce total facility as an organization
	Orient to specific operational aspects of a department or unit
Education program forms	Document additional inservice education
Performance appraisal forms	Encourage improved performance in current role
	Provide growth opportunities for employees desiring promotions
	Provide the organization with individuals qualified for promotions to higher level positions
Discipline forms	Document instances of unacceptable employee behavior
	Plan to correct/change employee behavior
	Protect the organization against liability
Staff forecast charts	Forecast of human resources needed by the organization for present and future operations

employment history within the organization, educational and vocational qualifications for the position, a perspective regarding performance and professional growth, salary history, and promotion within the organization.

At the aggregate level, components of the information system can be utilized by various department managers for statistical reporting. For example, the nurse executive can use the division's composite salary information to make budget projections for the upcoming year and estimate the total cost to the division of future salary increases. For the nurse recruiter, aggregate data can pinpoint the "hard to fill" positions in various departments and identify target areas for recruitment campaigns. For the personnel manager, the personnel management data base augments affirmative action reporting and facilitates the development of labor force forecasts.

FORMAT DESIGN

Creating effective documents depends on appropriate format design for data collection and use. It requires awareness of the flow of information in individual settings. From a systems perspective, forms and formats serve as a vital communication link to facilitate collection of all types of data—about the patient, research, education, and other types of data needs. In turn, initial reports must lend themselves to incorporate secondary analyses at a later time that summarize or aggregate pertinent information.

Although the purpose of the form guides its design, a number of cultural factors must be considered. In English, we read from left to right and from the top to the bottom of the page. This should be a primary consideration in design. The readability component, along with the form's purpose, is a major concern. Similar groups of data (for example, patient identification data) should be placed together on the form. Design selection should facilitate ease in data collection, completeness, and error control. In designing forms, these primary questions should be kept in mind:

- Why is the information being recorded?
- What information should be on the form?
- Where does the form originate?
- What department introduces the form into the system or initiates data entry on the form?
- Who will be using the information on the form?
- Who determines the completeness of data entries?
- Who will receive copies of the form?
- Where will the form be filed?
- How long should this information be retained?

Guidelines for Designing Forms:*

1. Assess each form individually to:
   a. Evaluate its necessity
   b. Avoid duplication in recording
   c. Insure its integration with existing record systems
2. Determine the purpose of the form, which in turn, will determine information to be included on the form.

---

*Adapted from Waters K, Murphy G, *Medical Records in Health Information* pp. 4–5, with permission of Aspen Systems, Inc., Rockville, MD, copyright 1979.

3. Identify the benefits derived from introducing the form into the record system.
4. Design forms as simply as possible; avoid cluttering them with headings, instructions, or captions.
5. Consider use of multipurpose flow sheets to reduce chart bulk and eliminate the need for several special forms to monitor special care factors.
6. Design all forms in the record to be uniform in size.
7. Be consistent in the placement of patient identification and form titles on every form.
8. Include a space for:
   a. Full patient name
   b. File number of the health record
9. Use bold print to highlight headings and captions.
10. Align headings to provide an uncluttered appearance and to promote ease in finding desired information.
11. Consider logical sequence of subject headings.
12. Use white paper with color coded borders for quick identification of different forms; colored paper may be difficult to read or photocopy.
13. Select captions that clearly state what information is to be entered on the form.
14. Use a box arrangement for checklists to save time.
15. Plan spacing according to the specific method of documentation:
    a. Typewritten entries: set lines according to the number of lines per inch on the typewriter and to accommodate vertical spacing
    b. Handwritten entries: set lines far enough apart to ensure readibility
    c. Computer readout format: set margins, spacing, and punctuation clearly
    d. Consider the time period each side of the form covers
16. Identify certain portions of a form that are restricted for use by designated groups (eg, medical records committee, utilization review committee); those areas should be surrounded with bold lines.
17. Consider printing on both sides of the sheet to reduce chart bulk and to maximize paper use.
18. Consider printing on reverse side to facilitate referencing when a form is in the chart holder.
19. Utilize a rubber stamp on an existing form to eliminate the need for a special form.
20. Allow sufficient space for signatures of individuals making entries.
21. As newly designed forms often require revisions, print or photocopy a small supply for trial use.
22. Use good quality paper stock in final printing.
23. Avoid card stock since it is difficult to use, it creates bulk, and may complicate photocopy techniques.
24. Stock a 6-month supply of the form to prevent waste due to a revision or change in documentation protocols.
25. Always introduce a proposed new form before implementation, and prefera-

bly during the initial design phase to promote input by those making entries and using the data.

26. Complete final review and approval of the draft form prior to implementation; utilize a multidisciplinary forms committee which includes a medical records administrator.

27. If a form is to be used by various departments, simple printed instructions will ensure uniformity.

28. If instructions are detailed, prepare separate directions concerning:
    a. Purpose
    b. Use
    c. Completion instructions
    d. Staff responsibilities
    e. References, if any

29. For forms likely to be sent elsewhere, include the name, address and city of the facility on the form.

30. Identify all forms by:
    a. A descriptive and simple title
    b. Stock control number
    c. The month and year of first, revised, or last printing.

Format and Forms Appraisal

The adequacy of form design is contingent on multiple factors. The primary considerations in appraising the efficacy of a newly designed form should include a review of the following[†]:

- Is the form necessary or does some form exist which could be adapted to meet this need?
- Is there a need for a procedure regarding the use of the form?
- Is the time period covered by the form adequate? Or should it be lengthened?
- Are all copies of the form necessary? Could one copy be routed to various departments? If a computer is used, where should electronic copies be sent?
- Does the form clearly indicate its use?
- Have the users of the form provided input into its design?
- Has approval of the form been obtained from those responsible for it and other appropriate personnel?
- Does the form design complement the recording format?
- Are like items grouped together?
- Is all the required information printed, leaving only variable data to be filled in?
- Does the format of the form facilitate its use?
- Is the form a standard size and no longer than necessary?
- With a revision, can it be distinguished from an earlier form?
- Are the margins correct and spacing correct?

[†]Adapted with permission from the University of South Alabama Medical Center, Mobile, Alabama.

- Is there enough space for signatures?
- Are references properly placed?
- For outside use, could the form be designed as a self-mailer?
- Is routing of the form indicated on each copy?
- Has disposition of the old form been delineated?
- Has the minimal order requirement of the form been established?
- Are printing specifications complete?

Forms and formats will continue to be the primary means of communication regarding the information needs of the organization. Specific health care settings will need to select forms and formats that are most appropriate for their needs. Health information personnel will need to draw on existing resources and design new forms and formats as the kinds of information parameters required for their respective settings continue to evolve.

WRITING REPORTS

Regardless of whether health care information is computer generated or initiated via a written format, the nurse executive will use the data in proposing and substantiating decisions. Often this is accomplished via written reports. It is imperative that these reports transmit the intended meaning. For example, a report sent from the occupational safety department informing the nursing department that there were 20 employee needle stick injuries in the month of October would be difficult to interpret without additional facts. How many needle stick injuries were there in September—is it an increase or decrease? On what nursing units did these injuries occur—is the incidence evenly distributed or grouped on one or two units? Without this additional information the nursing department would not be able to respond with an appropriate action plan.

When writing a report, it is important to identify the direction of the communication flow. Is the report being sent from the nurse executive to department heads? Is the report providing information to the board of directors? Is the report transmitting information laterally between department heads? In addition, information meaningful to one receiver may be puzzling to or misinterpreted by another. An awareness of the level of understanding of the individual receiving the report, as well as the purpose of the report should be considered for information to be distributed.

The purpose of the written report and its intended use must be carefully reviewed. Is the report intended for internal use only or can the information be published? If it is only for internal use, what are the ramifications if the information became public? For example, information on negative patient outcomes supporting the need for additional staffing in an intensive care unit is "discoverable" information (can be used by a prosecuting attorney in a malpractice case) unless it is published in the context of a quality assurance program.

Reports can be categorized as informational, analytical, or a combination of both. By thinking of reports in this manner, the writer is less likely to wander from his or her original purpose. When the writer's sole purpose is the presentation of data and no interpretation occurs, the report is considered to be informational. When a writer is comparing, contrasting, discovering, or evaluating relationships among factors, the report becomes analytical. In this type of report, the writer must substantiate the conclusions with facts.

Informational reports generally present information without drawing conclusions from the facts presented. The writer provides the data necessary for the decision maker to draw the conclusions. For example, the nurse executive considering expansion of an affiliated child care facility as part of a nurse retention program, may ask for data regarding the number of nurses in the institution requiring preschool care for their children. The nurse executive wants to assure that strategic decisions optimize the effective use of limited financial resources. The writer of the report will need to clearly identify the purpose of the information to be gathered. The writer should consider what the nurse executive needs to know about the subject. Identifying only the number of nurses with preschool age children may not be enough information. How many nurses on staff already have adequate preschool care? How many nurses work evenings and nights? Do the nurses consider the rates charged by the child care facility affordable? The identification and collection of critical data for informed decision making is the writer's responsibility.

The analytic report compares data related to the topic of the report rather than simply presenting information, and provides recommendations based on the results of the analysis. The more effort or expense a recommendation requires, the more likely the writer will need to support the recommendation by presenting a thorough analysis. The writer must have a clear understanding of the process leading to the conclusions or recommendations drawn from the report.

- What data did the writer review to arrive at his or her conclusion? Are the data relevant?
- If the writer is projecting into the future, has the individual provided adequate evidence of the hypothetical future or trend?

In selecting background material, the writer should consider whether the material needs to support a judgment, serve as a buffer, or catch the interest of someone needing persuasion. The data must be displayed in a manner that clearly supports the analysis and conclusions. When writing the report, the relationship between the issues and conclusions must be made clear.

The writer's credibility in report writing is supported by a careful and unbiased analysis of the available information. Inclusion of weaknesses as well as strengths in the report is a useful method of defusing potential critics of the report. Encouraging feedback suggests to the reader that the writer is confident in the presentation of the material. If others assisted in the development of the report they should be acknowledged. This technique assists in establishing the credibility of the report because the writer has not operated in a "vacuum."

An effective opening sentence or paragraph is essential for a successful report. It should establish contact by clearly stating the purpose of the report. The opening remarks emphasize the importance of the issues to the receiver, and should summarize key facts, findings, and recommendations. The need for a closing along with the type of closing chosen will vary according to the nature of the report. A closing may summarize the content of the report, it may call for action, it may identify who has the next move, or it may be omitted entirely.

If a report is longer than three pages, plan to write a one-page summary. Include the body of the report as an attachment. In the summary the writer should:

1. Establish contact and state the subject. State the purpose, worded as a statement of the problem, an objective, or a question.
2. Summarize key facts. State any important assumptions and any standards, tests or rules used in analyzing the problem(s). Show the alternatives considered.
3. State key findings and recommendations. State the benefits to be expected.
4. Refer to detailed discussion, either by summarizing the material or by listing the section headings to refer to for the detailed discussion.
5. Close the one-page summary by making it clear who has the next move.

In this age of information overload, a one-page summary is a useful tool to draw attention to the report and improves the chance of getting action.

A careful, honest writer does not need to worry about style. As one becomes proficient in the use of the language, a style will emerge. However, a few ground rules should be observed as the "new" report writer begins the process. Initially, the writer should write in a way that flows easily and naturally, using words and phrases that are familiar. Prior to composing the report, a basic structure or design should be developed. For some it will be an outline; for others only a rough scheme is needed. It is suggested that one use nouns and verbs. It is the nouns and verbs that give good writing its toughness and color. During the review and editing process, flaws in the report can be identified and changed.

Overstatement of one's position concerning the issue often puts the reader on guard. Unless there is a good reason for the writer's opinion to be included in the report, it should be avoided. Opinions scattered indiscriminately throughout the report leave a mark of egotism and bias on the work. The content of the report should be clear, concise, and to the point. Graphs and charts should be properly labeled using standard techniques.

Well-written reports become the most effective way to deal with information overload. Identification of information essential for decision making becomes the earmark of a "good" report.

SUMMARY

The nurse executive faces a formidable challenge in facilitating the flow of information within the institution. The informational needs of the nurse executive will continue to grow as automated systems become more sophisticated in providing access to a myriad of information with relative ease. Legal, financial, and accreditation/regulatory requirements will continue to have a profound influence on the types of information health care settings are required to have available for review.

The nurse executive needs to remain sensitive to the timely presentation of information, so that he or she can sustain a position where there will be "no surprises" when asked to discuss nursing care delivery with other top level administrators in the organization. In this age of information overload, the nurse executive must articulate what her needs are regarding the types of requisite data elements which are unique to nursing and critical to corporate operations in order: (a) to facilitate informed decision making; (b) to substantiate claims concerning the quantity and quality of nursing services provided; and (c) to document the resources utilized in the provision of nursing care.

REFERENCES

Doughty D, Mash N. *Nursing audit.* Philadelphia, FA Davis Co, 1977

Gibson S, Rose MA. Managing computer resistance. *Computers in nursing.* 4:5, 201, 1986

Health Information Policy Council. *Background paper: Uniform minimum health data sets.* (Unpublished). Washington, DC, US Department of Health and Human Services, 1983

Heidler B, Damrosch S, Romano C, & McCarthy, M. Graduate specialization in nursing informatics. *Computers in Nursing.* 7:2, 68, 1989

Hodge M. *Medical Information Systems: A New Source for Hospitals.* Rockville, MD, Aspen Systems, 1977

Kline N. Principles of computerized database management: Considerations for the nurse administrator. *Computers in Nursing.* 4:2, 73, 1986

Kovner C. Using computerized databases for nursing research and quality assurance. *Computers in Nursing* 7:5, 228, 1989

Lindauer J. *Communicating in Business,* 2nd ed. Philadelphia, WB Saunders Co, 1979

Mongale J. *Risk Management: A Guide for Health Care Professionals.* Rockville, MD, Aspen Systems, 1985

Morris J. *Make Yourself Clear.* New York, McGraw Hill Book Co, 1972

National Library of Medicine. *Long-Range Plans for Medical Informatics* (Report of Panel 4). Washington D.C.: US Department of Health and Human Services, 1986: 8–10

Raco R. Leveraging the hospital executive. *Computers in Healthcare.* 28, August 1988

Rowland H, ed. *The Nursing Forms Manual.* Rockville, MD, Aspen Systems, 1985

Rowland H, Rowland B. *The Nursing Administration Handbook.* Rockville, MD, Aspen Systems, 1985

Silva N. R.N.s Rx for H.I.S. *Computers in Healthcare.* 38, April 1988

Skurka M. *Organization of Medical Record Departments in Hospitals,* 2nd ed. Chicago, IL, American Hospital Publishing, Inc, 1988

Strunk W. *The elements of style,* 3rd ed. New York, MacMillan Publishing Co, 1979

Waters K, Murphy G. *Medical Records in Health Information.* Rockville, MD, Aspen Systems, 1979

Werley HH, Lang NH, eds. *Identification of the Nursing Minimum Data Set.* New York, Springer Publishing Co, 1988

Organizing The Work

CHAPTER 22

Staffing and Scheduling

Sandra Robertson
Mary K. Pabst

Key Concept List

Staffing plans and process
JCAHO standards
Nursing shortage
Workload and requirements of care
Scheduling
Absenteeism

Hospitals today are looking to decrease costs. Since nursing is a significant portion of the health care organization's labor expense, it has become a prime target. Therefore, effective and efficient use of the nursing salary budget is a major concern of the nurse executive. It is important that the staffing system not only meets requirements of external accrediting agencies and is responsive to internal budget restraints but also assures that nursing services delivered are appropriate to the patient's need and nursing care is scientifically and technologically sound. In such an environment, nurse staffing of a patient care area is by no means a simple task.

Staffing can be defined as a process which provides an appropriate quantity and quality of nurses to deliver safe, competent care to patients. Staffing should have as a focus both quality and cost which has to be balanced at some predetermined level. A master staffing plan documents the need for staff using an established staffing standard for each nursing unit and serves as a general statement of the number and skill mix of staff needed and how the needed staff are allocated to meet the forecasted workload. The master staffing plan is implemented as a master schedule. Although scheduling is a major part of the staffing process, it is not staffing. Effective scheduling ensures that the appropriate number of nursing personnel are available on units to meet patient care needs. The workload of a unit is an estimate of the total amount of nursing care required of the staff. In most institutions, workload is determined as a result of a patient classification system.

The staffing plan is integrally tied to budgeting activities. The budget can be defined as a statement of the financial resources necessary to acquire needed staff to meet the nursing department's goals (see Chapter 14). Since financial resources are so closely tied to staffing requirements, nurse executives need to carefully assess the current management of their human resources in all aspects of the operation.

Staffing plans developed must be based on information that is valid, reliable, and justifiable to the financial officers of the institution. The key to a meaningful staffing plan for a nursing service starts with the actual nursing care provided at the unit level and centers around the nursing needs of the patient. The chief nurse executive is responsible for supplying the resources necessary to meet the identified nursing care requirements. Determining how patient needs are met depends on external requirements as well as multiple organizational components (see Fig 22–1).

This chapter focuses on the multiple variables that impact human resource requirements to help nurse executives plan for nurse staffing and scheduling of patient care services.

EXTERNAL REQUIREMENTS

A staffing plan must comply with the Joint Commission on Accreditation of Healthcare Organizations (JCAHO) as well as with the American Nurses Association (ANA)

```
External requirements
  JCAHO nursing standards
  ANA standards
  State codes
  Consumer expectation
Organizational components
  Nursing service philosophy
  Nursing service structure
    Delivery of care system
    Staffing policies
    Nursing characteristics: education, qualifications, experience
Support systems
  Medical distribution
  Material supply system
  Food distribution
  Patient care information system
Workload
  Patient needs
  Requirements of care
```

Figure 22–1. Variables Affecting Staffing

standards and individual state requirements. Consumer expectations must also be considered especially since nursing care has a major impact on patient attitudes toward a particular health care organization and quality nursing care is frequently used to market the organization.

JCAHO Standards

The accreditation survey process by JCAHO is theoretically voluntary but most hospitals elect to participate because federal funding is tied to accreditation. JCAHO standards place emphasis not only on delivering safe, effective patient care but on factors involved in the process of care. The most current JCAHO standards must be carefully reviewed and evaluated in relationship to the staffing requirements of the patient care units.

ANA Standards

There are a number of similarities in the standards set by ANA and JCAHO. The ANA standards focus on nursing practice in all patient care settings and, in essence, form the basis for professional practice. Nursing service departments can use the standards as a model for developing their own standards of practice and care guidelines. As they proceed to develop standards or guidelines for patient care, however, there must be a commitment by administration to provide the necessary support to meet expectations expressed in the standards. The relationship between standards of care and patient care unit staffing is crucial. Nursing executives must be able to express effectively to hospital administrators the long range effects of understaffing. The risk a hospital takes when a patient care unit is not staffed appropriately to meet external standards must be considered in light of legal and financial aspects. Hospital legal departments are often questioned as to adequacy of staffing when untoward events occur. If an institution does not have written standards, practice will be measured against the standards or practice patterns of comparable hospitals. The external pressure of meeting current practice patterns within nursing departments must be carefully considered when staffing plans are developed.

State Codes

In addition to the JCAHO and ANA standards that support the need for effective nurse staffing plans, nurse executives also need to examine codes pertaining to patient classification and staffing patterns in order to assure that their departments are in compliance with state and local requirements.

Consumer Expectations

Patient satisfaction has become a key element in an institution's financial viability. Although patients are admitted to an institution by a physician, when provided a choice, they will choose to be admitted to one perceived as being "patient friendly" and where the reputation of the quality of nursing care is good. Quality of nursing care is frequently mentioned in the promotional material of the organization.

ORGANIZATIONAL COMPONENTS

Nursing Service Philosophy

The philosophy of nursing service provides the basic framework for activities within the organization's nursing department. A philosophy is a statement of beliefs and values that directs day to day practice. The philosophy and practice should be consistent. If real-life practice is not consistent with the written philosophy, one or the other must change. In light of the changes occurring in the health care arena, the philosophy of the nursing department can be a guide in choosing alternatives in the delivery of patient care.

Nursing Service Structure

A nursing care delivery system is developed within the context of the whole organization and is directed by the philosophy of the nursing department. Staffing policies of the nursing department should support the philosophy and the nursing care delivery system. (Also, how nursing is organized plays a large part in determining how the nurse provides care.) Nursing characteristics, such as education, qualifications, and experience are the key elements in the determination of staffing numbers. Many hospitals have developed career ladder systems with the stated purpose as being to keep "experienced" nurses at the bedside. Such systems are also used to improve nurse satisfaction and thereby improve retention of experienced nurses.

Nurse executives must ask several questions. Do I have the resources in today's health care environment to realize the expectations of the delivery of care system adapted by our nursing department? Are there alternatives to the delivery system that would be more efficient or effective without threatening the standards of care adopted by the nursing staff? Do we need to explore other models of nursing care delivery? The challenge is to provide quality care in a cost-effective way. The key in today's health care environment is the efficient and effective use of the nurse who is in short supply but is an essential part of the system.

Support Systems

Nursing activities not directly related to patient care must be built into staffing components. The higher the efficiency of the support systems, the lower the nurse staffing needed to provide a given amount of direct care. In order to maximize support services, nursing activities not directly related to patient care should be examined.

Nurses in many institutions are treated as all-purpose workers. It is not unusual for nurses to assume the function of other professionals when these persons leave at 5:00 PM or on weekends and holidays thus decreasing their caregiving activities. Also attempts of administrators to curb costs in the past several years have produced cuts in general support activities. For example, in one institution linen packs formerly supplied were stopped due to cutbacks in laundry room personnel. The impact of that cutback was felt by nurses on the units when they had to spend time preparing their own linen packs.

The nursing shortage has forced hospitals to examine how the nurse is being utilized. Attention has been directed to the study of the nurses role in the current health care environment. Questions being asked are: Do we really need more nurses?

What type of support services would free the nurse to concentrate on direct patient care? Before an institution can answer these questions it must determine what the nurse is actually doing in its institution.

Work sampling methodology can be useful in the analysis of where nurses spend their time. It can identify: (1) how much time is spent by head nurses, staff nurses, practical nurses, student nurses, nursing assistants, and unit clerks on activities requiring their own level of skill; (2) how much time nurses actually spend with patients and; (3) how much time goes into activities that could be performed by other classes of personnel (Chapter 12 also describes job analysis in detail).

Once the activity pattern of nurses has been clarified, certain options are open. Enough nurses can be hired to enable staff to function in their current role or appropriate changes in support services can be made to allow the staff to function at their skill level.

WORKLOAD—PATIENT NEEDS AND REQUIREMENTS FOR CARE

Since different patients require varying amounts of nursing care (Bermas, 1984; Giovanetti, 1984), a patient classification system is necessary to identify the workload and as a major source of data for a staffing plan. Data supplied should include not only an indicator of the patients' needs for nursing care but how that care should be distributed across the 24 hour period. It should also identify the appropriate skill mix for the patient population on the unit. The patient classification instruments in use today fall into two basic categories: prototype evaluation or factor evaluation methods (Reinert & Grant, 1981). The prototype evaluation method determines nursing resource requirements through the assignment of patients into predetermined categories based on a description of patient care needs. The factor evaluation method identifies pertinent patient care attributes with predetermined weights or relative value units. The assigned weights of the pertinent care attributes are summed to classify the patient into one of several homogeneous groups.

A major issue regarding patient classification is whether the system should identify care that is actually delivered or the optimal care that could be delivered based on the identified needs of the patient. One side of the debate maintains that it is unrealistic to classify patients according to optimal needs if sufficient staff cannot be provided for optimal care. Otherwise staff will feel they are not meeting the needs of patients and become discouraged. The other side argues that the nursing care goal should be to provide optimal care.

While both sides have legitimate points, the purpose for which the instrument has been designed should be considered. If the purpose of the classification tool is to determine staffing needs, it is desirable to use an instrument that identifies patient needs rather than one that reflects nurse activity. A tool that focuses on nurse activity may have difficulty responding to changes in the delivery system, such as introduction of new technology, elimination of old or creation of new positions, and support systems. The value or weight assigned to an individual nursing activity may need to be changed when new equipment is acquired. For example, when intravenous monitoring pump devices are introduced, nurse activities related to monitoring IV administration change. The patient's need for monitoring has not changed but the nursing activity surrounding that patient need has.

Ledwidge (1988) suggests that the patient classification instrument is a means of identifying the impact of changes in the health care system on the patient's need for nursing services. Although patients are being admitted at a more acute stage of their illnesses than in the past, it is not totally correct to interpret the resulting increase in workload as simply due to sicker patients. For example, the nursing needs of a patient who has coronary bypass surgery have not changed significantly over the past 2 years. What has changed is that most surgical patients no longer come into the hospital preoperatively for laboratory tests and x-rays. Instead they have the preoperative workup done on an outpatient basis and are admitted on the day of surgery. Also patients no longer stay in the hospital 6 to 7 days after surgery. Those who once would have been discharged with a low need for nursing care are being discharged while they still need fairly complex nursing care, and therefore require extensive discharge instruction and often, home health or nursing home care. Due to these changes in surgical admission and discharge patterns, most hospitalized surgical patients require more nursing. As a result, there is a concentration of more patients requiring more nursing care. Table 22–1 shows the acuity level of a surgical unit. One can see an increase in overall acuity and a compression in the range of acuity.

In today's changing health care environment, a classification instrument that focuses on patient need is a reasonable choice. It monitors "patient need" for nursing care without having to make frequent adjustments to accommodate the changes in technology and nursing activity. Whichever patient classification methodology is used in determining nurse staffing, the instrument must be validated and the patient attributes or nurse activity data reliably captured.

A valid and reliable classification instrument is an essential part of the staffing process and provides a comprehensive, accurate, objective data base that can be used in developing a staffing plan. A patient classification instrument focuses on elements of patient characteristics but not, however, on the nurse's functioning in relation to organizational support and nursing resources.

The Staffing Process

The actual staffing process should occur at least once every year. Since the budget is so integrally connected to the staffing requirements, most institutions coordinate the

TABLE 22-1. ACUITY SHIFTS IN A SURGICAL NURSING DEPARTMENT

	Average Acuity (Range)[a]
1985	1.54(1.4–1.6)
1986	1.52(1.3–1.7)
1987	1.67(1.5–2.0)
1988	1.74(1.6–1.8)
1989	1.86(1.8–1.9)

[a]Acuity range: .5 (low need for nursing care) to 5.0 (high need for nursing care)

staffing process with the budget cycle. Tied into the budgeting cycle at the corporate level is the forecasting of what is expected to occur in the next fiscal year. Some of the decisions that impact the staffing process include the following:

1. Projection of patient days
2. Addition of new programs, eg,
   A. Specialty physicians such as renal, oncology, and transplant
   B. New technology
3. Increase or decrease in services, eg,
   A. Cutback in transfusion therapy services
   B. Additional staff added to chest physical therapy
4. Closing and/or relocation of units for remodeling

Corporate decisions should be communicated to the nurse managers before the actual staffing process begins. The first step of the staffing process should be an evaluation of the current staffing plan. Did the plan provide for the effective and efficient delivery of nurse care? Were there enough staff to meet the patient care requirements? Was it necessary to make significant changes to the staff mix during the year to accommodate an increase in patient acuity? This evaluation process should occur at the unit level and be reported to the department. To assist in this evaluation process, it is essential that nurse managers have a concurrent, comprehensive variance reporting system in place and functional. At the departmental level unit information can be used to identify problems in the overall staffing plan. This type of review helps the nurse executive to identify the differences and similarities between units. At this point in the planning stage, decisions regarding any changes in the care delivery system need to be implemented and/or evaluated.

The unit manager uses the following information to forecast staffing requirements at the unit level:

1. Evaluation results of current staffing plan
2. Historical staff requirements
3. Projected patient acuity
4. Impact of new programs and technology
5. Availability of staff
6. Educational and experiential level of staff
7. Historical trends related to patient census and acuity level

Using this information, the unit leader can predict daily staffing needs for the average patient mix for the unit. The staff mix, number of registered nurses, licensed practical nurses, nursing assistants, is totaled into daily staffing needs. When this type of systematic assessment approach is used in determining staffing needs for patient care areas, it is probable that the standard will vary from unit to unit. The standard is defined as the average hours per patient day needed to supply the unit with appropriate coverage to meet patient needs. The formula for calculation of the standard hours is the total number of staff needed each 24 hours times 8 hours per shift divided by the averaged daily census. The standard hours per patient day and the projected yearly census are then used to project the staffing requirements for the unit (see Fig 22-2 for an example of a staffing plan worksheet).

Once the total staffing requirements for the unit have been determined, the next step is to distribute staff requirements to appropriate shifts which is dependent on patient acuity. In an intensive care unit one would expect the staff to be fairly equally distributed across shifts while transplant or general surgery units would require more staff on the day shift (see Fig 22-3).

The staffing plan for the nursing department is a summary of the individual unit plans and represents the average daily staffing needs by staff level and shift assignment. This plan is then the basis for the budget development for the nursing department. Once the daily staffing requirements are determined, the resources necessary to supply the daily staffing needs is calculated. Factored into that calculation are vacation, holiday, off days, and sick and absence time.

Also included in the staffing process should be a method to monitor concurrently throughout the year whether or not the staffing plan is effective and being applied appropriately. Since the staffing plan is based on a forecast of the needs in the coming year, the information that should be monitored should reflect whether or not the forecasts were accurate and how the variances were explained. See Figure 22-4 for an example of a variance reporting form.

The key element in the staffing process is the identification of an appropriate standard for each nursing unit. Since the standard may vary from unit to unit, nurse executives must be able to show in a quantifiable way that the standards set by the patient care area are justified. They need to demonstrate the impact of deviation from the standards on the quality of patient care (outcome measures), patient satisfaction, and nurse satisfaction (eg, turnover, sick days, and absenteeism).

SCHEDULING

Once the staffing plan has been devised, the manager can redirect energies to the process of scheduling staff. In many institutions, scheduling is a time-consuming process. Many full-time equivalents (FTEs) are expended annually just in generation of time schedules! These FTEs are often filled by senior professional staff whose talents may better be utilized in other activities. Scheduling need not be a time-consuming, frustrating process. By giving careful thought to the parameters underlying the schedule and logically applying decision rules to the personnel, the process can be streamlined and performed by non-nurses in a manner that is efficient and highly satisfactory to the professional staff. When the schedule is effectively done, it should balance both patient care needs and nursing resource availability. While the administrator's fundamental obligation is to meet the needs of the institution, the wishes of the staff must also be considered to maximize retention. To do this, a process must be defined that is fair and allows staff maximum control over their work schedules. When the scheduling process is understood by staff and perceived to be fair, most nurses are willing to be flexible enough to accommodate the needs of the institution.

UNIT	PROJECTED CENSUS	STANDARD HR/PT. DAY	TOTAL HOURS/YEAR	HOURS/DAY	STAFF 8 HR/DAY	12 HR/DAY
Transplant Unit	10,766	5.71	61,474	168	21.0	14.0
General Surgery	12,520	4.31	53,961	148	18.5	12.3
Surgical Intensive Care	7,729	18.66	144,223	395	49.4	32.9

Figure 22-2. Sample Staffing Plan Worksheet

Unit	Shift Staff Allocation			(8 hr shifts)
	7 AM–3:30 PM	3 PM–11:30	11 PM–7:30 AM	Total
Transplant unit	8	7	6	21
General surgery	8	6	5	19
Surgical intensive care	17	16	16	49

Unit	Shift Staff Allocation		(12 hr shifts)
	7 AM–7:30 PM	7 PM–7:30 AM	Total
Transplant unit	8	6	14
General surgery	7	5	12
Surgical intensive care	17	16	33

Figure 22-3. Sample Staffing Plan Worksheet B

Before beginning the process of actually assigning shifts to employees, a number of factors must be considered. Careful consideration of these issues will allow the manager to design a schedule that is fair to all employees and facilitates matching of unit needs and available resources. There are multiple solutions to many of these issues; therefore, the scheduling process need not be the same for all institutions or even all units within an institution. What is important is that all the issues be considered and policies generated by nursing administration. Implementation of these policies and actual schedule generation can be done in a satisfactory manner only if proper attention has been given to the dimensions that underlie the process.

Scheduling practices should reflect the nursing service philosophy, selected nursing care delivery, and the average length of stay for patients on a given unit. Policies on the use of temporary personnel as well as those regarding "floating" of staff to and from other units will also affect the way that resources are scheduled and the length of time for which a schedule is generated.

Scheduling may be done in a centralized or decentralized manner. Some institutions have found it advantageous to have all schedules generated from one central office. Advantages include development of significant expertise in scheduling and maximum knowledge of resource availability throughout the department. Disadvantages include perception of lack of control by the staff or unit mangers over work schedules and some increased rigidity in scheduling policies. When centralized scheduling is utilized, variations can still be made to account for differences in patient populations on selected units. Many institutions that utilize a centralized scheduling system also employ full-time float nurses to cover for days off, vacations, and illnesses of regular staff. The need for these nurses can be calculated and will be discussed.

Institutions may delegate the responsibility for scheduling to individual unit managers. When a decentralized system is in place, the nurse executive should make

Unit _____ Date YTD _____ to _____ Period _____ to _____

	YTD			PERIOD			
	Budget	Actual	Variance	Budget	Actual	Variance	EXPLANATION OF VARIANCES
Patient Days (PD)							
Acuity							
Budget Hours/PD							
Positions (FTEs)							
RN							
Other							
Agency							Reason for use of outside agency nurses
Overtime							
Total							

Figure 22-4. Variance Reporting Form

certain that all managers have a good understanding of the scheduling process. Likewise, the nurse executive should examine variations in scheduling practices by unit to make certain that those variations can be justified by the patient populations. Inequities in scheduling policies on a given unit can damage morale and retention for the department as a whole. When units in a department utilize different scheduling patterns, communication to a centralized person or office is essential so that assistance can be given across units for short-staffing situations.

Dimensions in Scheduling

The schedule can be generated only when three underlying dimensions are defined: personnel requirements dictated by the staffing plan, policies established for the entire unit (unit dimensions), and variances that have been granted for individual staff members (staff dimensions).

Unit dimensions include (1) basic shift length for the unit, usually 8, 10, or 12 hours; (2) maximum work stretch; (3) shift rotation patterns; and (4) weekend patterns. The maximum number of consecutive days that a nurse will be scheduled can be expected to vary as a function of the shift length chosen. Absentee rates of employees can be used to identify work stretch length problems.

Weekend and shift rotation patterns must be clearly defined. The staffing plan will dictate the number of staff necessary on weekend shifts. These patient care requirements and the total number of staff will determine the number of weekends off per schedule that each staff member can expect. Efficient utilization of part-time staff will maximize the number of weekends off for staff. Hansen (1983b) presents a more complete discussion of this process.

Like weekends, rotation patterns are determined by the number of staff needed on evening and night shifts as well as the number of staff who have agreed to permanently work these shifts. While permanent shifts are desirable, it can be difficult to recruit sufficient staff to nonday shifts. A growing number of managers are considering the assignment of most staff to weekday positions on permanent shifts and filling the weekend positions with other staff who work only weekends. This approach necessitates paying significant compensation packages to nurses working all but weekday day shifts. When the cost of these packages is less than the fees paid to temporary staffing agencies for unfilled positions, the approach is justified. If rotation is necessary, it should be of sufficient length to allow the nurse to adjust to working at a different time of day. This may mean a longer rotation at less frequent intervals (eg, 1 month of night shift every 4 months rather than 1 week of nights each month). If the decision is made to vary the amounts of rotation expected of staff, rules governing the rotation must be carefully set.

Decreased rotation has been used as a means to reward longevity on a nursing unit. It is tempting to use number of years of service as an absolute guideline. However, if all staff remain for that amount of time, they will expect to rotate less and yet the shifts will remain to be covered. Rescinding a rule at that time could be demoralizing and could result in unwanted staff turnover. It may be more advantageous to select the number of positions that could qualify for decreased or no rotation. As these positions become vacant, staff can be moved into them according to a predetermined protocol. Well-defined rotation and weekend patterns can be a powerful re-cruitment and retention tool.

Individual nurse managers must decide if staff will be scheduled for the unit as a whole or for subsections within the unit. Scheduling for subsections may be advantageous for implementation of a nursing care delivery system, but it can make the scheduling process more difficult. It actually is generation of a second time schedule for the same unit.

It is often necessary to consider the individual needs of some staff. This should be done with great care, balancing the needs of one nurse with the greater good of the entire staff. If large numbers of exceptions need to be made each month, the manager should re-examine the unit policies. Well-defined unit dimensions should reduce the number of staff dimensions to be considered.

All staff can be expected to have special requests. These can be for single dates or short-term situations as well as long-term fixed arrangements. Individuals may request a fixed pattern for a number of reasons, including child or elder care arrangements, coordination with a spouse's schedule, or additional education. The key to success in deciding which of the requests to grant is a thorough understanding of the staffing plan and the number of requests that can be granted before the plan becomes compromised. The number of FTEs assigned and filled on a roster dictate the total number of shifts available in a given time period. Subtracting the number of shifts needed to meet the staffing plan will provide the number of additional shifts available for granting requests for paid time off. Likewise, the amount of paid time off available to staff in any given year can easily be calculated. Doing so will enable the manager to know the minimum number of staff who should be on vacation at any given time as well as the maximum the unit can afford to have away on paid time off. Publication of this information will assist staff in their planning as well.

While it would be hoped that staff requests would not overlap, it is well known that conflicts can and do occur. The administrator should have policies for handling such conflict when it occurs. The wise administrator builds in interstaff negotiation into these policies. All staff on a unit are responsible for a schedule, not just the manager. Encouraging staff to take responsibility for coverage reinforces this fact. Some managers will grant blocks of paid time off before honoring requests for single days while others look at all requests on a seniority or "first-come first-served" basis. The effect of a paid holiday should also be factored into the planning process. Often, fewer vacations can be granted during a payroll period that includes a holiday due to the number of staff who must be granted an additional day off. Whatever the policies are, they should be made clear to all staff. Those policies should also state how far in advance requests must be made. As policies become more clearly defined, staff find it easier to plan and often the number of requests that are difficult to fill diminish.

Finally, careful attention must be paid to any labor laws or collective bargaining agreements that may govern all or some of the staff. These documents may specify such things as work stretches, weekend patterns, number of days worked in a calendar week, floating policies, or nurse-patient ratios.

The primary source of data for any time schedule is a complete and accurate data base containing information about the unit personnel. The process of updating the data base need not be time consuming, but it should be constant and methodical. Essential elements of this data base include FTE status; weekend, shift, and rotation patterns; agreements for fixed work days; paid time off balance, and special work needs. Requests and arrangements for days on duty are as important as those for days off. It is often the planned days on duty for things such as committee meetings or special patient care assignments that the nurse manager tries to commit to memory, yet often forgets when creating the schedule. Trying to switch the schedule after it has been posted to accommodate these plans is difficult and frustrating. A separate schedule listing just fixed work schedule days can be a valuable asset to the manager (see Fig 22-5). When it is possible to view the weekend patterns, planned days on duty, and promised days off for all personnel, it becomes readily apparent when unit staffing plans can no longer be met or if special requests can be granted.

The Scheduling Process

Once the issues discussed above have been given careful consideration, the actual schedule generation can begin. Schedules can be generated as often as every 2 weeks or as infrequently as every 6 months, depending on the type of the schedule created and the needs of the unit staff. The length of schedule should be a multiple of payroll period length for efficient calculation of paid work time and for reconciliation of the schedule with financial data. Schedule generation itself is a process where the unit's policies are applied to the personnel data base. The entire process is represented schematically in Figure 22-6.

There are multiple approaches to the scheduling process including cyclical staffing, controlled variables staffing, self-scheduling, and automated scheduling. The choice of approach can vary by unit, depending on the stability of the staff and the patient care requirements of the unit. Regardless of the method chosen, it must meet the requirements of the staffing plan and provide for a fiscally prudent use of resources. The time taken to actually generate the schedule may vary from minutes to many hours per month, depending on the complexity of the unit. Schedule creation time that is unusually lengthy often results when (1) insufficient attention has been paid to underlying scheduling policies or (2) policies have been set up that conflict with one another.

Traditionally, schedules have been generated manually. A list of available personnel for a shift is made; weekends and special requests are assigned; and nonpaid days off are assigned to each staff member to prevent long work stretches or single days on duty. The numbers of staff on duty each shift are matched against the staffing plan and then days off are adjusted to balance the totals with the desired numbers and to correct maldistribution of staff. It is this last process that is time consuming and frustrating. It is also during this time that managers often change planned days on or requested days off inadvertently. It is important to mark these days differently so that they will not be changed. There are limited numbers of patterns that allow one to work 10 days in a 14 day pay period. The challenge is to choose the best combination of patterns that both meet the staffing plan and are perceived as desirable by the staff.

Figure 22-5. Sample Master Work Agreement Plan

FTE	Name	Comments	MTWRFSS	MTWRFSS	MTWRFSS	MTWRFSS	MTWRFSS	MTWRFSS	MTWRFSS	MTWRFSS
1.0	RN1	cn	D DD	D XX	DD	D DD	DD	D DD	DD	D XX
1.0	RN2	cn	DD	XX	DD	XX	DD	XX	XX	EE
1.0	RN3	cn	EE	EE	XX	EE	XX	XX	XX	EE
1.0	RN4	cn	XX	XX	EEE	XX	EEE	EEE	EEE	XX
1.0	RN5	cn, no Thur pm	EEE	DD	XX	DD	XX	DD	XX	EE
1.0	RN6	cn	DD	XX	DD	XX	DD	XX	XX	DD
1.0	RN7	cn	RNN	RNN	RXX	RNN	RXX	RNN	RNN	RXX
1.0	RN8	cn	XX	NN	NN	XX	NN	XX	XX	NN
1.0	RN9	night shift								
1.0	RN10		XX	XX	XX	XX	XX	XX	XX	XX
0.6	RN11	weekends	----NN--	--NN--	----NN-	----NN-	--NN-	----NN-	----NN-	----NN-
1.0	RN12		R EE	R EE	R EE	R EE	R EE	R E	R XX	R EE
0.6	RN13	weekends	--NN---	----NN-	--NN-	--NN-	--NN-	--NN-	R XX	--NN-
1.0	RN14		R EE	R EE	R EE	R XX	R EE	R EE	R EE	R XX
1.0	RN15		XX	DD	DD	DD	EE	XX	DD	DD
1.0	RN16		N N	X XX	DD	XX	DD	N N	XXX	EE
1.0	RN17		XX	DD	XX	DD	XX	DD	DD	EE
1.0	RN18		DD	XX	DD	XX	DD	XX	DD	XX
0.4	RN19		----DDD	--D--	---DDD	--D--	----DDD	N N	----DDD	--D--
0.4	RN20	no Tuesday	XX	DD	XX	DD	XX	DD	DD	DD

Code

X = scheduled day off
R = requested day off
cn = can be charge nurse
D = day
E = evening
N = night

Notes

1. RN1 needs to attend policy and procedure meeting each Wednesday, 11AM –1 PM
2. RN4 may need to be house supervisor on Friday evenings on even numbered weeks
3. RN2 has management meeting on 2nd Monday of each 4 week schedule 8–9AM

519

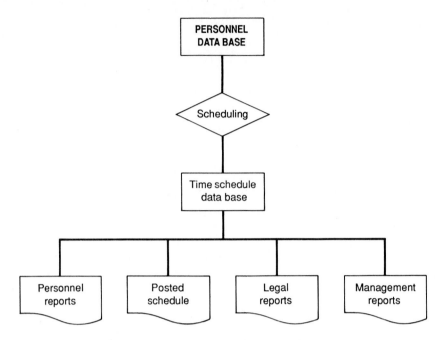

Figure 22-6. Schematic of Scheduling Process

Cyclical Staffing

In the early 1970s, nurse administrators began to see the advantage of finding the right combination of patterns for the staff and repeating these patterns over time. This approach is known as *cyclical scheduling,* and is used with considerable satisfaction by many nursing departments. Generation of the initial schedule is a time-consuming process, but the time is recovered as the pattern is repeated. As the pattern is developed, there is an attempt to evenly distribute work stretches or combinations that are perceived as less desirable among all staff. When the master pattern is posted, staff either request or are assigned a particular pattern. Since the pattern will repeat itself for an extended time, usually several months, it is assumed that employees can make arrangements more easily for personal activities, since days off are known so far in advance. If staff wishes to take vacations or needs other time away, the unit can be covered by a variety of mechanisms, such as use of an inhouse float pool.

Selected units may not realize the benefits of cyclical scheduling. These are units experiencing high rates of turnover where supplementary coverage is not readily available or units where staff availability varies frequently. This is often seen on units where multiple staff members have returned to school. They may be requesting different days off to attend class as often as every 10 weeks. Regeneration of the master schedule so frequently is not an efficient use of managerial time. It should also be noted that in institutions where use of float pools is essential to the success of a cyclical schedule, the unit schedules must be communicated to the float pool coordinator and anticipated requests made known well in advance so that they can be filled. This often necessitates institutionwide policies about paid time off to even out the demands made on the float pool.

Controlled Variable Staffing

In institutions where there is great variability in census or patient care requirements, it has become increasingly difficult to create schedules that consistently meet the staffing plan. Under these conditions, an approach known as *controlled variable* (Hanson, 1983a) staffing may be beneficial. Sufficient numbers of staff are assigned to units to meet the estimated daily workload. However, no additional positions are assigned to cover either the paid or nonpaid days off of the permanently assigned personnel. When needed, personnel are provided from a central pool. When the staffing plan is devised, the number of personnel needed to cover for the permanently assigned staff is calculated. Not all of these positions are filled with permanent personnel; rather, a fraction of the positions are filled with the assumption that some float staff will always be needed. The rest of the positions are filled by temporary personnel. This allows the manager to remain within the limitations of the personnel budget if the predicted patient days do not materialize or if there are wide variations in patient census. This type of schedule necessitates communication with a central staffing office and department wide policies for granting paid time off. Permanently assigned staff can usually be given satisfactory schedules within these departmentally established policies. Two drawbacks to controlled variable staffing are difficulty in finding sufficient numbers of staff to work in a permanent floating situation and salary requirements of temporary personnel that can make the approach fiscally undesirable.

Self-Scheduling

Many nurse managers have attempted to give staff more control of their schedule by instituting a system of *self-scheduling*. The manager lists the staffing requirements for each date and shift, and staff sign up for their desired shifts. Units that use this system successfully have clear guidelines for how staff select shifts. These guidelines may include the number of weekends and nonday shifts each staff member must cover as well as the order in which the staff may sign up for desired shifts. There are also unit policies for handling problems that arise with coverage or shifts that remain uncovered. Units that have reported success with this type of schedule tend to be relatively small with staff who are comfortable negotiating with their peers.

When some staff are working one basic pattern (eg, 8-hour shifts) and others are working another shift length (eg, 12-hour patterns), continuity of patient care must be considered as the schedule is generated. It is desirable, for example, to have equal numbers of day and night 12-hour personnel on any given day so that major adjustments in patient assignments do not have to be made in the middle of the evening shift. Careful attention to the numbers of personnel working 12-hour shifts as well as the weekend and rotation patterns of those personnel will make this task as easy as possible.

Automated Scheduling

Many professions have used automated processes for generating schedules but nursing has turned to the computer only recently. Multiple software packages are now available, and automated technology has been successfully applied in both centralized and decentralized scheduling situations. A basic understanding of how these programs work is essential before undertaking a selection and implementation process.

A computer generates a time schedule by a process known as linear optimization. An algorithm that contains instructions concerning scheduling practices is followed and repeated searches of the personnel data base made until the best possible combination of scheduling patterns is found. Programs differ in the number of instructions or constraints that can be handled. The number should be sufficient to meet the needs of the purchasing institution. Some programs address constraints but are limited in the number of individual requests that can be handled. For example, the staff member who wishes to request a Thursday evening off to attend a child's school play may need to settle for the only 2-week pattern that has that day off. This same pattern may contain a work stretch that is within unit parameters, yet undesirable to the individual staff nurse.

Not all programs that are described as scheduling systems contain optimization routines. Some do not consider individual staff requests at all. Instead, they generate master schedules that can be used for staff to select from when using a cyclical scheduling system. Still others are tracking systems only. The manually generated schedule can be entered and used to generate multiple reports.

If a department's manually generated schedules are fundamentally sound, the automated program should produce schedules that are of equal or improved quality. Even when improved schedules are produced in a more efficient manner, automated scheduling systems are not always implemented successfully. Staff often distrust the ''machine,'' believing that it will not permit attention to individual needs. Managers often experience a loss of control but they may find that the time formerly spent in schedule generation is now available for other management activities. If these other activities are more difficult or less satisfying than schedule generation, the manager may resist implementation of the new technology. All of these problems can be anticipated and addressed. Active participation by managers and staff is strongly encouraged.

Posting the Schedule

Once the schedule is generated, it should be carefully examined before posting. Criteria for evaluation of the schedule should be established. Sample criteria are shown in Figure 22-7. Personnel totals for each shift should be compared against the staffing

---

Number of shifts that equal or exceed the staffing plan
Extent to which scheduling patterns are in compliance with unit dimensions
Number of staff dimensions are met
Staff satisfaction with the posted schedule
Reasons for denial of staff special requests

Figure 22-7. Criteria for Evaluation of the Schedule

plan to see if any variations can be justified. If the schedule has been generated automatically, the manager should have the option to make adjustments before the final copy is printed. Charge nurse or other responsibilities that require professional judgment may also need to be assigned. If it has not been possible to grant all requests, the manager should be able to explain the reasons for the denial and should discuss the situation with the staff nurse involved rather than wait for the nurse to examine the schedule.

The generated schedule is also a data base and is often subject to considerable change as the time period proceeds. Illnesses and other unforeseen emergencies may necessitate changes that need to be recorded. This final data base becomes a source of information for multiple other management functions, including generation of the payroll, productivity reporting systems, and legal records that may be needed for reference for a lengthy period of time. It is essential then that any changes be reported completely and accurately.

The basic schedule, as well as any anticipated problems, should be made known to staff as far in advance of the starting date as possible. Posting 14 to 21 days before the start of a noncyclical schedule is usually sufficient for staff to make any arrangements necessary to plan their time effectively. If the central staffing office is responsible for supplying additional personnel to meet unit staffing plans, the schedule may need to be generated further in advance of the starting date to allow that office to schedule float or temporary personnel. If the lead time is too lengthy however, staff may not know days they need off. This can result in time-consuming schedule adjustment after the schedule is posted. Automated scheduling systems may assist in decreasing the time between schedule generation and schedule start date.

There may be times that the personnel available to schedule will not meet the staffing plan. Shortages of available personnel resulting in unfilled budgeted positions is the most common cause. There may be other times that serious illness or injury to staff members causes reductions in available personnel. Serious difficulties in scheduling to meet the staffing plan, should be communicated to the nurse executive as soon as this fact is known (Calafee, 1987). There are several possible approaches to handle this situation: re-adjustment of existing available personnel, utilization of temporary workers, or reduction in the number of available beds and operating hours in the institution. Each of these approaches has strengths and limitations.

The manager's responsibility does not end once the schedule has been posted. The staffing plan that served as a basis for schedule generation is usually made using historical or projected data. As real data regarding patient census, acuity, and nursing resources become available, the schedule must be re-examined for adequacy. Variation of the schedule can occur on either the demand or resource side of the scheduling equation. In some institutions, average census is found to be 60 to 80 percent of capacity on some units. This permits wide variations in demand that can strain the ability of even the most creative manager.

The patient classification system is usually the most readily available tool for estimating actual patient care requirements. This system may yield fairly precise estimates of staff requirements, but caution should be taken not to use it as an absolute rule. Qualifications and experience of the actual staff scheduled, the ability of the scheduled staff to work as a team, and types of activities planned for patients but not measured by the tool should also be considered. Decision criteria should be established for the amount of over or understaffing that may exist before the manager takes corrective action.

Absenteeism

Absenteeism is a significant concern for the nursing administrator. American workers have an absentee rate of 5.5 days a year (Statistical Abstracts of the United States, 1989). The administrator must attempt to pinpoint the causes of absenteeism and institute changes when possible to reduce the absentee rate to the lowest level possible. Some reasons for absenteeisms (eg, accidents, illness) are not under the control of the administrator. Even these situations should be viewed with an index of suspicion, however, to make certain that the work environment is not causing sufficient stress to contribute to these events. This will be especially important as the nurse labor force continues to age. Situations that are definitely under the control of the manager are scheduling practices that may encourage absenteeism.

Absenteeism is classified by the frequency, amount, and predictability of the work time lost. Examination of employee attendance records can reveal patterns and will assist the manager to determine the causes and implement solutions. Two types of absentee rates are usually calculated: the percentage of work time lost and the frequency rate. The formulas are shown in Figure 22–8.

When the causes are discovered, the manager has a range of options available. The current methods available can be described as either motivational or punitive in nature. Motivational methods include commending or rewarding good attendance; providing sick-child care facilities; or changing job descriptions to increase autonomy or task-variety. Punitive measures include making the call procedure more difficult; requiring medical verification of any illness; or disciplinary action. All methods have been used with varying levels of success.

Frequency Rate:

$$\frac{\text{Total number of absences/year}}{\text{Average number of employees}} \times 100 = \text{Yearly frequency rate}$$

Percentage of time lost:

$$\frac{\text{Number of days lost}}{\text{Potential work days}} \times 100 = \text{Percentage of time lost}$$

Figure 22-8. Two Types of Absentee Rates

Effects of Scheduling on Retention and Absenteeism

The US Department of Health and Human Services (1990) reports that 80 percent of registered nurses in the United States are working with over 95 percent employed in nursing positions. Those who are not working are not able to do so because of age, health, or family responsibilities. Over one third of the nurses who are working part time do not wish to add additional work hours. Only a small percentage of nurses wish to work shifts in addition to their full-time assignment on a regular basis (Roberts et al, 1989). Therefore, the need to retain current nursing employees is critical if the nurse manager wishes to meet the staffing plan. Exit interviews with departing staff often indicate dissatisfaction with scheduling as an important reason for changing positions. Nurses will often accept positions with lower salaries in order to increase control over their work schedules. Part-time nurses who are willing to add shifts indicate that control over their schedule would be essential for them to increase their work hours (Roberts et al, 1989).

Nurses who do not or are not able to work when scheduled have a highly significant impact on the staffing plan, the nursing budget, and the morale of the remaining staff. Staffing plans today rarely have more than the minimum number needed to meet patient care demands. When a nurse is not present, several undesirable situations may occur: A unit may need to operate understaffed; unprepared staff may be floated into the unit; or a more expensive temporary worker will be utilized. A temporary worker may not be available on short notice, resulting in additional stress and frustration for remaining unit staff members.

Ineffective scheduling practices can result in a time schedule that chronically does not meet the staffing plan. Other schedules meet the staffing plan but do so by making staff nurses work unreasonable patterns. These patterns may be ones that force the nurse to work many days before a day off or where the days off are poorly spaced. The nurse who has a day off, works only one day, and then has another day off will be tempted to call in sick on that isolated day on duty. The effects of shift rotation on employee health have been shown; managers need to be prudent in the way rotation patterns are defined. If there are not enough staff available to utilize a certain basic hours pattern (eg, 10-hour shifts), the staff may need to consider another pattern until more staff become available. If the basic hour pattern cannot be changed, several positions may need to be devoted to nontraditional shifts to meet peak workload times. For example, a surgical unit may experience increased demands early in the evening shift due to patients returning from the recovery room. Often, day shift staff have been asked to stay overtime to assist. It may be possible to schedule one day shift nurse to work from 10:00 AM to 6:00 PM on selected days to meet this need.

Many institutions have policies that in fact support absenteeism. In many situations, the employee may accrue a maximum number of sick time hours. This can combine with an organizational cultural characteristic that views sick time as a right rather than a benefit of employment. The result is a "use-them-or-lose-them" attitude that encourages that employee to call in sick when they are really available to work. Many institutions have adopted a paid-time off system that rewards employees' accrued sick time hours by allowing them to use the time for scheduled time off. This practice allows managers to better plan the number of days that employees will be available and they have been shown to decrease absenteeism (Scholtzhauer & Rosse, 1985). Other institutions require that an employee have a minimum balance of sick time hours before any can be used. Still others have compensated employees for either unused sick time or excellent attendance records.

If absenteeism is not controlled, increased turnover of staff may result. Individuals conducting exit interviews should attempt to determine if scheduling had any effect on the employee's decision to terminate. These data should be made available to both the individual nurse managers as well as the nurse executive, so that changes can be made at the appropriate level.

Process of Re-allocation

Readjustment is necessary when a unit is inadequately or inappropriately staffed. Both types of situations can occur and are handled differently. The number of staff scheduled may not be able to meet the current workload or sufficient numbers of personnel may be scheduled, but there may not be enough registered nurses. Also too many personnel can be scheduled for the actual patient care demand on a given day creating financial concerns. Solutions to all problems can be sought within the nursing department as well as from outside agencies. They include floating staff to other units, use of available temporary personnel, asking staff to work overtime, redirecting admissions, and closing beds. When selecting a solution, the legal risks of understaffing, the quality and continuity of patient care, and the stress placed on the scheduled staff by the solution chosen must be considered.

Because of the dynamic nature of patient care, isolated situations will arise. The manager should document the occurrence of any situation, and periodically review these records to see if the misallocation between patient needs and scheduled staff could have been prevented. Some of these changes happen insidiously. For example, operating room schedules may change, resulting in heavier workloads on different days than had been anticipated when the annual staffing plan had been done. Other patterns may be more general. For example, one unit may find that most understaffing occurs on Tuesday evening due to a number of the staff taking Tuesday evening classes. If a pattern can be identified, scheduling should be adjusted to fit the pattern or arrangements made to have more temporary workers available at those times.

If workers are floated, they should be cross-trained in advance whenever possible. Cross-training is not without cost, however, it can be done efficiently. A group of nurses may be trained for "partner" units—those with similar patient assignments such as medical-surgical units or psychiatric, chemical dependency, and stress disorder units (Rutkowski, 1987). A smaller number of nurses may be cross-trained to work many areas. Decisions regarding cross-training are based on the range of patient care assignments in the institution, the number of staff available to float, and the number of units that regularly require assistance. Floating is a difficult assignment for many nurses. The policy regarding floating should be made clear to employees as soon as possible, preferably prior to hire. In addition, staff should know the disciplinary consequences if they refuse a float assignment.

There will be times that the staffing shortage cannot be satisfactorily resolved. The manager should document what attempts have been made to resolve the problem. If the situation becomes chronic, the nurse executive should become involved. The decision to close beds and restrict income is never easy, yet the expenditures for legal actions resulting from patient accidents due to understaffing or inadequately prepared staff may far outweigh the income generated from admitting those patients.

SUMMARY

The outcome of the staffing process should result in providing an appropriate number and mix of nursing personnel while maintaining a stated level of quality care. The process of staffing is complex and depends on many variables and external conditions both internal and external to the organization.

Scheduling personnel to meet the staffing plan requires the manager to consider policies that will affect the unit or department as well as variations that can be granted for individuals. There are multiple techniques for scheduling. Those that are well understood by the staff and allow them maximum predictability and control given the needs of the unit are well accepted and keep absenteeism at minimum levels. Schedules are generated based on anticipated needs. Because of the dynamic nature of nursing workload, the schedule must be examined and adjusted as often as every shift.

REFERENCES

Accreditation Manual for Hospitals. Joint Commission on Accrediting Hospital Organization. Chicago, 1989

American Nurses Association. ANA commission on nursing services. Nursing staff requirements for in-patient health care service. NS-201-MR 6/78, 1977

American Nurses Association. Standards of nursing practice. Kansas City, Mo, American Nurses Association, 1973

August J. Strategies: Retention of nurses in hospitals. *Nurse Executive Management Strategies 12.* Chicago, American Hospital Association, 1988

Benner B. *From Novice to Expert.* Redwood City, CA, Addison Wesley Co, 1984

Bermas NF, VanSlyck A. Patient classification systems and the nursing department. *Hospitals.* 58:22, 99, 1984

Bille DA. Philosophy of nursing service as a control system. *Nursing Management.* 16:9, 1986

Calafee B. Understaffing: Do you know the risks? *Nursing Life.* 25, November/December 1987

Courtemanche J. "Gearing up" for an automated nurse scheduling system in a decentralized setting. *Computers in Nursing.* 4:2, 61, 1986

Giovanetti P. Staffing methods—Implications for quality. In: Willis LD, Linwood MI. *Recent Advances in Nursing—Measuring the Quality of Care.* pp. 123–149, New York, Churchill Livingstone, 1984

Glandon BL, Colbert KW, Thomasma M. Nursing delivery models and RN mix: Cost implications. *Nursing Management.* 20:5, 30, 1989

Hanson R. *Management Systems for Nursing Service Staffing.* Rockville, MD, Aspen Systems Publishing, 1983a

Hanson R. *Managing Human Resources: New Measures at Productivity.* Paper presented at the Nurse Educator/Journal of Nursing Administrating Conference, Chicago, 1983b

Hoffman F. *Nursing Productivity Assessment and Costing Out Nursing Services.* New York: JB Lippincott Co, 1988

Ledwidge L. Expanded utilization of the patient classification system. In: Scherubel JC, Shaffer FA. *Patients and Purse Strings,* 2nd ed. New York, National League for Nursing, 1988:150

Nutt PC. *Evaluation Concepts and Methods: Shaping Policy for the Health Administrator,* rev. ed. New York, Spectrum Publications Medical and Scientific Books, 1982

Panyan S, McGregor M. How to implement a proactive incentive plan: A field study. *Personnel Journal.* 55:460, 1976

Reinert P, Grant DR. A classification system to meet today's needs. *Journal of Nursing Administration.* 1:21, 1981

Reitz JA. Toward a comprehensive nursing intensity index: Part II testing. *Nursing Management.* 16:9, 1985

Roberts M, Minnick A, Ginzbert E, Curran C. *What to Do about the Nursing Shortage.* New York, The Commonwealth Fund, 1989

Rutkowski B. *Managing for Productivity in Nursing.* Rockville, MD, Aspen Systems Publishing, 1987

Scholtzhauer D, Rosse J. A five-year study of positive incentive absence control program. *Personnel Psychology.* 38:575, 1985

Shukla R. The theory of support systems and nursing performance. In: *Human Resource Management Handbook.* Chapter 5. EM Lewis & JC Spicer, eds, Rockville, MD: Aspen, 1987

Taunton RL, Krampitz SD, Woods CQ. Absenteeism—retention links. *Journal of Nursing Administration.* 19:6, 13, 1989

Statistical Abstracts of the United States, 10th ed. Washington, DC, US Government Printing Office, 1989

US Department of Health and Human Services. *Seventh Report to the President and Congress in the Status of Health Personnel.* DHHS Pub. No. HRS-P-OD-90-1. Washington, DC, US Government Printing Office, 1990

CHAPTER 23

Control Systems and Quality Assurance

Dennis Dossett
Carolyn H. Smeltzer

Key Concept List

Motivation theories
Control systems
Standards of quality assurance
Quality assurance program
Risk management

Organizational control ensures that planned activities produce desired results (Woodward, 1970). Since accomplishing planned activities in organizations requires that someone actually *does* something, we are faced immediately with the problem of motivation. Motivation theories provide different perspectives on the answers to two questions: (1) Why do people do what they do? (2) How do we influence that behavior in the future? The second question, of course, is a primary concern of organizational control systems. A brief review of the major approaches to motivation and their implications for organizational control systems is provided. Figure 23–1 presents an overall model of motivation (Dossett, 1992) which shows how the various theories are related.

There are two basic categories of motivation theories: (1) *content* theories which attempt to answer *what* motivates people. They share the basic notion that people have needs for certain things and that fulfilling these needs is the essence of motivation; and (2) *process* theories which approach the problem from the standpoint of *how* people are motivated.

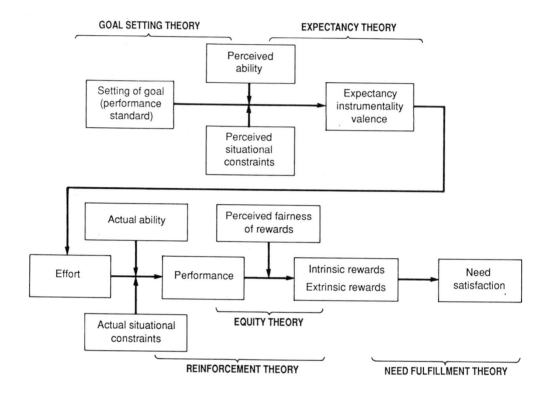

GOAL SETTING THEORY   EXPECTANCY THEORY

Figure 23-1. Integrated Model of the Motivational Process *(Dossett DL. Motivating Staff. In: Sullivan EJ, Decker PJ, eds.* Effective Management in Nursing, *(3rd ed.) Menlo Park, CA, Addison-Wesley, 1992. Reprinted by permission of Addison-Wesley)*

CONTENT THEORIES

The idea that motivation is instinctive dates from the late 1800s. By the 1920s, the list of specific "instincts" presumed to cause human behavior had grown to several hundred. Consequently, this general idea was replaced by a new class of motivation theories called *need theories*. Like instincts, the seemingly endless list of human needs led Maslow to develop a limited need hierarchy (Maslow, 1943, 1954). Some needs are more important than others and always take precedence in motivating and directing behavior. Thus, *physiological needs* (eg, hunger, thirst) took precedence over (bodily) *safety needs* which were considered more important than *belongingness or social needs* (eg, friendship, affection, love). These needs took precedence over *esteem needs* (appreciation, recognition, self-respect) and *self-actualization* (developing one's maximum potential). Behavior is directed to the satisfaction of lower-order needs before motivation to satisfy higher-order needs begins.

The concept of need categories and hierarchical relationships has gained little research support (Lawler & Suttle, 1972; Wahba & Bridwell, 1973); yet Maslow's theory was the first to clearly state that higher-order needs should be an important consideration in organizational life. Alderfer (1969, 1972) collapsed Maslow's five needs into three categories: *existence* (physiological and safety), *relatedness* (social), and *growth* (esteem and self-actualization). He postulated simultaneous operation of multiple needs and that frustration of higher-order needs emphasizes importance of lower-order needs.

Herzberg's *two-factor theory* (Herzberg, Mausner, Peterson, & Capwell, 1957; Herzberg, Mausner, & Snyderman, 1959) postulates a hygiene factor comprised of lower-order need satisfiers (eg, pay, job security, supervision) and a motivating factor comprised of higher-order needs stemming from the work itself. Thus, pay and promotions are necessary in work settings, but they may not lead to high work motivation. Herzberg contends that such extrinsic rewards motivate attendance rather than performance because they are sources of job dissatisfaction, not job satisfaction. Truly motivated workers have high job satisfaction because their work is meaningful and fulfilling.

Although Herzberg's theory gained wide popular acceptance among managers, it has not enjoyed much scientific support (King, 1970). Both hygiene and motivating factors are sources of job satisfaction and job dissatisfaction. Nevertheless, Herzberg's theory is important because it identifies the work setting as a major influence on motivation.

PROCESS THEORIES

Reinforcement theory postulates that behaviors followed relatively quickly by positive consequences (positive reinforcement) tend to be repeated while negative consequences (punishment) following a behavior decrease its occurrence. Thus, behavior is learned (motivated) by the environmental consequences of the behavior. If a behavior is not reinforced, it will soon *extinguish*. Reinforcement theory places the onus for employee performance directly on the organizational control systems which monitor, measure, and respond to performance.

With reinforcement, employees learn what leads to reward; with punishment, employees "learn" not to exhibit the punished behavior while the supervisor is monitoring the situation. The latter rarely leads to permanent change in employee behavior. It also produces ill feeling and mistrust between employees and the organization, so punishment should be avoided unless continued poor performance must be stopped immediately. Punished behavior may stop, but it must also be replaced with appropriate behavior. This is accomplished with positive reinforcement.

Basing reinforcement on the frequency of desired behavior (a ratio schedule) is far more effective than interval reinforcement schedules. Furthermore, many reinforcers lose their effectiveness on continuous schedules. Praise, for example, very quickly begins to sound mechanical if it occurs every time a nurse performs some aspect of the job correctly. Thus, *partial schedules* (less than 100 percent reinforcement) are generally more effective. If there is a brief lapse in reinforcement under partial ratio schedules, the desired behavior will be maintained longer (without reinforcement) than when maintained by continuous schedules.

A major caution is in order. With a *monetary* reinforcer, employees not only prefer continuous reinforcement but perform as well as or better than when using variable ratio schedules (Pritchard, Hollenback, & DeLeo, 1980). To optimize individual performance, the choice of schedule is dependent on the choice of reinforcer. Reinforcement theory is not very helpful when it comes to selecting among reinforcers. The manager must simply try different reinforcers to see what works! If a given reinforcer no longer works, try another one until an effective reinforcer (one which changes behavior) is found.

In addition *negative* or *avoidance reinforcement* can be used. In this case, one removes an undesirable consequence in order to reinforce desired behavior.

Expectancy theory is a process theory based on *anticipated* need satisfaction (Porter & Lawler, 1968; Vroom, 1964). It assumes that people make conscious, rational choices regarding their work behavior and performance to maximize personal outcomes. This includes both maximizing rewards and minimizing punishment.

Since some outcomes are more desirable than others, expectancy theory measures their relative attractiveness or desirability as *valence* (V). Outcomes gain valence because they satisfy human needs. Even a highly desirable (or undesirable) outcome will have little influence on behavioral choice if the individual believes it unlikely that the outcome will actually occur. The perceived probability that a given outcome will occur is called an *instrumentality* (I) because the behavior is instrumental to obtaining the outcome. It is also called a $P \rightarrow O$ (performance→outcome) expectancy because it reflects the degree to which a person expects a given performance or behavior to lead to valued outcomes. Valences and instrumentalities are multiplied and summed for each behavior alternative, the individual then "choosing" the behavior which is most attractive (ie, which maximizes the person's outcomes). The formula for attractiveness is:

Behavior attractiveness = (IV) (the sum of instrumentality × valence)

A third building block of the theory is *expectancy* (E), the perceived probability that a given level of effort will produce a given level of performance. Expectancy is sometimes referred to as $E \rightarrow P$ (effort→performance) because it represents the perceived linkage between effort and performance. Adding this component to (IV), the theory assumes that individual's consciously choose the amount of effort they will expend based on the outcome maximization principle. The expectancy for each possible effort level (there are usually several) is multiplied by the attractiveness of each performance level and summed as follows:

$$\text{Effort level attractiveness} = [E \times \Sigma\,(IV)]$$
$$[\text{expectancy} \times \text{the sum of the product of (instrumentality} \times \text{valence)]}$$

The level of effort with the highest attractiveness will then be chosen.

Although expectancy theory seems complex, the fundamental idea is simple and very powerful. If one considers the effort equation in simplified form

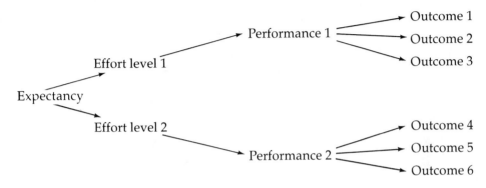

So, Effort $= (E{\to}P) \times \Sigma[(P{\to}O)(V)]$ for each effort level.

People choose to work hard if they think they can attain a performance goal which leads to valued outcomes.

Adams *process theory* (1963; 1965) deals with psychological equity, or perceived fairness in the ratio of organizational outcomes (eg, pay, status) to personal inputs (eg, effort, experience). This perceived ratio is compared to a similar ratio for a comparison person or co-worker. This theory has been included in later versions of expectancy theory (see Fig 23-1). Perceptions of unfair treatment destroy perceptions that rewards and punishers are linked to employee behavior (instrumentality). *Perceived reality* (versus objective reality) directs an individual's choice of behavior.

Goal-setting theory is one of the most practical and effective perspectives on human motivation available to managers. The theory posits that specific goals (ie, conscious intentions) produce higher performance than general goals such as "Do your best" (Locke, Shaw, Saari, & Latham, 1982).

Second, specific, difficult goals lead to higher performance than specific, easy goals. The higher the goal the higher the performance, provided the goal is accepted. Goals should be difficult, but seen as attainable (high expectancy) in order to produce high motivation and performance.

The third tenet of goal-setting theory is that goals mediate (literally, operate between) incentives and performance. In diagram form:

$$\text{Incentives} \to \text{Goals} \to \text{Performance}$$

Without specific, difficult goals, the chain of cause and effect between incentives and performance is broken. Except for very large sums of money, goals indeed appear to to mediate incentives and performance (Locke et al, 1982). Even with large monetary amounts, the influence of specific, difficult goals appears to be far more important than a monetary bonus (Latham, Mitchell, & Dossett, 1978).

The implication of goal-setting theory for practice are: (1) specific, difficult performance goals are the immediate precursors of high motivation and performance; and (2) incentives have little or no influence on performance independent of a person's conscious intention (goal).

CONTROL SYSTEMS

Control systems exist to ensure that planned activities produce desired results. Smaller, simpler organizations typically have fewer and less formal control systems while larger, more complex organizations depend upon a number of formal control systems. Without control systems of some type, organization would be impossible.

Organizations exist for the purpose of attaining goals which cannot be accomplished by individuals alone or which cannot be accomplished as effectively or efficiently by individuals. Collective goals require organizations, and organizations require control systems to ensure collective goal attainment.

Organizational control systems are used to ensure organizational goal attainment by organizations and by the individuals who comprise them. These involve both human systems (ie, supervision, management) and structural systems (eg, personnel policies, accounting procedures, quality control).

Function of Control Systems

Control systems are designed to organize and direct organizational functions. For example, some systems focus on organizational processes (eg, performance appraisal, accounting) while others specify particular content (eg, performance rating format, requisition/order forms). Thus, control systems are designed to perform different functions or to serve different purposes in an organization.

Some control systems are overtly coercive in nature. For example, policies which specify penalties for infractions of rules or procedures are designed to provide a deterrent against violation as well as punishment for offenders. A graduated disciplinary policy specifying successively more harsh penalties for continued infractions (eg, verbal warning followed in order by a written warning, suspension, and dismissal) is one example. Other control systems are neutral and serve such utilitarian purposes as proving an orderly, equitable basis for compensation (eg, job evaluation systems, systems for vesting or other perquisites based on tenure or job level). Still other systems provide positive reinforcement (eg, employee-of-the-month or other public recognition programs) or influence behavior through normative pressure (eg, organization culture, formal socialization practices).

Anatomy of a Control System

Control systems are analogous to the thermostat that controls a furnace (McKelvey, 1970). Such an analogy describes the major functions present in all useful control systems. A thermostatic control systems contains (1) an adjustable device which sets a *standard* (the desired temperature); (2) a *sensor* which measures the temperature of the room, (3) a *discriminator* compares the desired temperature (goal) with the actual temperature (performance); next, (4) an *effector* responds to the signal from the discriminator and turns the furnace on or off as necessary; (5) *communication* among system components; (6) the *activity* itself (furnace) is provided by electrical wires. Finally, the activity is powered by a source of (7) *energy*. Figure 23–2 illustrates these components in terms of a typical (supervisory) organizational control system.

Standards and Goals. No control system is possible without clear explication of organizational goals and the standards of performance used to evaluate progress toward goal attainment. Without clear goals, any effort toward goal attainment will lack guidance in both direction and amount.

Task Behavior and Output. Unless there is some identifiable outcome (either behavior or results) to measure performance, it is impossible to identify what has been accomplished.

Sensing Mechanisms. The sensing mechanism in organizational control systems is the administrator charged with supervising employees and their work activities. The actual comparative mechanism may be informal (supervisory impressions) or formal (eg, annual performance evaluation based on organizationally prescribed measurement criteria). Performance measurement is covered in more detail in Chapter 13.

Other sensing mechanisms also may be used to compare performance with goals

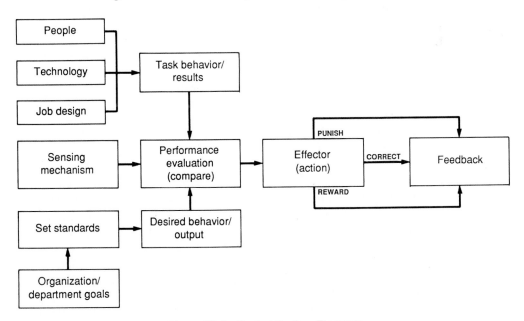

Figure 23–2. Control System Elements

or standards (eg, quality control, budgetary processes). These ''other'' mechanisms generally provide feedback to the manager responsible for an employee's performance evaluation.

Effectuating. Goal/performance comparisons are a primary managerial responsibility. They may be relatively automated by prescribed policies and procedures or much less formal, entailing greater managerial discretion. In general, penalties are more likely to be prescribed by organizational policies and procedures while allowable rewards are more likely to be influenced by managerial discretion.

Methods of Communication. Communication in a control system involves feedback. Feedback is necessary for goals to affect performance (Erez, 1977), especially over an extended period of time. For example, in the analogy of a thermostatic control system, the standards are produced by management. Unless individuals are given feedback regarding the degree to which current objectives have been attained, it will be impossible to set realistic and meaningful goals for the future. Similarly, unless the employee receives detailed feedback regarding behavior or results, it is difficult to adjust behavior to desired performance.

Types of Control Systems

There are many different types of control systems in organizations. Budgets and accounting mechanisms are financial control systems. Frequently, management information systems are used to track performance relative to defined organizational goals or standards. Formal policies, procedures, and rules may be automatically invoked when the control system indicates performance departing from standards. For example, a specified number of incidences of lateness may automatically result in a reprimand. Assuming a performance goal has been set (through task assignment or Management By Objectives system), a nurse manager (discriminator) compares the performance rating (sensor) of a nurse with the performance goal (standard) and either rewards or punishes (effector) the nurse. Performance feedback (communication) is provided to the nurse and a new performance goal (adjustable standard) is set for the next performance cycle.

Organizational policies, procedures, and rules also serve as control mechanisms as they set the standards against which employee performance is judged. The discriminator in this case may be the employee or a co-worker rather than a supervisor. Policies, procedures, and rules may also serve as effectors by indicating what action should be taken in response to employee behavior or performance. Similarly, organizations roles (eg, job descriptions, task assignments) and structure (eg, functional and liaison responsibilities) prescribe appropriate job-related activities.

Other formal control systems include socialization, mentoring, and sponsoring programs. Socialization may include formal training and orientation activities which convey expected behavior or performance standards (professionalism). Similarly, formal mentoring (eg, preceptors) or sponsorship activities (eg, inservice training, professional conferences) provide training in expected behaviors and may provide both social and tangible reinforcement for their enactment.

Not all control systems are organizationally or formally defined. The informal influences of social mores and group norms prescribe expected employee behaviors and frequently prescribe the social sanctions for violation.

Tying Control Systems to Reward Systems

Control systems specify both desired behaviors and performance levels. Extrinsic reward systems encourage people to engage in appropriate organizational behavior, especially when they probably would not exhibit such behavior on their own. Most people, for example, perform organizationally specified tasks in order to receive a paycheck. Thus, reward systems motivate people to engage in the behaviors specified by organizational control systems.

One potential disadvantage of tying control systems to extrinsic rewards is the potential *decrease* in intrinsic motivation, the motivation derived from interest and pleasure in the activity of performing the task itself (Deci, 1975). People stop performing the task because they like it; rather they do it for the extrinsic reward. This is not necessarily undesirable in that it potentially places more control over task motivation at the disposal of the organization. In addition, most jobs (even intrinsically interesting jobs) have some aspects which are neither desirable nor interesting. Caring for patients may be intrinsically rewarding, but it may also requires emptying bed pans! External influences on motivation through organizational control systems is clearly desirable and needed in most cases.

The basic principles for tying control systems to rewards are clearly specified by expectancy, reinforcement, and equity theories of motivation. Expectancy theory tells us that the valence of an outcome must be relatively large and (for a reward) positive. That is, unless people regard the reward as attractive (in both quality and quantity), it will not motivate behavior. Similarly, unless people believe their behavior is instrumental to obtaining rewards, one cannot expect those rewards to motivate desired organizational behavior. Reinforcement theory explains the same principle as follows: Unless rewards are made contingent on desired organizational behaviors, positive reinforcement of those behaviors will not occur. Finally, unless the rewards and the manner in which they are distributed is seen as equitable or fair, neither valence nor instrumentality perceptions will be high.

Dysfunctions of Control Systems

Bureaucratic Behavior. Control systems can result in rigid employee behavior which is dysfunctional with respect to organizational goals (Blau, 1955). This occurs when people behave in ways which make them "look good" on control system performance measures. The primary problem in such instances is that the performance criteria are deficient, contaminated, or both. Another manifestation of this problem is selective attention to standards of performance. Performance which is reinforced will tend to be repeated while nonreinforced behaviors will be extinguished or disappear. If the control system measure is not valid, bureaucratic behavior will result.

Other factors involved in bureaucratic behavior involve performance standards that are too high, especially when there is little or no involvement by the people expected to meet them. Unless employees see goals as attainable, they will simply "play it safe" by reacting in stereotypic (bureaucratic) ways which focus the blame for substandard performance on persons or entities other than themselves (eg, "That's not *my* job!"). Only a combination of valid performance criteria and realistic performance expectations based on factors over which employees have a considerable degree of control (including goal levels) will minimize bureaucratic behaviors when rewards are tied to control systems.

Provision of Invalid Data. Invalid data are frequently provided as input into control systems when the individuals being evaluated provide the data themselves. This takes two forms: (a) data regarding what is possible or realistic (planning criteria, especially budgets) and (b) data regarding what has actually been accomplished (especially when performance has been relatively poor). Contamination and lack of objectivity are probable when relying solely on self-report data. This is especially true when employees have a low level of trust in the organization (Mellinger, 1956). Invalid data are most likely to be provided (a) for the most important control system criteria; (b) when the data are subjective; and (c) when employees have little influence on performance standards.

Resistance. Control systems often meet with fierce resistance by employees, primarily as a response to perceived threat over loss of control. For example, control systems can automate expertise, bypassing the individual's ability to control what information is provided, how much, and to whom. Even if the data were always valid in the past, the loss of control over that data is regarded as a threat to the individual's professionalism. Similarly, control systems can create "new" expertise by handing an individual's control to someone else (eg, those who staff management informations systems). Of course, control systems can potentially measure performance more accurately, but one must be especially careful to ensure that "accuracy" in this means "relevant and objective" rather than only an increase in precision (eg, the number of decimal points).

Desire for Control Systems: Why Do People Want Control?

There are a number of personal reasons why people actually *want* control systems in organizations. First, well-designed control systems structure tasks and minimize sources of role ambiguity and role conflict. Uncertainty regarding what is to be done, how it is to be done, how the end product will be evaluated, and whether rewards really are contingent on job performance are common sources of stress in the workplace. Such stress not only decreases satisfaction but also undermines motivation and can (when severe) contribute to acute or chronic health problems.

A second reason why individuals often want control systems is to obtain feedback on performance. This is particularly important when the job itself provides little meaningful feedback. This may occur because of the lack of feedback channels from the work itself, because of isolation from social channels (eg, co-workers, clients, supervisor) or because of lengthy delays in the feedback process (eg, annual performance reviews). In addition, some tasks are performed in group settings where individual performance either is difficult to identify or is difficult to measure on an absolute scale. In these situations, a well-designed control system can provide comparative feedback on performance relative to other group members.

Finally, most people prefer rewards based on performance. Not only can such rewards provide a sense of satisfaction and competency, but the built-in contingency can give people a sense of control over their personal outcomes. Thus, contingent rewards can increase employee perceptions of empowerment. Of course, this is not possible if employees do not trust the organization to administer either control systems or reward systems equitably, or if they believe performance measures are invalid.

Designing Effective Control Systems

Behavior versus Output. A primary decision in designing control systems is whether to measure behavior or output. Many problems in implementing and operating control systems stem from this either/or mentality. Organizations are obviously concerned with output. It is inconceivable that boards of directors or administrators would be satisfied with "average" employee performance ratings as a measure of organizational effectiveness.

On the other hand, output measures are contaminated by a host of factors over which employees have little or no control. Employees contribute but one thing to organizations, their behavior. What they *do* on the job reflects *all* of their ability, motivation, and problem-solving activity in dealing with an unpredictable or uncertain performance environment. Thus, behavior is the least contaminated measure of employee performance possible. If performance measures focus clearly on behaviors *necessary* to attaining organizational goals, those measures (by definition) will not be deficient.

Different control systems serve different purposes (eg, financial performance for boards of directors and stockholders, performance feedback for employees) and may provide a logical choice between output and behavior. However, a nurse who performs technical tasks accurately but whose interpersonal interactions with patients is consistently poor is clearly a substandard performer (except in surgery). Similarly, a nursing supervisor whose unit exceeds all professional standards (output) but whose leadership style (behavior) produces staff turnover rates of 80 percent per year has a definite performance problem. Compare this nursing supervisor with a peer in another setting where staff performance is equally excellent, turnover is 80 percent per year due to low wages and poor working conditions, but the supervisor's leadership behavior keeps performance high and the turnover rate from going even higher! Clearly, focusing either on behavior alone or on output alone does not present the full picture of employee performance.

In short, there are many instances in which *both* output and behavior are legitimate and important control system data. The key problem is how to combine these data into an overall assessment of performance. The best answer to this problem is an a priori, mutually agreed on weighting system uniformly and impartially applied to all employees with the same job.

Influence of Uncertainty. The greater the reliance on output measures, the greater the employees' uncertainty because of their inability to control or influence the *measure* of performance through their own behavior. Consequently, one should expect an increase in "game-playing," bureaucratic behavior, and so on as uncertainty increases. When output measures of performance must be used, they should be used in conjunction with behavioral measures and should be weighted proportionately less as uncertainty increases.

Costs. Everything one does in an organization has a cost. The key to effective management is making wise "purchases" so that the benefits outweigh the costs. Control system costs include not only monetary and other material resources but also the human costs of time and cooperation. Unless a control system is built with the human costs constantly in mind (especially with an eye toward purchasing greater individual security, equity, and control), employees will respond by resisting the control system. The dysfunctions characteristic of poorly designed control systems can then be expected.

Influence of Professionalism. Professional employees present both unique opportunities and unique problems for control systems. Professionals have both explicit and implicit standards of behavior and performance which often exert tremendous influence on individual employee behavior. Usually, such professional standards are highly desirable because they provide strong pressures toward positive behaviors, at least according to the profession. On occasion, however, professional standards may conflict with organizational goals and expectations. For example, a hospital administrator might severely punish a nurse who publicly discloses evidence of improper contaminated waste disposal (ie, a "whistle-blower"). In short, "problems" with professional staff may indicate problems between organizational and professional standards than inappropriate employee behavior.

Control of Individuals versus Groups. Control systems should focus clearly on influencing either group performance or individual performance. When goals, measurement procedures, and performance consequences designed for groups are applied to individuals, employees perceive a loss of control over both their own behavior and their own outcomes. Consequently, motivation suffers and the dysfunctional aspects of control systems are likely to occur. Similarly, group performance is rarely the simple sum of individual efforts. Basing group-level control on individual goals and performance focuses individual efforts on related but *different* factors necessary for high group performance. This may occur because only some individual tasks contribute to overall group performance or because individual performance is dependent on other group members.

Number of Control Systems. Simplicity and efficiency argue for a single control system, but effectiveness does not. Expecting a single control system to meet all organizational needs is both unrealistic and naive. For example, performance ratings made for coaching and feedback purposes are quite different from performance ratings used to determine salary levels; other examples also abound (Bernardin & Beatty, 1984). Similarly, goal difficulty levels for planning purposes and for intrinsic motivation should be different from those used to maximize extrinsic motivation (Lawler, 1976). Thus, control systems should be tailored to specific purposes and should be carefully reviewed to avoid separate control systems requiring conflicting employee behaviors.

Substitutes for Formal Control. The notion of a substitute for formal control systems is appealing but misleading. The real issue is how well a given control system is integrated with other, relevant systems and the degree to which those systems systematically (formally) optimize organizational control or whether they allow unsystematic (informal) influences to determine the effectiveness of the primary control system. For example, selection, placement, and promotion systems range from highly formalized to haphazard, their utility largely determined by the degree of systematization and formality. "Professionalism" is really an adjunct to formal control systems. The key is to integrate their positive influences on employee behavior and minimize conflicts between professional and organizational criteria.

Even the notion of intrinsic motivation as something which "happens or not" and as beyond the ability of the formal organization to influence is a fallacious and (managerially) irresponsible position. Jobs *can* be designed to facilitate both intrinsic motivation and satisfaction (Griffin, 1982). Whose responsibility is the design of jobs if not that of the formal organization? Some may choose to say that job design "substitutes" for formal control systems, but the fact is that well-designed jobs constitute a very conscious effort to control both employee and organizational outcomes. In short, reliance on "substitutes" for formal control systems reasonably could be viewed as an abdication of managerial responsibilities.

QUALITY ASSURANCE: AN EXAMPLE

Quality assurance within a nursing department can be a scientific method to augment professional judgments when evaluating nursing care, developing or revising policies, developing guidelines for nursing care and generating knowledge for future nursing practice. It is a control system nonetheless.

The process of systematically analyzing health care is not new; quality assurance dates back to Florence Nightingale. She advocated that all nursing care be evaluated. During the Crimean War, she reported statistics comparing the mortality of civilian and British soldiers before and after changes in nursing practice. At one site, based on changes in practice, Nightingale measured a 2% decrease in mortality (Nutting & Dock, 1907). Her work was supported widely by the government and by relating new practices with rates of mortality; she was instrumental in determining the importance of similar health care standards and practices for both soldiers and civilians. Based on Nightingale's work, the government instituted a system for regular evaluation of health care.

Historically, in addition to nursing review, patient outcomes were also evaluated by the medical profession. Dr. Armory Grove, in the early twentieth century, studied and evaluated patient care based on a system to classify different disease processes. He developed a system to determine the needs for revisiting patients based on their classification (Bull, 1985).

Also during the twentieth century, the nursing and medical profession began evaluating their educational structure. The Flexnor Report of 1910 recommended structural changes in education. Nursing licensure and registration were recommended to protect the general public from unsafe practitioners.

Organizing, planning and evaluating health care services became a broad public concern in the late 1950s. The Joint Commission on Accreditation of Hospitals (now the JCAHO) was established in 1952 to provide standards and methods for hospital accreditation. The American Nurses Association and the National League for Nursing published manuals in 1959 which helped form standards and expectations about health care.

In the 1960s, the American Nurses Association (ANA) created a division of nursing practice whose major responsibility was to develop standards for nursing practice. These standards were designed to provide the basis for a quality assurance program. The ANA further developed a process to evaluate the quality of patient care.

Regulatory agencies developed guidelines for evaluating selected aspects of health care. The Social Security Act in 1972 mandated professional review of health care delivery through the Professional Standards Review Organization (PRSO). The purpose was to determine whether the health care offered met professional standards within an appropriate health care setting.

JCAHO, in its initial quality assurance standards, required audits of care delivered. In 1975, they increased the number of multidisciplinary audits required and nursing became a major contributor to the evaluation of documentation. Currently, JCAHO has stated that the nursing department must examine a nursing care problem quarterly, document its assessment of the problem, develop and implement a plan for correction, and evaluate the effectiveness of the action taken (Smeltzer, 1983).

Although instruments for measuring nursing care were developed particularly in the 1970s, limited data were generated and published in quality assurance studies. Some process and outcome quality assurance instruments were developed including the Slater Rating Scale of Nursing Competence; the Quality Patient Care Scale (Qual-Pacs), which measures the quality of nursing care concurrently; and the Medicus tool, which evaluates structure, process, and outcome components of nursing care, emphasizing nursing process (Smeltzer, 1988a).

JCAHO in 1988 revised its nursing quality assurance standards for nursing care. The standards state that care needs to be evaluated objectively against pre-established standards and criteria and that results need to be analyzed to determine the problem areas in nursing practice. Furthermore, a plan has to be developed to correct practice deficiencies with a method to re-evaluate the effectiveness of the corrective action.

Administrative Support

It is common knowledge that health care is in a constant state of flux with the exception of one basic principle: Quality of care needs to evaluated, maintained, or improved, while cost is maintained or decreased. Currently, the public is comprised of educated health care consumers. Patients satisfied with their care are important in attracting patients, physicians, and third-party payors to a particular health care organization. Administration now realizes that institutions have to be competitive and gain "market share" in order to survive while, at the same time, assuring quality. The nurse administrator is in a unique role of maintaining accountability for nursing practice and for attracting patients to the institution. A quality assurance program supported by nursing administration can be one mechanism that recognizes and accomplishes both goals.

A quality assurance program can only be effective if the nurse administrator is committed to an environment where nursing care is questioned and evaluated. The nurse administrator must provide systems that support and study nursing issues, recognize the need for change in nursing practice based on the results, and identify accountability for initiating and evaluating change (Smeltzer, 1988b).

Standards

In order to assure quality, structural process and outcomes, nursing standards must be identified and articulated. Nursing department standards are based on nursing values, research, professional standards, nursing philosophy, and institutional goals in providing patient care to a specific population. Structural standards of nursing practice encompass the setting in which care occurs, as well as conditions in which the nurse and patient interaction happens. Structural standards need to be based on the philosophy and objectives of the nursing department and profession, as well as the fiscal resources, equipment and working conditions of the nurses. Process standards concentrate on activities or behaviors of the nurse in rendering patient care. The process standards are based on the nursing process: assessment of the patient, identification of patient problems, the development of a plan of care to correct patient problems, the method of implementing the plan, and the system for determining the patient response. Outcome standards may or may not be directly related to the nursing intervention. These standards include the patient's health status, knowledge, compliance with treatment, and satisfaction. Standards of care in terms of process, structure and outcome and their interrelatedness must be determined to assure that the quality assurance program validly reflects the quality of patient care.

Designing a Quality Assurance Program Plan

Once the standards have been determined, criteria to measure the standard and a method of evaluation must be determined. Quality assurance committees should review developed quality assurance tools to determine their applicability in the institution. If a tool is not applicable, criteria or questions to indicate whether the nursing standard is being met need to be devised. The criteria must be pre-established, objective, valid, and reliable. Each statement or question used as a criterion must be clear, easy to answer with yes, no or nonapplicable, and should be specific and objective.

The effectiveness of the quality assurance program rests with the validity and reliability of the criteria. Data collection may include patient observation and/or interview, nurse observation and/or interview, and review of documentation. Data collection should require that 60 percent of the data be collected on days, and 40 percent on evening and weekends. Ten percent of the patients should be evaluated monthly.

Collection of Data

The criteria will help determine who collects the data. This depends on the availability of resources, cost, and credibility of the individuals doing the data collection. For quality monitoring, a staff member should possess a comprehensive knowledge of nursing; demonstrate clinical expertise; feel comfortable on the nursing units being evaluated; be interested and committed to nursing; demonstrate good interpersonal skills; be comfortable interviewing patients and nurses; and understand quality assurance (Smeltzer, 1988a).

Interpretation, Follow up and Reporting Mechanism

Guidelines for interpretation of the quality assurance data must be well-defined through policies, procedures, and organizational charts. These guidelines must be evaluated continually for effectiveness. Nursing administration must make a clear statement about who is responsible for receiving and analyzing quality assurance information and making recommendations for changes. At what level in the organization does the analysis take place? To whom do the data analyzers report their analyses and recommendations? Staff nurses should know who reviews the evaluation of their care. If administration does not delineate these functions, there is less chance for the program to be effective.

Nurses must interpret data critically. Choosing an effective course of action to correct problems depends on the results of the analysis. Actions should be chosen to improve patient care, not punish the nursing staff. Action may include offering continuing education or inservices, changing head nurse management style, changing chart forms, changing nursing support systems, as well as continuing to determine the source of the problems. Appropriate action must be chosen and implemented. If this does not occur, the quality assurance program will not be effective. That is, this standard needs to be re-evaluated after the change has occurred to determine whether the standard has been met.

Evaluating Effectiveness of Quality Assurance

A quality assurance program can benefit the nursing profession if the concepts of the program are understood, operationalized appropriately, and evaluated. The quality assurance program provides a systematic method of evaluating nursing practice. Some criteria that must be met to have a successful quality assurance program are:

- Quality assurance must be a priority in the institution.
- Those responsible must implement the program, not just use it as a tool for data collection.
- Roles and responsibilities for implementing quality assurance must be delineated.
- The staff needs to be adequately educated about the intent and uses of quality assurance.

- Nurses must be informed about the quality assurance process and the results.
- Data collectors must be adequately oriented.
- Quality assurance data must be reliable and valid.
- Quality assurance data should be analyzed and used for nursing decisions and reflected in committee meeting minutes.
- Quality assurance programs need to be evaluated continually for effectiveness (Smeltzer, 1988a).

Criteria for a successful quality assurance program are:

1. Quality assurance must be a priority.
2. Appropriate standards and criteria that are measurable, reliable, and valid must be developed.
3. Those responsible should implement a program, not just collect data.
4. Roles and responsibilities should be delineated for accountability in terms of quality assurance.
5. Nurses are to be informed about the process and the results of the program.
6. Quality data must be analyzed and used by all nursing personnel for decisions concerning patient care, when appropriate.
7. Strategies for change must be utilized in implementing quality assurance.
8. Quality assurance activities should be evaluated for effectiveness in changing nursing practice process to improve patient care.

Risk Management

Risk management is one aspect of a quality assurance program (see Chapter 21). It is a process established to determine where the liability risks are in the organization. This includes hospital employees, visitors, and patients. The program includes a system to identify risk, control the risk, and reduce or prevent future safety issues and loss to the institution.

A risk management program includes control and knowledge of professional liabilities, recognizing environmental issues, safety issues, security measures, infection control, and identification of potential safety or financial risks that may occur while providing patient care.

A risk management program includes the evaluation, treatment, and financing of present or future loss while trying to control the possibility for loss. A successful risk management program identifies and analyzes risk, but also develops an environment to prevent risk to patients as well as employees. A risk management program, even though financially driven, has the purpose of patient welfare and is an integral aspect of improving the quality of patient care (Colp, Boemaeret, & Miller, 1985).

Quality Assurance and Research

Nursing research and quality assurance programs are both systems and methods that can change nursing practice. The steps in research and quality assurance appear similar, but differences exist (see Chapter 27). Both nursing quality assurance and nursing research can broadly be defined as the systematic testing or evaluation of nursing practice to generate data enabling nurses to make informed decisions concerning nursing practice and ultimately to improve patient care.

Quality assurance can be defined as setting standards of care, developing a system for evaluating the standards, assessing the standards, analyzing the assessment, and improving or changing nursing practice based on the analysis. The research process can be defined as a systematic method for gaining new knowledge that can be verified and generalized beyond the study sample. The purpose of the research process is to verify or provide new knowledge to expand or revise existing theories and develop new theories.

> The major differences that exist between the quality assurance and research process basically concern the purpose of the studies and how the study results are utilized. The purpose of a quality assurance program is to assure the public that a system for evaluating and correcting nursing care problems is in place. The purpose of research is to answer a question in order to add to knowledge. The results from a quality assurance program are used to give direct patient care modification, while results from the research process may be used to correlate variables or develop a casual link between variables which might ultimately contribute to theory development. Finally, results from a quality assurance study might be patient population-specific or hospital-specific, while results from research should be generalizable (Smeltzer, 1988a, p 212).

Computerization and Quality Assurance

Computerization can decrease time-consuming tasks involved with quality assurance. Several questions determine the effectiveness of a computer in a quality assurance program. These include:

1. Relevance and use of present forms
2. Information flow of data
3. Potential for the data to be automated
4. Type of storage necessary
5. Format of the data for effectiveness of interpretation
6. Data to be inputted
7. Accountabilities for inputting reliable data
8. Commitment for data to be manipulated for statistical purposes
9. Mechanism to report results that can be understood

Computerization is one mechanism that decreases the time commitment in certain aspects of quality assurance (Wilbert, 1985), facilitates processing data and produces information in a meaningful manner (Wilbert, 1985, p 236).

SUMMARY

Content theories maintain need satisfaction is the basis of human motivation. Reinforcement theory emphasizes the consequences of behavior in both decreasing undesirable behaviors and increasing desirable behaviors. Expectancy theory posits the anticipated value of rewards and punishers and their perceived linkage to future performance in conscious choices of both behaviors and performance levels. Equity theory adds the perceived fairness of rewards and punishers relative to perceived employee input variables. Goal-setting theory posits a person's conscious intentions as the immediate determinants of behavior and performance.

Organizational control systems designed on the basis of well-established principles of human motivation are necessary to effective and efficient organizational functioning. Such systems not only influence employee behavior and performance, they can also contribute to the quality of organizational life through enhancement of individual satisfaction and perceptions of control over personal outcomes. Control systems which are not carefully designed around effective principles of employee motivation lead to dysfunctional employee behavior and to decreased satisfaction and trust in the organization.

A quality assurance program provides nursing with a systematic method of evaluating nursing practice. Quality assurance programs can only be instituted and integrated into a nursing department as effectively as the manager believes in the system, assumes accountability, and are motivated to change behavior to improve care. Motivational theories and control systems, therefore, need to be addressed in detail.

REFERENCES

Adams JS. Toward an understanding of inequity. *Journal of Abnormal and Social Psychology*. 67: 422, 1963

Adams JS. Injustice in social exchange. In: Berkowitz L, ed. *Advances in Experimental Social Psychology*, vol 2. New York, Academic Press, 1965:267–299

Alderfer CP. An empirical test of a new theory of human needs. *Organizational Behavior and Human Performance* 4:142, 1969

Alderfer CP. *Existence, Relatedness, and Growth: Human Needs in Organizational Settings*. New York: The Free Press, 1972

Bernardin HJ, Beatty RW. *Performance Appraisal: Assessing Human Behavior at Work*. Boston, Kent, 1984

Blau PM. *The dynamics of bureaucracy*. Chicago, University of Chicago Press, 1955

Bull M. Quality assurance: Its origin, transformation and prospects. In: Meisenheimer CS, ed. *Quality Assurance*. Rockville, MD, Aspen, 1985:3

Culp B, Goermaire N, Miller, E. Risk management: An integral part of quality assurance. In: Meisenheimer CS, ed. *Quality Assurance*. Rockville, MD, Aspen, 1985:169

Deci EL. *Intrinsic Motivation*. New York, Plenum, 1975

Dossett DL. Motivating staff. In Sullivan EJ, Decker PJ, eds. *Effective Management in Nursing*, 3rd ed. Menlo Park, CA, Addison-Wesley, 1992:179–208

Dossett DL. Dimensional characteristics of behaviorally based performance ratings. *The Journal of Management Systems*. 1:51, 1989

Erez M. Feedback: A necessary condition for the goal setting-performance relationship. *Journal of Applied Psychology*. 62:624, 1977

Griffin RW. *Task Design: An Integrative Approach*. Glenview, IL, Scott, Foresman, 1982

Herzberg F, Mausner B, Peterson RO, Capwell DF. *Job Attitudes: A Review of Research and Opinion*. Pittsburgh: Psychological Service of Pittsburgh, 1957

Herzberg F, Mausner B, Snyderman BS. *The Motivation to Work*. New York, Wiley, 1959

King NA. A clarification and evaluation of the two-factor theory of job satisfaction. *Psychological Bulletin*. 74:18, 1970

Latham GP, Mitchell TR, Dossett DL. The importance of participative goal setting and anticipated rewards on goal difficulty and job performance. *Journal of Applied Psychology*. 63:163, 1978

Lawler EE. Control systems in organizations. In: Dunnette ME, ed. *Handbook of Industrial/Organizational Psychology*. New York: Rand McNally, 1976

Lawler EE, Suttle JL. A casual correlational test of the need hierarchy concept. *Organizational Behavior and Human Performance*. 7:265, 1972

Locke EA, Shaw KN, Saari LM, Latham GP. Goal-setting and task performance: 1969–1980. *Psychological Bulletin*. 90:125, 1982

Maslow AH. A theory of human motivation. *Psychological Review*. 50:370, 1943

Maslow AH. *Motivation and Personality*. New York, Harper, 1954

McKelvey WW. *Toward a Holistic Morphology of Organizations*. Santa Monica, CA, Rand Corporation, 1970

Mellinger GD. Interpersonal trust as a factor in communication. *Journal of Abnormal and Social Psychology*. 52:304, 1956

Nutting M, Dock L. *A History of Nursing*. New York, Putnam, 1907:142

Porter LW, Lawler EE. *Managerial attitudes and performance*. Homewood, IL, Irwin-Dorsey, 1968

Pritchard R, Hollenback J, DeLeo P. The effects of continuous and partial schedules of reinforcement on effort, performance, and satisfaction. *Organizational Behavior and Human Performance*. 25:336, 1980

Smeltzer CH. Organizing the search for excellence. *Nursing Management*. 19, 1983

Smeltzer CH. Evaluating a successful quality assurance program: The process. *Journal of Nursing Quality Assurance*. 2(4) 1, 1988a

Smeltzer CH. Quality assurance and the evaluation research process. In: Stull MK, Pinkerton S, eds. *Current Strategies for Nursing Administrators*. Rockville, MD, Aspen, 1988b:205

Vroom VH. *Work and Motivation*. New York, Wiley, 1964

Wahba MA, Bridwell LG. Maslow reconsidered: A review of research on the need hierarchy theory. *Proceedings of the Academy of Management*. 514, 1973

Wilbert C. Computers: Quality assurance application. In: Meisenheimer CS, ed. *Quality Assurance*. Rockville, MD, Aspen, 1985:207–239

Woodward J, ed. *Industrial Organization: Behavior and Control*. London, Oxford University Press, 1970

CHAPTER 24

Conflict Management

Marlene K. Strader

Key Concept List

Interpersonal and organizational conflict
Antecedents and consequences of conflict
Interdependence
Differentiation
Conflict management

Conflict is an inevitable outcome in social interaction. Organizational interfaces bring together individuals with the potential for compatible as well as incompatible behavior. Conflict can range from a simple misunderstanding between people about the time of a meeting to a battle between physicians and hospital administrators over the purchase of new equipment. Long-term conflict becomes a source of increased stress and decreased productivity for managers and employees and almost always ends up affecting quality of service. Managers spend 25 to 60 percent of a working day dealing with conflict (Robey, 1986). If we use a conservative 25 percent estimate to calculate time spent in conflict resolution, a head nurse earning $40,000 per year will have an annual conflict cost of $10,000. Thus a hospital with 100 head nurses spends $1 million annually on management time alone. Staff nurses' time, increased turnover, recruitment, orientation, and closed beds must also be considered to arrive at actual conflict cost. It is in an institution's best interest to resolve conflict in the quickest manner possible and with the best possible outcome for the institution. If ignored or denied, conflict will fester and become more serious. Nurse administrators must actively manage conflict by maintaining and strengthening cooperative links between individuals or groups with divergent interests.

DEFINING CONFLICT

Deutsch suggests, "conflict exists whenever incompatible behavior occurs" (Deutsch, 1973, p. 10). A conflict is potential to the extent that incompatible behavior is likely to occur. Incompatible behavior refers to individual acts intended to oppose or frustrate another person. Incompatible behavior has many levels ranging from passive lack of support, explicit disagreement and sabotage, to violence in open battle.

Conflict Development

Over the years many attempts have been made to describe conflict development. It has been described on the basis of its sources and levels (context) or on the underlying forces of perceived and experienced realities which lead to subsequent conflict behavior (process). In this chapter an integrated context/process model will be used describing conflict on the basis of antecedent conditions, various levels from which it arises, contributing cognitive processes, subsequent behavior and, lastly, consequences that occur (Fig 24–1).

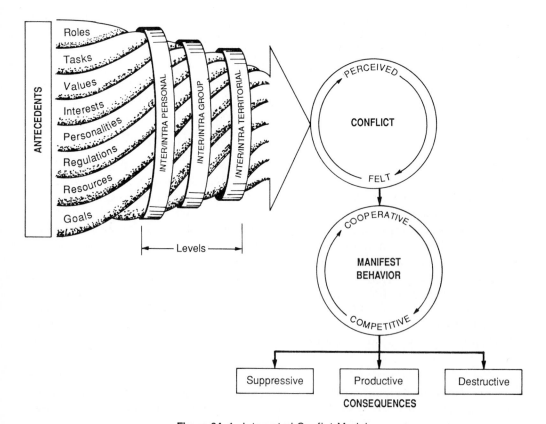

Figure 24–1. Integrated Conflict Model

Antecedents

Conflict may develop from a number of antecedents sources such as role ambiguity, values, interest, or goals. To understand the nature and implications of conflict more clearly it is appropriate to describe conflict on the basis of the following antecedent sources:

1. *Conflict of goals* develops when the desired outcome of socially interactive individuals is incompatible. It may involve divergent preferences in all decision outcomes, presenting a no-win situation for all.
2. *Conflict in distribution of resources* develops when resources are scarce and individuals have high expectations of rewards.
3. *Conflict of regulations* develops when some individuals have high needs for autonomy and self control while others have high needs for regulating mechanisms.
4. *Conflict of personality* develops when traits, attitudes or behaviors of one individual are not acceptable to another individual.
5. *Conflict of interest* develops when there is discrepancy between individuals' preferences for recognized and unrecognized outcomes that are affected by the interaction of individuals.
6. *Conflict of values* develops when socially interactive individuals differ in their values or philosophies regarding certain issues.
7. *Conflict of roles* develops when two individuals have equal responsibilities but actual boundaries are unclear or when they are required to fill simultaneously two or more roles that present inconsistent or contradictory expectations.
8. *Conflict of tasks* develops when outputs of one individual or group become inputs of another individual or group or where outputs are shared by several individuals or groups.

Levels

Conflict can develop on any of these various levels: intrapersonal, intragroup, intraterritorial, interpersonal, intergroup, or interterritorial. Territory in this context can refer to organizations, hospitals, nations, or other entities. Conflict may originate within one person, group, or territory; such conflicts are called *intra*personal, *intra*group, and *intra*territorial. For example, an intrapersonal conflict exists when a nurse is required to provide tube feedings to a brain dead child while believing that withholding treatment would be a better choice. When conflict occurs between two or more persons, groups or territories, such conflict are called *inter*personal, *inter*group, or *inter*territorial. Conflict between staff nurses and nurse managers regarding floating patterns is an example of intergroup conflict. Levels of conflict most commonly investigated are interpersonal, intergroup, and interterritorial (interorganizational).

Perceived or Felt Conflict

Conflict may develop according to an individual's perception of existing conditions. Perceptual processes contribute to conflict in several ways. First, they provide a valid or invalid assessment of existing conditions. Second, they affect the extent to which an individual views a situation as one resulting in a potential loss (Filley, 1975). For example, a conflict situation developed between nurses who did not smoke and some who did regarding the use of a small lounge. Both sides held valid perceptions of the room's inadequate ventilation system, however the situation of incompatible interests and scarce resources led to overt conflict behavior.

Individual feelings also contribute to conflict development. Feelings that set the stage for conflict development arise from individual personality characteristics that have their origins in cultural background, developmental, and personal experiences, as well as perceptual processes. Whatever the source, these feelings become important determinants in conflict development, and explain many situations of felt conflict under conditions which do not seem to present conflict.

Manifest Behavior

Manifest behavior of individuals, based on antecedent conditions, occurring on various levels, and resulting from perceived or felt conflict may be exhibited as either cooperative or competitive. Cooperative behavior exists when goals for an individual or separate participants can only be achieved if all individuals under consideration can also enter their respective goal regions. Competitive behavior, on the other hand, exists when goals for the individual or separate participants can only be achieved by blocking all individuals under consideration from entering their respective goal regions (Deutsch, 1962). An example of competitive behavior is seen when two nurses from the same unit are being considered for a head nurse position and one candidate, the scheduling coordinator of the unit, uses this influence to acquire letters of recommendation from staff nurses.

The inherent organizational ideology that competition fosters greater motivation to be productive, more than other forms of social relationships, has been studied extensively (May & Doob, 1937; Deutsch, 1962; Johnson & Johnson, 1979). It has been found, however, that productivity in interdependent groups is greater when the reward structure orients the group toward intergroup cooperation rather than competition. More recently, Cosier and Dalton (1988) found that individuals not only performed better under a cooperative reward plan but also exerted more effort. They also found that persons who highly value helping behavior in organizations may work better if given a cooperative environment.

The last step of the integrated conflict model examines consequences which may be suppressive, productive, or destructive. With suppressive consequences, an individual may have antagonistic feelings that merely set the stage for further conflict development. On the other hand, productive consequences can produce expanded understanding of issues, mobilization of individual resources and energies, and enhanced ability to work together in the future. An example of a productive conflict consequence occurred when a difference of opinions (interests) arose between laboratory and ICU staff (interpersonal) regarding maintenance of arterial pressure monitoring systems (perceived conflict). ICU nurses vehemently opposed laboratory technicians drawing blood culture specimens from arterial lines while lab technicians argued that subjecting patients to multiple venipunctures causes unnecessary pain and bruising (conflict behavior). The conflict led to a small funded research study with results that both sides accepted and implemented (productive resolution).

By contrast, destructive consequences of conflict reduce cooperation and teamwork. Little productivity takes place because of the high energy required to sustain antagonistic attitudes. Its bitterness and hostility destroy the status quo without replacing it. This leads to a breakdown or destruction of social progress. As an example, in a hospital with a particularly busy operating room, nursing service required the OR supervisor to advise operating room nurses of mandatory overtime. A destructive conflict situation quickly emerged. Surgeons who arrived late for afternoon cases expected all OR nurses to stay until their cases were finished. The supervisor and nurses felt it was an unnecessary burden on their personal lives to be required to meet the needs of physicians who were not honoring elective time commitments in the OR (conflict of values, interests and tasks on an intergroup level). Hostile feelings began to be exhibited by both physicians and nurses, the conflict escalated and the OR supervisor and twelve nurses resigned (perceived or felt conflict resulting in competitive conflict behavior). The hospital was forced to intervene and call-staff plans were instituted, too late, however, to avoid the loss of experienced nurses (destructive consequences).

ORGANIZATIONAL CONFLICT

Organizations can be identified as having either cooperative or competitive operations that compel individuals to interact because of a powerful third party. Conflict then is rooted in the organizational structure. Organizational conflict can be described as an outcome of the organizational structure that can largely be managed through changes in organizational design. Three structural factors that contribute to organizational conflict have been identified and described: differentiation, interdependence, and resource-sharing. Antecedent conditions and levels of conflict interface with structural factors contributing to subsequent conflict behavior.

Differentiation

Differences between departments occur naturally when the organization's overall goal is accomplished through specialization. This division of labor allows individuals to work on one particular aspect of a job and to use specialized skills in a supportive environment. As a result, individuals in various departments perform tasks differently from those performed in other departments. Differences exist in working methods, personalities, training, and education as well as in the very process of thinking. These differences are necessary for successful operation of the organization; however, it is because of these differences that problems develop. Departmental differences usually mean less tolerance and sympathy for the problems other departments encounter.

Differentiation makes communication a problem by reinforcing group identity and by creating a special vocabulary that cannot be understood by people in other departments. For example, nurses describe patients' needs in a much different way than do pharmacists. Working together to design a system to more efficiently deliver medications to nursing units on holidays and weekends presents a conflict when pharmacists and nurses do not communicate well. Differentiation also creates potential for conflict because individuals are partitioned off within the organization and physical separation of departments reinforces group differences.

Origins of Differentiation

Many organizational differences between groups can be traced to technologies used within different departments as is so often true in health care settings. A postpartum floor uses highly predictable and familiar technologies to deliver routine care. But in an emergency room a great deal of uncertainty exists and appropriate care has been designed to match the degree of task uncertainty. The result is a high degree of differentiation between these two groups and potential for intergroup conflict over multiple antecedent conditions. Differentiation in hospitals is exemplified when nurses are asked to ''float'' between departments. Differences in tasks, personalities, and roles contribute dramatically to conflict behavior in this example.

In other cases differentiation occurs because some departments face outward while others face inward. Outward facing departments experience demands and situations different from those of an inwardly oriented one. The laboratory department in a hospital faces inward with interactions taking place between or among employees. The public relations department faces outward. The nursing department faces both inward and outward. Outward facing departments are more susceptible to uncertainty. Nurses must interact with patients and families who are external to the institution as well as other hospital employees and physicians who are internal to the institution. Demands placed on each department are different and consequences of these arrangements can contribute to intergroup conflicts.

Other departmental differences have been described in many ways. Lawrence and Lorsch (1967) found departments differed in four ways: (1) managers' goal orientation (eg, nurse executives versus nurse managers); (2) time orientation (long- versus short-term); (3) interpersonal orientation (task- versus relationship-oriented); and (4) formality of the organizational structure (bureaucratic versus systematic).

Differentiation comes from aspects of structure and design as well as personal characteristics of individuals involved (Lawrence & Lorsch, 1967). The psychological development of department personnel is very much influenced by the tasks and structures within respective departments. For example, ICU nurses who perform highly specialized life-saving skills could develop superior attitudes toward nurses who work on general medical floors. A good administrator will realize that conflict analysis must include assessment of underlying departmental differences as well as individual personality types.

The number of different departments in an organization is also affected partly by the size and diversity of the external contacts an organization experiences. A large metropolitan hospital, because of its various services, has more departments than a small community hospital. Each new demand forces the hospital to increase its differentiation to remain competitive. As more uncertainty develops over the services a hospital can or should provide, new departments are created to accomplish the many tasks. Territorial differences arise between departments and potential intraterritorial (intraorganizational) conflict increases. High degrees of differentiation alone are not sufficient to cause conflict. When differentiation is combined with high degrees of interdependence, however, conflict potential is enhanced.

Interdependence

The more groups are interdependent on each other, the more the potential for conflict exists. If individuals did not have to work together, conflict could be avoided by either accepting or ignoring differences. This type of tolerance is difficult to maintain, however, when departments are interdependent. Job interdependence, the second origin of conflict within the organizational structure, creates opportunities for disturbance and goal-blocking that normally would not exist.

There are three types of interdependence, which range from minimal to maximal. These are: (1) pooled; (2) sequential; and (3) reciprocal. As the continuum shifts from pooled toward reciprocal interdependence, there is a greater demand for coordinated effort. Conflict develops when the coordinating efforts become strained and fails to produce the desired degree of cooperation.

Pooled interdependence involves situations wherein each part contributes and is supported by the whole but there is little or no direct contact between them. For example, the home health service of a hospital is relatively independent regarding actual work flow. The major purpose of pooled interdependence in this case is to develop standards and continuity of client care at home. Once information from the discharge planning nurse is integrated into the plan of care by the home health nurse, direct contact is minimal. There is little conflict in this type of interaction because interdependence is not direct.

Sequential interdependence is sometimes called the one-way work flow. There is direct interdependence between units and the direction of flow is one way. As stated previously, the greater the interdependence the greater the potential for conflict. Assembly line workers usually operate in sequential interdependent work situations. In addition to regulations and standards, rigid schedules are enforced. Individuals working on an assembly line often must produce consistently according to a set of standards and strict rules. There is much frustration and conflict of regulations, roles and tasks develop when deadlines must be met and machinery breaks down, or some component that was produced earlier violates production standards. Managers must be able to coordinate sequentially interdependent functions to prevent potential conflicts between departments. An example of sequential interdependence in a hospital is when emergency room patients must be admitted to an ICU on an urgent basis. Conflict arises when emergency room nurses are forced to ''hold'' patients until ICU beds are ready.

Reciprocal interdependence refers to situations in which departments provide each other with information regarding job performance. Each department completes its work independently, but information flows both ways. Mutual adjustment is necessary in addition to standardization and scheduling to coordinate reciprocally interdependent departments. Direct contact among team members is the best way to achieve coordination. This includes regularly scheduled meetings, informal discussions, and impromptu gatherings. Social service and nursing have a reciprocal interdependent relationship. The social service department receives information from the nursing department about patients' social needs. Social service accepts input from the nursing unit and provides new input to the same unit. If the situation becomes more uncertain, however, and mutual adjustments are no longer sought, a potential for conflict exists.

Resource Sharing

The third origin which contributes to conflict within the organization is shared resources. Scarce resources such as money, time, space, personnel and equipment that must be shared among different departments produce a wide variety of conflicts. For example, allocations of budget dollars to departments in a large medical center is a highly political process. Departments such as surgery or opthalmology, which bring in large amounts of revenue, make demands for new costly equipment. A burn unit or neuroscience division, perhaps a source of losses, demands support on the basis that they are essential for the institution to offer complete care. A new office building for physicians will stimulate conflict over allocation of office space. Shared photocopy machines, word processors, and lounges produce conflict situations. The need to share resources may stimulate considerable conflict even where pooled interdependence exists.

Cochran and White (1981) found greater conflict occurred in nonroutine, high-cost purchase transactions than in routine, low cost ones. Larger transactions were not covered by existing budget categories since they were usually new expenditures. Large purchase decisions required greater internal justification and greater interactions among those involved in the decision. Outside vendors also exerted direct sales pressure on individuals involved in decision making. With smaller transactions, these salespersons only went to a single purchasing agent in the hospital. Thus the common resource of money invokes conflict when those who must share an institution's financial resources see an opportunity to have those resources spent on them.

CONFLICT MANAGEMENT

When describing conflict management, most recommendations are to eliminate or reduce conflict. The trend today is away from resolution of conflict and toward management of conflict (Robey, 1986). However, the literature on conflict management does not indicate what set of guidelines are most effective or when managers should intervene. In addition, it is difficult to measure productive and destructive consequences of conflict management. Thus each organization must set up criteria to evaluate their conflict management. Typical outcome criteria to measure productive consequences are productivity, turnover, profitability, satisfaction (which decision outcomes), and conflict recurrence. Conflict management is a process which involves steps similar to those used in the nursing process, ie, assessment, diagnosis, planning, intervention and evaluation (see Fig 24–2).

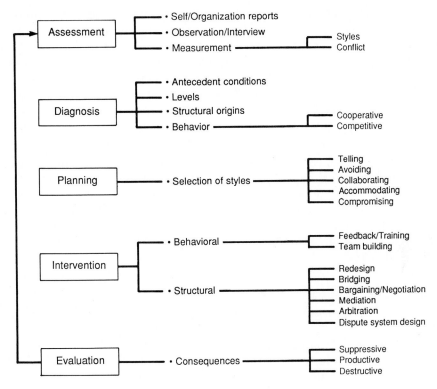

Figure 24-2. Conflict Management Model

Assessment

Often managers will intervene before correctly assessing the conflict situation. A systematic approach is needed to correctly diagnose the cause of conflict in an organization. In many conflict situations primary issues are concealed. If managers intervene before assessing real conflict issues, solutions will not be appropriate nor effective. Assessment includes self and organizational reports, observations, and interviews as well as measurement of conflict styles and the amount of conflict.

Measurement includes: (1) amount and source of interpersonal or intergroup conflict and (2) type of conflict management used by nurse managers. The Rahim Organizational Conflict Inventory-I (ROCI-I) measures the amount of conflict at intrapersonal, interpersonal, and intergroup levels (Rahim, 1983a). There are also a number of instruments that have been developed to measure individual's preferences for conflict resolution styles (Lawrence & Lorsch, 1967; Hall, 1972; Putnam & Jones 1982; Rahim, 1983b).

Conflict management styles identified by Blake and Mouton (1964) made a significant contribution to understanding interpersonal conflict management. The five-style classification of interpersonal behavior for managing conflict are: competing, collaborating, compromising, avoiding and accommodating. Thomas (1976) interpreted these as reflections of two dimensions. The first dimension, concern for production, explains the degree (high or low) to which an individual attempts to accomplish tasks. The second dimension, concern for others, explains the degree (high or low) to which an individual attempts to satisfy another person's concerns. These dimensions describe the motivational orientations of a given individual during conflict. Kilmann and Thomas (1978) superimposed on the two-dimensional model a five-category mode representing behavior an individual might use for meeting concern for production compared to concern for others. Figure 24–3 represents the five style category along the two dimensions adapted from Blake and Mouton (1964) and Thomas (1976).

Telling. With high concern for production and low concern for others, individuals pursue their own needs and goals to the exclusion of others. This style means that an individual attempts to gain power or influence by the use of open confrontation. Frustration, anger, or argument may be observed during conflict situations. Individuals who engage in this type of behavior are likely to be distant from the conflict scene due to their position or other social or organizational pressure. This is a highly assertive style.

Compromising. In this style there is intermediate concern for production and others. Individuals who compromise realize that in conflict situations no one is always satisfied. Neither party has all needs and goals met but both get something. Compromising reflects a willingness to trade or bargain with another individual and to search for a middle ground. This is a pragmatic style that involves negotiating and searching for a relatively quick solution to a problem.

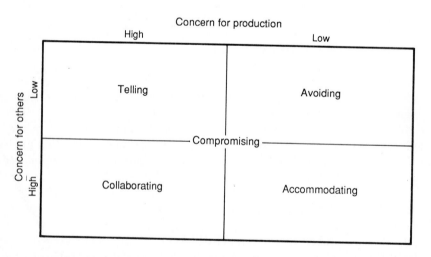

Figure 24–3. Description of Dimensions and Styles of Interpersonal Conflict Management *(Adapted from Blake RR, Mouton JS. The Managerial Grid. Houston, TX, 1964. Gulf LA and Thomas KW. Conflict and conflict management; Dunnette MD, ed. Handbook of Industrial and Organizational Psychology. Chicago, Rand-McNally, 889, 1976)*

Avoiding. In this style, there is low concern for production and others. This style tends to be characterized by a negation of the issue at hand in the belief that any attempt to either discuss or challenge the behavior of another individual is hopeless or futile. Avoiding involves putting the issue to one side so that the immediate onset of conflict is avoided in hopes that there will be a better time for individuals involved to deal with their differences. This style puts resolution of the issue into the future with a view that time may in itself solve the problem or that people will be more agreeable later. Avoiding may involve withdrawing from the conflict, agreeing to put it aside or successfully side-stepping the issue.

Collaborating. In this style, there is high concern for production and others. The collaborating style typically involves an effort on the part of an individual to actively seek effective problem-solving activities so that all parties can achieve a mutually satisfying conclusion. For this method to be successful, individuals must be able to find a resolution to the problem satisfactory to all. Collaborating requires exploring a disagreement in depth and requires considerable sharing of views and information in an atmosphere that encourages confrontation with integrity. This style demands creativity in order to be successful.

Accommodating. In this style, there is low concern for production and high concern for others. The accommodating style is essentially a cooperative interaction in which the individual is not assertive. Typically, the individual gives up personal needs for another's point of view. Accommodating may involve attempts to soothe another's feelings in order to prevent further conflict or to achieve an appearance of being reasonable and receptive. There is high need for acceptance and approval from others. When situations of conflict do arise, the accommodating individual is likely to take a middle of the road approach, not wanting to risk disruption of interpersonal relationships and at the same time unable to express a firm opinion.

Diagnosis

Diagnosis of conflict should be made after assessment data have been reviewed and analyzed. This involves examination of antecedent conditions and determinants of the levels on which conflict takes place, ie, interpersonal or intergroup. If competitive behavior is manifested, further analysis is needed to determine if hostile attitudes are developing. DuBrin (1972) suggests managers prepare a conflict matrix, which identifies levels of conflict, contributing antecedents and levels, structural origins and type of conflict behavior exhibited as well as the intensity of the conflict (see Fig 24–1).

Planning

The five conflict management styles involve various degrees of manager and employee interactions. Given the five styles, Table 24–1 lists characteristic situations in which the styles may be applied.

In theory, collaborative conflict management is the best intervention in interpersonal conflict. However, in practice any one of the five conflict management styles

TABLE 24–1. CONFLICT MANAGEMENT STYLES AND APPLICABLE SITUATIONS

Telling

Simple issue
Immediate action necessary
Inexperienced employees
Assertive individuals taking control
Issue important to nurse manager
Unfavorable outcome costly
Threatening situation
Unpleasant conditions
May be acceptable for conflicts of resources, interests, roles, tasks, and regulations
Competitive behavior manifested

Compromising

Complex issue
Cooling off period needed
Individuals share common authority
Other styles have failed
Possible temporary resolution
May be acceptable for conflicts of interests, resources, personality, tasks, and regulations

Avoiding

Noncritical issue
Cooling off period needed
Employees willing to defer a decision
Individuals unwilling to reach consensus
Agreement not possible
May be acceptable for conflicts of goals, values, and personality

Collaborating

Complex issues
Sufficient time for problem solving
Individuals able to synthesize ideas
All individuals concerned with outcome
Acceptance of resolution critical for implementation
Individuals share organizational goals
May be acceptable with conflicts of task, roles, regulations, and resources
Cooperative behavior manifested

Accommodating

Complex issues
No time for problem solving
Manager does not have adequate information
Issue more important to other individual
Manager dealing from a position of weakness
Preservation of relationships important
May be acceptable with conflicts of personality, values, interests, and goals
Competitive behavior manifested

may be appropriate depending on the circumstances. Marriner (1982) studied actual conflict situations, frequency of conflict management styles used by nurse managers and percentages of successful conflict resolutions. The style most frequently used was collaboration with a successful conflict resolution rate of 74 percent; followed by avoidance, 17 percent; telling, 27 percent; compromising, 76 percent; and accommodation, 60 percent. In other words, the style chosen most frequently by nurse managers did not necessarily give the highest success rate. Findings provide some support for using various styles, especially those of collaboration, compromising, and accommodating.

Intervention

The two basic methods of intervention in conflict management are: behavioral and structural. The behavioral method is recommended for improving intrapersonal and interpersonal conflict involving antecedent conditions such as values, personalities and goals. Behavioral approaches encourage individuals to examine their values, feelings and goals so that situations which elicit irrational or self-destructive behaviors can better be understood.

Structural methods attempt to improve organizational conflict by changing certain characteristics of the organization, eg, degrees of differentiation, dependency situations, communication and reward systems. These approaches are recommended for interpersonal, intergroup and intra/interorganizational conflict.

Behavioral interventions include *feedback and training* sessions which help individuals become assertive, confrontational and better communicators and listeners. One such method is the Johari Window exercise (Luft, 1961). This training method involves communication and listening skills and helps individuals phrase verbal messages to prevent misunderstanding. *Transactional analysis* (Berne, 1961; Harris, 1969) has also been used to understand interpersonal dynamics of conflict.

Transactional analysis encourages two-way communications in which messages exchanged are examined to determine whether communication is direct and appropriate (adult-adult) or crossed and inappropriate (adult-child) or (parent-child). Couch (1965) found supervisors who participated in these types of training sessions learned to alter their behavior through reasoning processes and observations while other supervisors learned by trial and error. Training methods therefore may affect fixed and/or resistant behavior and allow managers to see disparity between what they say and what others hear, often the real source of conflict. Workshops which use the Myer-Briggs type indicator (Myers, 1962) or other personality inventories to explain individual differences may also reduce conflict by reducing personal threats and preventing critical judgments and defensiveness among individuals. The Myer-Briggs type indicator (MBTI) approach is mainly designed to enable individuals to understand personal differences in a nonjudgemental framework, allowing cooperative action to take place.

Team building involves changing attitudes and behaviors of groups to improve overall organizational effectiveness. Beckhard (1967) describes team building as a process in which assessment of interpersonal relations, leadership styles, communication skills and motivational levels takes place. Individuals simultaneously work on changing group attitudes and behavior while developing new goals to be implemented. Blake and Mouton (1964) found that when intergroup problem solving methods are used to manage conflict, groups develop higher level goals and more effective strategies to reduce conflict. (Chapter 17 explores team building in more depth.)

Structural interventions are used when conflict develops from antecedent conditions, occurs on interpersonal, intergroup or interorganizational levels or involves factors such as differentiation, interdependence and resource sharing. Through organizational redesign, underlying factors (differentiation, interdependence, and resource sharing) contributing to conflict can be altered to reduce conflict potential. Differentiation can be decreased by making departments more alike and by providing cross-training.

Floating, a conflictual issue among nurses, is a direct result of differentiation. Many hospitals do not want nurses to become generalists because they believe that specialists perform specific tasks more productively. Thus cross-training may not be an acceptable strategy for this issue. Nurse managers have searched for solutions to resolve the floating issue and through collaboration with staff nurses and nurse executives, some restructuring has taken place. In many hospitals, nurses float only to similar environments. Such approaches have produced successful resolutions where intense specialization is a necessity and fluctuations in patient census is an ongoing problem.

Redesign offers another advantage: reduction of the degree of interdependence between groups. In the situation presented earlier regarding emergency room transfers to ICU, this might be solved by making each department less dependent on the other. This can be done in several ways. Each department could be self-sufficient; direct contact between the conflicting departments could be avoided by creating a buffer or shared supervisory position. One function of nurse managers is to handle direct conflicts between levels. With this type of conflict, a physical buffer, such as a holding room, could reduce conflict between the two groups. While this is a classic example of interdependent conflict on an intergroup level, the intervention, a holding room, involves more than one level.

Sharing resources also contributes to conflict potential. Such conflict can be reduced if the resources for all departments are increased or sharing is decreased. Resource allocation increases or decreases personnel, information, or other resources relevant to conflict management. Two approaches for reallocation of resources are: (1) to change the nature of interdependence between individuals or (2) to change resources available for conflict management. Resource reallocations are usually expensive but have a powerful impact when resources are linked to important conflict issues. Because nursing represents labor intensive costs without identifying direct revenues, nurses have less power to determine resource allocation. A major conflict among nurses is expectations of housekeeping duties on evening and night shifts. Since interdependence between nursing and housekeeping is not easily changed, resource allocation to establish coverage for housekeeping duties on these shifts is one means to reduce conflict.

The structural configuration of an organization can be redesigned to reduce conflict. For example, an ailing high-low (eg, physician-nurse) relationship can be brought closer to equilibrium or an out of control equal-equal (BS nurse-nurse) relationship can be altered by giving one individual a greater power base. This generally is a laborious process but altering power and dependency relationships through redesign should be considered as a potential solution.

Bridging

Another technique used for conflict intervention is bridging. This technique involves devising creative solutions to serve the primary interests of disputants in a conflict (Fisher & Ury, 1981). Bridging is a type of tradeoff; both parties make concessions on low priority interests. This method creates a new element, the bridge, which becomes part of the negotiation. For example, in a conflict between nursing and maintenance at a satellite surgery center, the center lost money which led to a cutback in maintenance employee hours. Prior to the cutback, one of the maintenance services was to exchange empty oxygen tanks for filled oxygen tanks. After the cutback, nurses were expected to move the tanks; they refused. The head of maintenance refused to approve travel to and from the surgery center as hours over budget. Conflict escalated until some nurses threatened to quit. The medical center decided to bridge the gap with an onsite housekeeping employee willing to exchange the tanks.

Bargaining and Negotiation

Bargaining and negotiation are aspects of conflict resolution in which disputants attempt to reach mutually acceptable outcomes. The terms "bargaining" and "negotiation" are often used interchangeably, however, they have somewhat different meanings. Bargaining is the technical process by which two or more individuals attain a mutually agreeable contract concerning limited resources. Bargaining should be used when disputants are not competitive, for example, when disputants would prefer to reach an agreement on a contract or problem rather than do nothing and a decision cannot be made unilaterally. For compromise to occur, all disputants must concede and any outcome must have the support of all disputants.

Negotiation involves human interactions which form the environment of the bargaining process. Negotiation is an art rather than a science. To differentiate, labor-management bargaining involves bids and concessions leading to a final contract while negotiations involve personal interactions between the labor leader and management.

Bargaining is primarily descriptive. The question to be answered is: What will be the best solution for this particular bargaining problem? Negotiation on the other hand is primarily prescriptive: What should a particular individual do in order to achieve his or her best outcome?

The negotiation process has two distinct time frames, *strategic* and *tactical*. Negotiation occurring over long periods of time, allowing individuals to reflect and decide on various courses of action, is strategic negotiation. Negotiation occurring rapidly and requiring quick decisions by participants is tactical negotiation.

Strategic negotiation involves planning and strategy selection when there is ample time to examine a variety of possibilities. The negotiator's task is to achieve a superior position for the individuals represented while at the same time ensuring that an outcome is achieved. Nurse administrators may develop successful strategic negotiation techniques with practice and the study of experienced negotiators. Administrators who use negotiation must be able to take a hard line, have and use power bases, correctly assess the opposition, and formulate strategies for negotiation.

Tactical negotiation refers to techniques required when quick decisions are needed without opportunity for conflict analysis. The nurse executive must be able to react in an intelligent and productive manner to unexpected actions of disputants. Tactical negotiation skills arise from inherent ability and experience (Karrass, 1972; Nierenberg, 1973). However, good technique goes beyond experience and requires understanding of the problem and the dynamics of negotiation. Familiarity with organizational concepts (eg, aspiration level, power, coercion, and threats) facilitate the assimilation of facts and development of tactics. In addition, the negotiator must be aware of the skills and preferences and foresee options and potential outcomes.

Mediation

The use of a third-party to clarify issues, circumstances, and alternative courses is mediation. In health care settings, the use of a mediator is more likely to succeed when individuals are unequal in status and power, for example, the interpersonal conflict between a physician and nurse. It has also been used in intergroup conflict. All disputants involved in conflict must accept the mediator. This implies all disputants are motivated to resolve the conflict and willing to do so with the mediator. If the mediator becomes identified with one particular group, if a personality conflict develops, or if one group is resistant to the mediator, the success of the process is in doubt. The mediator must set up contacts with both groups, provide a clear description of the process and set up a method of communication. It helps the mediator to understand the structure of the groups involved. If there is no structure, the mediator helps the groups develop one to facilitate the exchange of information. The mediator should identify formal and informal group leaders and determine their willingness to participate in conflict management.

The mediator maintains equilibrium among groups. The greater the power differences, the greater the chance that more powerful groups will resolve the conflict by imposing their demands on the weaker groups. The mediator intervenes at an impasse or deadlock when the groups are unable to move and attempts to lead the groups to a higher level of problem solving.

A mediator always tries to prevent conflict escalation. If the level of conflict is out of control, the mediation process is ineffective. Acute crises can sometimes be handled by a cooling-off period in which the status quo is temporarily maintained until the groups show some willingness to communicate. If conflict is chronic and the groups learn to live with it, there is little chance for a constructive compromise.

The mediator has disputants explain the grievances, the background and the consequences. In this differentiation process the mediator identifies substantive and emotional issues and confronts the groups with these issues. The object is to clarify perspectives for both sides. The result of this confrontation of perspectives should be synthesis of solutions, understanding, and compromise. This is known as *integration*.

If an impasse is reached the groups again go through the process of differentiation until integration occurs.

The mediator's interventions are guided by attainability, urgency and movement. Solutions should be attainable, of quality, and comprehensible. A forceful and resolute manner in the mediator provides structure and direction. The mediator also establishes procedures for the groups and, when necessary, clarifies and defends them. This provides the calm atmosphere necessary for conflict resolution. Ambiguity or lack of confidence conveyed by the mediator creates mistrust and confusion. Disputants feel threatened if the mediator cannot regulate group interactions and a hostile atmosphere can easily erupt into a new conflict.

Arbitration

Arbitration is a process which involves the use of a third-party to reach an agreement. (Chapter 18 discusses arbitration in the context of labor relations.) In mediation, the third-party serves as an adviser, while in arbitration, the third-party has the power, granted by the organization or by mutual agreement, to impose a settlement upon the groups. Arbitration is used when a potential emergency is likely to occur. Rarely does arbitration eliminate recurrence of the issue or reduce anger, distrust and resentment.

Dispute Systems Design

Dispute systems design attempts to reduce costs of conflict and realize its benefits by changing how people handle their disputes. It assumes conflict is inevitable in organizations and often a sign of need for change. This intervention is applicable to interpersonal and intra/interorganizational conflict. Dispute systems design is similar to bridging but is much more comprehensive.

Conflict resolution based on this method involves interest-based rather than rights-based negotiations. Reconciling interests often involves identifying underlying concerns, prioritizing them and devising tradeoffs in which the parties concede on low-priority interests in order to receive satisfaction on high-priority interests (Raiffa, 1982). Interventions that reconcile interests often provide all disputants with much of what they wanted. In addition, information shared in the process of searching for resolution may increase mutual understanding and benefit the relationship. Studies comparing interest-based negotiations with rights-based negotiations have shown that disputants prefer interest-based procedures, especially with grievances, (Brett & Goldberg, 1981), small claims (McEwen & Maiman, 1981), and child custody disputes (Pearson, 1982). An additional benefit of this type of negotiation is that conflict recurrence is low and consequences are productive (Pearson, 1982).

The method involves using negotiation cooperatively rather than competitively. Essential to interest-based intervention is commitment by the organization to this method of conflict resolution. Without active support by all parties, it is difficult to make any substantial changes or evaluate the results. Powerful parties in the health care system who have been winning with old procedures may be reluctant to cooperate with dispute systems designers. Less powerful parties, eg, nurse managers and staff nurses, may have to champion dispute systems design. Several elements are needed to facilitate this method: formal forums to encourage discussion of conflict; feedback; veto power of nurses; and third-party mediation if needed.

When interest-based negotiation takes place, groups must focus on maximizing joint gains rather than individual gains. Most individuals negotiate over a single issue, for example, the purchase price of a car. The seller makes a high initial offer, the buyer makes a low initial offer, and the two make concessions until they reach agreement or impasse. However, by examining mutual interests and reaching agreements each party may receive more than they would in a compromise.

While interest-based negotiations have been successful in getting groups to take their disputes through to resolution instead of fighting them out, often groups are so emotionally involved with the issues they need to vent emotions before they can negotiate successfully. In such situations, an advisory third-party mediator may be needed to help reach an agreement. If no resolution can be attained at least the mediator can encourage disputants to think about an agreement they both can accept.

Evaluation

Evaluation of results is the final step in conflict management. Were the sources of conflict accurately determined? Was the intervention style appropriate? Interventions should be evaluated on whether they resulted in suppressive, destructive or productive consequences. With suppressive behavior, individuals may feel defeated and express negative feelings by becoming less trusting, personalizing the situation, and exhibiting distorted communication. Such individuals manifest low level commitment to the solutions.

Destructive consequences occur when disputants direct their energies against each other rather than toward a common solution. Individuals assume fixed positions to emphasize an obvious or accessible solution rather than defining the problem. Communication is judgmental and accusatory rather than factual. Differences rather than similarities are emphasized. Oftentimes isolated issues become generalized in an atmosphere of bitter dispute. Intergroup warring may develop into intragroup warfare.

Outcome criteria of organizational effectiveness (productivity, acceptance of the decisions, turnover, profitability, etc.) measure productive consequences. Then all individuals experience feelings of success with the outcome and a high commitment to the solution. Individuals also have positive feelings toward the conflict management process which increases their ability to problem solve in future conflicts.

SUMMARY

Conflict management is costly to organizations. Conflict exists whenever incompatible behavior occurs. Conflict development can be described on the basis on antecedent conditions, levels of origin, and types of conflict behavior observed. Consequences of conflict can be suppressive, destructive, or productive.

Three structural origins of organizational conflict are differentiation, interdependence, and resource sharing. As group differences increase, greater potential for dissension and conflict exists. As interdependence increases, conflict is more likely. If resources are shared, disagreements tend to develop. Conflict management requires that managers determine structural origins of conflict and develop methods to bring individuals together interpersonally.

Styles of handling interpersonal conflict can be classified as telling, compromising, avoiding, collaborating, and accommodating. Management of organizational conflict involves knowledge of the various styles and appropriate applications. Conflict management requires assessment, diagnosis, planning, intervention, and evaluation. Assessment includes self and organizational reports of conflict, observations and interviews, measure of styles, and the amount of conflict. Diagnosis includes identifying sources and levels of conflict and conflict behavior. Planning involves selection of intervention styles. Intervention is indicated when conflict becomes dysfunctional or when the conflict management style does not match the situation. There are two types of interventions, structural and behavioral. The behavioral approach manages conflict by encouraging participants to develop conflict management styles and promote effective communication. The structural approach manages conflict by changing an organization's structural design, or using a structural intervention. Evaluation is essential to determine whether conflict management has been (1) suppressive, which increases the likelihood of future conflict; (2) destructive which causes antagonism that sets the stage for new conflict; or (3) productive which contributes to harmony and cooperation.

REFERENCES

Beckhard R. *Organizational Psychology*. Boston, Allen and Bacon, 1967

Berne E. *Transactional Analysis in Psychotherapy: A Systematic Individual and Social Psychiatry*. New York, Grove Press, 1961

Blake RR, Mouton JS. *The Managerial Grid*, Houston, TX, Gulf Publishing, 1964

Brett JM, Goldberg SB. Grievance mediation in the coal industry: A field experiment. *Industrial and Labor Relations Review*. 37:49, 1983

Cochran DS, White DD. Intraorganizational conflict in the hospital purchasing decision-making process. *Academy of Management Journal*. 24:324, 1981

Cosier RA, Dalton DR. Competition and cooperation: Effects of value dissension and predisposition to help. *Human Relations*. 11:823, 1988

Couch PD. *Some Effects of Training and Experience on Concepts of Supervision*. Unpublished doctoral dissertation, University of Wisconsin-Madison, 1965

DuBrin AJ. The practice of managerial psychology: *Concepts and methods of manager and organization development*. New York, Pergamon Press, 1972

Deutsch M. Recurrent themes in the study of social conflict. *Journal of Social Issues*. 33:222, 1973

Deutsch M. Cooperation and trust: Some theoretical notes. In: Jones MR, ed. *Nebraska Symposium on Motivation*. Lincoln, University of Nebraska Press, 1962

Filley AC. *Interpersonal Conflict Resolution*. Glenview, IL, Scott, Foresman, 1975

Fisher R, Ury W. *Getting to yes: Negotiating agreements without giving in*. Boston, Houghton-Mifflin, 1981

Hall DT. A model of coping with role conflict: The role behavior of college educated women. *Administrative Science Quarterly*. 17:471, 1972

Harris TW. *I'm OK-You're OK; A Practical Guide to Transactional Analysis.* New York: Harper, 1969

Johnson KW, Johnson R. The instructional use of cooperative, competitive and individualistic goal structures. In: Walberg HJ, ed. *Educational Environment and Effects: Evaluation, Policy and Productivity.* Berkeley, McCutchon, 1979

Karrass CL. *The Negotiation Game.* New York: World Publishing, 1972

Kilman RH, Thomas KW. Four perspectives of conflict management: An attributional framework for organizing descriptive and narrative theory. *Academy of Management Review.* 3:59, 1978

Lawrence PR, Lorsch JW. *Organization and Environment.* Boston, Harvard University, Graduate School of Business, 1967

Luft J. The Johari Window. *Human Relations Training News.* 5:6, 1961

McEwen CA, Maiman RJ. Small claims mediation in Maine: An empirical assessment. *Maine Law Review.* 37:237, 1981

Marriner A. Managing Conflict. *Nursing Management.* 13:6, 29, 1982

May MA, Doob LW. Competition and cooperation. *Social Science Research Council Bulletin.* #25, New York, 1937

Myers IB. *Manual: The Myers-Briggs Type Indicator.* Palo Alto, CA, Consulting Psychologist Press, 1962

Nierenberg GI. *Fundamentals of Negotiating.* New York, Warner Books, 1973

Pearson J. An evaluation of alternatives to court adjudication. *The Justice System Journal.* 7:420, 1982

Putnam LL, Jones T. Reciprocity in negotiations: An analysis of bargaining interactions. *Communication Monographs.* 49:171, 1982

Raiffa H. *The art and science of negotiation.* Cambridge, MA, Harvard University Press, 1982

Rahim AM. Measurement of organizational conflict. *Journal of General Psychology.* 109:189, 1983a

Rahim AM. A measure of styles of handling interpersonal conflict. *Academy of Management Journal.* 26:2, 368, 1983b

Robey D. *Designing Organizations,* 2nd ed. Illinois, Richard D Irwin, Inc, 1986

Thomas KW. Conflict and conflict management. In: Dunnette MD, ed., *Handbook of Industrial and Organizational Psychology* Chicago, Rand-McNally, 1976:889–935

CHAPTER 25

Leadership and Project Management

Mary Kay Hermann
JoAnn S. Alexander
Joan T. Kiely

Key Concept List

Leadership
Power
Motivation
Delegation
Team building
Behavior modeling
Project management
Project manager
Project checklist
Network planning techniques

With rapid changes in health care environments, health care institutions are finding it necessary to function more efficiently. Many institutions are therefore adopting organizational designs such as project management to selectively market their services. Executives and managers at many levels may be involved in development or management of project teams. Thus, nurse managers must have a clear understanding of the role of leadership, delegation, team building, and effective project management.

Effective leadership is crucial for promoting organizational goals at all levels of nursing administration. Leadership, the product and process of influencing goal attainment, occurs in an open system through interpersonal interactions between leaders and followers. These interactive processes involve the use of power in creating and altering the direction of change, managing resources, and motivating others to achieve desired goals. Leadership is an essential factor whenever coordinated efforts of people are desirable, such as in project management.

Leadership is increasingly important to health care institutions under conditions of uncertainty. Leaders must predict the effects of dynamic social, political, and economic environments upon institutional services. They must recognize the need for change and must manage the process of change to promote institutional vitality. The rapidity of change and interdependence with the environment increase the complexity of the leader's task.

Effecting change through project management demands team leadership which may modify leader-follower roles and functions. Trends such as increased health care costs, prospective payment systems, emphasis on quality control, and advancing technology challenge today's leaders. Under these conditions of constraint and competition, project management may be an effective strategy for coping with environmental change. Thus, project managers must be effective team builders with interpersonal, human relations, and group process skills in order to utilize a diversity of human talent.

Project management may involve nurse managers at various organizational levels. The chief nurse executive may recommend needed services to be offered through project management, may launch product lines, and may select and appoint nurse project managers who collaborate with other professionals in the design or implementation of a project. It is therefore necessary for all nurse managers to have a clear understanding of various leadership and related theories and processes.

PROJECT MANAGEMENT

What is it? Project management is a decentralized organizational approach to achieve unique objectives within a specified time. The goal is integration and coordination of efforts for a specific purpose. Projects usually require diverse specialists who may be drawn from various locations in the organization. Thus, team membership may cross vertical and horizontal lines in order to achieve project goals. Vertical lines are managed by line managers while horizontal functions are managed by project managers. Products may be outcomes of projects which are components of programs within organized systems. Thus, project management may be referred to as product line management, service line management, or program management (Kerzner, 1982).

Project management is not new. It is an organizational approach initially applied in industry in the creation and development of a new product (Gaddis, 1959). What is new is its increasing acceptance by health care institutions. A fresh look is being taken at services offered in the context of needed, marketable, and profitable products.

This new perspective may enhance and generate other services that the institution can offer. For example, an institution may decide to promote health care for a specific group such as infants, adolescents, or aging individuals. The focus of care might become more comprehensive, for example, wellness programs in addition to illness care. Educational programs for hospitalized patients might be expanded and marketed to the entire community. Specific diagnostic groupings could be selected as a product line or therapies might be targeted for increased emphasis. For example, cardiovascular health could be marketed to include primary prevention, acute care, and rehabilitation. Considering all levels of care, all age groups, and therapies for all health problems in a new perspective unrestricted to the immediate setting has the potential of identifying other services as products.

Clinical specialties, managed by a unit business team of physician director, nursing director, and administrator, are designated product centers at The Johns Hopkins Hospital (Nackel & Kues, 1986). Also organized by product line management is Canada's Comprehensive Cancer Program (Wodinsky, Egan & Markel, 1988). Oncology's multiple disciplines, specialties, treatments, and types of cancer are cited for its appropriateness as a product line. The wide representation of necessary project members is credited for contributing to the program's support and identity.

Project management evolved from systems analysis as a means of functioning dynamically in a changing environment. Derived from a total view of the organization in its environment, project management may be selected to restructure an organization across one or many organized departments when rapid change is needed. The demands associated with changing technology have increased its acceptance (Kerzner, 1982; 1984).

The integration of departmental and project lines on a large scale may evolve into a more permanent structure referred to as matrix management (Kerzner, 1982; Cleland, 1984). For example, Dixon (1978) describes how matrix organization is applied in the British health care system using multidisciplinary teams in managing and planning within health districts. The district team includes an administrator, physician, nursing officer, and financial officer individually responsible to the overall district authority. The teams depend on horizontal organization both for planning approaches to specific health problems and for delivery of services although vertical organization also co-exists (Dixon, 1978).

Case management is a form of managed care in which service is a product. Currently expanding to control costs in acute care and community settings in the United States, case management also utilizes a cross-disciplinary approach. This model alters the traditional hospital organization to meet specific outcomes in patient care (Zander, 1988). The patient's physician and nursing representatives from various functional nursing units where the patient is to receive care function as a team to formulate and monitor desired outcomes with the patient and family. The selected nurse manager for the case has authority across nursing units to promote the achievement of outcomes. The product in this instance is the quality of care based on established protocols and cost outcomes and evaluated by the health care team. In addition to multidisciplinary collaboration, extending the management of care across the entire system is considered essential for comprehensive care in further developing case management (Togno-Armanasco, Olivas & Harter, 1989). Case management may be selected as the modality of care in a product line, and establishing a case management program can itself require project management.

Project management requires that identified criteria and defined deadlines be met with allocated resources (Gaddis, 1959). The participants in the project include a manager with responsibility for the project and specialists selected for their particular expertise (Longest & Klingensmith, 1988). Thus, the uniqueness of the project determines the needed mix of professionals and, in turn, influences the leadership approach.

Although project managers are responsible for meeting deadlines with allocated resources, departmental managers provide the project team members. Since project team members may report to two managers, it is essential for the managers to collaborate in order to accomplish their goals. Conflict management and negotiation may be required. In addition, knowledge of departmental operations and professional skills, management skills, effective communication and interpersonal relationships are essential for the project manager (Kerzner, 1982).

Why Use It? Strategic planning within the total system is critical to an institution's well-being. It requires examination of the institution's relationships with present constitutents, the impact of current legal, ethical, financial, and political trends in order to identify needed and desirable change within the organization. As a participant in long-range institutional planning, the chief nurse executive has an important leadership role in identifying nursing services that may be marketed in creative ways to selected populations. Project management may be selected to market a particular product line (Jones, 1988).

Project management is a change strategy. It can facilitate needed change in one or more parts without permanently changing the total organization. Changes can be evaluated, successful endeavors can be continued, and unprofitable programs can be discontinued. The organization can adapt its structure to environmental demands while diversifying its services and controlling its risks.

By crossing vertical lines to include those best prepared to accomplish specific goals, project management provides a method to accomplish tasks within a defined time limit and budget. Analytical tools may be used to visualize the various tasks and deadlines that must be met in order to reach the intended outcome. When the total project is broken into specific tasks to be accomplished, needed resources can be identified, tasks can be delegated, and accountability for assigned functions is possible.

LEADERSHIP IN PROJECT MANAGEMENT

Leadership is essential in project management because it involves managing people as well as project activities. Project managers must know what changes are needed and must use selected strategies to achieve results, but the ability to motivate others will determine if project goals are reached. The project manager's power base will be instrumental in motivating team members to accomplish project goals. Moreover, the quality of manager-member interaction will influence the project's success. Hence, power, motivation, and leadership theories will be reviewed.

Bases of the Project Manager's Power

If the manager can induce members to focus on a common goal and purpose, the team can move in a common direction. Thus, French and Raven's (1960) bases of power will be examined:

1. *Reward power.* The manager must not only be perceived as having the ability to obtain and grant rewards but must also be able to control rewards.
2. *Referent power.* The manager's ability to reward strengthens the member's identification with the manager which may eventually result in the member's compliance without additional reward.
3. *Coercive power.* The manager has power to the extent that the potential recipient perceives that the manager can and will punish.
4. *Legitimate power.* The recipient believes that the manager has the right to expect certain behavior with the obligation of compliance.
5. *Expert power.* Recognition of the manager's knowledge and skills in a specific area increases the manager's credibility, trust, and influence.

Bases of power are derived from organizational, positional, or individual sources.

Major questions that project managers should ask to determine their power sources as shown in Table 25-1 include the following: What is the organizational structure for project management? Does membership cross disciplines? Is the project subject to accreditation standards that must be met? Does the project manager control the project budget? Is there a position description for the project manager? Is the project manager responsible for developing position descriptions for other members involved in the project? Is the project manager responsible for evaluation of team members participating in the project?

Since power is the currency of the leadership process, it can be accumulated, used, exchanged and shared to accomplish the organizational goals of project management; yet, coercion may result in resistance, withdrawal, or even resignation. Using power that is not legitimate or using expert power outside the specific area of expertise decreases power. Project managers must be aware of resources that may be used to influence project goals but must also understand members' and colleagues' receptivity to various kinds of influence. Motivation theories assist in understanding this receptivity.

Theories of Motivation

Theories of motivation describe and explain factors that may assist the project manager in building productive relationships necessary for reaching project goals.

Dossett's Integrated Model. Need, incentive, and expectancy theories including that of Vroom (1964) are synthesized by Chung (1977) and by Dossett (1988) to describe and explain motivation (see Fig 25-1).

TABLE 25-1. SOURCES OF POWER, DERIVED POWER, AND POSSIBLE RESOURCES FOR THE NURSE PROJECT MANAGER

Sources of Power	Derived Power	Possible Resources

Organization	Legitimate/referent	Institutional philosophy
		Organizational structure
		  departmental units
		  project lines
		Committee structure
		  representation
		Accrediting agencies
		  criteria

	Reward/punishment	Institutional policies Employment contracts Personnel policies Merit policies
Position	Information	Budgetary allocation Access to administrators Formal and informal communication Statistical data
	Legitimate	Organizational charts Administrative support functional authority project manager Position description Policies/procedures Project member evaluation

Personal	Expertise	Credibility/trust
		Timing
		Knowledge
		  understanding of values
		  professional knowledge
		  corporate functions
		Education
		Experience
		  professional
		  political

	Referent	Superiors, colleagues
		  project members
		    individuals
		    groups
		Image
		  personal
		  positional

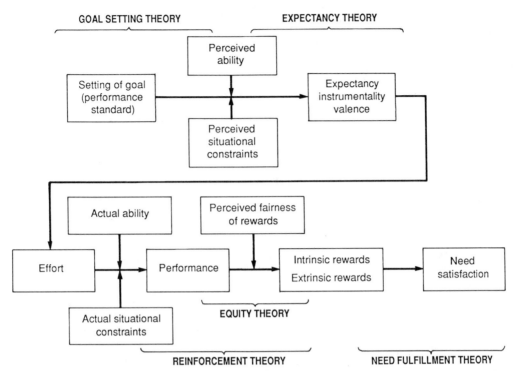

Figure 25-1. Dossett's (1988) *Integrated Model of the Motivational Process (Source: Dossett DD. Motivating staff. In: Sullivan EJ, Decker PJ, eds.* Effective Management in Nursing, *3rd ed. Menlo Park, CA, Addison-Wesley, 1992)*

Chung's Integrative Expectancy Model. In Chung's (1977) approach (see Fig 25-2), motivational effort, nature of the task, the magnitude of incentives, the strength of needs, and linkages between these factors interact to determine motivation. It is the combined effect of need, incentive, anticipated effort and perceived ability to perform a task, the expectation that task performance will lead to the desired incentive, and the ability of the incentive to fulfull a perceived need that determines motivation strength.

Chung (1977) suggests that effort is a function of ability for undertaking a task, the performance of which will lead to organizational rewards and need satisfaction. The nature of the task, the magnitude of the incentive, and the strength of the need influence the motivational effort (Chung, 1977). For example, if a project team member is motivated by growth needs, participating in the project may be viewed as an opportunity to develop certain skills or to gain specific experience. Motivation may be enhanced by offering incentives that provide challenges and intrinsic motivation.

In applying this approach, the project manager should consider the importance of these factors in selecting staff, in team development, and in delegating tasks. For example, what are the most rewarding activities in the project? What interactive and organizational rewards should be available to the project development team? What

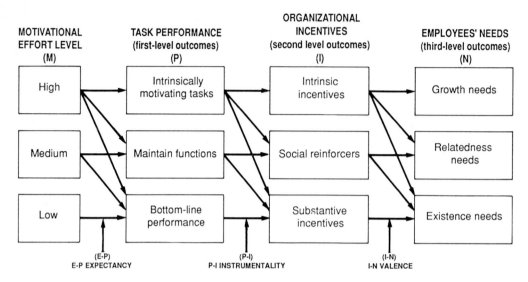

Figure 25-2. Chung's (1977) Integrative Expectancy Model *(Source: Adapted from Chung KH. Motivational Theories and Practices. Columbus, OH, Grid, Inc, 1977: 98–99)*

needs can the project meet for involved project members? How important are different levels of needs to the participants? What is the relationship between performance and reward? Is the reward great enough to obtain the desired level of performance? These questions may be considered in relation to the various factors influencing motivation. Examples of these factors are included in Table 25-2.

Project managers must recognize factors that may be motivating for project team members and must be aware of the potential power for influencing team members. However, utilizing power to enhance motivation occurs through the process of leadership. The project manager-member interaction also influences team members' performance.

Theories of Leadership

Fiedler's Contingency Model. Fiedler (1969) found that high performance of various groups occurred with different patterns of leader-group interaction. The effectiveness of the leader reflects how well the group performs and is contingent upon the interaction of the group, the task, and the leader within a given situation (Fiedler, 1967).

Based on Fiedler's model, variations in leader-group relations, task structure, and position power determine whether or not the situation is favorable for the leader. The conditions and preferred leadership styles based on Fiedler's model are shown in Figure 25-3.

According to Fiedler's model, if the task is unstructured and the goals and solutions are unknown or unclear, then the leader must make a greater effort to involve, to consider, and to gain members' participation. For example, positive relationships with group members will be needed if the project manager wishes group members to

TABLE 25-2. ACTIVITIES AND PREREQUISITE ACTIVITIES FOR IMPLEMENTATION OF A PROJECT

Activity	Prerequisite Activities
A. Select project team	
B. Establish budgeting system	A
C. Establish management information system	B
D. Contract for construction and for furnishings/supplies/equipment	B, C
E. Develop marketing plan	B, C
F. Develop managed care approach	B, C
G. Order construction materials/furnishings/supplies/equipment	B, C, D
H. Establish community support	B, C, E
I. Adopt standards of care	B, C, F
J. Delivery of construction materials	B, C, D, G
K. Develop care protocols	B, C, F, I
L. Develop staff position descriptions	B, C, F, I, K
M. Determine staff mix	B, C, F, I
N. Begin construction	B, C, D, G, J
O. Begin community education	B, C, E, H
P. Establish staffing plan	B, C, F, I, M
Q. Establish quality assurance program	B, C, F, I, K
R. Recruit staff	B, C, F, I, M, K, P, L
S. Hire staff	B, C, F, I, M, K, P, L, Q, R
T. Staff education	B, C, F, I, K, M, L, P, Q, R, S
U. Complete construction	B, C, D, G, J, N
V. Delivery of furnishings/equipment/supplies	B, C, D, G
W. Orientation of staff	B, C, F, I, M, K, L, P, Q, R, S, T
X. Furnish facility	C, D, G, J, N, U, V, X

initiate a plan for marketing selected services. The project manager needs members' participation because the exact outcome cannot be specified by the project manager. Creativity and sharing of beliefs will be required, and project members will make their greatest contribution in a climate of trust, encouragement, and acceptance. The task-oriented project manager will be effective when the task to be accomplished is not very clear and the method for completion has not been standardized. Project managers will be most effective when the situation is favorable for their individual leadership styles. The most favorable situation results when the leader's orientation to people is matched with the type of task structure and group atmosphere (Fiedler, 1967).

The Vertical Dyad Leadership Theory. The *dyad* as conceived by Dansereau, Graen, and Haga (1975) is an exchange model in which a leader and individual subordinate interact. The quality of the relationship influences the leader's behavior and affects the autonomy that the subordinate is permitted in the work role. Those members

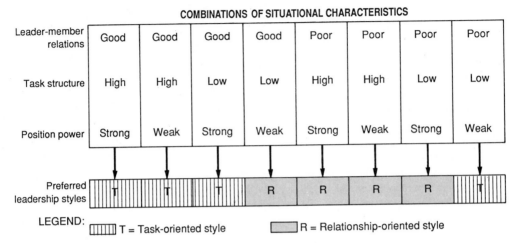

Figure 25-3. Preferred Leadership Styles Based on Fiedler's (1969) Model *(Source: Dossett DK. Motivating Staff. In: Sullivan EJ, Decker PJ, eds.* Effective Management in Nursing, *3rd ed. Menlo Park, CA, Addison-Wesley, 1992)*

with favorable relationships with the leader constitute the ''in-group.'' In contrast, other members are directed by the leader's formal authority. Thus, relationships with individual members may influence leader behavior, and dyad as well as group relationships need to be considered in the leader's approach (Landy, 1989). It is interesting to consider whether favorable relationships are a consequence of the leader's referent power and whether leader selection of members, for example for a project team, has positive benefits for the project manager. However, further study of dyad influences on general leadership style is recommended (Landy, 1989), and development of other tools for identifying group membership of dyads is encouraged by Vecchio and Gobdel (1984).

House and Mitchell's Path-Goal Theory of Leadership. From the perspective of path-goal theory (House & Mitchell, 1974), the leader is successful when she helps members obtain rewards in their work. House and Mitchell's theory of leadership involves defining a goal, clarifying the means of obtaining it, and convincing the member that it can be reached. The leader must actually increase the member's awareness of and desire to obtain the goal which will benefit both leader and member. House and Mitchell (1974) propose that satisfaction and motivation of the member correspond to the leader's ability to interpret what to do and how well to do it in order to reach an expected goal. Moreover, the leader must guide members toward goals that are not only valued by them but that actually can be rewarded by the leader (House & Mitchell, 1974).

Helping members identify and value possible goals, removing obstacles, and providing support and encouragement are functions of the leadership process (House & Mitchell, 1974). However, group members differ in their acceptance of leader direction. Leader direction is more satisfying with highly structured than with unstructured tasks. Leader orientation, varying along a continuum from direction to achievement, will need to be adapted accordingly (House & Mitchell, 1974).

The Vroom-Yetton Normative Model. Vroom and Yetton (1973) recommend the use of decision rules for selecting leadership styles. They propose that autocratic leadership is feasible only if the leader knows all of the solutions and doesn't need members in implementing them. However, this is rarely the case, and the leader must consider methods that enhance the quality of decision making. This model was shown and discussed in Chapter 17. It shows choices to be considered in arriving at the most feasible leadership strategy.

DELEGATION

Delegation is also an essential leadership strategy in team building. Effective delegation requires granting authority to team members who share responsibility and accountability for task completion. Delegation is thus a critical tool for managing time and goals.

Delegation gives managers increased flexibility by freeing them from routines and allowing them to plan; the result is increased productivity. In addition to increased productivity, delegation facilitates participation, develops the potential and confidence of team members, makes them feel a part of the team, increases creativity through diversity of ideas, and helps to accomplish goals efficiently. Delegation promotes better use of resources, saves time, and allows members to become more proficient in handling future tasks. Opportunities arising from delegated tasks may also promote a sense of accomplishment within the team.

In delegation, *authority* must be granted in order for someone to perform, and project managers must consider the resources and authority required for completion of project goals. *Responsibility* should also be shared when a task is delegated. Although the ultimate responsibility belongs to the manager, the team member accepting the task accepts responsibility for completing the task appropriately and is *accountable* to the manager. Thus, managers must be well informed about team members' abilities and must provide controls for safe and acceptable performance.

Too much delegation can overburden team members; too little delegation can overburden managers. Managers must know not only that the task to be delegated is consistent with the team member's job description but also that the member has the ability to actually perform the task. The ability to know when help is needed and willingness to ask for help are also important considerations.

Requirements for success in delegation include matching the right person to the right task, providing authority and resources for task completion, and establishing accountability for correct achievement. Thus, project team members must know the expectations—the specific results to be obtained—if delegation is to be effective. Information needed to complete the task, the time frame for completion, opportunities for clarification, and validating standards of accountability with the project member are necessary elements for success.

Obstacles to effective delegation may include personal barriers that limit managers' ability to delegate. For example, managers may be reluctant to delegate because of fear of failure, fear of losing control, or fear of being replaced. There may be apprehension that someone else will not do the job as well or will do it too well, or managers may enjoy certain activities and wish to continue performing them. However, managers must recognize that what feels most comfortable is not necessarily the best use of time.

Obstacles to effective delegation may also result because of managers' choices when delegating. Managers may delegate inappropriately by overloading particularly competent project members. However, a history of unsatisfactory work by a member should also alert managers to a possible obstacle to be avoided. Delegating too much to members who are already overburdened may overwhelm them, create resentment, and adversely affect performance.

TEAM BUILDING FOR PROJECT MANAGEMENT

Although team building is an ongoing process in project management, efforts are especially indicated when the group is initially formed (Dyer, 1977). A project team is usually temporary and often functions under unstable organizational conditions which prompted the need for the project. Project team members will not have functioned together previously as a working group, and their loyalties and their time may be divided between the project and their functional departments. However, project team members are selected for the project because of their special and diverse abilities and skills. Accomplishment of the project goal is dependent on coordinated team contributions.

Involvement of team members as early as possible in the project is desirable to permit their participation in project planning and to establish group standards that will promote effective team function. Graham (1985) recommends that the project manager involve the team members in network planning to plan activities, deadlines, and their contributions to the project goal. This involvement provides the team members with a total view of the project as they develop as a team.

Since project team members will interact with functional departments and other project team members from diverse backgrounds, good interpersonal interactions are necessary for effective problem solving. Modeling the interactions needed in problem solving with diverse members, as described by Decker and Nathan (1985), may be a helpful approach to promote the desired social learning required in team building.

Social learning may also assist in achieving high standards of team performance. The Pygmalian effect (Livingston, 1969) can be useful in team building. Based on this phenomenon, it has been shown that performance will depend on the manager's treatment of subordinates. When the manager expects success of group members, the expectations are more likely to occur. Livingston (1969) observed that being able to inspire success in group members depended on the manager's self-image, realistic goals, and the manager's sincere confidence in members that was evident to them. Successful experience in management, knowledge of tasks to be accomplished, and rapport and support by administration are factors that enhance the project manager's self-confidence to facilitate team function.

Team development will need to continue throughout the project. The diversity of member characteristics and conditions involved in projects will require project managers who can effectively manage both team members and activities. Situations will arise that require problem solving within the group. Knowledge of departmental operations and professional skills, management skills, effective communication and interpersonal relationships are thus essential for the project manager. Political skills will also be required.

New norms will emerge as the team develops. Thus management approaches will be contingent on the prevailing conditions and will vary as the project proceeds. Since the purpose of a project is usually innovation, it is important to recognize that there is not a standardized method to accomplish the project goal. An environment fostering creativity is needed. Imagination, flexibility, and cooperation are team assets that need to be rewarded.

Teamwork is essential for progress and survival of any organization but is particularly important in effective project management. Farley and Stoner (!989) describe team building as an integral function of corporate nurse leaders. They acknowledge that leadership has been necessary in managing teams for patient care, but other skills are now needed to establish and maintain executive teams between disciplines. Group process skills must include skills needed in power relationships. The leader may need to establish relationships to support team efforts and may have to negotiate conditions in order to promote team functioning. See Chapter 17 for more information on group process.

PLANNING IN PROJECT MANAGEMENT

Project management requires the effective use of time in order to accomplish all that is expected. Thus, it is essential to utilize personal organization and self-management. This process includes setting goals, establishing priorities, objectives, and deadlines. In order to improve time utilization, it is important that project managers utilize strategies to plan project activities and to meet required deadlines.

Project Proposal

An initial step in planning for a project is the development of a proposal for the project. After the need is identified, the proposal is submitted to secure the approval and resources for proceeding. Let us suppose that a potential need for rehabilitative services has been identified in a private, acute care, city hospital. Before a rehabilitation unit could become a reality in the setting, the need would have to be justified prior to development of a specific project plan. The following activities could be achieved through a preliminary project directed by a corporate nurse leader.

1. Submit the initial proposal to the administrator, usually the chief executive officer (CEO) of the institution to obtain approval for detailed exploration of the need.
2. Select professionals within the institution to collect data to begin developing the formal proposal to be submitted to the institution's governing board by the administrator. The team could be selected from medicine, nursing, physical therapy, social work, and other related areas.
3. Explore funding sources for possible grant funds to conduct the feasibility study and for sources of funds for construction or start-up costs.
4. Develop a market feasibility plan with the team to demonstrate the specific demand for the unit and to justify expenditures. Statistical support for projected needs should be available. Examples of data collected include: How many patients are referred elsewhere for rehabilitative services? Do other regional institutions refer patients to other facilities at great distances? Would patients in smaller outlying facilities utilize rehabilitation services in this institutional setting if available? What recurrent patient problems exist because of a present lack of available services? How will provision of services in the planned location be cost effective for patients? Are adequate specialists (eg, neurologists, neurosurgeons, othopedic specialists, nurse clinicians) available?
5. Select other specialists to project the potential budgetary implications of offering the services. What would be the usual length of hospitalization? Would outpatient services be needed? What mechanisms for reimbursement of services exist? What case mix of personnel would be needed for staffing? Are needed and qualified staff available?
6. Determine the budgetary implications of constructing or converting a physical unit to provide rehabilitation services. What location is needed for accessibility to consumers and other needed services? How many patient rooms would be required? What additional space such as therapy facilities would be needed? What additional equipment are required? What are the projected capital and operational costs for construction, equipment, personnel, and supplies?
7. Review appropriate guidelines such as state and local health rules and regulations, building codes, licenses, sanitation and environmental codes and regulations, and safety regulations. Is compliance possible for the potential project? Consult the institution's attorney to review all necessary legal criteria and guidelines.
8. Submit the formal proposal with justification for the proposed project.

The previous hypothetical proposal illustrates preliminary planning that would be needed before a decision on a project could be reached. A specific action plan for implementation is then needed.

Project Plan and Checklist
In the planning phase of project management, the approved project is developed as a project plan for implementation and the project manager is selected. In health care

settings, physicians, nurses, social workers, or other professionals may function as project managers. The nurse project manager's clinical knowledge is an advantage in interacting with other health professionals in a variety of health settings. Nurses with clinical, administrative, and management qualifications are especially suited as project managers (Orsolits, 1988).

The project manager's position should be depicted in an organizational chart for the project. Using a chart similar to the rehabilitation product line shown in Figure 25–4, the project manager's position would indicate team representation from various functional areas and direct accountability to the CEO.

Project team members should be involved in planning how to meet the project goals. Program documentation including project goals, policies, procedures for action, budgets, and plans assists in control of the project. This information should be included in a project manual which is developed as the project evolves.

Cleland and King (1968) recommend the project checklist for periodic evaluation by a review team and by the project manager. Representatives from the project can serve as the review team using the checklist to determine the project's status and progress. These reviews permit identification of difficulties such as improper sequencing of activities and allow needed readjustments. Depending on the scope of the project, the checklist may explore areas such as reporting, staffing, communication, management, and budgeting. See *Systems Analysis and Project Management* (Cleland & King, 1968) and *Project Management for Executives* (Kerzner, 1982) for detailed treatment of the project checklist.

Network Planning Techniques

Planning tools for project management are often referred to as network planning techniques. These techniques require that activities of a project be identified so that they can be scheduled, coordinated, and controlled within projected time periods. The project manager may select techniques such as Gantt charts, PERT, CPM, and LOB which are included in the following descriptions.

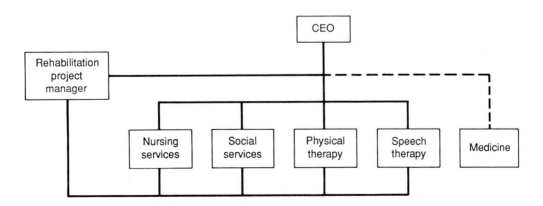

Figure 25–4. Organizational Chart for the Project Manager *(Source: MK Hermann)*

Gantt Charts. The Gantt chart, one of the first planning tools developed, is especially useful to display schedules and deadlines. Desired time periods can be shown on the horizontal axis with activities, events, or items listed along the left vertical side of the chart. Symbols such as the bar may indicate work schedules for designated periods of time (Longenecker & Pringle, 1981). Figure 25–5 shows the use of a Gantt chart for displaying activities in developing the rehabilitation proposal example. Activities and deadlines are easily visualized to monitor completion of projects by a target date (Gilles, 1989). Because of this advantage, Gantt charts and network charts may both be used for planning a project (Graham, 1985).

PERT. Program Evaluation Review Technique (PERT) is a more complicated technique than the Gantt chart but may be desirable when many activities must be coordinated in a project. PERT has been widely used in government, military, and industrial projects since its development by the Navy (Miller, 1962). PERT permits the project planner a total view of the activities involved in the project. This is possible because PERT requires the project to be broken into individual activities from which prequisite activities are selected and sequenced to achieve the desired outcome. Time estimates must be projected for each activity to plan for completion of the project. When those variables are diagrammed in a PERT chart, the total requirements and interrelated activities can be seen.

After the activities of the project are identified, they are labeled according to the sequences and time in days needed for completion. Although there are many variations, when using the ''activity on arrow'' notation, circles represent events which are connected to other dependent events by an arrow which shows the end of that

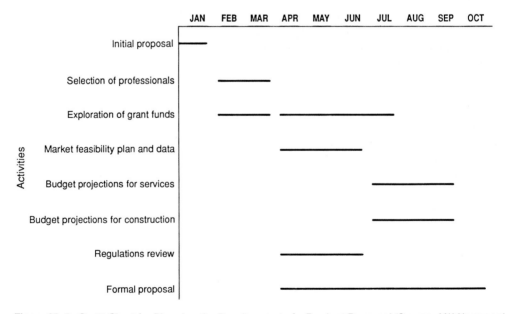

Figure 25–5. Gantt Chart for Planning the Development of a Product Proposal *(Source: MK Hermann)*

activity. Numbers inside the circles may be used to show the progression of events from node to node. Letters symbolizing activities may be placed above the arrow, while numbers below the arrows indicate estimates of time for completion of the activity (Graham, 1985).

Completion of two or more activities may be required prior to an event which may require more than one activity for its completion. This may result in several arrows converging on or emerging from an event. This results in different tiers of events that eventually merge to achieve the final goal. Hayden (1986) recommends no less than 10 and no more than 100 events in a PERT network. However, some projects may contain thousands of events. When a project is extremely complicated, he recommends a summary network for major tasks of the overall project and detailed networks for smaller parts of the project.

The probable time needed for completion of each activity is projected to obtain the least, average, and longest time that may be required. Formulas may be used to calculate the *critical path time* and the *slack time* to permit readjustment to meet final deadlines. Examining the network reveals the critical or longest time it will take to complete the project.

The scenario that follows will be used to illustrate network planning and use of the PERT chart. Returning again to our hypothetical rehabilitation project proposal, we will continue with the project plan to develop these services as a product line. Rehabilitation services will be offered by constructing a new hospital unit and will utilize existing support systems in the institution. The institution's governing board has approved the proposal based upon the feasibility study and has allocated funds for construction and staffing using a managed care approach.

As the newly appointed nurse project manager, your task is to coordinate the activities of project team members and to collaborate with construction and engineering representatives to implement a two-year completion schedule.

The institution views its mission as an important service to the community. Thus, community education will be important to communicate the services that will be offered. Both quality and cost standards must be met. Fortunately, there are experienced and capable nurse clinicians, physicians, and other health professionals who are available and challenged by the opportunity to participate in the project. You are an experienced clinical nurse with previous head nurse, quality assurance, and nurse management experience and are also qualified for the position by your business background and graduate education. The chief nurse executive recommended you for this position and has offered support if needed. Top management recognizes the importance of this development to the institution and has provided the necessary authority for your position. You will be reporting directly to the CEO although you will work closely with directors of all departments and with managers of functional units and support services. The institutional commitment has been widely shared to acquaint all levels with the planned project.

Your beginning objective is to select the project team members, eg, physicians, nurse managers, clinicians from other nursing units, a finance officer, construction and engineering representatives, and representatives from other health professions. Once the team is selected, you will involve them in developing appropriate aspects of the project plan for implementation. Consultants may be sought as the plan proceeds, and additional members may be recruited to accomplish discrete tasks identified by the primary team.

With your project team, you analyze the outcomes and deadlines for initiating rehabilitation services as a product line. Managed care with multidisciplinary teams has been selected for the delivery of comprehensive services for this unit. This means that a future care management team will be involved not only for patients admitted to the rehabilitation unit but also for other patients that may need rehabilitation services. A team member may be notified, for example, when a patient arrives for emergency care (eg, patient with head injury), for a patient in an intensive-care unit (eg, following a craniotomy for brain tumor), or for a patient on a general unit who has or develops a condition requiring rehabilitation services (eg, a patient with hemiparesis related to cerebral hemorrhage).

With these background requirements, your approach is to involve the project team in network planning. The team identifies the activities for the project and estimates the time for their completion. Since these activities must be implemented in the appropriate sequence, the team also identifies those that must be completed first and the needed sequence for scheduling them. The project activities and their prerequiste activities are shown in Table 25–2.

The identified activities are then depicted as letters on a PERT chart with the average expected time in weeks below the arrow representing the activity. As shown in Figure 25–6, the PERT diagram provides a visual overview of the entire project showing the major events for establishing the hypothetical product line. The critical path is the longest time (8 + 8 + 6 + 4 + 4 + 2 + 48 + 3 + 3 = 86) in weeks.

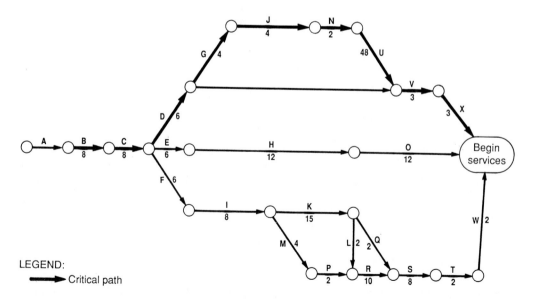

Figure 25-6. Project Planning Using a PERT Chart

CPM. The Critical Path Method (CPM) is similar to PERT since it also uses events and projected times for completion of activities. However, CPM uses only the longest time estimate which is obtained from those experienced with the activity (Longenecker & Pringle, 1981). Being able to closely judge the time required for separate activities is more likely for previously implemented activities than for the implementation of a new project. Thus, CPM may be especially useful for detailed parts of project planning. A current application of critical path technique is in case management with the use of critical paths for planning and evaluating patient outcomes (Zander, 1988; Togno-Armanasco et al, 1989).

LOB. Line-of-balance (LOB) has been used in various applications since its development in 1941 (Mundorff, 1963). LOB provides an expected standard for a designated time against which production is measured. According to Enrick (1965), LOB is a method for forecasting and evaluating progress that requires: (a) identifying necessary events; (b) using a flowchart to show the sequence and priority of events; and (c) showing the time required for each event. LOB also can be used for cost monitoring, and periodic reports can indicate progress toward scheduled events. When there is imbalance between planned and actual outcomes, later events may then be delayed. This technique can be adapted for monitoring research and development progress (Mundorff, 1963).

LOB uses information from a chart to display the expected and actual level of accomplishment (Murdoff, 1962). The line of balance may be designated by a dotted line with actual values plotted to show comparison with the LOB. Although LOB has been used widely to monitor or report production units, it could be used to show the number of services projected and delivered or to visualize projected and actual utilization for designated time periods. Figure 25–7 illustrates the planned budget as the LOB for a project and the actual expenditures for each month.

Comparing Network Planning Techniques. Gantt and LOB charts require fewer people, less training, and less consultation than do PERT and CPM methods; computer analysis is usually required for PERT and CPM which provide more information for planning and adjusting schedules (Glaser, 1963). PERT is considered especially suitable for research projects while LOB is ranked highest for production and subcontracting projects (Glaser, 1963).

Planning techniques such as Gantt charts, PERT, CPM, and LOB facilitate planning projects and therefore result in more efficient and objective plans and outcomes. Network tools also facilitate improvement in structure and communication, save time, and are particularly useful for task force or project forms of organizations as well as for specific projects.

SUMMARY

Health care institutions are finding project management useful in adapting to rapidly changing conditions in their environments. Corporate nurse leaders have a

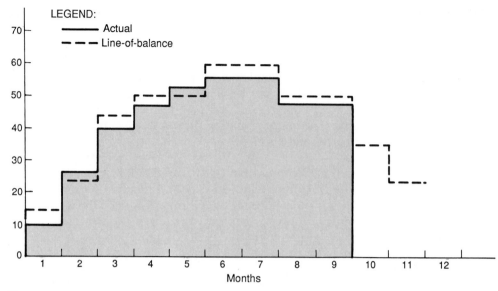

Figure 25-7. Budget Allocation for a Project and Actual Expenditures Using Line-of-Balance (LOB).

significant role to play in initiating and implementing various health care services provided through project management organizational structures. Nurse managers may serve as project managers and inevitably will be involved directly or indirectly with some form of program, product, or service line management.

Project management demands continued and increasing attention to the process of leadership. Using influence to motivate others in leader-follower interactions is requisite to goal accomplishment. Developing others through delegation and planned team building will facilitate the combined team efforts needed to meet organizational demands.

In-depth analysis and detailed planning are required for corporate nurse leaders and nurse managers participating in project management. These leaders are uniquely destined to utilize and refine their skills to meet the challenges demanded in dynamic organizations. These challenges generate new opportunities for leadership in the health care field.

REFERENCES

Amabile TM, Gryskiewicz SS. Creative human resources in the R & D laboratory: How environment and personality affect innovation. In: Kuhn RL, ed-in-chief. *Handbook for Creative and Innovative Managers* (pp. New York, McGraw-Hill, 1988:501–524

Chung KH. *Motivational Theories and Practices.* Columbus, OH, Grid Inc, 1977

Cleland DI. A kaleidoscope of matrix management systems. In: Cleland DI, ed. *Matrix Management Systems Handbook.* New York, Van Nostrand Reinhold Co, 1984

Cleland DI, King WR. *Systems Analysis and Project Management.* New York, McGraw-Hill, 1968

Dansereau F, Graen G, Haga WH. A vertical dyad linkage approach to leadership in formal organizations. *Organizational Behavior and Human Performance*. 13:46, 1975

Dixon M. Matrix organization in health services. In: Knight K, ed. *Matrix Management, A Cross-Functional Approach to Management*. England PBI-Petrocelle Books, 1978:82–90

Dossett DL. Motivating staff. In: Sullivan EJ, Decker PJ, eds. *Effective Management in Nursing*, 2nd ed. Menlo Park, CA, Addison-Wesley, 1988:179–207

Dossett DL, Jenkins RL, Decker PJ, Sullivan EJ. Leadership skills. In Sullivan EJ, Decker PJ, eds. *Effective Management in Nursing*, 2nd ed. Menlo Park, CA: Addison-Wesley, 1988:209–237

Dyer WG. *Team Building: Issues and Alternatives*. Reading, MA, Addison-Wesley, 1977

Enrick NL. *Management Operations Research*. New York, Holt, Rinehart and Winston, 1965

Farley MJ, Stoner MH. The nurse executive and interdisciplinary team building. *Nursing Administration Quarterly*. 13:24, 1989

Fiedler FE. Leadership: A New Model. In: Gibb CA, ed. *Leadership, Selected Readings*. Baltimore, Penguin Books, 1969:230–241 (Original published in 1965)

Fiedler FE. *A Theory of Leadership Effectiveness*. New York, McGraw-Hill, 1967

French Jr JRP, Raven B. The bases of social power. (Reprinted from D. Cartwright (Ed.), *Studies in Social Power*. Ann Arbor, MI, Institute for Social Research. In Cartwright D, Zander A, eds. *Group Dynamics: Research and Theory*, 2nd ed. Evanston, IL, Row, Peterson, 1960:607–623

Gaddis PO. The project manager. *Harvard Business Review* 37:89, 1959

Gilles DA. *Nursing Management*. Philadelphia: WB Saunders, 1989

Glaser JJ. Critical Path Method (CPM). In: Heyel C, ed. *The Encyclopedia of Management*. New York: Reinhold Publishing Corporation, 1963:142–144

Glaser JJ. Integrated project management. In: Heyel C, ed. *The Encyclopedia of Management*. New York, Reinhold Publishing Corporation, 1963

Graham RJ. *Project Management, Combining Technical and Behavioral Approaches for Effective Implementation*. New York, Van Nostrand Reinhold Co, 1983

Hayden C. *The Handbook of Strategic Experience*. New York: Free Press, 1986

House RJ, Mitchell TR. Path-goal theory of leadership. *Journal of Contemporary Business*. 81, (Autumn 1974)

Jones KR. Strategic planning in hospitals: Applications to nursing administration. *Nursing Administration Quarterly*. 13:1988

Kerzner H. *Project Management for Executives*. New York, Van Nostrand Reinhold Co, 1982

Kerzner H. Matrix implementation: Obstacles, problems, questions, and answers. In: Cleland DI, ed. *Matrix Management Systems Handbook*. New York, Van Nostrand Reinhold Co, 1984

Landy FJ. *Psychology of Work Behavior*, 4th ed. Pacific Grove, CA, Brooks/Cole Publishing Co, 1989

Livingston JS. Pygmalion in management. In: Shtogren JA, ed. *Models for Management: The Structure of Competence*. Woodlands, TX, Teleometrics, Inc, 1969:39–53

Longenecker JG, Pringle CD. *Management*, 5th ed. Columbus, OH, Charles E Merrill Publishing Co, 1981

Longest Jr BB, Klingensmith JM. Coordination and communication. In: Shortell SM, Kaluzny AD, Associates, eds. *Health Care Management, A Text in Organization Theory and Behavior*, 2nd ed. New York, John Wiley & Sons, 1988:234–264

Miller CC. *Project Management. How to Make it Work*. New York, AMACOM, 1976

Miller RW. How to plan and control with PERT. *Harvard Business Review*. March-April 1962

Mundorff GT. Line of balance. Its value in manufacturing operations. In: Stilian GH, et al. *PERT*. New York, American Management Association, 1962:164–171

Mundorff GT. Line of Balance (LOB). In: Heyel C, ed. *The Encyclopedia of Management*. New York, Reinhold Publishing Corporation, 1963:420–428

Nackel JG, Kues IW. Product-line management: Systems and strategies. *Hospital and Health Services Administration*. 31:109, 1986

Orsolits M. Product line management: Third generation decentralization. In: Stull MK, Pinkerton SE, eds. *Current Strategies for Nurse Administrators*. Rockville, MD, Aspen Publishers, 1988:51–63

Togno-Armanasco VD, Olivas GS, Harter S. Developing an integrated nursing case management model. *Nursing Management*. 20:26, 1989

Vecchio RP, Gobdel BC. The vertical dyad linkage model of leadership: Problems and prospects. *Organizational Behavior and Human Performance*. 34:1984

Vroom VH. *Work and Motivation*. New York, John Wiley and Sons, 1964

Vroom VH, Yetton PW. *Leadership and Decision-Making*. Pittsburgh, University of Pittsburgh Press, 1973a

Vroom VH. A new look at managerial decision-making. *Organizational Dynamics*. 66, Spring, 1973b

Wodinsky HB, Egan D, Markel F. Product line management in oncology: A Canadian experience. *Hospital and Health Services Administration*. 33:221, 1988

Zander K. Nursing case management. *Journal of Nursing Administration*. 18:5, 23, 1988

Optimizing the Organization

CHAPTER 26

Nursing Marketing

Douglas Fugate
Germaine Freese

Key Concept List

Origins of marketing
Exchange relationships
Marketing mix
Development of a marketing orientation
Market segmentation and target marketing
Market research
Marketing of nursing services

For most nursing administrators, the practice of marketing might seem to be a low priority item on an otherwise crowded managerial agenda. The traditional understanding of marketing implies some sort of business activity like packaging or advertising. These commercial practices must seem far removed from the primary mission of planning, organizing, staffing, and directing for the care of patients. However, recent changes in the health care industry suggest that marketing has become an important managerial tool for nursing executives. This chapter explores the origins of marketing, explain basic marketing concepts, shows why marketing can be important to nursing administrators, and demonstrates how various market planning tools apply to the practice of nursing.

ORIGINS OF MARKETING

Prehistoric peoples lived in small, self-sufficient groups. Typically, group members produced goods (eg, cooking vessels) or performed services (eg, gathering firewood) for immediate consumption by the primary living group. There was little thought of creating inventories and economic wealth.

Later on, someone recognized that goods produced by one group could be traded for useful objects produced by another group. However, exchanging things of value necessitated producing goods in excess of that needed by the immediate living group. Workers had to work more efficiently and effectively to create surpluses. Eventually, this shift in thinking resulted in a new economic order: one based on exchange, specialization of labor, and speculative production.

Exchange required a communication system so communal groups could inform each other about what was available. It also required a pricing system so parties in an exchange relationship would have a sense of what kind of value was given and what kind of value was received. It is axiomatic that one only trades when one perceives a net gain in total wealth.

Over time, trading between communal groups became more institutionalized. Recognized trading rules and trading locations were observed by many people. Certain places were selected as market places because of their proximity to land routes, river navigation, prominent features or other considerations. Many of those ancient trading locations still exist today as modern cities.

Exchange Relationships

The basic requirements for a marketing exchange are two parties, each with something of value that the other desires, information about these objects, a pricing system to establish their worth, and a place or mechanism whereby things of value can be exchanged. These elements of product (something of value), promotion (information), price (worth of the product as perceived by the parties), and place (where the product is received) are commonly called the 4 P's of marketing; collectively they are called the *marketing mix.* The conscious planning of these variables to achieve a goal is called *marketing management.*

The Concept of Utility

The elements of the marketing mix are largely responsible for manifesting the economic concept of utility. Utility means usefulness. Activities which increase the functional usefulness of a product adds form utility. For example, biodegradable medical supplies have more form utility than those that are not. Activities which overcome the problems of time and distance between producers and users of a product add time and place utility. For example, medications manufactured in Massachusetts are not of much use to a nurse in Los Angeles unless someone arranged for transportation and storage in California where they are needed. Activities which facilitate the ability to own, possess, or otherwise control the use of a product creates possession utility. For example, billing procedures which allow products to be purchased on credit or on some sort of automatic order/payment system increases possession utility. Marketers who are able to provide the greatest bundle of utilities or satisfactions are usually most sought out by customers. Marketing managers must create and consistently maintain an offering of need satisfying products or services.

DEVELOPMENT OF A MARKETING ORIENTATION

Until recently, the elements of the marketing mix were planned for the benefit of the manufacturers or sellers of products. The American economy operated for many years with a production orientation—a system which primarily benefited those who controlled productive factors. Rapid population growth, western expansion, the Industrial Revolution, and the lack of effective laws governing business power and practices practically ensured domination by manufacturing interests. Americans were pleased to have affordable, mass produced products widely available. Manufacturers gave little thought to the wants and needs of individual consumers.

Increased competition, a relatively high standard of living, and a slackening of demand brought an end to the production orientation in the early 1900s. This period was followed by a relatively short sales orientation era. This was a time when producers made many unsubstantiated claims in order to stimulate consumption. Since goods no longer sold themselves, high-pressure sales tactics, radio advertising, and sales promotions were used extensively. Many of our consumer protection oriented laws were passed in response to these practices.

With the articulation of the marketing concept consumers, not producers, of goods were given primary consideration by enlightened managers. The marketing concept, a simple yet powerful philosophy, states organizations should exist to serve its buyers or markets; organizations should be goal directed; and organizations should integrate marketing with the other management functions.

The marketing concept was revolutionary because it placed the consumer in the center of the consumption cycle. In a very real sense, the desires of consumers became the device which allocated the use of land, labor, and capital resources of this country. Customers no longer were faced with purchase options that could be manufactured efficiently but provided limited satisfaction. Customers no longer were obligated to transact many kinds of business activities at locations or times that were convenient only to the producer. Marketing oriented organizations were willing to provide new product shapes, new locations, new times, and new purchasing alternatives. In other words, marketers were willing to increase the form, place, time, and possession utilities associated with most products and services.

Since greater utility (in a relative, not absolute sense) means greater satisfaction with the purchase, those organizations who provide the greatest satisfaction are rewarded with sustained patronage or customer loyalty. Health care in America has belatedly followed this marketing evolution. Traditionally, the health care market was self-driven by producers of medical products and medical services. However, insurance companies, governments, and consumers have begun applying pressure on those producers to keep health costs down and to be more responsive to consumer demands. Health care organizations are being forced to create more utilities in order to survive.

MARKET SEGMENTATION AND TARGET MARKETING

In a complex society, it is unlikely that all prospective buyers will perceive the same quotient of utility in any given purchase. Different groups of people will desire different combination of product attributes or characteristics. This means marketers must take a large heterogeneous group of prospective buyers and divide them into smaller, more similar groups who want approximately the same thing. This process is called *market segmentation.* Each subgroup is called a *market segment.* Useful segments are those which exhibit intragroup homogeneity and intergroup heterogeneity, possess identifiable product needs, can be readily reached through available channels of communication, are large enough to service efficiently, and are permanent enough to justify the allocation of limited organizational resources.

There are many ways to segment a market—for example, demographic variables such as age, sex or income; psychographic variables such as lifestyle; or behavioral variables such as quantity used or occasion used. Some marketers use a single variable to segment markets (eg, all customers between 18 and 25 years of age) but most often two or more segmentation variables are used (eg, all males between 18 and 25 years of age who live in rural areas). A nursing division of a hospital is often divided into subunits based on disease entities (eg, cardiac care), body systems (eg, neurology) or other patient characteristic, such as age (eg, pediatrics).

Marketers are typically not interested in serving all market segments. Each segment should be evaluated according to a set of predetermined criteria. For example, some segments are not attractive because they are already being satisfactorily served by another firm. Some segments are eliminated because the organization does not possess the factors required to successfully satisfy that segment. Assessing each segment against this weighted (since all criteria are not equally important) list of evaluation criteria should identify the natural target markets of the organization. Selecting the largest segments as your target markets is often a poor decision. These segments will typically be the most crowded with competitors and be most subject to price competition because supply is greater than demand. Seeking the largest segments is called the majority fallacy.

If a single target market is chosen, the organization is practicing a concentration strategy. It is a high risk strategy since all objectives must be satisfied from a single source. However, it does allow for specialization and accompanying benefits such as an accelerated learning curve and high level of expertise. If two or more target markets are chosen, the organization is practicing a *multisegment* strategy. Obviously it is less risky but requires more resources, encounters more competition, and is more difficult to manage.

Failure to segment and target markets leaves an organization in the position of practicing *mass marketing.* This simply means an organization offers its products to all potential buyers without any consideration given to the differences that may exist between these customers. Mass marketing is a very high risk strategy since almost any competitor can offer segment members a more satisfying product. Eventually, the organization practicing mass marketing may have no customers except those who have no freedom to choose otherwise. The practice of mass marketing health care is too expensive in terms of utilizing health care resources to be viable in today's economy.

NEED FOR MARKET RESEARCH

Market segmentation and targeting requires the marketing manager to have a good understanding of the market. Marketers need to know what product attributes will satisfy each segment, what promotion efforts will reach each segment, where exchanges should take place to provide place utility, and how much customers are willing to pay for the total bundle of satisfactions they receive. It also requires a thorough understanding of how consumers make purchase decisions, knowledge of competitors, and an awareness of a host of environmental variables which could influence the organization's ability to provide satisfying products.

The process of gaining the information necessary to operate any business is called *market research*. The research process can range from very informal to very formal. Informal research techniques often rely on personal observations, chance meetings, networking opportunities, and other unprogrammed actions which give managers some idea of their markets. Formal research techniques rely on more systematic gathering of information from sources both inside and outside the firm. Surveys, experimental designs, expert panels, and subscriptions to proprietary or syndicated research reports are typical of the formal research effort.

Information which is routinely gathered, codified, analyzed, and stored is part of a *marketing information system*. The MIS becomes a ready source of information for decision makers. Nurses frequently use the data collected into the MIS to analyze current and projected acuity levels. When the MIS cannot provide sufficient depth or detail, managers often request a specific market research project. This effort is very narrow in its focus since it is intended to answer a one-time question. If the same question arises frequently, the information needs should be built in the MIS system.

MARKETING MIX

Once an organization has decided which segment or segments to serve, the manager begins the task of putting together a *marketing mix*. The marketing mix is much like a recipe. The individual ingredients are not nearly as important as the outcome. Managers must constantly work to ensure that the marketing mix elements are highly complementary.

Product

The product, whether it be a physical product or an intangible service, or some combination of both, is a bundle of attributes which help satisfy consumer's consumption problems. These attributes are product manifestations or outcomes which consumers use to compare one alternative with another. The marketer must carefully select which attributes belong in the product and then ensure that consumers are aware of those attributes and their utilities to the user.

Until recently, the health care consumer was not actively involved in choosing health care products. The free market principle that product information is readily available to both consumers and producers was not characteristic of the health care arena. As a result of this and other market forces, consumers made little use of product attributes in their decision processes.

In some cases, consumers choose to ignore evaluating product attributes, assuming that all products are nearly identical. These products are known as *convenience goods*. The buyer is unwilling to invest much time and effort in choosing between alternatives since there is little expected gain. In some cases, consumers can be informed that all products are not the same and that distinct satisfying differences do exist. However, if no bona fide differences exists, marketers of convenience products must rely on lower price, better distribution, or other marketing mix decisions to help market their product. One special case of convenience goods is *emergency goods*. These are unplanned purchases where immediate availability is the primary consideration. An emergency room visit is an example of emergency goods. Under normal conditions, consumers would make these purchases using a different set of criteria.

Sometimes, products are similar but still possess a unique set of product attributes. There are many brands of automobiles, all provide basic transportation, but all have distinct design features, images, options, and other characteristics which set them apart. These are called *shopping goods*. This simply means that consumers will compare each set of attributes or product offering to find the one that most clearly matches their needs, including affordability. This is an area where consumer knowledge is paramount. Without knowing which features are valued, marketers may fail to satisfy enough consumers to stay in business. Obstetrical services, while offering the same basic delivery service, have expanded and begun marketing specific product attributes which attract certain categories of buyers (eg, home-like birthing centers).

The customer who seeks out a product and will accept no substitute is seeking a *specialty product*. Specialty products possess some combination of unique satisfying characteristics. Marketers who can successfully turn their products into specialty goods can usually command higher prices and more desirable outlets.

Branding

To help consumers readily find products that they have used before, marketers often brand their products. Brand names identify a particular seller's products and may enjoy legal protection. Besides identification, brand names can convey product benefits (eg, "Sick Bay," day care for children who are too ill to go to school). Brand names should be easy to remember, distinctive, and identifiable with the product category (eg, "The Stork Club" for a maternity program).

Packaging

Packaging is an important part of product development. Just as a brand name suggests the product benefits, a package can also symbolically or tangibly convey important product attributes. Pancake syrup comes in attractive, table ready containers. We do not eat the package but it makes it more useful to us. Strong detergents come in boldly colored packages; this signifies strength. Mild detergents come in pastels and white, signifying gentleness. Packaging primarily must protect but beyond that packaging can communicate much product information, extend the utility of the contents, increase the value of the purchase by having a usable package after the contents are gone, serve as a visible reminder of the purchase, and even stimulate repeat buying by some system of refunds or reuse. The attire of a nursing staff is a form of packaging for nursing care. Numerous institutions are switching from the classical white uniforms to a ''package'' representative of the institution.

Price

Price has two basic roles: information and allocation. The information role, besides providing the price, acts in a variety of ways. Low prices suggest value or perhaps low quality; high prices suggest exclusiveness or perhaps high quality. It is a perception or surrogate indicator rather than an absolute piece of information. For example, patients might not have much confidence in a cut-rate physician or hospital. The allocation role tells potential consumers what portion of their limited resources this purchase will require. This allows consumers to determine how to get the greatest quantity of satisfaction from various combinations of purchases.

There are many pricing objectives. However, nearly all will have to be related to profitability in the long run. Pricing is the only business activity that generates revenue for the organization. In the short run, pricing may be used to increase volume (in a growing market), to shift consumers from one product to another, to increase market share (in static or growing markets), to help sell complementary goods (eg, sell cameras near cost in order to sell higher margin film and film processing), or to introduce new products (low introductory price to reduce risk).

Whatever pricing strategy is chosen, the marketer must estimate demand at that price level and forecast the response of competitors. The first tells the marketers if the pricing objectives can be reached and the second allows the marketer to anticipate and plan for future competitive reactions.

Place

The distribution of a product greatly influences its ability to provide time and place utility to the buyer. For example, automatic bank teller machines permit consumers to access banking services at convenient locations and convenient times. Banks that do not provide this service are at a greater competitive disadvantage.

Marketers typically create channels of distribution to move the product from producer to user. In the case of small, easily handled, and/or shelf stable products, this channel may be quite long (many intermediaries between producer and user). In the case of services, the channel is typically quite short (few intermediaries between producer and user). In some cases, where there is a fixed service facility (eg, an amusement park, hospital, or a laundromat), the user must go to the provider. Health care institutions have operationalized new channels by providing home health care services within catchment areas, mobile treatment units, and free standing outpatient clinics.

Channel members must focus on the needs of the final consumer as well as their own needs. The individual success of any channel member is unimportant if the final consumer is dissatisfied. Channels often are highly integrated in order to maintain the kind of channel control in order to provide consistent time and place utility. Channels also influence price—storage, transportation, materials handling, insurance, security, documentation, order processing, and risk taking can become quite expensive for certain products.

Promotion

Target markets cannot evaluate and purchase product offerings, no matter how well conceived and satisfying, unless they are aware of their existence. The generic role of marketing promotions is to inform, persuade, or remind customers about a product.

Promotion management begins with an understanding of the target markets the firm has chosen to serve. This means one must know which media (eg, newspapers, television, and so on) they use to get information and understand how they process information and make decisions. Without such basic information, any promotion efforts are expenditures with only random chances for successful communication.

Basic active promotion objectives are to attract new customers, to encourage more consumption of the product among existing customers, or to attract a larger share of existing customers. However, not all promotion efforts are intended to result in short-run behavior by the target market. Sometimes, promotion objectives are set to create awareness or to inform potential customers. Perhaps they are designed to bring about a favorable attitude changes. Often, the intent is to create a favorable image among important and interested public groups (eg, stockholders, government officials, suppliers, and professional organizations). This is called good will advertising.

Health care organizations have traditionally communicated their ability to treat illnesses to health care consumers who were ill (Porter-O'Grady, 1990). Today, health care providers are attempting to attract business by communicating their ability to maintain or enhance health and wellness.

Health care facilities have increasingly assumed sponsorships of health-based activities such as fun runs, sporting events, and nutrition fairs. This shift in promotion focus is a key strategic shift for nursing. Although most nurses work in illness care, they have been educated to provide health care and, in this expanding arena, can exercise the expertise their education has provided.

Whatever the objectives, the organization must then develop a promotion strategy consisting of specific goals, plans to achieve them, an adequate budget to support this effort, and a method for evaluating results. The promotion plan will include some combination of promotion tools. This combination is commonly referred to as the *promotion mix*. Like the marketing mix, it is a synergistic blend of elements. The four groupings of promotion tools are advertising, sales promotion, public relations/publicity, and personal selling.

Advertising is the impersonal messages sent through a paid medium with an identified sponsor. Advertising media frequently used include television, radio, newspaper, magazine, transit and highway billboards, telephone and business directories, and a wide variety of direct advertisements (sometimes called specialty advertising).

Sales promotions are an unstructured collection of activities which are typically designed to stimulate some kind of direct action by the receiver. Contests, sweepstakes, demonstrations, free samples, coupons, hot air balloons, banners, point of purchase displays, and brochures are generally classified as sales promotions.

Public relations and publicity are closely related but yet different activities. Every organization has *publics*, or outside groups who have or potentially have an impact on the organization's success. Activities which are designed to foster good will, understanding, forgiveness, or acceptance among any of these groups is called public relations. For example, a free blood pressure screening at the local shopping mall is public relations for a hospital or clinic. If that activity was reported in the local newspaper as a legitimate news item, then publicity has been generated. Publicity is "free" advertising in the sense that the organization did not have to pay for broadcast time or newspaper space because the creation of newsworthy activities can be very expensive. Also, publicity is not always favorable. Published or broadcast incidents of medical malpractice or mistreatment, whether actual or alleged, is a form of publicity health care organizations do not want.

Personal selling is the only promotion tool which provides for face-to-face contact and a two-way exchange between the sender and receiver of a message. It is also the most expensive channel. However, in those situations where customers engage in extended decision making, personal selling may be the only effective tool. Nurses are positioned closest to the patients and, by virtue of this positioning, can promote the selling of quality care.

Each medium has its advantages and disadvantages. It is up to the sender to determine which medium is most appropriate for the message to be sent to the receiver. The constraints of the message, characteristics of the receiver, the budget, the time allowed, and other competing messages makes this a very difficult task.

Product Positioning

The task of the marketing mix is twofold. First, it must make a clear statement about what the seller has to offer to prospective buyers. Second, it must make a clear statement about what the seller has to offer compared to other sellers. This second point is called *positioning*. Marketers should carefully delineate the differences between themselves and others offering somewhat or even very similar products. For example, Hallmark Greeting Cards has built their business by positioning their product as the one to send "when you want to send the very best" or a hospital may advertise itself as "the only level 1 trauma facility in Eastern Oregon."

ORGANIZING FOR MARKETING

Marketing oriented organizations usually place all marketing related activities under someone at the vice-presidential level. This ensures that marketing is no less visible or influential than other functional activities such as personnel or accounting. Below the vice-president, the organizational structure varies widely. The usual structures focus on managing individual products through product managers or managing individual functions such as advertising, research, sales, or customer relations.

The primary difference between the two basic structures is in the scope and authority of the managers. Product managers are only concerned with marketing their products or product line. However, they have no real authority. They must lobby for functional support and justify the resources they request. Functional managers allocate their resources to various products under the direction of a manager who has simultaneous responsibility for all products offered. Both systems have strengths and weaknesses. Often, some combination scheme is used instead of exclusively one or the other.

MARKETING MANAGEMENT

All management operations follow the same basic format. Someone assumes responsibility for monitoring marketing results and comparing them against marketing goals. In those cases where performance standards are above or below expectations, an analysis of nonconformance should be performed and remedial action taken. Careful record keeping of all administrative actions is helpful in future planning and execution of marketing plans.

MARKETING FOR NURSE ADMINISTRATORS

Nurse administrators might be tempted to agree that marketing is an interesting business phenomenon but question its relevance to the profession of nursing. Nurses, like accountants or entertainers, are in the business of offering a service to potential consumers. All service businesses must compete for customers just as organizations that sell more tangible goods.

Nursing and marketing share similar philosophy and processes (Smith & Pinkerton, 1988). The philosophy of serving the consumer is inherent in the philosophy of nursing. Also, the steps in the nursing process parallel those in marketing. In many health care settings nursing is the basis of all the services provided. Therefore, nursing and marketing recognize the needs of consumers and the responsibility to serve them so all their requirements are met.

Services
By definition, *services* are something that are experienced, a performance or activity performed for the customer by someone else. Services cannot be owned by the purchaser. However, the benefits of the service can be purchased and consumed by the consumer, for example you are allowed to purchase a long-distance telephone call but you do not own or possess any of the service production equipment or personnel. Services can be associated with tangible goods (eg, a landscaping service which involves design and plants). In other instances, there is literally no physical goods to suggest a service has been consumed (eg, a marriage counseling session). A contin-

uum of service tangibility is shown in Figure 26–1. Nursing services use tangible goods but typically falls toward the "high intangibility" side of the scale. The education nurses provide is generally "low" intangibility but the written educational materials provided are viewed as "high."

Do Nurses Need to Market Their Services?

Nurse administrators might argue that nursing is a profession and is much too serious to package and promote like potato chips. A decade ago, physicians, lawyers, dentists, optometrists, and others advanced the same position. They thought marketing would be harmful to their image, would lower the standards of their profession, would sacrifice quality for volume, and would shift decision making power to a public ill qualified to make those decisions. Today, many professional groups use marketing effectively to increase their sensitivity to consumers needs and desires and to increase consumers awareness of their services.

Rapidly escalating health care costs and a constraining economic environment has created a shift to wellness or health-based activities and, at the same time, an emphasis on cost containment. Consumers are demanding to be involved in health care decisions (Christensen & Inguanzo, 1989). Progressive health care organizations have begun providing information to consumers to assist them in making informed choices. Institutions that can market and regularly implement marketing plans are likely to have a larger, more satisfied clientele than those institutions who do not.

Nurse administrators may argue that nursing is an integral part of the health care package provided by a hospital. Nursing care is a major component in the production of health care services delivered. As such, the admission of a patient to a hospital by a physician automatically requires nursing care; there is no separate demand for nursing care so there is no need for marketing nursing.

However, this derived demand argument fails to recognize the complexity of the consumer decision-making process. In a service organization, everyone and everything that comes in contact with the customer is the product. Consider the following analogy. Domestic airlines fly essentially the same airplanes, land at essentially the same airports, connect with the same ground transportation, and charge competitive prices. Airline passengers do not judge the quality of their flight on the basis of ground acceleration, aeronautical hardware, or the skill of the airline employees they do not see. Passengers have a good flight when their needs are quickly and courteously satisfied by flight attendants. The attendant's performance is immediate, it is

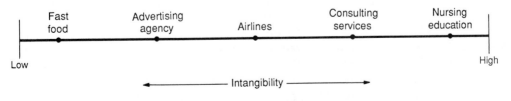

Figure 26-1. Continuum of Service Tangibility

observable, it is relevant, and it becomes the core of the flying experience (barring some misfortune).

Nurses occupy much the same role as the physician who sets broken arms, an attorney who prepare wills, or the bank officer who approves the loan. No matter how technically proficient and accurate the service might be, the satisfaction gained from the service purchase depends largely on the purchasers' face-to-face qualitative perceptions of the provider's (or the provider's employee's) behavior. These perceptions become the basis for favorable word-of-mouth communications about the hospital experience, the basis for stored information for future decision making, and greatly affects the probability that this hospital will be selected again in the future.

Patient satisfaction is an integral component of the marketing program. Costello (1985) reports the primary sources of patient dissatisfaction are: discourteous nurses; discourteous staff attitudes, confusing bill statements, and room appearance. Patient satisfaction is the key to repeat business and positive word of mouth. Organizations measure potential sources of dissatisfaction using patient surveys.

Surveys routinely demonstrate that patients are increasingly asking physicians to admit them to specific hospitals. Patients are choosing hospitals based on previous experiences, recommendations, or perceptions based on the image of a particular hospital. However, due to third-party payment systems, the health care consumer is not always free to choose a specific hospital. In some cases, the consumer is the payer. Lack of consumer choice, consequently, should not be assumed and hospitals must be concerned with consumers' perceptions of the institution.

When two or more hospital facilities are presumed to be similar by potential patients (or the family member making the decision for the patient), evaluations of nursing care often are an important decision influence. This criterion and other key service characteristics are called *determinant attributes*, the comparison of determinant attributes provides a means to choose between available alternatives. Thus, consumers' perceptions of the quality of nursing provided by competing hospitals can help determine the volume of current and future business for a healthcare facility. In this regard, the marketing of nursing helps ensure the continued existence of the hospital.

NURSE ADMINISTRATORS ARE MARKETING MANAGERS

If one accepts that nursing services should be marketed to help create and sustain demand for hospitals services, the logical question is to ask how? First, the marketing concept philosophy requires a systematic approach to marketing. This means that all parts of an organization are expected to maintain consumer satisfaction while also achieving other organizational goals. Quality nursing in this decade will be clinically correct as well as satisfying to consumers if the organization is to prosper. Nurse administrators who manage both dimensions of nursing are good marketing managers.

Second, nursing personnel are the most highly visible providers of health services in most institutions. Economic pressures have decreased occupancy rates of hospitals by switching inpatient services to an outpatient basis and shortening the length of stay. As these events occur, the average acuity level of remaining hospitalized patients is increasing. With the increasing acuity levels and high technological levels of care needed, there are fewer patient activities which can be properly delegated to LPNs or ancillary personnel (Cleland, 1990). It is imperative that nursing administrators have the support staff necessary to deliver care. It is also imperative that nursing administrators demonstrate to consumers that the organization can provide efficient and effective quality care.

Third, nursing care should be viewed as part of a hospital's product mix. It is one of the product lines offered by the organization and, like all product lines, it must positively contribute to overall organizational goals. Under current billing practices, nursing service costs are not used directly to generate revenues. Johnson (1989) has called for treating nursing as a revenue center instead of a cost center. This would mean determining costs so a recovery and contribution price could be placed on nursing services delivered. This would quantitatively demonstrate what nursing contributes to the organization as a whole.

Currently, nursing staffs can indirectly generate revenue by helping increase return hospital stays. This is accomplished by producing satisfied customers (patients) who tell others of their experiences. More hospital stays generate more revenue.

UNIQUE CHARACTERISTICS OF SERVICES

Before the question of how to market nursing services can be addressed, it is necessary to examine the four unique characteristics of services: intangibility, perishability, simultaneity, and homogeneity. These four characteristics influence how a service such as nursing can be marketed.

Intangibility means the service cannot be examined separately from the organization that produced it. Goods have physical properties that can be touched, smelled, tasted, or otherwise evaluated in some place and time distant from the point of production. Goods have some kind of permanence, some evidence that they exist. Services typically have no physical properties, no lasting evidence of existence, and cannot be compared side by side since they are consumed entirely. Often this means that a service business is built on a promise offered by the service provider. If there is sufficient confidence in that promise, the service will be purchased. When the service promise is delivered and compared to expectations, satisfaction or dissatisfaction will occur. Initial lack of confidence in the service provider's promise will result in nonpurchase of the service since the consumers believe that their needs will not be satisfied.

Intangibility also means that services typically cannot be sampled before purchasing. Without any actual service to examine, potential consumers rely heavily on others' recommendations and use whatever judgment and prior experiences to assess the quality of a service offering. In the former case, favorable word-of-mouth recommendations and the reviews of critics heavily influence the decision of theatergoers to attend a particular play or stage production. In the latter case, cues that make the service more tangible help consumers make those assessments. For example, Prudential Insurance uses "the rock" to help consumers visualize the strength and dependability of their company.

The second characteristic is *perishability*. Perishability means that the service cannot be stored up until it is needed. Services exist only at the time of creation and cease to exist once they have been created. For example, unsold theater seats for the 3:00 PM matinee cannot be held until 7:00 PM and then sold. Perishability creates tremendous problems balancing supply and demand since inventories cannot be used to buffer against anticipated or unanticipated needs. Electric utilities face this problem constantly. Providing sufficient generating power potential to meet peak demand loads is very expensive. Having less than peak demand capability means that many electricity consumers will experience "brownouts" or worse, "blackouts." Likewise, services cannot be returned by dissatisfied customers nor can they be repossessed by service providers when they are not paid for.

The third characteristic is simultaneous production and consumption. *Simultaneity* means that services are created and consumed within the same time frame (eg, a physical therapy session). Simultaneity also means that production and marketing of services cannot be optimized in isolation from each other and they should not be separated from each other in an organizational sense. Simultaneous production and consumption mean that the service provider and service user often have to interact on a face-to-face basis. This is also referred to as the customer always being in the service "factory." This means that customers are always "factory workers" and passively or actively participates in the creation of the service. Teaching service consumers to be better workers (eg, use the service better) is one of the tasks of most service marketers. Teaching patients to be good workers (eg, follow care regimens) is one of nurses' tasks.

Simultaneity creates a number of logistical problems which must be resolved by making the customer go to the service provider or taking the service to the user. Services cannot be sold to wholesalers or retailers to provide convenient locations for the service consumer. Simultaneity means that the service producer and user often have to work together. Service providers must agree to help create a positive exchange environment. If a harmonious relationship is not possible, the quality of the service product usually suffers or cannot be performed.

The fourth characteristic is *heterogeneity*. Factories can produce one or one thousand items. The items can be made identical because they can be quality controlled before they leave the factory for storage or delivery. However, it is very unlikely that any quantity of service products will be identical. Differences in services occur because the creation of services depends upon human performances. Humans can be tired, thoughtless, careless, and forgetful. Machines are not. In those situations, quality control becomes a problem of personnel training (see Chapter 15) and administration.

Lack of consistency may be due to variations in the ability or willingness of consumers to participate in the service encounter. The diabetic patient who will not follow the diet may not achieve the same results as one who does.

Finally, heterogeneity may be due to the variance found in the conditions under which the service is performed. Crowding, time constraints, and interruptions by other customers are just a few of the possible variables which might affect service performances and homogeneity of results.

STRATEGIC RESPONSES TO THE UNIQUE CHARACTERISTICS OF SERVICES

Service characteristics pose unique managerial problems and require well executed strategic responses. The following discussion provides helpful strategies.

Dealing with Intangibility

Since services are not material and cannot be evaluated ahead of time, it is important that nurse administrators teach their staff to project an image of providing quality care to potential consumers. This helps build patient confidence and relieves the perception of risk of uncertainty that usually accompanies purchases of the unknown, especially in a threatening situation such as illness.

Nurse administrators must manage the peripheral evidence which indicates that the service exists. This evidence might be a symbol or cue that is normally associated with the service promise you are trying to project. By constantly pairing the symbol with the service, the service takes on the characteristics of the symbol. This is known as classical conditioning. For example, nurses in an obstetrical unit might wear a pelican on their uniform since the pelican is known to take extraordinary measures to take care of their young. If that symbolism is not well known, it can be taught through other promotional programs.

It is important that the nursing service be consistent. Many service providers have been successful, not because they were the best, but because they were predictable. One major motel chain recently built a whole campaign around the theme of "when you stay here there are no surprises." This reduces perceived risk about the type of nursing care that will be provided. It also permits nursing care to become a determining attribute in making hospital choices.

One way to deal with intangibility is to carefully manage the essential evidence— that is, objects that are associated with production of the service but cannot be possessed by the consumer. Tangible objects used or found where services are being provided become part of the service product. Therefore, actions should make equipment look less threatening, more comfortable for the patient, or suggest quality, high technology, or effectiveness. Nurses who wear teddy bears on their stethoscopes are able to make equipment less threatening to their pediatric patients.

Another way to deal with intangibility is to manage the environment within which the nursing service is delivered. Many restaurants command high prices for their food service (which isn't any better than anyone else's) because they deliver it in a satisfying environment or atmosphere. The tangible elements of lighting, furniture, or decorations, help consumers define and evaluate the total dining experience. Nurses can increase patient satisfaction if they ensure quality nursing services are delivered in a need satisfying environment. When nurse administrators encourage their staff to make suggestions about managing the tangible, physical surroundings, patients can use those cues to help define and evaluate their nursing care.

Dealing with Perishability

Unfortunately, nursing care cannot be stored on the shelf until it is needed. This means that each nursing shift must have as many nurses on duty as might potentially be required or run the risk of not having sufficient staff to meet patient care needs. Entirely meeting the potential demand is very expensive and not particularly efficient although satisfying to consumers. Not meeting actual needs might result in customers lost to competitors or worse, have tragic human results.

As marketing managers, nurse administrators are responsible for balancing supply and demand. This accomplishment generates consumer satisfaction and meets organizational goals. One technique to accomplish this is to decouple services. This means separating a normal service performance into those component parts which the nurse must provide and those which others (including the patient) can provide. Performing only predetermined nurse-delivered services, but seeing that other service components are delivered, help balance demand against supply. Nurses' time needs to be utilized performing nursing duties. Tasks that can be done by ancillary health care providers, (eg, housekeeping, pharmacy) need to be delegated to the appropriate personnel. Nurses need to be utilized to provide *nursing* care.

Another possibility is to shift demand from peak time to off-peak times. The telephone company tries to shift users away from heavy weekday use to weekend use by offering lower prices. While there are definite limitations to this technique, nurse administrators might be able to get patients to agree to receive routine procedures at off-peak times in exchange for other inducements. This provides more discretionary time for the nursing staff and allows them to re-allocate their time resources.

The inability to inventory nursing services means that patients often have to wait to receive care. Waiting causes dissatisfaction for patients and others who are protecting the patient's interests. However, research suggests that real time and perceived time are quite different. Customers typically overestimate the time spent waiting (eg, to be seated, served). Service providers have been able to reduce the perception of waiting time by making waiting more comfortable and pleasurable. To the extent possible, nurse administrators should investigate typical waiting areas (eg, examination rooms, clinic seating areas) and determine if they can be made more pleasant.

Nurse administrators need to teach the value of flexibility to their nursing staff. Flexibility means the willingness to vary a work routine as the situation requires. Service providers must be willing to improvise around peak demands and not permit self-imposed (and personally preferred) work routines to interfere with the balance between supply and demand. Flexibility becomes the administrator's creative challenge where nurses are employed within a contractual agreement.

Supply can be increased with part-time help as well. Nurse administrators might want to consider maintaining a pool of nurses who do not want to work full-time but would consider filling in during periods of high demand. This technique poses its own set of problems but should at least be considered as an option to the problem of perishability. Institutions have on-call nursing personnel for high demand but often these are nurses who hold another job.

Dealing with Simultaneity

The characteristic of simultaneity is particularly applicable to nursing care; at least in auto repair, you can leave your car and pick it up later. Nursing does not happen that easily. The core of nursing practice is the patient (Torres, 1985). It is from the patient's needs that the other three concepts (environment, health, and nursing) and all nursing theories are built.

Nursing is an active process which requires a patient. Because the patient must be in contact with the nurse, the nurse should consider the patient as an "employee in the nursing care factory." This philosophical point of point has several practical implications. First, simultaneity affects nursing productivity so any human resources that the patient can provide for his or her own care decreases demands on the nursing staff. Second, perceived loss of control is dissatisfying to most patients. The loss of control may be behavioral, cognitive, or decisional. If the patient is part of the nursing process, it is likely that satisfaction will increase because of user involvement. Perceived risk should be reduced as well.

The nurse administrator encourages the staff to teach scripts and schemas to their patients. A script is a sequence of verbal (or other communicative) exchanges which leads to the appropriate transmission of information between sender and receiver. A schema is a time-ordered sequence of behavioral exchanges that leads to an appropriate completion of a task. Patient education consists of scripts and schemas. Nurses teach health related behavior that helps in health promotion (eg, the impact of lifestyle in preventing heart disease). Nurses also instruct patients on maintaining health. Patients who are able to self-catherize after instructions from the nurse have used a schema.

It may be necessary to reward nurses who adopt the "consumer as producer" position since there may be some who do not accept that nursing is something that is done *with*, not to, the patient. Also nurses are typically the ones who need to indicate when scripts and schemas need to be changed.

Depending on the circumstances, simultaneity means that the nurse is the primary contact person with the patient and the patient's significant others. Hence the nurse might have to interpret tangible cues and manage expectations for the patient. This key communication role is very instrumental in generating consumer satisfaction. In a similar way, simultaneity means that the nurse is a major part of the service product and thus must be able to interact well with the patient.

Dealing with Heterogeneity

Most human performance-based services are subject to the problem of heterogeneous performances. It is difficult to obtain "cookie-cutter" repetitions due to the complex interaction of provider, receiver, and situation. The typical business response in this situation is to limit customization efforts, to standardize performances, and to utilize equipment or technology whenever possible as a substitute for human labor. Unfortunately, using these solutions can be depersonalizing to patients and may reduce satisfaction with the services received. Consumers are demanding consistent performances from health care providers and simultaneously demand personalized care. Thus, nursing administrators have to weigh the tradeoff between consistency and patient satisfaction and find an appropriate combination for the organization.

Technology use includes both hard and soft technology. Soft technology includes standardized systems, processes, and preplanned programs that remove much variance that occurs when the decisions are left up to individual discretion. Except in life-threatening situations, soft technology is a means of reducing heterogeneity. Hard technology is the use of equipment to reduce variability that occurs when humans perform a task. While this may increase the consistency of the service performances, it is at the price of impersonality.

The best solution to heterogeneity is to select, hire, train, and retain the best nurses available. High quality workers will provide a more consistent performance over time. Consistency, given the likelihood that a patient will receive care from a variety of nurses, is particularly important in shaping patients' perceptions. Inconsistent nursing care, even if technically acceptable, will create patient doubt and likely result in unfavorable word-of-mouth communications. It follows that personnel policies that reduce employee turnover are an effective means of controlling heterogeneity.

Nursing care encompasses many different types of patient and health care environments. Services will always possess these unique characteristics. Some recommendations for dealing with these characteristics will not be appropriate. In those situations, the nurse administrator has to carefully analyze what kind of response would be most appropriate to meet both patient and organizational goals.

NURSING MARKETING MANAGEMENT

A true marketing-oriented approach would result in a marketing plan for nursing services. Such a plan would depend, however on an overall marketing orientation of the organization since most of the key marketing decisions are made by top hospital or health facility administrators. The nurse administrator's role is to adapt operations to contribute to overall organizational goals. This task is much easier if management uses internal marketing. Internal marketing means top management informs everyone in the organization of institutional priorities and goals.

Assuming a marketing-oriented institution, all employees would know that nursing is not a support service like financial administration, but is part of the service product that patients and their significant others are comparing and evaluating against competitors or expectations. Nurse administrators should consider the following steps if they wish to manage a marketing-oriented function.

First, they would adopt these critical cultural values for services firms: a strong commitment to customer satisfaction, a willingness to be flexible, a willingness to innovate, and a concern for employees.

In order to implement the first value, the nurse executive would use both formal and informal research techniques to understand the dimensions of consumer satisfaction. Where do they get health care information? How are expectations formed? Who significantly influences satisfaction? What causes dissatisfaction with nursing care? Information should be systematically gathered, analyzed, and stored on all aspects of the patients' collective consumer behavior.

Addressing the last three values requires the nurse administrator to be a good personnel and operations manager. While this might not sound like marketing, it is impossible to separate personnel and operations from marketing in the service sector.

Second, nurse administrators should influence the process of segmentation and target marketing whenever possible. Nurses cannot be all things to all people (mass marketing approach) but a nurse can be many things to some people. Thus the nurse administrator should identify what the nursing staff can do well (within the limits set by top management) and offer that service product to that part of the health care market that wants those services more than any others.

Third, the nurse administrator should develop a marketing mix specifically for the chosen target market or markets. The elements of the marketing mix are product, place, price, and promotion.

The nursing product is the bundle of satisfactions derived from receiving nursing care. It is far more than just the core benefit of a nursing procedure or act: it includes satisfaction across a broad spectrum of activities and responses. A patient can have a very unsatisfactory experience if the patient disagrees with the problems being addressed in the individualized nursing care plan (nurse-centered versus patient-centered).

To propose that a nurse's job is to assist in health recovery whether the patient agrees on the problems identified or not is to assume that the product orientation is still a viable way of doing business. The product approach only works when the patient has no choice. Patients of this decade will exercise choice and health care providers who do not recognize the importance of providing satisfactory bundles of service product satisfaction will be contributing to the declining occupancy and financial position of their institution.

Nursing cannot do much to influence the real price of health care presently. However, nurse administrators can influence the perception of price by increasing the bundle of benefits the patient receives. Possible actions to make prices seem more reasonable include explaining the intangibles of the care received, reducing perceptions of risk, reducing loss of control, removing dissatisfiers, and otherwise generating patient satisfaction.

The issue of promotion is more accurately called impression management since nurse administrators typically do not plan the promotion mix of advertising, sales promotion, personal selling, and public relations/publicity. However, the quality of nursing available could be part of the facility's overall positioning strategy if that were a determinant criterion for targeted market segments. In those instances, the nurse administrator might become involved with message creation.

More often, the nurse administrator must ensure that nursing personnel and tangible evidence communicate the right messages to the patient and significant others. All employees who come into contact with patients must have communication competence. The staff who delivers care is the institution's informal advertisements. It behooves nurse managers and nurse executives to clearly communicate and assist the staff in developing this behavior. Communications that flow from former patient to other potential patients can be influenced through staff development too. Favorable word-of-mouth communications is one of the most credible and influential forms of promotion available for target markets who cannot make expert judgments about service alternatives.

Fourth, the nurse administrator should implement a program of control and evaluation. This means that the nursing administrator should specify goals which have both magnitude and some time frame. Progress toward accomplishment of these goals should be measured on a periodic basis. Corrective action is needed when there is an unacceptable discrepancy between actual and desired achievement levels. Lessons learned during one planning and execution period should be used to set goals for subsequent periods.

SUMMARY

The health care industry continues to change rapidly and, as it does, marketing is a key function to ensure survival. Nurses are the largest group of health care providers and as such, are in a position to influence health care consumers' decisions regarding choice of health care providers.

Nursing is an action that occurs with the patient. Therefore, nurses are in a prime position to affect satisfaction of services delivered. The patient's perception of services delivered is a key element in returning for later services. Nurses do affect the whole organization and the need for nursing to be a key marketing element is timely.

REFERENCES

Christensen M, Inguanzo JM. Smart consumers present a marketing challenge. *Hospital.* 63:16, 42, 1989

Cleland VS. *The economics of nursing.* Norwalk, CT, Appleton-Lange, 1990

Costello MM. Patient satisfaction is often ignored by health marketers. *Marketing News.* 8, October 25, 1985

Johnson M. Perspectives on costing nursing. *Nursing Administration Quarterly.* 14:1, 65, 1989

Porter-O'Grady T. *Reorganization of Nursing Practice: Creating the Corporate Venture.* Rockville, MD, Aspen, 1990

Smith GA, Pinkerton S. Formation of the consortium. In: Pinkerton S, Schroeder P, eds. *Commitment to Excellence: Developing a Professional Business Staff.* Rockville, MD, Aspen Publishers, 1988:243–250

Torres G. The place and concepts of theories within nursing. In: George JB, ed. *Nursing Theories: The Base for Professional Practice.* Englewood Cliffs, NJ, Prentice-Hall, 1985:1–13

CHAPTER 27

Institutionalizing Research in Nursing Services

Roma Lee Taunton
Diane K. Boyle

Key Concept List

Institutionalizing research
Nursing research committee
Research networking
Clinical research
Administrative research
Multisite studies
Field research
Research utilization
Resource allocation
NIH National Center for Nursing Research

INSTITUTIONALIZING RESEARCH

Nursing engages in research to support and improve its practice. Participation in that research is important to nurses because they and the public expect that future decisions about nursing care and its delivery systems will be grounded in research as is the case in other professions. As well as ensuring the delivery of care, nurse executives face the challenge of fostering clinical and administrative research. Leadership in institutionalizing research will be critical in the future.

Research is institutionalized when it characterizes an organization. Another view is that research is institutionalized by putting it into the care of an organization. Examples of institutes recognized nationally for their commitment and productivity in nursing research include the University of Arizona; Beth Israel Hospital, Boston; and Barnes Hospital, St. Louis. Such institutions encourage, nourish, and support nursing research. Research is incorporated into their formal organizational systems; consequently, the public associates the respective university or hospital with nursing research.

Hinshaw and Smeltzer (1987) identify two outcomes of effective institutional nursing research programs: provision of (a) information for policy decisions and (b) knowledge to enhance the discipline's science. Hospitals must be well-managed to survive over the coming years and institutionalized nursing research will be an important factor assisting with effective management. Such research results can be utilized to generate and evaluate innovations in nursing practice, to assess new service markets, and to facilitate management. Research-based practice can be stimulating and satisfying, and such quality-of-work-life concerns are very important to nurses.

Stevenson (1989) describes three key ingredients for a successful research program: (a) people; (b) equipment; and (c) resources. Many nurses are talented, knowledgeable, and committed people, but nurse executives must create a vision that integrates research into organizational and departmental goals, provide needed support, and gain commitment to the research goals. Several different structural models have been effective frameworks for institutional research programs (Hinshaw & Smeltzer, 1987; Stevenson, 1989), but all reflect a common theme—leadership and commitment of resources by the chief nurse executive.

Leadership includes establishing and promoting research goals for the nursing department; assuring that performance expectations for managers and staff nurses incorporate research; and assuring that research is accommodated in workload estimates, assignments, and performance appraisal. The institution's CEO also must be supportive of the nursing department's goal for research. Resources such as facilitators, consultants, library support, and special equipment are essential for success. External funding is useful from a variety of perspectives, but much research and related activities can be conducted with minimal internal funding. The more critical issue usually is nursing staff availability to participate in or conduct research. Busy nurses become overloaded and burn out quickly when committee work, team meetings, data collection, and other research activities are superimposed on an already full workload. Such problems are avoided by carefully designing the research program to fit the organization's characteristics and goals, with specific input from interested nurses who will be involved.

Planning an institution's research program requires a clear view of the desired outcomes. Nurse executives must deal with the need to evaluate and utilize research findings as a basis for practice policies and protocols as well as the need to respond to investigators' requests to conduct research. Consultation with nurse executives and scientists who have successful research programs facilitates decisions about placement of the program in the administrative structure and assigning responsibility for its development. Having a nurse scientist develop and administer the institution's research program indicates strong commitment and enhances credibility; however, other models have been successful. Arrangements that allow an initial period for planning and input from nursing staff are useful. Egan, McElmurray, and Jameson (1981) share their experiences in determining the feasibility of a nursing research program. Stetler (1984) describes the Massachusetts General Hospital Nursing Studies Program in detail, including philosophical beliefs, organizational structure, and policies, procedures, and guidelines.

Four elements are common across organizations recognized for nursing research productivity: (a) a nursing research committee; (b) research networking; (c) investigation of administrative and clinical issues; and (d) research utilization. A nursing research committee and research networking foster a supportive environment, whereas investigation of administrative and clinical issues and research utilization involve conducting research. Nurses may participate in research conducted by external researchers or researchers from other departments, conduct replication or evaluation studies required for appropriate utilization of research findings, conduct studies to generate knowledge for administrative or clinical decisions, help drug and equipment manufacturers evaluate their products, or collaborate in multisite projects. Each common element for research productivity is discussed in a subsequent subsection, as are the resources required to support research.

THE NURSING RESEARCH COMMITTEE

Nursing research committee responsibilities depend on the long-term goals and structural model chosen for the institution's research program. This committee provides leadership in sustaining a supportive climate, gaining acceptance, and eliciting participation. It is a visible focus for the institution's research program and a formal mechanism for dealing with issues. The research committee advises the chief nurse executive about the program, recommends policies and procedures, plans and conducts staff development activities, and approves investigator proposals to conduct nursing studies. Assuring consultation and colleague review is an important service for nurses who are developing proposals and research reports. The committee also may conduct research utilization projects and other studies needed to support the nursing department goals.

Nurses interested in research and committed to building and maintaining a successful institutional program of research are the most effective committee members. Success rests on the support and participation of staff nurses, and at least half the members should come from that group. The membership also should reflect administrative responsibility and support. Expertise and previous experience are very useful qualifications, but should not limit participation on the committee. Development experiences can assure that members have a common beginning knowledge base.

Overlapping membership with the organization's research review board and human subjects' review committees can help ensure that nursing proposals are evaluated equitably and that nursing's viewpoint will be presented. Such membership also ensure access to information about other research activities within the institution. Proposals for studies conducted by investigators other than nurses may not come to the nursing committee for review, even though patients or nurses are involved. Nurses appointed to both groups can facilitate communication, liaison, and problem solving.

RESEARCH NETWORKING

Colleague support is an essential part of institutionalized research—within the institution, locally, regionally, and nationally. The responsible persons need opportunities to exchange and discuss ideas, problem solve, and expand beyond agency boundaries. Hunt and several co-authors (1983) describe The Nursing Research Network of Boston, and Dahlen-Hartfield (1989) has reported the establishment of the Washington Metropolitan Area Nursing Research Consortium. Other local networks have been established in St. Louis (Potter, 1990) and Milwaukee (Jenkins, 1989) and are an important resource in initiating and maintaining an institution's research program.

Local research networks serve several purposes, including bonding for professional growth; facilitating communication; promoting collaborative research; reinforcing and refining nursing knowledge; clarifying research standards of practice; sharing developed tools, techniques, strategies; sponsoring research conferences; and providing a creative outlet. Members of local networks willingly share information and materials (Dahlen-Hartfield, 1990). Networking with regional and national groups increases contacts with potential allies. Regional groups are a cost-effective opportunity for broader exposure to nursing research and researchers. The Western Society for Research in Nursing and the Midwest Nursing Research Society, long-established networks, influence research development considerably in their respective areas. Compared to national groups, membership of regional societies is somewhat more heterogeneous, and participation, including presentation of posters or papers, is less intimidating.

Most national groups are more specialized than regional research societies. Notable exceptions are the American Nurses Association (ANA) Council of Nurse Researchers and the National Research Development Conference, an informal group that has met annually for more than 20 years. Increasing numbers of hospital-based research facilitators participate in the National Conference, and research facilitators meet informally at ANA Council conferences. The Association for Health Services Research offers unique opportunity for multidisciplinary interaction about organizational issues such as quality of care and effectiveness.

Participation in External Studies

Networking institutions are more likely to be approached by researchers seeking access to subjects. Participation in research conducted by external investigators may require only inclusion of relevant performance expectations for nursing staff, nursing research committee approval, and the institution's human subjects committee approval of proposals. Appointing a member of the administrative nursing staff to facilitate communication with the investigator and coordinate in-house activities is helpful. A letter of support confirming access, conditions, and the staff contact usually is sufficient documentation of agreements.

More complex arrangements are important when investigators want nursing staff involvement in conducting research or to collect data from staff during work hours. The Washington Metropolitan Area Nursing Research Consortium participant packet (Dahlen-Hartfield, 1990) includes several examples of institutional policies and procedures for participating in research. Collaboration may include assistance with data collection, liaison activities that persist over time, and nursing staff participation in implementation of an experimental protocol. An investigator seeking funding from a government agency or private foundation needs letters of support, evidence of review for protection of human rights, and other documents. Formal agreements may extend to contracts when the clinical agency is reimbursed for services.

INVESTIGATING CLINICAL AND ADMINISTRATIVE ISSUES

Researchable questions can be formulated for every aspect of nursing practice and vary from one health care setting to another. Researchers in long-term health care institutions are concerned with such patient problems as impaired physical mobility, alterations in bowel elimination, and potential for injury. Questions of interest in acute care settings relate to such topics as alterations in cardiac output and fluid volume deficit. Nonetheless, these types of problems are common to all health care settings as are issues related to productivity, quality of care, and costs.

Clinical Research

The NIH National Center for Nursing Research has seven priorities (Table 27–1) for clinical research. These priorities incorporate a wealth of issues from which to develop researchable questions. Each volume of the *Annual Review of Nursing Research* (Fitzpatrick, Taunton, & Benoliel, 1990) includes recommendations for studies needed on specific clinical topics.

Clinical research has the greatest potential for impacting the quality of patient care. Research findings from replicated studies have immediate application to nursing practice. Examples of replicated findings include interventions to assist patients in coping with the threatening event of surgery (Johnson et al, 1985) and the effects associated with nasogastric tube feeding and parenteral nutrition (Martyn et al, 1984). These studies are important because they advance nursing knowledge, are reproducible, and provide models of clinical research for nurses. Nurse executives encourage improved clinical practice when they promote these types of research studies and their application to practice.

Administrative Research

Administrative research provides support for establishing policy and allocating resources, thus increasing the organization's likelihood of survival in a competitive market. In reporting findings of the National Nursing Administration Research Priorities (NNARP) study, Henry and colleagues (Henry et al, 1988) compare ten topics of

TABLE 27-1. EVOLVING CLINICAL NURSING REASEARCH PRIORITIES, NATIONAL CENTER FOR NURSING RESEARCH

Low birth weight—mothers and infants. Research related to: preconceptional and prenatal nursing care, with a focus on preventing the delivery of preterm or growth-retarded infants; care of low-birth-weight infants in the acute care setting, with a focus on prevention of complications; and models of care delivery after discharge from the institution.

HIV infection—prevention and care. Study of: ethical issues, prevention of transmission, physiological and psychosocial factors, and issues relating to delivery of care to persons with HIV infection or AIDS.

Long-term care for older adults. Developing research areas focus on both the older adult and the family, and include: clinical problems encountered in the long-term care of older adults residing in institutions or in the community; and issues related to the delivery of long-term care services such as continuity of care and transitions across clinical settings.

Symptom management. This area of research focuses on the development of effective assessment measures and intervention strategies for pain and other symptoms associated with acute and chronic illness, with an emphasis on bio-psycho-social parameters.

Nursing informatics—support for patient care. This area of research is designed to strengthen patient care. Priorities will be selected from research into the collection, organization, processing, and dissemination of information for clinical practice, including the design and development of databases, classification systems, computer models, and expert systems.

Health promotion for children and adolescents. This area of study will focus on understanding health behaviors in childhood and adolescence, a critical developmental period; and on testing theory-based interventions to facilitate health-enhancing behavior patterns and to reduce health-compromising ones.

Technology dependency across the lifespan. This research addresses technology used to support or replace lost function of body organs or systems when it is an essential element in the treatment of chronic disease. Included are the study of individual and family responses, prevention of complications, bioethical issues, and demand for resources.

Source: NIH National Center for Nursing Research, 1991. For more information contact the Office of Information and Legislative Affairs, National Center for Nursing Research, Building 31, Room 5B03, Bethesda, MD 20892; (301) 496-0207.

nursing administration research in progress in hospitals and schools of nursing with priority topics identified through a NNARP Delphi Study.

The Delphi panel was comprised of members of the following groups respectively: nursing service administrators, administrators of university hospitals, deans of nursing, nursing administration faculty, health administration faculty, and experts located in government, universities, and public and private foundations. Henry et al (1988) reported that research in progress in hospitals focuses on patient care classifications, retention of personnel, and improvement of productivity. In nursing schools emphasis is on understanding nurse administrator characteristics and job satisfaction, recruitment, and retention of faculty. Seven of ten priorities of the Delphi experts are foci of studies most frequently in progress in hospitals or schools. Ongoing program announcements from the National Center for Nursing Research (NIH, 1988b) address important public policy questions such as nursing resources and retention. These announcements, together with the NNARP Delphi study, provide fertile sources of administrative research issues for years to come. The *Annual Review of Nursing Research* also includes administrative topics, for example, interorganizational research (Krueger, 1983) and costs of nursing care (Sovie, 1988).

Multisite Studies

The benefits of investigating clinical and administrative problems increase as nurse executives and nurse researchers reach outside the bounds of their institutions and collaborate with researchers in other settings. Conducting studies in multiple sites increases resources available to researchers, such as money, materials, subjects, technical services, consultative services, and information. Further, conducting research in multiple sites allows replication, which involves reproducing the study design and methods with a new group of subjects in order to determine whether findings will be similar. Finding similar results from the same study conducted in different settings and with different subjects increases confidence in the findings, and leads to the expectation that the situation is the same in unstudied populations and samples (Taunton, 1989).

Taunton (1989) also suggests that nurses collaborate in multisite studies to address clinical problems in their practices. For example, complications associated with positioning of patients for tube feeding not only can be studied simultaneously within the same hospital in neonatal, medical, and surgical intensive care units (ICUs), but also in ICUs across several hospitals. Finding one patient position associated with fewer complications across multiple units in multiple hospitals increases confidence that proper positioning would benefit patients in other settings.

The nurse executive must consider three critical factors when embarking on multisite research: The research-oriented attitudes of other chief nurse executives, the research environment in other nursing departments, and the values and flexibility of both other hospitals' and nursing departments' organizational structures (Chance & Hinshaw, 1980). For multisite research to be successful, all involved nurse executives must value research and all environments must be conducive to the use of and participation in research activities by both administrative and clinical staff.

Each institution and researcher may have different goals for a multisite study. An academician-researcher may have, as a priority, the pure knowledge to be produced, whereas clinicians and administrators in the agency may be concerned with applicability of results to the immediate clinical setting (Hinshaw, Chance, & Atwood, 1981). Therefore, clarifying goals and resolving differences among them upfront is imperative for a successful collaboration. Resolution and agreement about each issue posed in Table 27–2 before the start of a multisite study increases success and enhances the research environment at each cooperating institution.

Special Problems of Field Research

Because health care studies generally occur in natural or field settings, nurse executives must be aware that nurse researchers rarely are able to use true experimental designs. Also, nurses who study human subjects must consider ethical issues around freedom from harm that limit research designs, for example, withholding treatment likely to be beneficial from a control group. Practical considerations such as subjects being available only as intact groups may prevent researchers from assigning subjects to experimental and control groups at random. Researchers in health care settings cannot insulate and isolate groups of subjects from each other as is possible in a laboratory.

TABLE 27-2. ISSUES TO RESOLVE BETWEEN INSTITUTIONS AND RESEARCHERS IN MULTI-SITE RESEARCH

1. Who will maintain oversight for the implementation of the research protocol?
2. What will be the linkage between the sites?
3. What commitments about resources will be required from each site?
4. What will be the roles of respective site players?
5. Exactly what is the intervention to be tested—can it be delivered identically in each site?
6. Who will have access to study data?
7. To whom and how will findings be disseminated?
8. What, if any, written policies will govern relationships among sites?
9. What will be the process of decision making?
10. What written procedures will there be; what standardized training of staff will occur?
11. What working subcommittees will there be, and who will be involved in these committees?
12. What political and cultural organizational issues must be dealt with?
13. What arrangements are to be made for authorship on publications and presentations?

Source: Katz DG, McCormick P, Mitchell PH, Valanis B. (1989). Alternative Models for Multi-Site Studies. American Nurses Association Council of Nurse Researchers. 1989 Nursing Research Conference. Chicago, 1989.

Nurse executives should assure that developmental activities for the research committee emphasize special problems of field research. Networking provides opportunity for the nursing staff to learn about issues and problems confronted by other researchers, possible solutions, and the reactions of the scientific community. Networking also facilitates identification of consultants who have expertise and experience in designing field research.

UTILIZING RESEARCH

Research utilization is basing nursing practice on research findings substantiated through replication. Several novel projects promote research utilization. Funk has conducted a series of focused conferences at the University of North Carolina to disseminate research findings related to mobility, nutrition, and pain. Outcomes of those conferences include recommendations about research utilization. The model developed at the University of Michigan in the Conduct and Utilization of Research in Nursing (CURN) Project (CURN, 1980–1983) is used most widely. The CURN model (CURN, 1980–1983) emphasizes planned institutional change, whereas Stetler (1985) focuses on the individual nurse as a critical thinker who uses research findings or the research process to provide or manage care more scientifically. The two viewpoints are not mutually exclusive. As Stetler points out, an action application such as a nurse's research-based decision to avoid medical jargon when teaching patients about their postoperative medications improves her practice and does not involve the organization. Nursing administration must be involved, however, in an action application across nurses or patient care units. Leadership from the nurse executive promotes research utilization as an institutional value.

Research utilization requires identifying and implementing the *good* findings on a topic. A proposed practice innovation based on *good* research findings is tested through an in-house clinical trial prior to hospitalwide implementation. For example, utilization of research findings about structured preoperative teaching includes review and integration of findings from published studies, adaptation of a specific teaching protocol for in-house use with general surgery patients, clinical trial on one patient care unit, and finally, diffusion to all appropriate patient care units.

Identifying groups of nurses within the institution who share an interest in research on a single topic is a critical step in research utilization. Janken (1988) and Stark (1989) describe their experiences in developing such groups. Each group needs support, encouragement, and direction from strong leaders. Access to both scientific and clinical expertise is essential. Within the goals of the institution's research program, each group establishes its scope and objectives, membership, meeting schedule, and work style. Groups evolve differently, some limiting their scope to critiquing published research reports and others extending to conduct evaluation, replication, or original studies.

RESOURCES

Institutionalizing research requires personnel, consultation, library services, space, equipment and support services, and funding. Each of the common elements of research productivity—nursing research committee, networking, investigation of clinical and administrative issues, and research utilization—demands specific resources.

Personnel

Responsibility for administering the institutional research program and conducting research must be formalized in the nursing department structure, job descriptions, and performance expectations. Hinshaw and Smeltzer (1987) indicate that administrative studies take as long as 2.5 years for completion. Nurse executives who institutionalize research effectively recognize that it is time consuming and deal with that fact upfront. They assign authority, responsibility, and accountability for the program, and expectations of participants are clear.

Hiring a well-qualified nurse scientist assures that someone focuses on the development and administration of the institution's research program and is readily available for consultation or to direct a study. Government agencies and foundations expect qualified principal investigators. Joint appointments or other links with academic researchers promote peer support and intellectual stimulation for clinically located research facilitators.

Clinical specialists and staff nurses must have time allocated to conduct research and participate in research-related activities. Staff nurses are particularly vulnerable in that they have less control of their work time than clinical specialists, managers, or administrators. They need time for meetings and to complete their between-meeting assignments.

Secretarial support assures that valuable nurse time is not spent on maintenance tasks for the research committee or research teams. Additional personnel are needed for chart review, data collection and entry, or for participation in experimental protocols. Staff nurses may be assigned or research assistants hired for those tasks. In most instances, clerical personnel can be trained for data entry.

As noted earlier multiple models are used to institutionalize research (Stevenson, 1989). For example, University Hospital, Arizona Health Sciences Center, uses a collaborative model (Chance & Hinshaw, 1980; Hinshaw, Chance, & Atwood, 1981) that incorporates joint appointments of nurse scientists and clinicians. In contrast, the director of nursing practice at Barnes Hospital, St. Louis, (Hailstone, 1990; Potter, 1990) administers the research program, with clinical specialists accountable for conducting research as a basis for development and implementation of practice changes. Staff nurses at Barnes negotiate time for participation in research to earn contribution points for *Excel*, a salary leveling program designed to reward nurses for remaining at the bedside. Researchers obtain consultation from experts who participate in the St. Louis Research Consortium or from nationally known investigators who have specifically focused and established research programs.

Consultation

Multiple consultants assure access to appropriate expertise in substantive content, research design, measurement, statistics, and project management. Nurse researchers experienced with designated variables and populations are invaluable. Where there is no in-house research facilitator, it is expedient to retain a nurse scientist for general consultation who can assist nursing staff members on an as-needed basis to organize and express their ideas for projects and to identify the specific consultation they will need. Consultants are most readily accessible from schools of nursing and other departments in local and state universities or from other nearby organizations engaged in research. Extending existing contracts for student clinical experiences to include collaborative relationships for research is mutually advantageous. As noted earlier, local, regional, and national networking provides access to consultants with all types of research expertise.

Library Services

The nursing research committee requires computerized literature searches, timely interlibrary loans, and reference materials related to research. These needs are intensified when conducting research is part of the institution's program. Computerized data bases for literature searches are available for personal computers and searches also can be obtained on a fee-for-service basis from larger libraries. Nurse investigators require reference books and journals related to research methods. Having library support staff initiate literature searches and screen preliminary materials increases Barnes Hospital nurses' time for generating ideas, developing and reviewing proposals, collecting and analyzing data, and other critical components of the institution's research program (Potter, 1990).

Space

New personnel hired for the institution's research program require office space, of course, but other space needs are not so obvious. Work space assigned to clinical nurse specialists and nurse managers may not include adequate storage or be conducive to working without disruption. Staff nurses rarely have private work space or locked file space. Research interest groups and individual investigators need meeting and workspace as well as controlled-access storage with locked files to protect consent forms, data, and other project materials. Long-term storage of data is an important consideration.

Many nursing studies are conducted within patient care units with available space and equipment; therefore nurses have great difficulty assuring timely access to space to conduct interviews, perform physical examinations, or collect data from family members. Controlled space for diverse activities in planning the research program must be acquired.

Equipment and Support Services

Computer hardware and software for conducting data analyses are basic research equipment. Personal computers for which statistical software is available may be adequate. Laptop and hand-held computers facilitate on-site data entry, and individual access to word processing equipment expedites nurses' research work. Data analyses, including computer services, may be contracted to an external consultant when the necessary statistical expertise is not available in the nursing department.

Even though much of the equipment and related support services needed for clinical research is available within the institution, specialized technology may be required (eg, transcutaneous intermittent nerve stimulators). Patient care demands limit access to equipment and critical purchases may be necessary.

Existing Data

Patient records and institutional documents are rich data bases for nursing studies. In addition, physicians and other investigators collect information about patients that is not included in medical records. Nurses are aware of such information and can negotiate access for secondary analysis on variables of interest to nursing. Large multisite national data bases collected through federal programs or by other organizations can be purchased at nominal costs.

Funding

In considering funding for the institution's research program, the nurse executive must remain mindful of the aim to provide information needed for making decisions. Personnel are the primary resource needed, and a few thousand dollars often can assure timely results of a proposed study. Incorporating funding for research into the nursing department budget makes sense in light of the financial risks or advantages associated with decisions organizations make.

The nurse executive's challenge in budgeting for the institution's research program is protecting those monies from attack in the budget review process or from raiding for other purposes. Accurate perceptions of the organizational climate and politics are important. Informal interactions with colleagues experienced at institutionalizing research facilitate identification of potential budgeting issues and pitfalls.

Success in obtaining external funding for research requires a documented track record of completed projects. Time factors and the upfront expenditures of money and resources associated with seeking external funding are balanced against the prospect of bringing new funds into the organization. If external funding is a goal, specific resources must be allocated to monitor funding programs of foundations, government agencies, and other organizations. Such functions commonly are vested in a corporate development department, endowment association, or academic research office. SPIN (Sponsored Programs Information Network), a regularly updated, computerized funding data base, is available in most academic medical centers and major universities. Many newsletters are available, some of which are free, for example, the *NIH Guide to Grants and Contracts.* Foundations circulate announcements of funding programs directly to hospitals and other organizations. Information about federal and national foundation initiatives is captured by SPIN. Some detective work and specific networking will pinpoint regional, state, or local funding opportunities. Requisite conditions for receiving monies vary from one funding organization to another and must be taken into account. Processes and procedures also must be established for internal review and approval of grant applications.

Nurses obtain small research grants through Sigma Theta Tau, International, and the American Nurses Foundation. State and local organizations and businesses have vested interest in communities and their respective health agencies, and drug companies and medical supply firms have vested interest in health care generally. Sufficient funds for a given project often are secured more easily and in much less time from those sources than from the federal government or organizations like the Kellogg or Robert Wood Johnson Foundations.

SUMMARY

Nursing research is important because nurses and the public expect that decisions about patient care and its delivery will be grounded in research. Nurse executives institutionalize research by incorporating it into formal organizational systems and encouraging, nourishing, and rewarding research productivity. Their leadership and commitment of resources are key factors in developing effective institutional research programs. Research-based practice is stimulating and satisfying, and such quality-of-life concerns are important to nursing practice. By emphasizing research utilization, nurse executives enhance the quality of patient care through application of *good* research findings. Collaboration in multisite studies increases resources available to researchers and allows replication. The nurse executive's assessment of other organizations' values, attitudes, and goals is critical when considering participation in a multisite study.

Regardless of the model chosen, nurse executives clearly assign authority, responsibility, and accountability for the nursing research program. They assure consultation and allocate staff time, secretarial support, library resources, space, and equipment. In budgeting, they consider information needed for making decisions, organizational climate and politics, and protection of monies. External funding is available through public and private foundations.

REFERENCES

Chance HC, Hinshaw AS. Strategies for initiating a research program. *J Nurs Adm.* 10:3, 32, 1980

CURN Project. *Using Research to Improve Nursing Practice. Ten Research-Based Protocols.* New York, Grune & Stratton, 1980-1983

Dahlen-Hartfield RA, ed. *Clinical Agency and University Perspectives for the Nurse Researcher.* Unpublished Washington Metropolitan Area Nursing Research Consortium participant packet, George Washington University Medical Center, Department of Nursing, Washington, DC, 1990

Fitzpatrick JJ, Taunton RL, Benoliel, JQ. *Annual Review of Nursing Research,* vol VIII. New York, Springer Publishing, 1990

Hailstone S. Personal communication, 1990

Henry B, O'Donnell JF, Pendergast JF, Moody LE, Hutchinson SA. Nursing administration research in hospitals and schools of nursing. *J Nurs Adm.* 18:2, 28, 1988

Hinshaw AS, Chance HC, Atwood J. Research in practice: A process of collaboration and negotiation. *J Nurs Adm.* 11:2, 33, 1981

Hinshaw AS, Smeltzer CH. Research challenges and programs for practice settings. *J Nurs Adm.* 17:7, 8, 20, 1987

Hinshaw AS, Smeltzer CH, Atwood JR. Innovative retention strategies for nursing staff. *J Nurs Adm.* 17:6, 8, 1987

Janken J. Research roundtables: Increasing student, staff nurse awareness of the relevancy of research to practice. *J Prof Nurs.* 4:3, 186, 1988

Jenkins L. Personal communication, 1989

Johnson JE, Christman NJ, Stitt C. Personal control interventions: Short- and long-term effects on surgical patients. *Res Nurs Hlth.* 8:131, 1985

Lincoln YS, Guba EG. *Naturalistic Inquiry,* 4th ed. Beverly Hills, CA, Sage, 1985

Martyn PA, Hansen BC, Jen KC. The effects of parenteral nutrition on food intake and gastric motility. *Nurs Res.* 33:336, 1984

NIH National Center for Nursing Research. *National Nursing Research Agenda: Evolving Clinical Nursing Research Priorities,* Bethesda, author, 1988a

NIH National Center for Nursing Research. *Research Related to Nursing Resources and Delivery of Patient Care Announcement.* PT34; KW0785130, 0785035, 0730065, Bethesda, author, 1988b

National Institutes of Health. *NIH Guide.* Bethesda, Printing and Reproduction Branch, 1990

Potter P, Personal communication, 1990

Rempusheski VF, Chamberlain SL. Nursing research image at Beth Israel Hospital, Boston. *J Nurs Adm.* 19:10, 6, 1989

Rossi PH, Freeman HE. *Evaluation: A Systematic Approach.* Beverly Hills, CA, Sage, 1985

Sovie MD. Variable costs of nursing care in hospitals. In: Fitzpatrick JJ, Taunton RL, Benoliel, JQ, eds. *Annual Review of Nursing Research, vol 6.*New York, Springer Publishing, 1988:131–150

Stark JL. A multiple-strategy based research program for staff nurse evolvement. *J Nurs Adm.* 19:9, 7, 1989

Stetler CB. *Nursing research in a service setting.* Reston VA, Reston, 1984

Stetler CB. Research utilization: Defining the concept. *Image.* XVII:2, 40, 1985

Stetler CB, Marram G. Evaluating research findings for applicability to nursing practice. *Nurs Outlook.* 24:9, 559, 1976

Stevenson JS. Forging a research discipline. *Nurs Res.* 6:60, 1987

Stevenson JS. Resources and structures to promote research in nursing. In: Abraham IL. Nazdam DM, Fitzpatrick JJ, eds. *Statistics and Quantitative Methods in Nursing.* Philadelphia, Saunders, 1989:40–46

Taunton RL. Replication: Key to research application. *Dimensions of Critical Care Nursing.* 8:3, 156, 1989

CHAPTER 28

Innovation, Decision Making, and Problem Solving

Judith Jezek

Key Concept List

Problem solving
Decision making
Decision-making models
Bounded rationality
Creativity
Entrepreneurship

As part of his discussion of *Why Leaders Can't Lead,* (1989) Warren Bennis presents the idea that human organizations are designed to limit the potential for innovation and creativity. Individuals remain in the organization and advance to management positions because they feel and express values and beliefs which "fit" with those of the organization. But, since human organizations are open systems, there is a continual tension between the forces which strive to maintain the status quo and those which call for change and adaptation. Organizations that have the greatest potential for survival are those which balance the forces that contribute to stability and unity with those which facilitate creativity and innovation. Kanter (1983) studied ten companies and discovered that the most effective innovation models combined individual and team efforts in ways which encouraged the building of a strong organizational culture which allowed many to participate in the development and realize the benefits of innovation. Without a culture that encourages adaptation to the changes occurring within and outside, an organization becomes paralyzed and risks extinction.

In the current social, economic, and political environment, nurse executives are challenged to balance many contradictory forces. The health care industry, like all other forms of American business, is trying to reconcile and respond to the forces which present opportunities for innovation coupled with shrinking resources. The challenge is to develop better ways of doing things at less cost. Innovations which move nursing and health care organizations toward the realization of this goal will require that nurse executives and their management staff develop new ways of doing things. To be most effective in meeting the demands of the changing environment, those responsible for leading the change process must first develop new ways of thinking about things. Instead of approaching the challenges for innovation as the process of "building a better mousetrap," nurse executives must start by deciding if there is still a mouse to catch!

The charge to help the organization maintain stability and achieve its objectives in the midst of a constantly changing environment is one of the greatest tests faced by managers in any business. Sometimes the challenges presented are predictable and allow the manager to use past experience and established guidelines or decision rules. But, executives are often confronted with issues and challenges never before faced by the organization or they must take leadership in creating a new direction which will place the organization in a proactive rather than reactive position. In these situations, the ability to generate and implement creative approaches to defined needs or perceived opportunities is essential. Whether the manager is called on to deal with routine (previously experienced) problems or to generate novel approaches to new challenges, the process of choosing a course of action from two or more alternatives is a fundamental activity.

PROBLEM SOLVING AND DECISION MAKING

Managers are in the position to consciously (or sometimes less consciously) choose a course of action or prescribe a behavior which provides direction for the organization and its members. Those decisions may be part of the process of solving a problem or they may reflect making choices in situations where no problem exists but alternative options are present. A nurse executive may be confronted with the "problem" of a nursing staff shortage. Before selecting a course of action, the executive will most likely go through several steps which may include a clarification of the nature and extent of the problem, identification of possible causes or reasons for the problem, and generation of several approaches designed to solve the problem. The next step in the problem-solving process is to make a decision about which identified alternative to pursue. In another situation, several candidates are available to fill an existing staff vacancy. The decision to offer the position to the person who, in the judgment of the manager, is the most qualified does not require problem solving.

Although it is possible to conceptually differentiate between problem solving and decision making, the terms are often used interchangeably. In this discussion, decision making will be used because it can broadly be defined as *the process of choosing a course of action from two or more alternatives.* But, it must be remembered that a problem may be solved without making a decision. Sometimes a decision is made as an outcome of a deliberative process and other times it is dictated by predefined rules or past experience. Decision making situations can be divided into three distinct categories: *routine, adaptive,* and *innovative.*

A *routine* decision-making situation involves a well-defined, known problem. The circumstances are reasonably certain and represent relatively low risk to the manager and the organization. Solutions can often be found in established rules or standard operating procedures. If an employee reports to work late on three consecutive days, the manager will most likely be able to consult the personnel policy manual to determine the appropriate (and expected) decision in this situation. Following the outlined procedure (eg, verbal warning after the second tardiness and written warning after the third) represents low risk to the manager who can expect the support of the personnel officers if the employee protests the actions taken. Situations which fall into the routine category are most characteristic at the first-line management level. The majority of decisions made by head nurses and other unit level managers are routine.

Adaptive decision-making situations involve moderately unusual or partially known problems. Decisions involve less certainty and require a moderate level of risk to the manager and/or organization because solutions usually require the modification or changing of known or past practices. For example, the hospital's staff nurse recruitment plan has included advertising in local newspapers, participation in career days at regional colleges with nursing programs, and staff have attended several selected national specialty nursing conventions. Although that strategy has produced acceptable results in the past, the current and projected staffing requirements suggest the need to develop additional or alternative approaches. The director of marketing has asked nurse managers to consider subscribing to a new system which will allow expanding recruitment at a national level through the use of a computer network which has terminals at most of the large schools of nursing and state nurses association headquarters. The hospital will pay a fee to the computer service for each nurse who is recruited. Many of the decision situations confronted by middle and executive level nurse managers require adaptive decisions.

Executive level nurse managers frequently encounter decision-making situations which are most appropriately labeled *innovative.* These situations involve discovering, identifying or diagnosing ambiguous problems which require unique and creative solutions. Because the problems are less clear and solutions require movement into "uncharted territory," these situations involve a high level of risk and uncertainty. The nursing department, as part of the strategic planning process, has determined that fewer baccalaureate and master's prepared nurses will be available to fill staff nurse positions in the next five years. During that same time, anticipated changes in the patient population include a marked increase in the level of acuity and an expansion of applied technology, both of which suggest the need for high level professional nursing care. The nurse executive establishes a small task group to propose a model for nursing care delivery which clearly delineates professional and technical levels of nursing practice.

Although the types of decision-making situations can be designated as characteristic of particular levels in an organization, each type of situation may occur at all levels. Some executive decisions may be clearly defined as routine and some situations encountered by a first-line manager will be best approached with adaptive or innovative approaches. In many situations the type of decision approach is not clear. In the process of responding to an apparently routine problem, a manager may discover information which requires the adaptation of a previously successful approach. Or, a problem that appeared to require an innovative solution may, on clearer definition, be solvable using an existing procedure or policy. McCall, Kaplan and Gerlach (1982) summarized the lack of order and predictability in decision making by observing that:

> Solving important problems will never be the logical, orderly process that most of us strive for, no matter how orderly the plan. Defining problems will remain an evolutionary process affected by points of view, vested interests, and the bits and pieces of information available at any given time. Pressures will ebb and flow, shifting attention from one problem to another, changing definitions involving and excluding various individuals. Sometimes the real problem won't materialize until well into the decision making process; or maybe not until after some action has been taken. People will take hip shots when they should have been more thoughtful; relatively simple problems will at times end up in convoluted decision making cycles. Finding truth will remain problematic. (p 16)

STATES OF NATURE

The conditions, situations, and events over which a manager has no control are called *states of nature.* Decisions are embedded in and affected by the state of nature. This state will determine the degree of certainty and level of risk associated with making decisions and will suggest the types of information which can and should be used to make choices. In a state of nature characterized by a high degree of certainty and low risk, decisions can be based on *objective reality*. Facts will drive the decision process and point to an appropriate alternative. When circumstances are less certain and the degree of risk increases, the decision maker is forced to use information based upon personal knowledge, beliefs and experience to establish a more *subjective reality*.

FUNCTION OF OBJECTIVES

Objectives can assist decision making by clarifying expected directions and outcomes. Such statements can serve to reduce the uncertainty when selecting from among alternatives. Options can be evaluated based on their potential for moving the organization or the individual toward the preferred outcomes. This idea serves as the foundation for an approach to management called management by objectives (MBO). In this system, managers use the agreed on objectives as guides for decision making and action.

Although objectives may assist in reducing the uncertainty in many management decision making situations, they can lead to a false sense of security or direct the decision maker to use an approach which is inconsistent with the circumstances. Managers at all levels must continuously monitor the environment for information about the type of decision most appropriate and be ready to adapt and even adjust the objectives if necessary.

DECISION-MAKING MODELS

Four basic models of decision making have been described by students of organizational behavior: (1) rational decision-making model; (2) bounded rationality model; (3) garbage can model; and (4) political model.

The *rational decision-making model* is based on the assumption that people strive for economic rationality. That is, they objectively attempt to maximize every decision outcome. Choices represent movement toward optimal goal achievement and are the result of a deliberative, thorough process of problem solving.

The problem-solving process has been described widely. The number and labeling of steps may vary, but the sequence always includes some form of (1) problem identification; (2) clarification of objective(s); (3) designation of alternative objectives and solutions; (4) evaluation and comparison of alternative solutions; (5) selection and implementation of the ''best'' solution, and (6) follow-up evaluation and control. Students of nursing are taught the ''nursing process''; medical students read texts on ''clinical decision making''; and students of management learn about ''management decision making.'' By changing labels, this rational model can serve many in their quest for ideal decisions. To be most effective, the logical steps and the careful comparative process require a well-defined problem, motivation for achieving the ''best'' solution, and adequate time and effort to accomplish the process—a combination of elements seldom available simultaneously in most nursing management situations.

Research directed toward defining the process actually used consistently by administrators to make decisions finds that day-to-day decision making in most human situations involves some deviation from the ideal model learned by so many. This does not mean that the rational approach is not valued nor that it has little to offer the administrators. It does mean, though, that administrators must understand factors which interfere with the realization of the process and learn to use approaches which move them closer to rationality. Some of those approaches are included in the discussion of decision-making techniques.

Herbert Simon earned a Nobel Prize for his description of a model of economic decision making which is characterized by *satisficing, limited search,* and *inadequate information and control.* Simon's (1957) *bounded rationality model* has served as the base for research on decision making in a wide variety of settings. A major deviation from the rational model is the assumption that managers select workable rather than best solutions. To accomplish this end they conduct searches for alternatives which are limited by resource constraints and the absence of all of the information needed for a best-informed decision.

This model includes acknowledgment of two of the major factors which interfere with rational decision making: (1) time and money constraints and (2) lack of information. An effective manager will openly admit these deficits and establish decision making approaches that allow the discovery of solutions which, in their experience, will most likely produce a workable result. Simon coined the term *satisficing* to describe this search for acceptable rather than optimal solutions. To "hold out" for the perfect solution may require too much time and result in inertia. Implementation of the selected solution will either solve the problem or reveal the need to look for alternative solutions. One of the underlying assumptions of *bounded rationality* is that critical information is often not available to the decision maker until the organization begins moving in some direction so results are seen.

Another important limitation faced by managers is that most problems, especially those confronted at the executive level, are complex and only small parts can be handled at one time. Dividing problems into successive and manageable parts or parceling it out to individuals and departments increases the potential for movement and ultimate resolution. Waiting until everything can be known by one decision maker will result in the what some facetiously call "the no-decision decision." By the time a decision is possible, the opportunity has passed.

The success of bounded rationality is at least partially related to the administrator's ability to use past experience as a guide for selecting possible solutions. As alternatives are identified, the administrator looks for one which yielded a positive outcome in a similar situation. This process may be conscious or it may involve intuition. Although intuition is based on past trial-and-error experience, intuitive solutions are more likely to succeed if tested using a conscious analytical process before implementation.

The manager who acknowledges bounded rationality is freed from a potentially unproductive pursuit of "the perfect solution" and can approach decision making as an ongoing rather than final process. But, recognizing that perfection is impossible should not be an excuse for not searching for reasonable alternatives and the principle of satisficing should not stop the process of looking for a better solution.

In 1972, Cohen, March and Olson extended some of the ideas implicit in bounded rationality and described the *garbage can model* of decision making. This model suggests that organizational decision making involves the connecting and decoupling of problems, solutions, participants and decision opportunities based on the rate at which these various elements flow into the system. In more graphic language, the system (organization) serves as a receptacle (ie, garbage can) into which are thrown problems, potential solutions, players with varying agenda and abilities, and various recognition of opportunity for decisions. These elements bump up against each other causing connections or the breaking apart of previously connected elements. At any point in time, the system is filled with problems seeking solutions, solutions looking for problems, solutions and problems waiting for decision opportunities, and players who may or may not have the energy or the understanding to make things "happen." The experienced nurse administrator recognizes this scenario as descriptive of most health care delivery systems!

In this model the boundaries which inhibit the application of rational decision processes include the way in which the elements important in a decision are juxtaposed. All of the limiting factors described by Simon continue to operate. "The garbage can model of organizational choice implies that random or heterogenous outcomes should be expected because the connections between decisions and outcomes are determined by temporal factors, such as time of arrival or overall load on the system, rather than by causal connections between decisions and outcomes'' (Levitt & Nass, 1989).

The *political model* of decision making emphasizes the role of powerful stakeholders in the decision process. Political clout may be used to affect any step in the problem-solving process. This model is especially important in organizations like hospitals and universities which are made up of distinct constituencies. The various constituent groups have loyalties and values divided between the organization and the special interests the group represents. The major stakeholders in a hospital are the nursing staff, medical staff, hospital administration, patients and families, third party payers, and a governing board. Depending on the organizational structure and other environmental forces, additional stakeholders may be unions and other professional groups. The political decision-making process is characterized by coalition formation and bargaining.

Each of the models of decision making has value for describing decision processes in small groups as well as organizations or larger social systems. In complex organizations like hospitals and other health care institutions, managers must understand all types of decision-making processes and be able to use or participate in each approach. The rational model is often represented as an ideal. Nurse executives who have learned to use the nursing process as a basis for clinical decision making often extend this rational approach to other types of decision situations. In some cases, however, the controlled processes which lead to "rational" decisions are not the most effective means for dealing with the types of innovative decision situations often encountered by the executive.

Effective management decision making requires the ability to quickly recognize a decision opportunity, understand and adapt to the environment within which the opportunity is embedded, and select approaches that are most likely to produce decisions which move the group toward established goals. An important part of defining a decision situation is determining the type of decision most appropriate for the circumstances.

TYPES OF DECISIONS

Decisions which can be achieved by the application of established policies, procedures and rules are called *programmed decisions.* Explicit policies and procedures can be used by managers at all levels in organizations as a guide to responding to routine matters. The most important part of the administrator's role in programmed decisions is defining the problem. Appropriately defined problems are then solved by applying the prescribed response. Situations for which programmed responses are not available require *nonprogrammed decisions.* Executive decisions most often fall into the nonprogrammed category. All of the types of decisions listed below can be either programmed or nonprogrammed.

Organizational versus Personal

Decisions can be differentiated based on the interest being served by the selected outcome. Administrators should be aware of decisions that impact the organization but are made to first serve the individual. It is often difficult to totally separate self from the organization, especially at higher levels of the organization. Some administrators use this blurring to justify self-serving decisions which are not really in the best interest of the organization. Sensitivity to this potential problem and a willingness to test decisions with others can help an administrator who wants to keep the organizational interests first.

Operational versus Strategic

Operational decisions are made on a day-to-day basis as part of a short range plan and are most likely programmed. Strategic decisions are responses to new and complex problems which require nonprogrammed choices.

Research versus Crisis-Intuitive

The degree of urgency for a response determines whether decisions may be based upon careful research or require a more spontaneous response to a particular emergency. The "research" label suggests that decisions are based on extensive data gathered to suggest and support the best choice in the presenting situation. There is time to define the problem and follow the steps outlined in the rational decision model. Crisis intuitive decisions do not offer the luxury of time. In these cases, administrators with previous experience with similar decision situations are most comfortable.

Opportunity versus Problem Solving

Situations which present well-defined problems are most amenable to problem solving. In contrast, an opportunity requires the decision maker to exercise foresight in defining the problem and predicting potential long-term gains.

DECISION-MAKING APPROACHES

Administrators select from a variety of approaches to decision making. The approaches discussed below are not mutually exclusive. Rather, each represents one dimension of the decision process which can be portrayed on a continuum. The approach used to make a decision will contain some element of each category described. The combinations are many and allow the decision approach to be tailored to the unique combination of environmental characteristics present in a given situation and the various outcomes desired.

Centralized versus Decentralized

A centralized decision-making approach prescribes that as many decisions as possible are made by top management in contrast to the decentralized approach of pushing and/or allowing decision making to occur at the lowest possible level. The centralized model allows quicker decisions and ensures that common parameters and policies are used in the decision process. Because decisions are made at a central point and disseminated to other levels in the organization, there is more control and the potential for more uniformity. Centralized decisions do not, however, allow consideration of circumstances which are unique to a particular subunit in the organization nor do they promote personal investment in decision implementation at lower levels in the organization. They are also less responsive to the environment.

Decentralized decision-making models can lead to decisions which are more relevant to the persons at the implementation level and account for unique situational variables. There is an increased potential for variability, however, which makes measuring the impact of broad direction more difficult and promotes comparisons and possible competition between units of the organization. In implementing personnel policies, for example, it makes the organization more vulnerable to charges of discrimination and unfair management practices.

Given the pros and cons of each extreme point on the centralized-decentralized continuum, an ''ideal'' model might use a centralized approach to set broad direction and sufficient parameters to assure *efficiency* and allow decentralization to ensure investment and adaptation at the lower organizational levels to increase *effectiveness*.

Group versus Individual

The group approach to decision making is based on the assumptions that (1) groups make better decisions because of the potential for expanded data for problem identification and the generation of alternatives, and (2) group decisions are easier to implement because the affected parties have opportunity to participate in the choice. The expanded data base may, however, dilute the contributions of individuals who are especially insightful or creative if their input is too deviant from the groups' established values or expectations. In addition, high status individuals or a clique may dominate the process and limit options available for consideration. In some cases, norms may emerge which limit dissent and conflict and move the group toward making decisions in the best interest of the group and its survival rather than those which facilitate achieving organizational goals. This latter process was described by Irving Janis as part of his study of the decision making processes used by an elite group of advisors to President Kennedy. He called the phenomenon *group think.*

An individual approach to decision making may be more effective than the group model if decisions are needed quickly or the cost of group participation is high. An administrator who uses this approach can enhance the potential for effective decisions by incorporating a participatory process.

Participatory versus Nonparticipatory

A participatory approach to decision making is implicit in the group decision-making method. It also is possible to incorporate participation in a model which reserves for the administrator the right to make a final decision after receiving input from the parties who will be more affected by the choice made. Two hazards of the participatory/individual model of decision making are: (1) seeking input from parties who will not be directly affected by the decision leads to wasted time and confusion, and (2) the process of soliciting input may lead to expectations that the opinion offered will drive the outcome. A nonparticipatory approach to decision making keeps the whole process of problem definition, data gathering, alternative generation, and choice within the purview of the manager.

Vroom and Yetton (1973) have identified five decision styles for leaders. Each style reflects a different combination of the approaches discussed earlier. The basic approaches he describes are autocratic (A), consultative (C), and group (G).

- A1 = The manager/leader solves the problem or makes the decision using information available to them at that time (individual/nonparticipatory).
- A2 = The manager/leader obtains the necessary information from subordinates, then decides on the solution to the problem themselves (individual/participatory).
- C1 = The manager/leader shares the problem with relevant subordinates individually, gets their ideas and suggestions without bringing them together as a group and then makes the decision (individual/participatory).
- C2 = The manager/leader shares the problem with subordinates as a group, collectively obtaining their ideas and suggestions, then makes the decision (individual/participatory).
- G = The manager/leader shares the problem with subordinates as a group then serves as a chair while a group decision is made and implemented (group/participatory).

Any of these styles can be used with a centralized or decentralized model of organizational decision making and with programmed or non-programmed decisions. This model is discussed in more detail in Chapter 17.

Democratic versus Consensus

Democratic decisions are achieved through a process of majority rule. Consensus implies that the group process will lead to agreement by all about the best choice. In either model, dominant groups may control the decision process either by vote or by neutralizing the input of outsiders. Administrators should carefully evaluate the use of either of these approaches in situations where decisions will serve as the foundation for change and innovation. Alternative methods to encourage new ideas may need to be considered. Some alternative methods will be considered later.

DECISION-MAKING TECHNIQUES

Because the conditions of risk and uncertainty can lead to powerful emotional responses to decision-making situations, administrators may look for ways to balance emotion with a more rational perspective. Several techniques that allow the quantification of data and a more direct comparison of alternatives have been developed and designated as approaches to *normative decision making*. Some of these methods facilitate building models which allow the decision maker to manipulate variables and predict the influence of choices on outcomes, but none include any mechanism for factoring the potential influence of political forces either within or outside of the organization. Normative decision-making approaches are based on the assumption that objectives are known and clear and that the nature of the problem has been agreed on. There must also be some information about the problem available. Because of these conditions, normative approaches are often not useful in the nonprogrammed decision situations frequently confronted by executive level managers unless the problem can be broken down into smaller, sequential problems which can be more clearly defined.

For Routine Decisions

Two decision-making techniques for situations in which the problem and the choices are relatively well-defined are rules and standard operating procedures and artificial intelligence.

Rules and standard operating procedures prescribe how decisions should be made and usually indicate what decision is most appropriate in a defined situation. This approach assigns clear parameters for management decisions and assures the highest possible level of consistency. Most organizations have clearly prescribed rules for the administration of personnel policies. Managers and employees know how much sick time or vacation time is allowed and the parameters which surround the payment for time off in either situation. There are most often equally specific rules and procedures for employee evaluation and promotion and for the discipline of employees in selected situations (eg, sleeping on the job will result in the immediate dismissal of the employee). Similarly specific rules and procedures are often developed to guide decisions regarding the administration of equal opportunity requirements or the purchasing of new equipment.

Artificial intelligence allows the administrator to build a computer-based decision system. This approach requires that a system of if/then rules be developed. The administrator can then insert information and expect the program to suggest a "good enough" solution. Most of the spreadsheet computer programs provide this capability. For instance, the nurse administrator is asked to provide information about the potential cost to the organization of adding enough nursing personnel to open three more beds on a designated patient care unit. With information about the cost of staffing one bed on that unit or a comparable unit, simple arithmetic can be used to develop a projection. But, if the administrator has access to an appropriate artificial intelligence program, much more comprehensive information about cost can be provided. This includes considering additional variables such as salary levels based on hiring nurses with various levels of experience or hiring full-time versus part-time nurses with lower benefit costs.

For Adaptive Decisions

When problems are moderately ambiguous and solutions represent modifications of known or well-defined alternatives, more complex techniques may be required to facilitate rational decision-making. Two such approaches are: *break-even analysis* and *payoff matrix.*

Break-even analysis shows relationships between units produced (output), revenue, costs and profits for a defined situation. Using this approach, the nurse administrator who is asked to provide information about costs of opening three beds would use more variables to determine not only how much it would cost to hire nurses for the new beds but, also, to determine the probability that the increased revenue would offset the cost and ensure a higher level of profit. The variables used in break-even analysis include:

1. Fixed costs: those costs which remain constant over a specified time
2. Variable costs: costs which vary with changes in production but not necessarily with each unit of output
3. Total costs: sum of fixed and variable costs
4. Total revenue: total dollars received
5. Profit: excess of total revenue over total costs
6. Loss: excess of total costs over total revenue
7. Break-even point: point where costs and revenue cross

The value of break-even analysis may be limited by unpredicted shifts in variables. For example, a competing hospital has introduced a $10,000 bonus for nurses who agree to work full-time nights for one year. Following their lead might increase variable costs significantly. Or a physician whose practice represents 40 percent of the admissions to this unit accepts an offer as department head at the university hospital on the other side of town causing a sudden drop from the projected revenue for the unit.

If the decision maker can assign probability to various states of nature (degrees of risk) associated with the decision, the payoff matrix may help in the prediction of expected payoff for various combinations of strategies and states of nature.

For Innovative Decisions

In situations which require discovering or diagnosing unfamiliar and ambiguous problems and/or developing unique and creative alternative solutions, decision-making techniques require models to facilitate discovery and test multiple possibilities. Four model techniques are described.

A *decision-tree model* charts the steps in evaluating each alternative faced in decision making, allowing the outlining of future choices resulting from decisions in the present. Using this model, a branching chart is developed which identifies (1) the possible actions associated with each decision point; (2) the probability of occurrence for each key event; (3) the anticipated payoff associated with each action; and (4) the expected yield computed by multiplying the anticipated payoff with associated probability.

The *Osborn creativity model* defines three steps in the decision process: (1) fact finding; (2) idea finding; and (3) solution finding. At each step, novel ideas and curiosity are stressed over logical analysis, and participants are encouraged to find new ways to define problems and generate solutions. Creative modeling takes time and requires participants have freedom from pressures which will undermine creativity, two qualities almost never available in high pressure management situations. This type of approach is most effective when individuals are removed from the usual responsibilities of day-to-day management, presented with a problem or issue, and allowed sufficient time to focus on each step in the process. Fact finding can be facilitated by techniques which require individual(s) to generate a variety of definitions for the problem (eg, state the problem from at least three different perspectives, or define the problem in at least five different ways). For each problem the process of idea finding involves generating tentative ideas and leads. Brainstorming, or some other approach to generating alternatives with little or no analysis or judgement, should emphasize quantity rather than quality of ideas. Once sufficient ideas are generated, the solution finding phase allows testing of tentative solutions and adoption and implementation of a final choice. Testing options may involve the use of some of the techniques described earlier (eg, decision-tree, payoff matrices, or break-even analysis) which allow better comparison of the possible outcomes of various choices.

The *nominal group method* is a form of silent brainstorming. This approach allows group members to generate ideas silently and to present them without comment from other group members. Discussion does not begin until many ideas are on the table and dissociated from the person who generated the idea. Rating ideas also includes a silent, individual phase and decisions are based upon the accumulation of individual ratings. This approach is especially useful in situations where individuals or cliques tend to dominate discussion and ideas. (This method is discussed in Chapter 17.)

Structured debate uses various techniques to avoid the premature or too narrow definition of a problem. Individuals who participate in this approach may be assigned to represent and argue for various opposing views or alternatives. Some approaches which are useful in structured debate include (1) devil's advocacy in which an individual is assigned to disagree with the group and present alternative information; (2) multiply advocacy which requires that multiple alternative points of view be presented; and (3) dialectical inquiry in which an individual is assigned to question the underlying assumptions associated with various problem statements and formal debate is used to bring out different interpretations of the same information. These approaches are most useful in the problem definition phase of problem solving but can be used at other stages.

The *Delphi technique* is similar to the nominal group approach but individuals do not face each other. Written information is collected, collated, recirculated, and recollated until decisions are reached. This approach is often used when participants in the decision process are geographically separated. It can, however, be useful in situations when it is difficult to gather the parties together for an extended time period. For instance, instead of scheduling an all-day retreat for all head nurses to discuss a common problem, a delphi strategy may be used to collect and refine ideas. The major drawback of this approach is the amount of time needed to move through the various stages of problem refinement. (The Delphi technique also is discussed in Chapter 17.)

EXECUTIVE DECISION MAKING

The many approaches to decision making already discussed may be useful at all levels in an organization, from first-line manager to the top executive. There are, however, a few considerations which are especially relevant to decision making at the executive level. Most decisions at this level are responses to ambiguous (nonprogrammed) situations and require a special awareness of the political process operative within the organization. During the problem formulation phase, coalition formation may be critical to assure building agreement among key players about the definition of the problem to be solved. Solutions at this level are generally reached through the process Cohen, March, and Olsen (1972) call "muddling through." Solutions are tried and, if they don't work, other approaches are tested.

Many decision-making theories encourage the division of problems into small, more manageable parts to allow testing of pieces without jeopardizing the whole organization. This process of incrementalization can facilitate the use of more quantitative approaches (eg, decision trees) to solve the small pieces. Or the division of the problem into smaller parts can be used to give pieces to smaller organizational units for solutions. This process is called *segmentalism*. But, the risk-reducing advantage of incrementalization and the enhanced participation of segmentalism is not without hazard if innovative outcomes are desired. Breaking problems into segments increases the risk of losing site of the "big picture." Too often, reality is more than the sum of the identified parts. If solutions to segments are developed in isolation from each other the outcome may lack coherence and have no clear relationship to the original problem. Kanter (1983), in her study of innovative business organizations, found that the "entrepreneurial spirit [which produces] innovation is associated with . . . the willingness to move beyond received wisdom, to combine ideas from unconnected sources, to embrace change as an opportunity to test limits." She calls this approach *integrative* and differentiates it from the *segmentalism* which she found characteristic of most American business environments. Although no health care agencies were included in Kanter's study, a thoughtful nurse administrator will recognize that the predominant approaches used in the health care industry are more segmented than integrative.

Because executives are often in the position to participate in decisions which move an organization in a new direction, they are sometimes confronted with problems which arise when information suggesting that the decision was a mistake becomes available. Not infrequently, those who made the original decision become more firmly committed to the choice and begin to commit additional resources to the situation in an attempt to justify the original decision. When individuals are personally responsible for a decision and its negative consequences, they may block or distort negative information. Understanding this tendency, effective decision makers try to build checkpoints and outside evaluation into the implementation process, especially when responding to ambiguous situations for which pre-validation is so difficult.

Confronted with the special challenges of decision making in poorly defined or new situations, the executive has a unique opportunity for creativity and innovation. It is at this level in the organization that the momentum for constructive change begins. The nurse executive is more likely to have access to information from the external and internal environments and can play a pivotal role in identifying the need for new directions or solutions. Once the need has been defined, the administrator can take a leadership role in developing or initiating responses. Or the administrator may hand the problem to other creative individuals or groups within the organization and adopt the role of *idea champion* once an innovative approach is ready for implementation. Kanter (1983) identified three sets of skills needed to effectively manage integrative, innovation-seeking environments. Those skills are: (1) power skills which persuade others to invest information, support, and resources in new initiatives driven by an entrepreneur; (2) the ability to manage problems associated with the greater use of teams and employee participation; and (3) an understanding of how change is designed and constructed in an organization. A nurse executive with these skills is more likely to function comfortably and provide leadership in a creative nursing department.

A CREATIVE NURSING ORGANIZATION

In 1965, Steiner described three distinct characteristics of creative problem solvers. Although many years have passed, his description remains as relevant today as when he published his findings. Steiner found that creative problem solvers can be differentiated from the less creative by examining their motivation, orientation, and pace. In his analysis, the creative problem solver is motivated by an interest in the problem and its solution, gets very involved in the task, and works harder and longer without external incentives. The creative problem solver is oriented toward and identifies with the larger professional community and is less loyal to a single organization. (Highly creative problem solvers change jobs to pursue their interests, not change their interests to pursue their jobs.) In their approach to problem solving, creative individuals spend more time on the stage of problem formulation which usually leads to more efficient and effective solutions. In comparing the creative individual with a creative department or organization, some of Steiner's major descriptors are included in Table 28–1.

The creative nursing department is characterized by a high level of energy and enthusiasm and willingness to find new ways to think about things and better ways to do things. Problems represent challenge and opportunity and brainstorming and new ideas are welcomed. But the characteristics of a creative organization identified by Steiner are not usually found as descriptors for nursing departments or health care agencies. In fact, traditional nursing education focuses on developing behaviors which are standarized, exactly opposite from those of creative individuals. Traditional nursing departments are organized to minimize risks and maintain order. Although reducing innovation is not a goal in most nursing organizations, the preferred organizational structures lead to that outcome.

One of the greatest challenges faced by nurse executives is to develop an integrative and innovative environment. The forces for change in the health care industry are intense. Shifts in the external environment create demands for examining old patterns and responses and developing new (and usually less expensive) approaches to the delivery of nursing services. Technology is created so rapidly that new ways of doing things are necessary before the "old" ways have been perfected! The idea

TABLE 28-1

The Creative Individual	The Creative Organization
1. Originality	1. Assigns non-specialists to problems. Allows eccentricity.
2. Conceptual fluency	2. Open channels of communication. Contact with outside sources. Overlapping territories. Suggestion systems, brainstorming, nominal group techniques.
3. Less authoritarian. Independent.	3. Decentralized, loosely defined positions. Resource slack to absorb errors. Risk-taking norms.
4. Persistent, highly focused, highly committed.	4. Resources allocated to creative personnel and projects without immediate payoff. Reward system encourages innovation and challenge.
5. Playful, undisciplined exploration	5. Allows freedom to choose and pursue problems. Not run as tight ship. Freedom to discuss ideas.

Source: Adapted from Gary A. Steiner (ed.), *The Creative Organization*, 1965.

of a creative organization which takes time to study problems and challenges and mull over options and possibilities seems like an impossible dream. Keeping us is the goal. Why should any administrator consciously want to "create" change when the organization already feels overwhelmed by demands for new responses?

A creative nurse administrator will look for ways to turn the organization from a reactive change mode to a proactive stance. If feelings of being overwhelmed can be shifted to feelings of being in control, a nursing department can emerge with renewed energy and move as leaders within the organization and within the larger nursing community.

ENTREPRENEURSHIP

The value of persons with entrepreneurial spirit and skills has been recognized in most areas of business. Health care has been slower to accept and understand the potential benefits of encouraging entrepreneurship. Because physicians usually relate to health care organizations as independent, or at least semi-independent, agents, they have often been freer to challenge the status quo and garner institutional support for their entrepreneurial endeavors. An examination of many of the recent changes in hospitals will most likely reveal the commitment of significant amounts of institutional resources to an entrepreneurial physician who promises great returns for the organization as well as for themselves. Lithotripsy centers, substance abuse programs, and free-standing ambulatory surgery centers are only a few of the ideas being financed by hospitals. Less often, nurses develop and sell entrepreneurial ideas to hospitals. This difference may derive from many social and economic differences between nursing and medicine, including differences in the organizational relationships of the two groups within the institution and the basic socialization of the professions. While nursing makes major contributions to patient care and to the institution, institutional administrators and the public have been slow to recognize these contributions. Nurse executives are in a unique position to introduce truly creative approaches to patient care which can represent new solutions to the new problems—as well as some of the older, still unsolved problems facing health care today. They have the potential to be *entrepreneurs!*

Pearce and Robinson (1989) define entrepreneurism as *the process of bringing together creative and innovative ideas and actions with the management and organizational skills necessary to mobilize the appropriate people, money, and operating resources to meet an identifiable need and create wealth in the process.* In this definition they emphasize the need to combine the skills of the inventor with those of the manager to realize a truly new way to think about and do things. In some cases, an executive who lacks creative and innovative skills may develop and lead a truly entrepreneurial nursing department by using management skills to create an environment which nurtures individuals with creative skills and by helping provide the business know-how to make new ideas happen. The administrator can serve as the link between resources of the organization and the new idea. The administrator can act as the tester of ideas and the ''devil's advocate'' during developmental stages of innovation as well as the idea champion and promoter.

Becoming an entrepreneur represents a new direction for nurse executives. But, according to Pearce and Robinson (1989) most characteristics of successful entrepreneurs can be learned. The characteristics they identify are:

1. Endless commitment and determination (eg, willingness to jeopardize own personal economic well-being, invest time, tolerate lower standard of living)
2. Strong desire to achieve
3. Orientation toward opportunities and goals (focuses on unmet needs, goal-directed toward identified opportunity)
4. Internal locus of control (self-confident, believes they control own destiny, very aware of own strengths and weaknesses)
5. Tolerance for ambiguity and stress
5. Skill in taking calculated risks (shares risk whenever possible and plans for anticipated problems)
7. Little need for status and power (stays focused on opportunity, customers, market and competition)
8. Ability to solve problems (can be decisive as well as patient)
9. High need for feedback (nurtures relationships from which they can learn which often leads to an expanded network of useful contacts and influence)
10. Ability to deal effectively with failure (uses failure to learn)
11. Boundless energy, good health, and emotional stability
12. Creativity and innovativeness
13. High intelligence and conceptual ability
14. Vision and capacity to inspire

Health care, like all other American industries, is in need of entrepreneurs. Nursing is in a unique position to generate and implement new ideas which can transform the industry. But nurses must see themselves as potential agents, not only of change, but revolution. They must start by finding new ways to think about things such as roles and functions of nursing within the health care delivery system, organizational relationships of nurses and nursing to hospitals and other health care agencies, the potential for nurses to operate as *professionals* rather than *workers.* These are only a few of the areas where innovation is both possible and necessary.

The challenge to combine problem solving with managerial skills to be an innovator and entrepreneur is not without conflict for the nurse executive. Kanter (1989) identified many of the incompatible forces which need to be confronted by anyone who is trying to lead innovation. She suggests the following:

- Think strategically and invest in the future—but keep the numbers today.
- Be entrepreneurial and take risks—but don't cost the business anything by failing.
- Continue to do everything you're currently doing even better—and spend more time communicating with employees, serving on teams, and launching new projects.
- Know every detail of your business—but delegate more responsibility to others.
- Become passionately dedicated to ''visions'' and fanatically committed to carrying them out—but be flexible, responsive, and able to change direction quickly.
- Speak up, be a leader, set the direction—but be participative, listen well, cooperate.
- Throw yourself wholeheartedly into the entrepreneurial game and the long hours it takes—and stay fit.
- Succeed, succeed, succeed—and raise terrific children. (p 89)

REFERENCES

Bennis W. *Why Leaders Leaders Can't Lead: The Unconscious Conspiracy Continues.* San Francisco, Jossey-Bass, 1989

Cohen MD, March JG, *Leadership and Ambiguity: The American College President.* Boston, Harvard Business School Press, 1986

Cohen MD, March JG, Olsen JP. A Garbage Can Model of Organizational Choice. *Administrative Science Quarterly.* 17:1, 1972

Daft RL, Steers RM. *Organizations: A Micro/Macro Approach.* Glenview, IL, Scott, Foresman, 1986

Gardner JW. *Self-Renewal: The Individual and the Innovative Society.* rev ed. New York, WW Norton, 1981

Hellriegal D, Slocum J Jr. *Management,* 5th ed. Reading, MA, Addison-Wesley, 1988

Janis I. *Victims of GroupThink: A Psychological Study of Foreign-Policy Decisions and Fiascoes.* Boston, Houghton Mifflin, 1972

Kanter RM. *ChangeMasters: Innovation for Productivity in the American Corporation.* New York, Simon and Schuster, 1983

Kanter RM. *When Giants Learn to Dance: Mastering the Challenges of Strategy, Management, and Careers in the 1990's.* New York, Simon and Schuster, 1989

Koontz H, Weihrich H. *Management,* 9th ed. New York, McGraw-Hill, 1988

Levitt B, Nass C. The lid on the garbage can: Institutional constraints on decision making in the technical core of college-text publishers. *Administrative Science Quarterly.* 34:190, 1989

McCall M, Kaplan A, Gerlach L. Caught in the Act: Decision Making at Work. Technical Report #20. Greensboro, NC: Center for Creative Leadership, August, 1982.

Nutt PC. Types of Organizational Decision Processes. *Administrative Science Quarterly.* 29:414, 1984

Pearce JA II, Robinson RB. *Management.* New York, Random House, 1989

Simon HA. *Administrative Behavior,* 2nd ed. New York: MacMillan, 1957

Steiner GA. *The Creative Organization.* Chicago, The University of Chicago Press, 1965

Vroom VH, Yetton PW. *Leadership and Decision making.* Pittsburgh: U. of Pittsburgh Press, 1973

CHAPTER 29

The Future of Nursing Administration

Tim Porter-O'Grady

Key Concept List

Impact of economics on nursing
Future use of nursing services
Future costs of nursing care
Future delivery of nursing care

Much has been written on changes in health care. The fact that the health care system is experiencing turbulent times is no secret to the administrator who must lead and manage the enterprise through these uncertain times. Success in the effort will depend, for the most part, on the attention paid by the nurse executive to the constraints and opportunities that emerge during the next decade. The future of nursing administration will depend, for the large part, on four major considerations:

1. An ability to understand and apply economic and financial skills to the reality of nursing service delivery in a financially constrained market place.
2. Skill in developing and managing a continuing decentralization of health care into smaller units of service in frameworks that do not reflect traditional institutional structures and are more professional in nature.
3. Vision in leading the continuing of nursing in an increasingly diverse health system with shrinking human resources in the context of a maturing nursing profession.
4. Increasing influence of technology on the role of the knowledge worker and the executive function in the health care setting.

IMPACT OF ECONOMICS

Since the 1800s America has not experienced a time when it was not the single most significant economic nationality. Its embrace of enterprise and opportunity catapulted it into an enviable and unilateral position as an ascendant economy. For most of the years since the turn of the present century, the United States has controlled the economic agenda of the western world.

Since the 1970s the scenario has been changing. Consumption has outstripped productivity. Debt has been amassed in numbers beyond imagination, exampled by the more than $2 trillion foreign debt figures (Beatty, 1990). Other economies have emerged in both Europe and the Asian basin that can more than adequately compete in the world market place and can do so to the disadvantage of the United States (Kennedy, 1988).

Health care in the United States is just one single example of the fallout from the change in the economic underpinnings of the American nation. For the past 10 years concerted and direct attention has been paid to tightening the belt of health care providers following two decades of unparalleled growth in access, service and cost of health care services. At the same time technology and medical intervention capabilities have burgeoned, enabling health professionals to undertake treatments that approach the fantastic. However, these medical advances have come with steep price tags.

Nursing as a discipline grew at a high rate during the past two decades, the direct beneficiary of expansion in access and service. As hospitals grew in size and patient acuity levels rose, the need for nursing services accelerated faster than at any time in the history of nursing in America. Continuous efforts of nursing educational institutions to keep up with the demand for new nurses is something they have never quite been able to accomplish (Helmer & McKnight, 1988). The increase in the number of nurses is just one of a host of signs indicating the growth of the health care system in the country. Because of this unequaled growth of health care and the constraining economic realities confronting the United States, political leadership at all levels has begun to look very closely at how the health care dollar gets generated and where it gets spent. Because the health care sector of the economy has grown at a rate 10 percent higher than that of the general economy, health care has experienced a significant share of cost reduction and control activities in both the public and private sectors (Grace, 1990). During the past decade an average of about $2 billion a year have been cut from the federal health budget (Kimball & Ready, 1989). In the private sector the insurance company leadership has been as interested in cutting their expenditures and are looking very closely at increasing control over how the insurance dollar gets spent for health care services (Davis, Powell, & Gross, 1987). What has appeared on insurance companies agendas is a growing interest in creating a managed care environment where dollars and services are closely managed and monitored with parameters defined before services are provided (Drew, 1990).

What is vital for nursing administration leadership in the future is to keep in mind that the health care system operates in a larger economic framework. Perhaps one of the greatest problems in nursing leadership is the prevailing lack of economic understanding and the failure to incorporate economic and financial principles into decisions that affect the patient care delivery. One of the most important realities that a nursing leader must first come to terms with is that health care in America is an economic enterprise, not a humanistic endeavor. While at first glance this may appear as a trite and parochial observation, it becomes less so when the structural and decisional processes used in nursing administration fail to reflect economics in the practices and work of nursing organizations. The truth is that standards of care, criteria that relate to staff distribution and use, mechanisms which tie the outcomes of care to costs are still generally missing from the nursing service data base. Even though DRGs have been in place for a decade now, nursing leadership in the service setting still has not created a justifiable tie between nursing resource use and the price paid for the services provided. In the future, all service frameworks will have to more clearly relate work costs of the service to the pricing structure provided by the payer regardless of the prevailing payment structure.

While not often discussed openly and clearly, much of the emerging struggle in a constraining economic environment reflects the power equation operating in the health care system. The fact that health care today reflects a medical model of service delivery fuels the flames of the struggle. For example, evidence produced in a wide variety of service settings and clinical frameworks indicates that much of the higher costing medical services provided can be delivered with equitable outcomes and reduced costs by nurses prepared with advanced nursing skills (Fagin, 1986). In this case, there is no objective justification for a health care system to maintain the ascendancy role of the physician in all health service areas. Yet the economic and political realities inherent in implementing a more rational, cost-effective, and less medically driven delivery system is fraught with the trauma of difficult political and power clashes. The nursing leader of the future will have to recognize the need to advocate for restructuring that uses effective nursing resources in ways that provide competent services in a cost competitive manner. The leader must also be willing to risk undertaking activities necessary to make room for broadened roles for nurse providers in a political structure that may be opposed to either sharing or transferring practice roles. As past efforts have shown in this power equation, sufficient data to support the argument that nurses provide equitable levels of services when compared to physicians at much lower cost is not sufficient to make successful systems changes (Maraldo, 1988). The battle for effective change will have to be waged in the boardrooms, legislatures, policy arenas, and in the public forums. The political and economic savvy necessary to successfully undertake such actions must be in the nurse leaders armamentarium of skills in order to accomplish a viable and appropriate role for nurses in a health system that needs to reduce the cost, but not the quality, of service. The packaging and selling of nursing services in other settings and other ways will have to also fall under the aegis of nurse executives of the future as they lead the competition with other providers in seeking payment for providing health care services.

As a series of directors of the Health Care Financing Administration have indicated, dollars directed to hospitals and physicians will continue to be scrutinized with the overall intent to reduce federal health expenditures for inpatient services and physician services. This will continue for the next few years (Altman, 1990). Recognizing this reality, the wise nurse executive will create opportunities and scenarios where the cost effectiveness of nurse driven services becomes evident. This will require defining a new reality, restructuring the way care gets done including the form and style of care as well as remixing the service provider to more closely match the demand for the category of care giver as indicated by the need. Administrators will make sure that the market for such services is closely tied to the cost efficacy of the services provided. Contribution margins will reflect the viability and value of nursing service to the corporate fiscal and service health thereby tying nursing service tightly to the goals, purposes and activities of the organization. Besides changing the perception of nursing service in the eyes of the policy makers and power brokers, be they administrators or payers, these role changes and fiscal connections link nursing service to the success of the enterprise both for finance and service in a productive rather than a consuming context.

For the nurse executive, then, the age of unlimited resources is over. Judicious use of existing resources and appropriate application of cost control strategies as defined herein appears to be a part of the operational imperative for the role for the long term. The struggle in this enterprise will be founded in the nurse executive's attempt to integrate professional values for care with the economic realities which influence what can reasonably be expected. This will drive three main concerns for the nurse executive of the future: the use of nursing services, the cost of nursing care, and the delivery of nursing care services.

USE OF NURSING SERVICES

Any product for which there is a defined economic value has some parameters within which the product is elucidated and priced (Reynolds, 1988). Price depends on use of a mechanism for ascertaining or attaching some dollar value to the product or service being sold. There are very few business enterprises that are willing to buy a service or product whose value to them is unknown. The obvious questions of need, worth, and price drive the purchaser in considerations of how to spend money.

When there is plenty of money available, relationships between need and worth are more loosely defined. However, when dollars are scarce and options are many, the purchaser is more careful in selecting where and how to spend money. In both public and private expenditures of health care dollars this reality will continue to affect the role nurses will play in health care for the next two decades. There will be increasing scrutiny of nursing service expenditures and a stronger relationship demanded between the services nurses provide and the outcomes they obtain. No longer will it be presumed that extensive use of dollars for registered nurse services is automatically appropriate just because nurses say that is so. Evidence of the value of registered nurse care versus that of other providers will need to be manifest. Some objective measure of the need and appropriateness of levels of care will be a requisite for accessing that portion of health care dollars spent on nursing services. Services provided by nurse extender and assisting personnel may need to be better and more clearly incorporated into the nursing delivery models and achieved with no net increase in full time equivalents or salary dollars allocated for nursing services.

Support for the nurse's presence is not automatic. The registered nurse, at whatever level of preparation or service, will always have to be aware of the demand to prove the value of the role and the appropriateness of the manner in which it is used.

The nurse executive in the future will have to accomplish the following outcomes in the use of nursing resources:

1. Clearly articulate the expectation of the role of the registered nurse in the delivery of a broad scope of nursing services.
2. Differentiate the roles of various levels of nurse provider between technical and professional roles interpreting such roles not only as they address nursing work but as they articulate value and payment for those roles. Differentiated roles will mean differentiated cost and, ultimately, differentiating the price of those services.
3. More clearly determine work intensity and acuity relationships so that a stronger relationship between need and use is identified and attached to the pricing of nursing services. There must be a tight match, in the future, between the service provided and the service provider, in this case, the nurse. No longer will standards of service be generically defined for a class or category of patients. Not all critical care patients need one to one care but neither do all medical unit patients need only one to eight care. Current nursing service standards are broken down in too broadly based delineations. Future payment demands will require a more specific fit between resource use and service payment (Halloran, Patterson, & Liley, 1987).
4. As alternatives to costly hospitalization continue to emerge in the health care system, the role of nurses in other settings and roles continue to need definition. This creates a problem and an opportunity in the future. The problem is that higher intensities of care will continue to occur in the hospital setting demanding concentrated and well defined nursing services (McCloskey, 1989). Other service opportunities outside the hospital will attract more nursing resources stretching the already declining pool of nurses available for hospital service. Utilization and distribution of nursing staff will have to be more adequately delineated by nursing leadership and then matched with the availability of support and assisting services. Clearly, better allocated and used support services inside and outside the hospital will be necessary in order to make the best use of nurses in either environment, assuring that they are used as clinical providers rather than messengers, material gatherers or patient transporters, etc.

Clearer delineation of service and service provider will require a stronger data support system that more clearly matches kind, quality, and cost indicators as they apply to nursing care. In order to better understand the relationship of care to outcome, that relationship must be more tightly defined in the future. Generalized determinants of nursing care based solely on time and intensity as is currently the practice, without consideration to outcome, will miss the mark regarding appropriation of both income and resources. The use of standards-based practice in the delivery of nursing care in a broad variety of settings is fast becoming an expectation for nursing care. The nursing service that can more clearly delineate what the consumer and buyer of nursing services is getting for their dollar through a clearer articulation of the care received and the outcome achieved will be ahead of the competitor who cannot do so.

In addition to service and outcome relationships, as nursing care becomes increasingly noninstitutional and decentralized, practicing nurses will have to be more able to manage their own practice. They will have to be able to communicate and relate with practitioners in other disciplines with some degree of equity. Since most of those are prepared at the masters degree equivalency, more nurses in multidisciplinary practice settings will need and have the masters degree. Educational institutions are retooling the curriculum to accommodate fast track efforts to produce this clinical person through new ''RN to MN'' pathway programs (National Commission on Nursing, 1986). Nursing service settings will have to accommodate the need for independence and control over their own practices as this level of preparation infers. Data support the more creative use of these practitioners in highly variable settings and the resulting value to the consumer (Fagan & Maraldo, 1989). More innovative service structures and management models will have to emerge which relate to and support use of these advanced prepared nurses.

It should be clear by now that the definition of the work of nurses and nursing will continue to be redefined as the demand for nursing services shift and grow. The nurse executive must be flexible and sensitive regarding how to incorporate these roles into the future nursing organizational model. Indeed the administrator must actively seek opportunities for new service use and extension of the nursing organizational model. Either through contracting, joint venturing, community-based nursing service structures, collaborative practice arrangements, or other not yet conceived approaches, the nurse executive of the future will develop a broad management frame of reference adjusting management approaches to the service structures opportunity creates.

COST OF NURSING CARE

No issue will have a greater impact on the future of nursing and health care than the spiraling costs associated with providing health care services. While nursing services have been one step removed from direct management and control of cost generation, it has certainly played a major part in hospital costs. There is no service any larger than nursing services in almost any setting where health services are provided. In its traditional coordinative role nursing service touches, in one way or another, almost every other service provided in the health care setting. Also, nursing services consume the largest single component of service-based cost in the institution. While it has never traditionally been associated with revenue generation, nursing services contribute in no small measure to the financial success of the enterprise over the long term (Sherman, 1990).

In constraining times societies become more concerned than usual about where money comes from and where it goes. Since there appears to be either less of it around or more of it being spent on the same things, there appears to be great legitimacy for this concern. As costs go up and service remains the same, expenditures for patient care become the focal point of attention for the payers. In diagnosis related grouping (DRG) payment format, an attempt at a cost accounted approach to paying for clinical services has been pursued. To the participant in this payment system many problems can emerge related to categorizing of patients, parameters of care, intensity of service, and changing characteristics of the patient, all of which affect appropriateness of the DRG delineation.

Whether the DRG approach to payment remains in place as presently formatted, some cost control payment structure will operate in the health care system for some time. The nurse executive's goal in such a system is to incorporate the realities of cost control into the nursing system and to adopt a cost framework for nursing. In one manner or another, the cost of providing nursing service must be identifiable in the package of costs that make up a particular patient care event. To assume that nursing cost is similar to the fixed costs associated with the room rate is to shield both nurse and payer from the realities and complexities of resource use. This sentiment has been expressed for the past two decades, still, only demonstration projects have ever been undertaken to address this issue (Edwardson & Giovanetti, 1987). As the payers move inexorably toward payment for service packages, or bundled service structures, there is a need to identify those elements of service and cost which comprise the "package" (Flarey, 1990). That part of the services provided which is nursing, therefore, must be identified clearly enough to attach a price tag to it and determine its percentage or ratio amount to the complex of services provided in the package. While the need to address nursing costs is not new, the approach to incorporating those cost into the composite of costs per DRG or service unit and thereby seek payment for them along with other legitimate costs is new and will become increasingly important as every service and function is scrutinized by the payers and regulators of health care.

To confront this reality, the nurse executive will have to be increasingly involved in cost strategizing and gaming at the administrative level. Included in proposals for new or innovative services suggested by nursing leadership in any setting will be the need to identify specific service related nursing cost. This costing instrument will have to reflect not only the time spent in nursing intervention but also the economic value attached to intensity of resource use and level of service provided by the nursing entity. If intervention occurs along a continuum of care, the various units of service and intensity at these intervention points will have to reflect the attendant costs associated with providing nursing services.

In the past decade, nursing has done much to show the comparable value of nursing intervention when it is likened to other providers, most notably physicians (Rooks et al, 1990; Minor, 1989). While service quality, satisfaction, and lowered cost have often been evidenced in studies related to primary care by nurses, there has been a lack of acceptance of that data by payers as a basis for making decisions about how and whom to pay. All too frequently, nursing services have not been perceived as an alternative equal to those services provided by physicians. Rather, nursing services, no matter how effective, are looked at as additional services to those already being offered by physicians, no matter how innovative or appropriate they might be.

Instead of substitute services of comparable quality, emerging nurse provided primary care services have been looked at by payers as a supplement or extender to physician provided services for which they were already paying. In the payer's mind, additional services, no matter how cost-effective, are not likely to be acceptable unless they actually replace more costly current services and service providers, again most notably, physicians (Deatsch & Shaw, 1990).

The nurse administrator will need to develop two major strategies in a market-based approach to selling nursing services in newer frameworks and settings. The first strategy will relate to joining in mutually beneficial ventures with physicians and others in order to provide an aggregate of services in structures for which payment is likely and physicians also can be beneficiaries. In the next two decades nursing leadership must and will move past the more recidivistic view that physicians are the enemy and will actually join with them in clinical enterprises that are mutually beneficial and provide both meaningful and cost effective relationships. These collaborative models will continue to unfold as cost and service frameworks become increasingly constrained and alternative noninstitutional service frameworks emerge in the community.

A second key strategy relates to the creation of smaller units of service in a broader number of settings within which nursing practice unfolds. Self-managed teams directed to definable patient care services whether inpatient or outpatient will continue to grow in health care (Taft & Pelikan, 1990). Increasingly nurse-physician teams, which include other caregivers within cross-functioning or related roles, will work with a specified group of physicians and their patients in a variety of health service settings. In some cases, contracts for service relationships between physicians, nurses, and other providers on these focused teams may be the service and economic relationship of preference within which they function. In this scenario, the nurse administrator has a different set of management characteristics which influences the role. More integration, facilitation, and coordination of these relatively self-directed and self-subscribed professionals will unfold for this manager and will call for a more collaborative but focused management style.

Looking through the eyes of the purchaser of health care services, the unique relationships which emerge in delivery and costing of nursing care does not mean much if it is not reflected in the price to be paid for those services, no matter how they are packaged and bundled. A fundamental change in the cost basis for care will have to evolve if the payer of health care is to maintain a willingness to both participate and to pay. A move to lowest cost first, highest cost last strategies (managed care) will be essential to the seller in approaching the buyer of care. Not only does the ongoing cost of care have to be kept to the lowest possible level, the long term costs have to be controlled too. That means developing programs and packages of care services which will assure the payer and user that healthy life-style changes and health enhancing strategies will be as valuable to the provider as intervention services are when illness develops. Since the aging of the population is a central trend on the

American social horizon, chronic illness will loom as the greatest possible purveyor of cost in the future (Dychwald, 1986). Teaching the public how to manage their chronic illness and maintain independence and self-direction in personal health management is not only a good health strategy, it is also a great economic effort as well. Evidence that such strategies will actually result in a much more appropriate use of the dollar and reduce overall individual health related costs will be the best argument in the short term for a more cost-effective delivery system (Porter-O'Grady, 1990).

DELIVERY OF NURSING CARE SERVICES

Perhaps there will be no greater or dramatic change in the role of the nurse executive as those that are emerging in changes in the delivery of nursing care services. As hospital bed vacancy rates fluctuate around 40 percent, clearly, services once provided inside the hospital for many more patients are now being provided elsewhere. Clearly 60 percent of traditional hospital-based services by the year 2000 will be provided in other ways and other settings (Goldsmith, 1990). Therefore, the majority of health care services will be provided somewhere other than inside the hospital structure. It is not as important which hospital services move out or when they move; it is important to know that all services will be affected by this move. Readiness for a move into other settings and service models will be the major task of the nurse executive over the long term. This will create a major shift in role and focus for the nursing service and the executive who will lead it (Townsend, 1990).

Newer models, not representing present structures, create new concerns for the executive in preparing for the future of health care. Current perceptions and models may not be sufficient designs for the service arrangements of the future. Collaborative, joint, and group practice arrangements with other disciplines and providers will become more evident as the interrelationships between providers emerge. Package payment for services provided, rather than for specific service providers, will continue to be better defined and structured as a part of the payment system. As technology reduces the use of surgery and other interventions drastically, hospital based activities and procedures, once considered as only institutionally appropriate will be done in outpatient or nonhospital settings. Some will even be done in the home. Cardiac procedures which strip atherosclerotic plaques from the coronary arteries will soon become pharmacy procedures rather than technical interventions. Cancer treatments will become noninstitutional procedures administered at work and in the home with limited hospital-based activities. Even in this small sample of clinical activities, the nurse will likely be the logical provider of services and the natural connection of the patient to other services provided within the health care continuum. However, this nurse will not necessarily be tied directly to the hospital where 68 percent of nurses now work.

In the short term, the nurse executive will have to lead the rest of health care in the transition into newer care models and facilitate restructuring of nursing and health care in ways that do not depend on institutional care models. At the same time the executive will have to effectively manage these often disparate and far-flung nursing services in an effort to ensure that they meet service objectives and financial goals. Over the long term, the nurse executive will have to plan entire programs and structures for care provided by nurses and others in multiple service units and multidisciplinary settings. In order to manage the nursing component of these service settings, generate revenue and control costs the administrator must manage a sales and productivity framework that clearly indicates the services provided by nurses and the contribution they made to the financial health of the enterprise within which they offer their services.

To fulfill these obligations of a new focus on the role of the nurse executive, this person must operate effectively and creatively in the following ways:

1. Develop a model of care, which reflects a continuum of services from home to hospital to home with nursing services being provided along the full continuum, connected to the nursing delivery system throughout the patient's health care experience.

2. Negotiate relationships with physicians and other providers of health services for referring patients, caring for patients, and following patients into a variety of settings. Included are teaching both providers and patients, connecting patients to the complex of health care services, and evaluating the outcomes of both the relationships in patient care and the effectiveness of services.

3. Plan, appropriate, cost, package, and price a wide variety of nursing and other service relationships in a widely differentiated market place. Sell them to buyers who are businesses, insurers, consortiums, preferred purchasers, special interest organizations, and other health care practices needing nursing services as a part of their composite of health related services.

4. Create complex service information networks that are community based, rural, urban, reflecting public and private interests connected by a clinical and management information system. They will communicate the essential management and resource information, keeping the nurse executive abreast of the financial and service characteristics which influence service effectiveness and viability.

5. Increasingly utilize state of the art computer technology connecting components of the nursing delivery model to assure that elements of care are linked but still decentralized. This computerized clinical delivery system will be managed by the practicing nurse and will reflect clinical documentation, the critical flow of care services, patient care pathways, clinical activities, and cost and revenue figures at various points along the patient continuum. Portability and consistency of data will facilitate the aggregation of a data base that can be adjusted wherever the patient intersects the delivery system.

6. Enter into individual and collective financial and service arrangements with nurses and other providers that pay them for case load and predescribed outcomes. Payment for services and productivity will be more clearly related. Gainsharing of revenues produced in the clinical work and identified in contractual arrangements will ensure higher levels of quality and efficacy.

Methodologies of care services provided by nurses will be highly variable and will reflect the location and circumstances of where and how care is delivered. Predominant models of care delivery will not be as inflexible as in fixed institutional systems. There will be more negotiation of delivery models and roles as differing service structures and relationships emerge. In a differentiated and multidisciplinary system, roles of each of the providers will be delineated within specific service frameworks to reflect patient needs in individual care systems. Income, benefits, and service-related costs will all be negotiated by nurses within the context of the service framework. Nursing care modalities will, therefore, be highly individualized and service specific.

Because of the high human resource costs of professional nursing services, use of lower cost extenders of nursing care will continue to be expanded. While the complexity of hospital care will not permit broad-based use of more limited prepared caregivers, nursing team and partnership programs using these care assistants will continue to grow. In a number of service settings beyond the hospital, care aids or assistants will be used for a limited range of services. Demand for the professional nurse will continue to outstrip supply, therefore appropriate use of a variety of caregivers, supportive of the professional nurse, will increase dramatically over the next decade (Olivas et al, 1989).

GETTING FROM TODAY TO TOMORROW

If cares becomes more individual and increasingly noninstitutional and decentralized, how will the nursing professional culture and organization remain intact and influential? How will what is uniquely "nursing" be maintained so that the values and social commitments of the profession related to policy formation, clinical integrity and quality assurance are adequately dealt with? Clearly, an organizational structure should provide wide latitude for diversity in care yet sufficient centralization of control to assure that fundamental nursing values are sustained.

The future of nursing administration calls for an entirely different approach to the management of a highly diverse and complex clinical service. As nursing matures into full professional circumstance, it will demand alternative approaches to both its management and organization.

Some realities that will confront future nursing services relate to the following circumstances.

1. Discernible roles and obligations will support differentiated educational preparation for divergent categories of nursing care. Nursing education in the future will not prepare practitioners for the same roles. The more technically prepared nurse will assume roles in structured environments where supervised and highly technical activities will be the focus of the work. Those nurses prepared in a longer course of study, with a focus on the continuum of care and multifocal interventions, will provide care services in a wide variety of formats which will include supervising other nursing and assisting per-

sonnel. More of the noninstitutional and decentralized services will be provided by the more broadly educated nurse (Koerner, et al, 1989).

2. The obligation for more advanced education at the graduate level in nursing will continue to unfold in the health care system. As health care services continue to be offered in a number of different forums and in a host of unique ways, nurses will have to be better prepared to manage their own practices and to reflect comparable value to colleagues in other disciplines at an acceptable level of interaction and contribution. Increasingly, graduate preparation will be required for newer nursing roles. Educational institutions will, in greater numbers, make the achievement of graduate education easier and more meaningful (National Commission on Nursing, 1986).

3. Increasingly, nurses' roles in these decentralized settings will be tied to the productivity of nurses and their relationship to what is accomplished or returned as a result of their work. Productivity and income will be more directly aligned to output of the individual nurse provider. Much as other more independent disciplines align their income to the success of the enterprise, so too will the nurses' role. Economic and benefits opportunities will be more directly tied to the nurse's contribution to the service (Forté, 1989).

4. As managed care approaches become more inculcated into the American health system, the gatekeeper role will shift from the most expensive provider of health care (the physician) to include the role of the nurse who may be the care system's "agent," referring the patient in the managed care system to the most appropriate but lowest cost service required by the patient's condition. This facilitates the notion of lowest cost first, highest cost last as indicated in current data which support the efficacy of the nurse in this key role (Nornhold, 1990).

Broadening the nurses' roles and extending the circle within which their roles interact, increases the complexity of administrative and clinical relationships necessary to both facilitate nursing service and also to increase its opportunity to make a difference in providing health care services. As nursing becomes more professional in its activities and relationships to other providers, there will arise a need to organize the management of nurses differently from the past. In addition to the changing character of the profession, woman's expectation and roles are becoming quickly equated with those of men. Nursing, as a predominantly female profession, is beginning to reflect some of the same professional values as those of predominantly male professions, such as law and medicine (Schwartz, 1989).

The needs of the professional worker are clearly different from those of the vocational worker (Mintzberg, 1989). This includes the need to control the profession's practice, set standards for the profession's work, and play a part in the policy making which affects how the role is used and how the collective enterprise operates.

Newer models of organization and care delivery best exemplified today in case management models and shared governance structures will continue to unfold as management of the profession becomes more diverse and incorporates the practicing nurse in decisions which affects what she does. These management models will reflect the changing character of nurses' work and the necessary decentralization of authority required to provide latitude in the nurse's role to undertake service arrangements and relationships that best use nurse skills and provide broadest access to those nurses serve. Managers simply cannot be present in every service setting. There will, therefore, be increased opportunity for nurses to have more control over their own practices and be evaluated on the effective relationship between commitment to provide service and outcomes of that service. The nurse will be connected to those who manage nursing service or by contracts.

Computer systems will both communicate with the nurse and maintain files which document nursing activities. Even if the nurse is in multiple locations or undertaking a variety of activities, linkage to the management center or data center can be assured through portable communication systems which keep the practitioner connected to resource management at all times (Patti, McDonagh, & Porter-O'Grady, 1990).

In addition to computer networks which connect the track nurses and their activities, structured time for professional education and interaction with other clinical providers will be incorporated into the nurse's schedule so that the personal and professional interplay and affiliations are facilitated. In these models and settings the manager will be the central linkage between nurses to each other and to the service system and as a control point between the nursing organization and the nurse. In this way the values, roles, and responsibilities of nurses will be moderated against the aggregate values and expectations of nursing service, assuring consistency in both role and performance wherever the nurse may practice. Just as many far-flung multinational corporate systems now do, the nursing organization of the future will individualize their management, marketing, and service structures to the client being served. The manager can then evaluate the nursing service provider through computerized standards and performance indicators in any setting in which a nurse is practicing. Unquestionably, there must be an organizational and operational shift away from highly centralized and bureaucratic models of management to more organic and fluid models of organizing work and service to reflect a more market or service sensitive milieu (Haddon, 1990). In addition, the nursing organization will have to incorporate into their management strategies mechanisms to include clinical nurses in decisions that affect their actions.

While it is important that the nursing service organization be well structured to provide service and to be responsive to its nursing staff, it is equally important to be sensitive to the transitional character of the health care market. There are no certainties currently in any arena of health care about what can be done, where it can be done, and whether it will be paid. There is no strong integrated policy at virtually any level in the United States guiding health care except for federal control over public expenditures.

The nursing executive must be ever vigilant in the kind and character of service opportunities and ventures to which the nursing organization responds. The executive will have to maintain awareness on several fronts:

1. Maintain familiarity regarding the short-term, specified political thrusts and current emphasis of legislators and policy makers for providing and paying for health care services.
2. Identify first those health services for which there is either programmatic or cost-based payment for services, maximizing services for which there is no capped payment for as long as it is viable to do so. Many ambulatory and noninstitutional services fall into this category but such programs will continue to decrease as Congress and policy makers develop payment caps for them.
3. Be ready to change service structures or parameters relatively quickly as the rules for providing specific services shift as a result of congressional or policy actions. Responsiveness and fluidity to shifting service demand are characteristic of highly transitional times (Drucker, 1988).
4. Nursing services must be offered in terms the buyer can understand. The language of nursing must be translated into terms that can be accepted by the purchaser—indeed, encourage the purchaser to use nurse provided services. The nurse "seller" in this case must couch the language of sale in the buyer's frame of reference so the purchase can be made within the context of the buyers values.

SUMMARY

Americans are entering into a period in history that is extremely unfamiliar to most people of the latter twentieth century. The social and economic paradigm is changing radically from anything previously known. Since there has always been plenty in comparison to the rest of the world, and the average American appears moderately comfortable when compared to other western industrialized societies, opportunity has always appeared unlimited with resources to match.

Now the news reflects a different story: scarce resources; national debt, growing poverty rates; heavy and successful foreign competition in the global markets; pollution; drugs; morass; and a host of other concerns that seem incompatible with the American consciousness. The health care system simply reflects these same conditions within its own arena. Clearly, something is different now than in the past.

One can interpret the condition of the American society in a number of ways. The thinker can be optimistic or pessimistic and be correct either way. One thing is certain: Times are different. When placed in a global context the changes appear, at minimum, radical. And so they are.

Whatever comes of the intensity of these times and the fierceness of the rate and nature of the changes, some kind of response will be demanded. This requisite is no less importunate for nursing and its leadership. In fact, it may be a time of increasing opportunity to provide both leadership and direction that is more compatible with the values and apperception of nursing. The historic barriers of sex, education, and role are quickly falling away allowing the bright and capable in nursing to emerge and to assume rightful roles in writing new scripts and setting new directions for health care as the resource structures and service frameworks shift into newer delivery and payment models.

Because there is great dissatisfaction with the system as currently structured, opportunity to retool the delivery of health care has never been more apparent. The medical model as a delivery system is under severe strain and detailed examination. The advantage to adjust, redefine, and restructure health care to be more cost sensitive and broader based in its application has never been better for nurses.

On almost all fronts there is the challenge to change and build new structures and ways of working in America. In health care the demand for change has never been more apparent or necessary. Access and efficacy are clearly the key words for a system sorely in need of direction. The choice to retrench or to innovate lies before all players in the health care system. History, however, documents the effectiveness of nurses at such times and their key roles in ushering in new forms and formats for delivering health care services, especially in trying or constrained times (Haddon, 1989).

This chapter has focused on the conditions and processes associated with leadership activities in nursing and health care in these transitional times. Focus has been on the conditions, circumstances, and activities which redirect the aim and skills of nurse leaders at whatever place they find themselves in the health care system. It expands the range of thought and consideration for nurse leaders and hopefully, challenges them, out of more traditional frames of response in writing a new script for the future of health care.

There is no single person who can accurately address the future and all it portends. At best, our view of it is an informed guess. The chaos of entropy and serendipity plays too heavily in the experience of life to ensure perceptual accuracy in defining what will happen (Hawking, 1988). The trends of today, which are simply the culmination of our yesterdays, do give us a glimpse into the probabilities of tomorrow. They are simply indications, sometimes warnings, of what is to come. No one person has a corner on reality; therefore, the script for tomorrow is always subject to the view of the writer.

There will be no one person or group who writes the script for the future of health care. Nursing leadership will have to be clear on what it sees for the future and make sure that they are at the table when the script for the future of health care is written. Certainly there is much that nurses have to offer. Through careful consideration of the role of nursing in providing health care services, good social and political strategy, and viable service delivery models, there is no doubt that nurses will contribute significantly to whatever emerges from these transitional times in health care through this decade and well into the twenty-first century.

REFERENCES

Altman S. Health care in the nineties: No more of the same. *Hospitals.* 64, April 5, 1990
Beatty J. A post cold war budget, *Atlantic Monthly.* 74, February 1990

Davis C, Powell D, Gross M. The changing health care environment. *Topics in Health Care Finance.* 14:2, 1, 1987

Deatsch D, Shaw D. Physician reimbursement: The need for change. *Topics in Health Care Finance.* 16:3, 58, 1990

Drew J. Health maintenance organizations. *Nursing and Health Care.* 11:3, 145, 1990

Drucker P. The coming of the new organization, *Harvard Business Review.* 45, January–February, 1988

Dychwald K. *Wellness and Health Promotion for the Elderly.* Rockville MD, Aspen Publishers, Inc, 1986

Edwardson S, Giovanetti G. A review of cost accounting methods for nursing services. *Nursing Economics.* 5:3, 107, 1987

Fagin C. Opening the door on nursing's cost advantage. *Nursing and Health Care.* 7:7, 353, 1986

Fagin C, Maraldo P. Feminism and the nursing shortage: Do women have a choice? *Nursing and Health Care.* 10:9, 365, 1989

Flarey D. A methodology for costing nursing service. *Nursing Administration Quarterly.* 14:3, 41, 1990

Forté F, Prospering Nurse: Overcoming Oxymoron. *Nursing Economics,* 7:2, 87–89, 1989

Goldsmith, J. A radical prescription for hospitals. *Harvard Business Review.* 104, May–June, 1990

Grace H. Can health care costs be contained? *Nursing and Health Care.* 11:3, 125 1990

Haddon R. The final frontier: Nursing in the emerging health care environment. *Nursing Economics.* 7:3, 156, 1989

Haddon R. An economic agenda for health care. *Nursing and Health Care.* 11:1, 21, 1990

Halloran E, Patterson C, Liley M. Case mix: Matching nursing need with nursing resource. *Nursing Management.* 18:3, 27, 1987

Hawking S. *A Brief History of Time.* London, Bantam Books, 1988

Helmer T, McKnight P. One more time—Solutions to the nursing shortage, *Journal of Nursing Administration.* 18:11, 7, 1988

Kennedy P. *The Rise and Fall of the Great Powers.* New York, Random House, 1988

Kimball M, Ready T. Congress Settles On $2.8 billion Medicare cut. *Healthweek.* 7, 34, December 4, 1989

Koerner J et al. Implementing differentiated practice. *Journal of Nursing Administration.* 19:2, 13, 1989

McCloskey J. Implication of cositng out nursing services for reimbursement. *Nursing Management.* 20:1, 49, 1989

Mintzberg H. *Mintzberg on Management.* New York, The Free Press. 171, 1989

Minor AF. The cost of maternity and childbirth in the United States. *Research Bulletin.* Health Insurance Association of America. December 3–13, 1989

Maraldo P. The economics of women's health. *Nursing Economics.* 6:3, 128, 1988

National Commission on Nursing Implementation Project. *Invitational Conference Notebook,* November 7, 1986

Nornhold P. 90 predictions for the 90s. *Nursing 90.* 35, January, 1990

Olivas G et al. Case management: A bottom line care delivery model. *Journal of Nursing Administration.* 19:11, 16, 1989

Patti J, McDonagh K, Porter-O'Grady T. Streetside support. *Health Progress.* 60, June, 1990

Porter-O'Grady T. *The Reorganization of Nursing Practice.* Rockville MD, Aspen Publishers, Inc, 1990

Reynolds L. *Microeconomics: Analysis and Policy.* Irwin, Homewood, IL, 1988:31–60

Rooks J et al. Outcomes of care in birth centers. *New England Journal of Medicine.* 321:1804, 1989

Schwartz F. Management women and the new facts of life. *Harvard Business Review.* 65, January–February, 1989

Sherman J. Costing nursing care: A review. *Nursing Administration Quarterly.* 14:3, 11, 1990

Taft S, Pelikan J. Clinic management teams: Integrators of professional service and environmental change. *Health Care Management Review.* 15:2, 67, 1990

Townsend M. A participative approach to administrative reorganization. *Journal of Nursing Administration.* 20:2, 11, 1990